1991

Medical and Health Annual

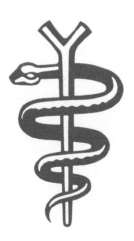

Encyclopædia Britannica, Inc.

CHICAGO

AUCKLAND•GENEVA•LONDON•MADRID•MANILA•PARIS•ROME•SEOUL•SYDNEY•TOKYO•TORONTO

1991 Medical and Health Annual

Editor	Ellen Bernstein
Senior Editor	Linda Tomchuck
Contributing Editors	Charles Cegielski, Barbara Whitney
Editorial Adviser	Drummond Rennie, M.D. Professor of Medicine Institute for Health Policy Studies University of California, San Francisco; Deputy Editor (West), *The Journal of the American Medical Association*
Creative Director	Cynthia Peterson
Operations Manager	Marsha Mackenzie
Senior Picture Editor	Holly Harrington
Picture Editors	Kathryn Creech, Katharine W. Hannaford, Cathy Melloan
Art Production Supervisor	Richard A. Roiniotis
Illustrators/Layout Artists	Kay Diffley, John L. Draves, John J. Mahoney, Stephanie Motz
Art Staff	Patricia A. Henle, Margaret Liebezeit, Diana M. Pitstick
Manager, Copy Department	Anita Wolff
Senior Copy Editor	Barbara Whitney
Copy Staff	Cheryl L. Collins, Ellen Finkelstein, David Gottlieb, John Mathews
Manager, Production Control	Mary C. Srodon
Production Control Staff	Jacqueline Amato, Marilyn L. Barton, Stephanie A. Green
Manager, Composition and Page Makeup	Melvin Stagner
Coordinator, Composition and Page Makeup	Michael Born, Jr.
Composition Staff	Duangnetra Debhavalya, Carol Gaines, John Krom, Jr., Thomas Mulligan, Gwen Rosenberg, Tammy Tsou
Page Makeup Staff	Griselda Cháidez, Arnell Reed, Danette Wetterer
Director, Corporate Computer Services	Michelle J. Brandhorst
Computer Services Staff	Steven Bosco, Ronald Pihlgren, Philip Rehmer, Vincent Star
Manager, Index Department	Carmen-Maria Hetrea
Senior Index Editor	Edward Paul Moragne
Index Staff	Kathy M. Howard
Librarian	Terry Miller
Associate Librarian	Shantha Uddin
Curator/Geography	David W. Foster
Assistant Librarian	Robert M. Lewis
Yearbook Secretarial Staff	Dorothy Hagen, Kay Johnson

Editorial Administration

Philip W. Goetz, Editor in Chief
Michael Reed, Managing Editor
Karen M. Barch, Executive Director of Editorial Production
Elizabeth P. O'Connor, Director of Financial Planning

Encyclopædia Britannica, Inc.
Robert P. Gwinn, Chairman of the Board
Peter B. Norton, President

Library of Congress Catalog Card Number: 77-649875
International Standard Book Number: 0-85229-527-8
International Standard Serial Number: 0363-0366
Copyright © 1990 by Encyclopædia Britannica, Inc.
All rights reserved for all countries.
Printed in U.S.A.

Foreword

Just a few of the features . . . The World Health Organization has targeted two major infectious diseases for extinction by the year 2000. One is guinea worm disease (dracunculiasis), caused by a parasite that affects 10 million people in Asia and Africa annually. The other is poliomyelitis, a more familiar disease to Westerners—especially those old enough to remember the merciless summertime epidemics of the 1940s and '50s—before a vaccine was available. But in many parts of the world, polio is still a major crippler and killer. The effort now under way to make polio one of the next two diseases consigned to the history books is the subject of the opening feature article in this volume. (Next year the *Annual* will report on the progress of the campaign to eradicate guinea worm disease.)

There are many people who equate a diagnosis of cancer with a death sentence and the treatments—*i.e.,* radical surgery, chemotherapy, and radiotherapy—with a fate worse than death. That is unfortunate. The feature article "Breast Cancer in Perspective" stresses that continuing intensive research has made possible both early diagnosis and effective treatment of the cancer women fear most. Often, however, the information they get comes from scattered news reports that are difficult to fit into a whole picture. The intention here is to provide a framework for more critical understanding of the scientific findings that are reported in the news and a basis for appropriate self-care. Probably, if the facts were widely known and if women were encouraged to act on them, the breast cancer death rate could be halved.

A true medical miracle of our time is the cure of childhood cancer—a triumph made possible by children whose families have allowed them to participate in daring human experiments. But while treatment benefits have been evident for years, only now are physicians learning that some cured patients may experience physical and psychological complications—sequelae that were previously unforeseen. "Children with Cancer: Odds in Their Favor" examines both the miracle of the cure and the potential problems facing young cancer survivors.

"Nowhere a Promised Land," describing the plight of refugees and "internally displaced" people, was completed well before Iraq invaded Kuwait on Aug. 2, 1990. Its message, however, is all the more poignant in light of what has become the world's latest refugee crisis. The article makes it quite clear that historically the world community has been ill-equipped to meet the needs of uprooted people. Indeed, by the end of August there were no fewer than 100,000 suddenly homeless victims of Iraqi aggression—Kuwaitis, Egyptians, Turks, Palestinians, Indians, Pakistanis, Bangladeshis, Sri Lankans, Filipinos, and others—subsisting in squalid desert encampments in unrelenting heat. Sorely lacking were medical aid, food, water, shelter, and, perhaps most notable of all, human compassion. The president of the Paris-based *Médecins sans Frontières* (Doctors Without Borders) described the situation facing the "hostages of the desert" as one that was "unparalleled" in his 20 years as a medical relief worker. Even well-off people, he noted, had been reduced to a level of mere subsistence literally overnight. At this writing, no one knows how or when the present situation will be resolved. Already the human toll is immeasurable.

Human health is not the only topic addressed in these pages. "Healing Pooch and Puss—from Angst to Ulcers" looks at "alternative therapies" for human ailments that are now benefiting veterinary medicine. Acupuncture and homeopathic remedies are examples; they have cured vomiting in poodles, diarrhea in felines, and lameness in horses. More surprising, however, is that a wide range of animal behavior problems—*e.g.,* separation anxiety and aggressiveness—are now being treated with remarkable success by a new kind of specialist: the pet psychologist.

Medical news from A to Z . . . An express purpose of the alphabetically organized "World of Medicine" (pages 229–415) is to put health-related stories covered in the media in the past year in perspective. This is no easy task, considering that each day brings reports of new methods of treatment, new diagnostic techniques, and new causes for alarm and anxiety—about environmental threats to health, what is (or is not) safe to eat, and what constitutes a healthy life-style. The *Annual,* therefore, turns to authorities—physicians and medical scientists who are among the most knowledgeable in their fields—to evaluate "breakthroughs" and assess risks.

We always try to report on matters that seem to be much on the minds of the public. Thus, this volume includes a report that reviews the evidence to date linking cholesterol to heart disease, examining recent and controversial findings; an assessment of the very popular very low-calorie liquid-formula diets; and Special Reports on electromagnetic fields and human health and the ethical implications of the massive and costly scientific project to map the entire human genome. Several "World of Medicine" articles have as their focus socioculturally induced health problems. Some people, for example, become "addicted" to shopping as a way to fill an emotional void or defend against deeper psychological problems. Others desperately seek to alter their appearance, having repeated cosmetic surgery, often with a disastrous outcome. Still others develop life-threatening eating disorders in their effort to achieve a standard of slimness projected by the media.

Of course, daily developments in the field of medicine mean that there have been important advances since this text was prepared. Our "AIDS" report, for example, covers developments through the June 1990 Sixth International Conference on AIDS. To be sure, subsequent progress and consequential issues concerning acquired immune deficiency syndrome that have not been addressed in this volume will be included in the 1992 *Annual*.

Information you can use . . . The principal aim of the 14 articles that constitute the "Health Information Update" (pages 416–481) is to reflect current medical practice and thinking, providing information for the layperson that is both instructive and useful.

Special thanks . . . Considerable gratitude is owed to the following individuals who lent their time and expertise to review manuscripts: George P. Canellos, Chief, Division of Clinical Oncology, Dana-Farber Cancer Institute, Boston; Stephen Lock, Editor, *British Medical Journal,* London; and George H. Pollock, Ruth and Evelyn Dunbar Distinguished Professor of Psychiatry and Behavioral Sciences, Northwestern University Medical School, Chicago. The editors also wish to acknowledge the tremendous assistance provided by *Encyclopædia Britannica* picture editor Katharine W. Hannaford, who met with the author of the feature article "Do Frescoes Make You Faint?" in Florence and served as a translator when Italian resources were consulted in the editing of the article.

Finally . . . We hope this is a book that will help readers keep pace with the exciting developments in medicine and health today. I have mentioned only a few of the articles contained in the pages that follow; turn the page for the complete contents.

Ellen Bernstein

—Editor

Contents

POLIO:

Conquest of a Crippler

by Donald R. Hopkins, M.D., M.P.H.

Following the global eradication of smallpox in 1977, public health authorities began to consider other diseases that might also be eliminated from the face of the Earth. A little over a decade later, the World Health Organization (WHO) selected two diseases as the next targets: guinea worm disease, or dracunculiasis, caused by a particularly loathsome, crippling parasite and affecting some 10 million persons annually in parts of Asia and Africa, and poliomyelitis.

In 1988 an International Task Force for Disease Eradication was established under a grant from the Charles A. Dana Foundation to the Carter Center of Emory University in Atlanta, Georgia. The charge was to systematically evaluate potentially eradicable diseases. Members of the task force, which included scientists and representatives from the Dana Foundation, WHO, UNICEF, the United Nations Development Program, the World Bank, the U.S. Centers for Disease Control (CDC), the Institute of Medicine, the Swedish Academy of Sciences, the Carnegie Corporation of New York, the Rockefeller Foundation, and others, agreed that guinea worm and poliomyelitis, or polio, were the two diseases most vulnerable to the kind of concerted global campaign that banished smallpox, given the tools that are currently available.

The task force also considered six other diseases (measles, rabies, river blindness, tuberculosis, leprosy, and yaws) in its first two meetings. The eight diseases were considered partly because each was already being promoted for eradication in some way or other. It was concluded that though none of the other diseases appeared to be eradicable at present, even now it should be possible to eliminate urban rabies and the blindness caused by the parasite responsible for onchocerciasis (river blindness), though not the infection itself, and to interrupt the transmission of yaws, a disfiguring bacterial infection spread by skin-to-skin contact among children in tropical areas where hygiene is very poor. The task force's first meeting at the Carter Center was attended by its founder, former president Jimmy Carter, who pledged his personal support in enlisting the cooperation of leaders of countries where major disease-eradication efforts are to be focused.

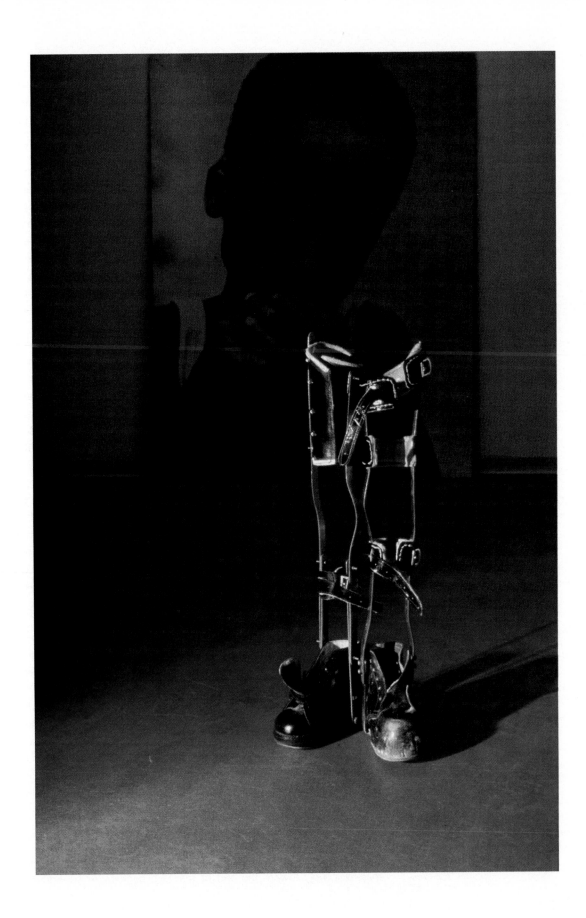

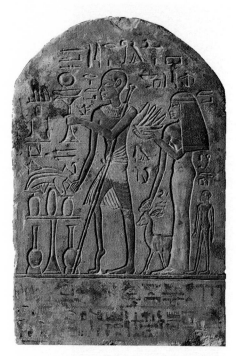

Although cruel epidemics of paralytic poliomyelitis began only about a century ago, sporadic cases are known to have occurred as far back as the 16th century BC. A carved stone stele from the 18th dynasty of ancient Egypt (1570–1342 BC) quite clearly depicts an unfortunate polio victim with characteristic withering of his lower right leg.

Donald R. Hopkins, M.D., M.P.H., *is Senior Consultant to Global 2000, the Carter Center, Atlanta, Georgia.*

(Overleaf) World Health Organization photograph by Jean-François Chrétien with the collaboration of Terre des Hommes, Lausanne

To appreciate why WHO has targeted polio for global conquest, one should know something of its unique history, its control, and the present efforts under way to eradicate it. If the current campaign is successful, the disease polio will soon join smallpox as one confined to the history books.

The disease polio

According to WHO, there are presently an estimated 10 million people in the world who have been disabled by polio, and each year another 250,000 persons are added to this number. Polio is an acute viral infection that often causes general symptoms (fever, headache, nausea, tiredness, muscle pains and spasms) that may or may not be succeeded by the more serious and characteristic flaccid paralysis of muscles in one or more limbs, the throat, or the chest. For every infected person who has symptoms, however, there are about 100 others who are infected but do not feel or appear to be ill. About 2–10% of polio victims—25,000 per year—with acute paralysis die.

Poliomyelitis means "gray marrow inflammation," referring to the virus's propensity to attack certain cells in the spinal cord and brain stem. The virus usually spreads by direct contact, from fecal contamination of food or fingers resulting in oral ingestion of the virus, or through inhalation of droplets expelled from the throat of an infected person who is talking, sneezing, or coughing. New victims may become ill about 7–14 days after ingesting or inhaling the virus. Infected persons may shed the virus from their throats for a week, beginning a day or more before suffering any symptoms themselves, and may shed the virus in their feces for a month or longer.

After it is inhaled or swallowed, the poliovirus multiplies in lymph nodes of the intestinal tract and spreads throughout the body via the bloodstream before it begins its assault on certain nerve cells in the brain and spinal cord. The virus can also spread directly in the elongated bodies (axons) of peripheral nerves to reach the spinal cord or brain. Human cells have a specific receptor for this virus that permits them to be infected by it. However, why the poliovirus reserves its most devastating effects for specific kinds of nerve cells is still unknown.

Infections may be abortive (without symptoms), nonparalytic (with symptoms but no paralysis), or paralytic. The risk of paralytic disease increases with increasing age, with pregnancy, or if, during the infection, injections are given or surgery is performed, especially tonsillectomy.

The virus can sometimes be recovered from modern sewerage systems, but there is no natural reservoir of infection besides humans. In countries with temperate climates, epidemics have a tendency to occur in the summer months and in the early fall. There are three main types of poliovirus (types I, II, and III), and persons who recover from an infection caused by one type are permanently immune to reinfection by that type of virus, regardless of whether they had symptoms.

History: ancient Egypt to modern epidemics

Polio is an ancient disease, although it began to cause outbreaks, or epidemics, only toward the end of the 19th century. A well-known stele

The elimination of smallpox from the world in 1977 proved that infectious disease eradication is feasible. An international task force that subsequently considered eight diseases for possible global eradication by the end of the 20th century deemed that only two were realistic candidates for complete conquest: guinea worm disease (dracunculiasis) and polio. For an eradication campaign to be successful, there must be international cooperation on a vast scale and, inevitably, mighty obstacles must be surmounted.

Candidates for eradication			
disease	current annual toll worldwide	chief obstacles to eradication	conclusion
poliomyelitis	250,000 cases of paralytic polio; 25,000 deaths	no insurmountable technical obstacles; increased political determination needed	eradicable
guinea worm	10 million people infected; few deaths	lack of public and political awareness; inadequate funding	eradicable
yaws and endemic syphilis	2.5 million cases	political and financial inertia	could interrupt transmission
onchocerciasis	18 million cases; 340,000 blind	high cost of vector control; no therapy to kill adult worms; restrictions in mass use of newly available drug ivermectin	could eliminate associated blindness
rabies	52,000 deaths	lack of effective way to deliver vaccine to wild animal disease carriers	could eliminate urban rabies
measles	2 million deaths (mainly children)	lack of suitably effective vaccine for young infants; cost; public misconception of seriousness	not now eradicable
tuberculosis	8 million–10 million new cases; 2 million–3 million deaths	need for improved diagnostic tests, chemotherapy, and vaccine and for wider application of current therapy	not now eradicable
leprosy	11 million–12 million cases	need for improved diagnostic tests and chemotherapy; social stigma; existence of potential animal reservoir in armadillos	not now eradicable

*goal = elimination of transmission—not eradication—because individuals may be infected for decades, and the organisms cannot be distinguished from those that cause venereal syphilis

Adapted from Report of International Task Force for Disease Eradication, *Morbidity and Mortality Weekly Report*, vol. 39, no. 13 (April 6, 1990), p. 211

from the 18th dynasty (1570–1342 BC) of ancient Egypt clearly depicts an unfortunate priest with a typical paralysis and withering of his lower right leg and foot. The mummy of the pharaoh Siptah from the late 19th Egyptian dynasty (1342–1197 BC) shows a similarly characteristic deformity of that ruler's left leg and foot. Owing to the sporadic appearance of the infection, the absence of epidemics until relatively recent times, and the nonspecific nature and infrequency of the acute illness, however, there is hardly another recognizable trace of the disease until the 18th century.

The writer Sir Walter Scott (1771–1832) was rendered lame in infancy in Edinburgh by an acute illness that appears to have been polio. In 1789 a pediatrician in London, Michael Underwood, published the first clear description of the paralytic disease of infants in a medical textbook. (Polio is also known as infantile paralysis.) In the early 19th century, small groups of polio-afflicted patients began to be reported in the medical literature, but still only as sporadic cases.

The tiny poliovirus has a unique propensity to attack specific nerve cells in the brains and spinal cords of humans. In some individuals infection causes no symptoms; in others symptoms may include fever, headache, nausea, and muscle soreness; the most serious cases are paralytic, and for 2–10% of those afflicted the disease is fatal.

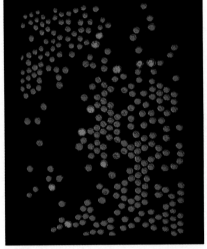

Peter Arnold, Inc.

9

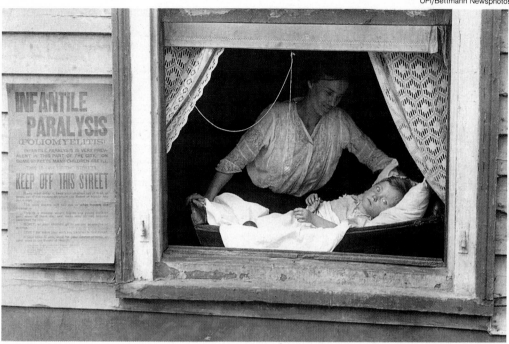

During the summer of 1916, New York City was in the grip of a merciless polio epidemic; the home of an infected child in a particularly hard-hit neighborhood was under quarantine. The notice posted outside by the Board of Health read: "Infantile paralysis is very prevalent in this part of the city. On some streets many children are ill. This is one of the streets. Keep off this street."

The first epidemics appeared in the form of outbreaks of at least 14 cases near Oslo, Norway, in 1868 and of 13 cases in northern Sweden in 1881. Not surprisingly, the idea that the hitherto sporadic cases of infantile paralysis might be contagious began to be suggested around the same time. That idea was firmly stated by a French physician, Sylvain Cordier, in 1888. The next significant epidemic, 10 times larger than previous outbreaks, with 132 recognized cases, erupted in the United States (Vermont) in 1894. During an epidemic of 1,031 cases in Sweden in 1905, Ivar Wickman first recognized the spread of disease from nonparalytic cases. By then the infection was well on the way from being an obscure, endemic, perennial but sporadic occurrence to becoming the familiar periodic epidemic phenomenon that was so widely known and feared in North America and Europe during the first half of the 20th century.

During its transformation to an epidemic disease in North America and Europe at the turn of the century, polio also began to strike older children and adults. This transformation occurred only in those industrialized countries that experienced significant improvements in hygiene. In earlier times the infection was common, and people were exposed and infected (in typically unhygienic environments) at very young ages, when they were less likely to suffer permanent paralysis as an outcome. As hygiene improved, the certainty of young people of successive generations being exposed to the virus was gradually reduced; in the new situation it was not until enough susceptible children and adults had accumulated that large numbers of cases, or epidemics, resulted when the virus appeared in their communities. The pre-19th-century sporadic, obscure pattern of polio still characterizes its status in many less developed countries. In fact, polio was not even recognized to exist in Third World tropical regions until World War II, when

10

susceptible British and U.S. troops stationed in the Philippines and Egypt began to come down with the disease.

The virus identified

The poliovirus itself was first discovered in 1908 by the Viennese immunologist Karl Landsteiner (who later won the Nobel Prize for Physiology or Medicine for his work on blood-typing) and his assistant, Erwin Popper. During the next large Swedish epidemic (3,840 cases) in 1911, Carl Kling and his colleagues at the State Bacteriological Laboratory in Stockholm recovered the poliovirus from healthy carriers as well as paralytic cases. In studying several fatal cases from the same outbreak, they found the virus in the victims' throats and in tissues of their small intestines. The existence of telltale specific antibodies to the virus circulating in the blood of infected persons had been discovered only two years after discovery of the virus itself. During the second decade of the 20th century, it became known that the number of people who had been rendered naturally immune to polio during the epidemics as a result of their having harbored silent asymptomatic infections was far higher than the number whose immunity was the result of their recovery from overt disease.

It was two Australian researchers, Franklin Macfarlane Burnet and Jean Macnamara, who in 1931 discovered the immunologic difference between strains of the poliovirus. Then, after the team of John Enders, Thomas Weller, and Frederick Robbins at Harvard Medical School in 1948 showed how the virus could be grown in large amounts in tissue culture (they shared the Nobel Prize for Physiology or Medicine in 1954 for this advance

In 1938 children with polio at the Warm Springs Foundation in Georgia entertained a special visitor, Pres. Franklin Delano Roosevelt. After Roosevelt was stricken with polio in August 1921, which left him paralyzed, he became determined to conquer his disabilities. At Warm Springs he undertook a systematic program of therapy that included swimming in the town's mineral waters. Subsequently, he established the Warm Springs Foundation, a not-for-profit rehabilitation center for polio patients, in order to share with others the benefits he had derived from his own therapy. Although FDR never achieved his greatest wish—to be able to walk again—his own obvious vitality testified that paralysis need not preclude an active and productive life.

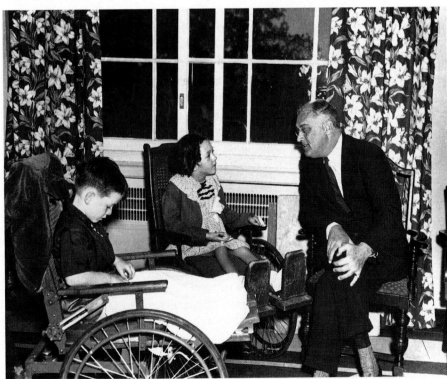

UPI/Bettmann Newsphotos

FDR's heroic efforts to mobilize the American public and the scientific community in the fight against polio perhaps were best realized in his founding of the National Foundation for Infantile Paralysis. The March of Dimes was NFIP's vastly successful public appeal for small contributions. In 1944 dimes flooded the White House mail room, where nimble-fingered workers counted the coins that would mean new strength for thousands of polio-afflicted youngsters. In 1946 the campaign featured its first "poster child," young, rehabilitated Donald Anderson.

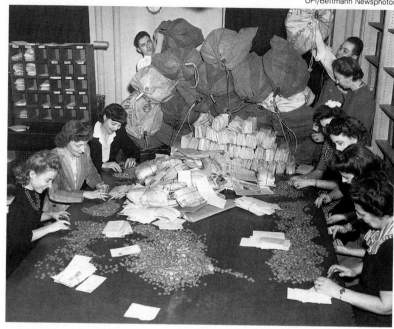

in the understanding of the virus), it was a short but painstaking step to the announcement by Jonas Salk at the University of Pittsburgh, Pennsylvania, of the efficacy of his killed-virus vaccine in 1953.

Vaccine trials

Salk's vaccine (inactivated poliovirus vaccine, or IPV) was put to a massive, successful nationwide test that involved 1.8 million children in the first, second, and third grades across the U.S. in 1954–55, after which it began to be used worldwide. Two weeks after the successful conclusion of this "Francis Field Trial" (named for Thomas Francis, Jr., the University of Michigan physician who directed it), faulty laboratory procedures at one manufacturer, the Cutter Laboratories in Berkeley, California, resulted in 204 vaccine-associated cases of polio. Had it not been for the rapid identification and recalling of the specific batches of faulty vaccine by Alexander Langmuir and other epidemiologists at what was then known as the Communicable Disease Center (CDC) in Atlanta, this "Cutter Laboratory incident" would have been a disastrous setback for the drive to prevent polio.

In the years 1961 and 1962, a new polio vaccine developed by Albert Sabin at the University of Cincinnati, Ohio, and using attenuated live viruses was licensed. This live, orally administered poliovirus vaccine (OPV) soon became the predominant vaccine used in the U.S. and most other countries.

FDR: a patient fights back

When the poliovirus attacked the 39-year-old progressive New York Democrat Franklin Delano Roosevelt in August 1921, leaving him confined to a wheelchair for the rest of his life, a series of events occurred that contributed mightily to the eventual defeat of the disease. Six years after he became a victim, FDR, using much of his own considerable fortune, established the

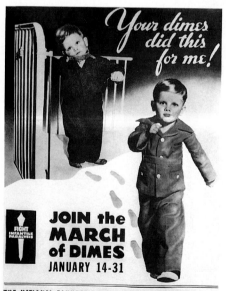

Georgia Warm Springs Foundation, an institution that became the premier establishment for rehabilitation and physical therapy of persons paralyzed by polio. Roosevelt, of course, went on to be elected president of the United States four times. Not the least of FDR's enormous contributions was his personal demonstration daily in his own very public life of the fact that the limitations imposed by paralytic polio could be triumphed over.

Soon after his first inauguration in 1933, an annual President's Birthday Ball appeal took place in order to raise funds for the fight against polio. In 1938 the National Foundation for Infantile Paralysis (NFIP), under the energetic direction of Roosevelt's former law partner, Basil O'Conner, was launched. This remarkable pioneering private institution effectively mobilized both the American public, which was increasingly alarmed at the growing size and impact of epidemic polio, and the American scientific establishment. NFIP began a public appeal, the March of Dimes, soliciting millions of small contributions. It also sponsored an influential series of international conferences on the disease and established several scientific committees of experts to address key polio issues. The collaborative interuniversity effort that typed the strains of poliovirus circulating in the U.S. in 1953, for example, was coordinated and conducted with funds appropriated by an NFIP committee. Work toward Salk's killed vaccine was also underwritten by the NFIP. Between its founding in 1938 and its disbanding in 1962, the NFIP raised an average of $25 million a year. Since then, the key role of funding and coordinating laboratory research on high-priority diseases has been assumed by the federal government, through the National Institutes of Health of the U.S. Public Health Service.

The terrible summertime polio epidemics that struck North America and Europe throughout most of the 1940s and into the early '50s are still well remembered. In 1952, when epidemics reached their peak incidence in the U.S. and 21,000 paralytic cases were recorded, children in iron lungs filled a hospital ward in Hondo, California, to capacity. Because polio attacks not only limbs but also breathing muscles, many victims needed respirators to prevent them from suffocating; iron lungs, or tank ventilators, saved the lives of those whose infections left them unable to breathe. The ventilators consist of a metal housing that repeatedly fills with air, then pumps it out. The entire body is encased in the airtight rigid tank, leaving only the head exposed. As the tank empties, air flows into the patient's lungs; as it fills, the air presses down on the body, forcing the patient to exhale. Some who were stricken by polio were dependent on iron lungs only while their own lungs revived; others needed ventilator assistance for the rest of their lives.

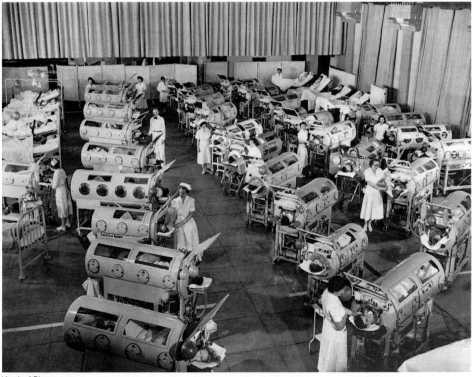

March of Dimes

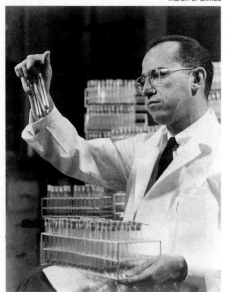

In 1953 Jonas E. Salk at the University of Pittsburgh, Pennsylvania, announced the efficacy of the first vaccine against polio, made from a killed, or inactivated, poliovirus (IPV). Polio's demise began when the Salk vaccine was released for general use in 1955, after vastly successful trials involving over a million U.S. schoolchildren.

Era of panic and fear

The summertime terror engendered by nearly annual polio epidemics in North America and Europe in the 1940s and early 1950s will always be remembered by those who experienced that era but may be hard to imagine for those who did not. At its peak incidence in the U.S., in 1952, approximately 21,000 cases of paralytic polio (13.6 per 100,000) were recorded. These were concentrated in the summer and early fall, and they were reported prominently in local and national press. Children were kept away from swimming pools, movie theaters, and other crowded places where they might be exposed to the dreaded virus. Polio victims encased in iron lungs (introduced in 1929 to assist their breathing), displayed in public areas such as department stores as part of the NFIP's effort to appeal for donations from the public, also added to the terror with which the disease and its seasonal appearances were regarded.

Thus, the announcement of the successful outcome of the trial of Salk's vaccine on April 12, 1955, the 10th anniversary of Franklin D. Roosevelt's death, was widely hailed. It was welcomed by some as a mid-20th-century "miracle." On that date polio's demise began.

Vaccine era: industrialized countries

Over four million doses of Salk's vaccine were given in the U.S. in less than a month after it was released for general use in 1955. During the next four years, more than 450 million doses of the IPV were distributed, and the incidence of the paralytic form of polio fell from 18 cases per 100,000 persons to less than 2 per 100,000. Sabin's OPV predominated in the U.S. soon after it was introduced in 1962. By the early 1970s the annual incidence of polio in the U.S. had declined 1,000-fold from prevaccine levels, to an average of only 12 cases a year.

In 1957 hundreds lined up for vaccination at a high school gym in Protection, Kansas. By 1960 more than 450 million U.S. children and adults had received IPV injections, and the incidence of paralytic polio had dropped from 18 cases per 100,000 persons to less than 2 per 100,000.

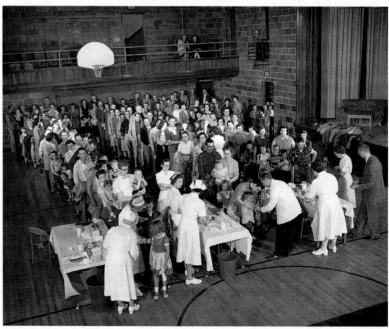

Finland began limited vaccination with the Salk vaccine in 1957 following two major outbreaks in 1954 and 1956. Some 1.5 million persons were then vaccinated in a mass campaign in 1960–61, which eliminated the disease altogether in that country. Sweden's experience was similar, as was that in The Netherlands—the latter achieving zero incidence in 1972; these countries, too, used only the killed vaccine.

Belgium began using the Salk vaccine in 1958 and the Sabin vaccine in 1963; as a result, polio disappeared as an endemic disease in the late 1960s. Denmark introduced IPV to its population in 1955 and the OPV in 1963 and experienced only sporadic cases of the disease after 1962.

Even before the Sabin vaccine was licensed for use in the United States, two Soviet researchers, Mihail Chumakov and Anatolij Smorodintsev, adapted strains of the OPV virus sent to them by Sabin for manufacture and testing in the U.S.S.R., and a live polio vaccine was introduced for public use. Whereas the Salk vaccine had been used on only a small scale in that country (some eight million doses), a massive immunization campaign with the live vaccine reached 77.5 million persons, or over 36% of the Soviet population, in 1959–60. The incidence of reported paralytic polio in the U.S.S.R. fell from 10.6 cases per 100,000 in 1958 to 0.43 per 100,000 in 1963. After 1964 rates fluctuated between 0.01 and 0.1 cases per 100,000.

As the fear and memories of polio epidemics faded rapidly in many European and North American communities after mass vaccination programs greatly reduced or eliminated the incidence of polio, the failure of complacent parents to have their children vaccinated soon led to lower overall rates of routine immunization. One important consequence of the failure to maintain adequate levels of immunization was the occasional spread of poliovirus, with appearance of paralytic cases again following importation of virus by travelers from regions where the disease was still endemic. Compulsory laws requiring the immunization of infants and school-age children were then introduced in various countries, with varying success.

The danger of this residual vulnerability in many industrialized countries was illustrated in particularly spectacular fashion by a multinational outbreak in 1978–79. The epidemic first came to attention in The Netherlands, where 110 cases, 80 of them paralytic, suddenly occurred in an unvaccinated religious community in 1978. Later evidence suggested the virus probably had been introduced there from a Middle Eastern country at the start of the outbreak. From The Netherlands the virus spread to a religious group of Dutch descent in Canada, where it caused another two cases, and then to Amish groups in the United States. A new laboratory technique called oligonucleotide mapping, which permitted the virtual "fingerprinting" of individual strains of poliovirus and which was far more sophisticated and sensitive than the simple typing into three groups, was used to trace the polio strains in these epidemics.

Two other problems attained prominence in some industrialized countries as polio incidence declined. A postpolio syndrome is recognized to cause new symptoms of disease in former polio victims whose original disease had been stabilized for years or even decades. This rare syndrome may

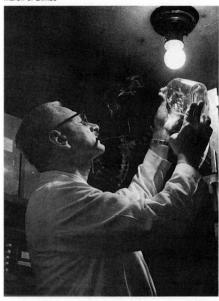

In the late 1950s Albert B. Sabin at the University of Cincinnati, Ohio, was at work developing a vaccine for polio using live attenuated, or weakened, virus. His orally administered poliovirus vaccine (OPV) was licensed for use in 1961–62 and soon became the predominant form used in the United States and most of the world. Debate about which of the two rival vaccines, IPV or OPV, is best continues to this day.

15

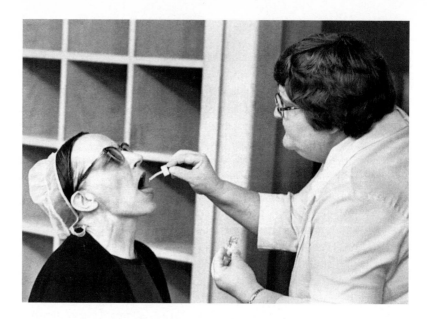

manifest itself as increased weakness, muscle atrophy, or other symptoms involving the originally affected muscle groups or different groups of muscles. The cause of the disorder is unknown, but it is suspected to be due to an altered, pathological immune reaction. The other problem (also rare) is the risk of vaccine-associated polio, which occurs when the live-virus vaccine causes disease in recipients or in one of their close contacts (often a member of the same family). The estimated frequency of paralytic disease from this complication is on the order of up to one such vaccine-associated case in a recipient and one in a contact per four million doses of vaccine.

For all the residual problems, however, the introduction of polio vaccines in the mid-1950s led inexorably to the decline and eventual disappearance of indigenous paralytic polio in many industrialized countries over the next quarter century. With very few exceptions, notably Cuba, this was not the case in the mostly tropical countries of Asia, Africa, and Latin America.

Polio in less developed countries: a very different course

As noted earlier, the very existence of polio in less developed tropical countries was not widely recognized until the early 1940s, when paralytic cases appeared among U.S. and British troops. Even up to the 1970s, polio was not considered a significant problem. Reporting of cases was very poor, as it still is for the less developed world; moreover, it was erroneously thought that poor sanitation caused infection by polioviruses in infancy, rendering indigenous populations permanently immune.

Immunization against polio was included in the Expanded Program on Immunization (EPI), launched by WHO in 1974, with the goal of ensuring vaccination against six diseases (diphtheria, whooping cough, tetanus, tuberculosis, measles, and polio) for all the world's children by the year 1990. At the time this courageous initiative began, fewer than 5% of children in less developed countries were receiving routine immunizations.

One of the early efforts of the EPI was to clarify the impact of the target diseases in the less developed countries. When "lameness surveys" were conducted in several tropical countries, it was learned, to considerable

16

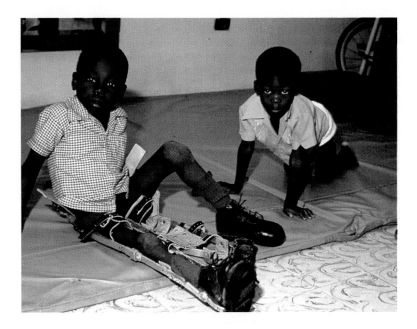

surprise, that from 5 to 9 of every 1,000 schoolchildren had evidence of lameness due to paralysis caused by polio. This kind of information helped to change the perception of polio in the tropics and provided stronger political support and justification for inclusion of polio vaccine in national immunization programs.

There were many obstacles that had to be overcome if the EPI's goal was to be achieved, despite the then-impending success of the global smallpox-eradication program. Smallpox was easily diagnosed; the vaccine against it needed to be given only once or twice; and the hardy vaccine remained stable under tropical conditions. By contrast, the polio vaccine is extremely vulnerable to heat; therefore, it requires careful refrigeration from the time of manufacture until the time it is administered. Further, it needs to be administered at least three or four times. The live attenuated Sabin vaccine was usually used since it was simpler to administer: it could be given by mouth, without the need for needles or syringes. Polio vaccination was also a more daunting task because the EPI sought to help countries develop a

The course of polio infection in the less developed parts of the world has differed markedly from that in industrialized nations. When leg braces had become a relic of the past in the developed world, polio remained rampant in tropical countries of Asia, Africa, and Latin America. The polio-afflicted youngsters above are from Malawi. Paralysis has left the Mexican youth below confined to life in a wheelchair. Rehabilitation services for young people handicapped by polio have not been adequate in most less developed countries. Recognizing the need to rehabilitate polio victims so that they can be integrated into society and live productive lives, the World Health Organization has established a Rehabilitation Program.

Photographs, Rotary International

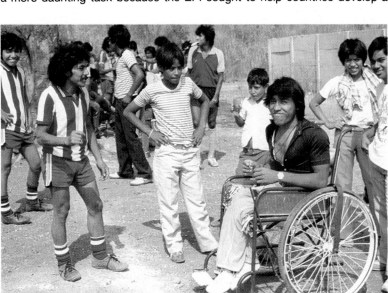

World Health Organization; photograph, J. Littlewood

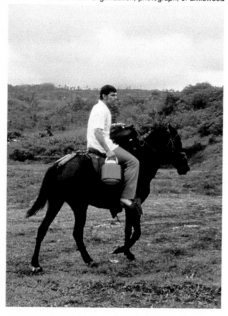

A health worker in Costa Rica carries polio vaccine in a special insulated container. A major hurdle to the success of immunization efforts in tropical countries has been the extreme vulnerability of the vaccine to heat. It requires careful refrigeration from the time it is manufactured until it is administered. Poor transportation networks have also impeded delivery of vaccine, especially to remote villages.

Sustained efforts that began with the Expanded Program on Immunization in the mid-1970s have been highly successful in nearly eliminating polio from Western Hemisphere countries. By mid-1990 only 3 confirmed polio cases had been recorded, compared with 45 cases at mid-1989. The campaign must now concentrate its efforts on the Eastern Hemisphere, particularly the tropical regions of Africa and Asia, where significant rates of infection yet prevail.

system that could ensure that all children would be routinely immunized as they came of age rather than only in a single mass campaign. In addition to the exacting need for adequate refrigeration (*i.e.*, a "cold chain" maintained from the manufacturer to the recipients), numerous other conditions needed to be addressed. These included overall poverty, the very poor state of the health systems in most countries, poor transportation networks, lack of vehicles, high cost of fuel, apathy toward health issues at local and national levels, and managerial weaknesses.

By painstakingly emphasizing improvement in surveillance of the diseases, training of national health workers and managers, and development of national plans of action and by encouraging practical research based on needs in the field, the EPI slowly laid the groundwork for sustainable immunization programs over the first decade of its existence. Beginning in the mid-1980s other international agencies, especially UNICEF, added their considerable energies to helping ensure the availability of sufficient external resources for the program. By late 1989 the proportion of children being immunized had increased from less than 5 to about 67%, and polio had been singled out for total eradication.

Toward global eradication

In May 1985 the Pan American Health Organization, WHO's regional body for the Americas, announced an initiative to eradicate indigenous transmission of polio from the Americas by the end of 1990. This followed the success of Canada and the United States in eliminating the disease, as well as the successes of Cuba and Brazil, among others. Cuba began its highly successful annual mass vaccination campaigns in 1962. Whereas an annual total of 214 cases was reported between 1955 and 1961, only five sporadic Cuban cases were recorded between 1963 and 1978. Brazil

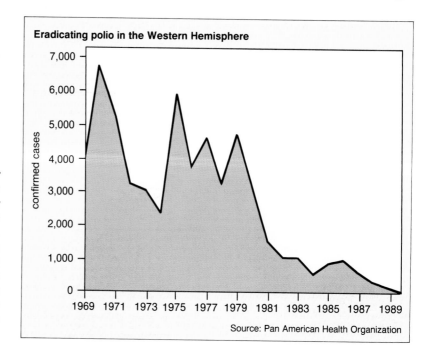

Eradicating polio in the Western Hemisphere

Source: Pan American Health Organization

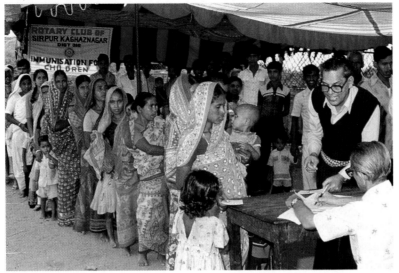

In 1985 Rotary International undertook its PolioPlus campaign, an unprecedented effort to raise funds that would provide polio vaccine to all parts of the world where it is needed. (Left) Rotarian volunteers assist national health workers in vaccinating villagers in India. The poster below announces an "immunization day" in Brazil. From 1980 through 1982 immunization days twice a year provided OPV to 20 million Brazilian children under the age of five. In each successive year dramatic drops were seen in the numbers of reported polio cases, and extremely low infection rates have been sustained.

began an extraordinary effort in 1980 of administering oral polio vaccine to all children under five years of age in a single day, twice a year. Over 20 million children were vaccinated in each of the six campaigns conducted in 1980, 1981, and 1982. Brazil's reported number of cases of polio dropped from an average of 2,330 per year in the years 1975–80 to 122 cases in 1981 and 69 in 1982.

 · Results of the effort in the Americas have been impressive. Only 335 confirmed cases were found in all the Americas in 1988 (a decline of 64% from 1986), and there was a provisional total of only 132 cases in 1989. More importantly, transmission of the wild virus (in contrast to vaccine strains) was confined to increasingly smaller geographic areas. Only 1.9% of the counties or districts in the region reported any confirmed polio cases in 1988.

Progress toward achievement of the 1990 goal set by the Americas was a major factor in the decision by the World Health Assembly in May 1988 to set the goal of global eradication of polio by the year 2000. The European Region of WHO had already announced its goal of eliminating indigenous polio by 1995. UNICEF, the U.S. Agency for International Development (USAID), and Rotary International, which were major supporters of the pioneering effort in the region of the Americas, pledged their support for the global effort as well. In an unprecedented display of private initiative, Rotary International announced its PolioPlus campaign in 1985, with the goal of raising $120 million to provide all the polio vaccine needed for the next five years. By the time this organization held its annual convention in 1988, the staggering sum of $219 million had been raised, in addition to the mobilization of countless Rotarian volunteers to assist in many countries' national immunization activities.

The final countdown

As the countdown to polio eradication progresses, laboratory services and research have critical, exciting roles to play. Confirmation of each suspected

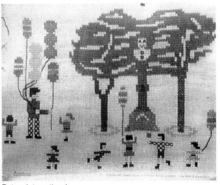

19

case by isolation of the poliovirus, linkage of cases epidemiologically, and detection of virus in the environment are increasingly important. Newer techniques have yielded more and more sophisticated ways to trace and link strains of wild poliovirus and to distinguish potentially infective naturally occurring wild strains of the virus from vaccine strains, which are rarely associated with paralytic disease. In the process of oligonucleotide mapping, the poliovirus strain is partly digested by an enzyme, then subjected to an electric current in two dimensions to elicit its characteristic "fingerprint" of spots from component fragments. This technique has been hailed as a particularly elegant example of molecular epidemiology used to trace connections between cases and outbreaks.

More recently, scientists have begun using a process called nucleic acid hybridization in combination with polymerase chain reaction techniques to detect incredibly small amounts of poliovirus in sewage or other specimens. These latest methods exploit a characteristic of the genetic material in the virus to specifically amplify any poliovirus that is present in a specimen, thereby increasing the amount of virus to more easily detectable levels, even though the original amount of virus may have been extremely small (e.g., one viral particle).

Other important research efforts continue to seek ways to improve the potency of the killed Salk vaccine (so as to reduce the number of injections required) and increase the stability of the live Sabin vaccine (to reduce the stringent requirements of the cold chain). Another effort is to create extremely pure hybrids of the live vaccine strains through genetic engineering techniques so as to eliminate the small risk of vaccine-associated paralytic disease altogether.

The debate about the two types of vaccines—and the rivalry between their progenitors, Salk and Sabin—continues. The live Sabin vaccine has been the one most widely used, mainly because it (1) is simple to administer (by drops placed in the mouth rather than by injection), (2) prevents circulation of wild poliovirus by creating immunity in the intestine as well as in the blood of vaccinees, and (3) is naturally spread to others in the family and community where hygienic levels are low. However, this form of vaccine is not perfect. Apart from the logistic requirements of the cold chain and the risk of vaccine-associated disease (especially in industrialized countries), other enteric viruses circulating in tropical communities (causing frequent episodes of diarrhea) appear to interfere with the live vaccine strain's ability to produce immunity in some persons. Thus, in recent years increasing attention has been given to the possibility that the killed vaccine may be preferable in some situations, especially if it could be effective after fewer doses. At present, both vaccines need to be given three times at intervals of about a month, beginning in early infancy. A fourth ("booster") dose of live vaccine is recommended at about six years of age; a booster of killed vaccine should be given about 6–12 months after the third dose. Some vaccine specialists advocate using both vaccines in the same children (two or three doses of killed vaccine followed by a similar series of live vaccine). When or whether one regimen or the other is clearly better in specific circumstances is still not known.

A crippler's road to extinction

c. 1475 BC: polio victim depicted on Egyptian stele

1789: first clinical description of polio (England)

1840: polio recognized to attack spinal cord (Germany)

1868, 1881: first epidemics recognized (Scandinavia)

1886: polio recognized as an infectious disease (France)

1894: major epidemic in Vermont (first in North America)

1905: importance of nonparalytic cases in spread of the disease recognized (Sweden)

1908: poliovirus discovered (Austria)

1911: virus isolated from paralytic cases, healthy carriers, and wall of small intestine (Sweden)

1927: Franklin D. Roosevelt establishes Georgia Warm Springs Foundation for polio victims

1931: differences in strains of poliovirus recognized (Australia)

1938: National Foundation for Infantile Paralysis founded (U.S.)

1948: poliovirus grown in tissue culture (U.S.)

1953: Jonas Salk publishes results of killed vaccine studies (U.S.)

1955: success of Salk vaccine trials (U.S.)

1961–62: Albert Sabin's live oral vaccine licensed (U.S.)

1974: WHO launches Expanded Program on Immunization

1985: Pan American Health Organization announces initiative to eliminate polio from Americas by 1990

1988: 41st World Health Assembly resolves to eradicate polio from world by 2000

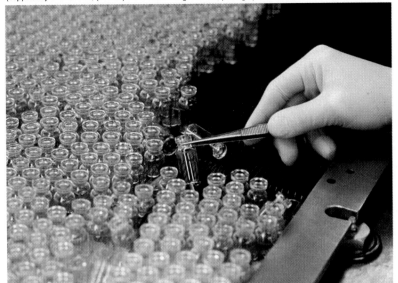

In the final countdown toward global eradication of poliomyelitis, research has a vital role to play. Newly developed tools of molecular biology now make it possible to delineate among the three types of poliovirus and to identify wild virus strains that are potentially infective. At the same time, because immunization remains the key to achievement of the goal, new efforts are being made to improve both IPV and OPV and to determine the best regimens for giving the vaccines. Certainly every remaining obstacle should be vanquished for the sake of the generations of young people the world over who will not have to suffer paralytic polio's lifelong consequences.

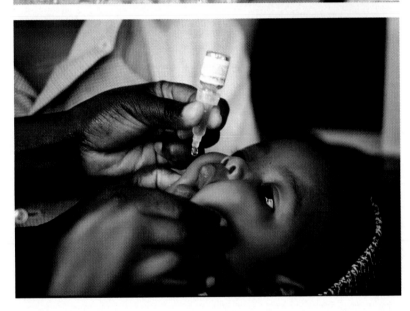

WHO estimates that between 1989 and 2000 the polio-eradication initiative will cost about $150 million in addition to the costs of the EPI itself. Virologist T. Jacob John, a leader in the polio-eradication effort in India, points out, however, that "the total financial loss due to one case of polio is sufficient to immunize 10,000 children and prevent 100 cases of the disease." According to the CDC, the U.S. alone is currently spending over $50 million per year in public sector costs in order to maintain its current polio-free status. Thus, the achievement of total polio eradication will bring not-insignificant financial benefits. But the greatest benefits of eradicating polio will surely be to those who will not suffer the lifelong consequences of paralytic poliomyelitis. As expressed by Ralph Henderson, who served as director of the EPI from 1977 to 1989, the eradication of polio will be a fitting gift from the 20th century to the 21st century.

21

A Less than
Loving Look
at
DOCTORS

by William H. Helfand

You often read a symptom wrong,
And never keep a patient long;
But after all—you do your best:—
The undertaker does the rest.

So reads the verse on a comic valentine, *c.* 1885. Such affronts to the doctor have been around since the time of the ancient Greeks. Plato, for example, wrote in the *Gorgias* (*c.* 460 BC): "The surest sign of bad government and social anarchy is to find many judges and many physicians." And Nicocles, ruler of Salamis, the principal city of ancient Cyprus, commented in the 4th century BC that the physician was fortunate, for the Sun exploits his successes and the Earth conceals his errors. Through the ages the specific targets of medical satire have varied with the times and the state of the art of medicine; the sharpness of medical faultfinding has been determined by the status of the physician and the way in which society has been served. Since the late 19th century, notable advances in the practice of medicine may have altered the direction of medical satire but by no means have caused its elimination.

The art of irreverence

Perhaps the most often-used and successful vehicles for attacks on medicine have been caricatures and cartoons. (The terms are often used interchangeably.) The word *caricature* derives from the Italian verb *caricare,* meaning "to overload," as with exaggerated detail. These graphic presentations are distorted in such a way as to hold persons, types, or actions up to ridicule. Caricatures as a form date to the Renaissance and the Reformation, with their emphasis on the importance of the individual. In its necessary distortion, caricature assaults an individual or an issue, seeing only the grotesque and negative. *Cartoon* in its original meaning was a full-size preparatory design for execution as a painting, a tapestry, a fresco, a mosaic, or other art form. In the mid-19th century the term acquired a new meaning, and cartoons thus came into being as pictorial parodies. Using the devices of analogy and ludicrous juxtaposition and frequently highlighted

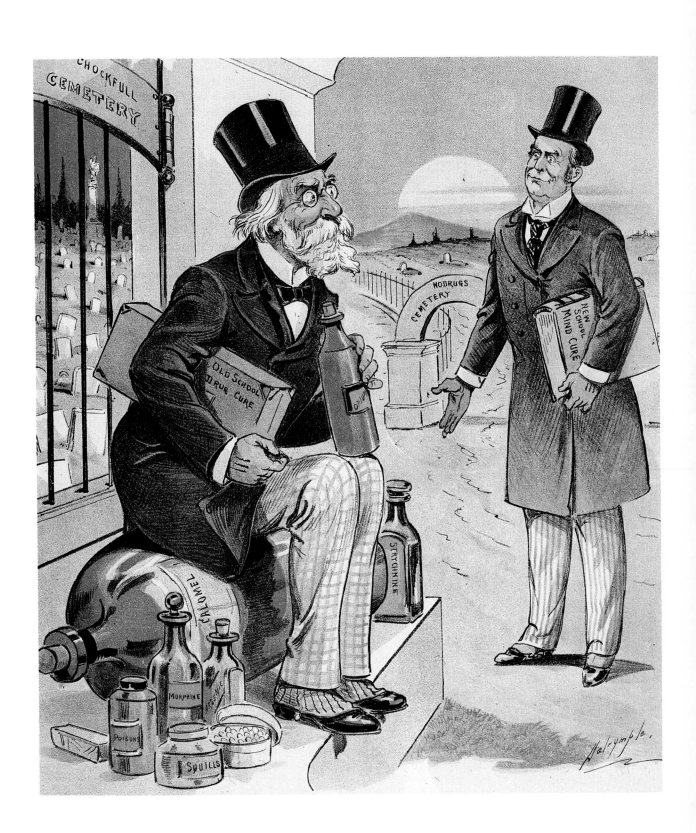

William H. Helfand is a consultant to the National Library of Medicine, Bethesda, Maryland, and the Philadelphia Museum of Art. He has lectured and exhibited portions of his personal collection of prints and ephemera in the fields of medicine and pharmacy in the United States, Canada, and Europe and is the author or coauthor of several books on medicine and pharmacy. Presently he is completing a book on medical and pharmaceutical posters.

(Overleaf) An 1898 American cartoon by Louis Dalrymple; photograph, The Granger Collection

by written dialogue or commentary, these drawings serve to sharpen the public view of a contemporary event or trend. Normally humorous, they can at times be positively savage.

It is easy to understand the widespread use of caricatures and cartoons to attack medicine in general and its practitioners in particular. Because they have always occupied necessary and important positions in society, doctors have offered ripe targets for observations by social critics. Attacks on medicine and the physician give a layperson's view of wrongs and situations to be changed; they can as such be perceived as having a positive purpose in their desire to improve. Backhanded though they may seem, by pointing to the limitations and deficiencies of such an estimable—indeed exalted—science and art, these attacks can be considered a tribute to medicine's achievements.

The character of the physician, like that of the clergyman, is expected to be above reproach, and any minor deviation from high moral standards is bound to be magnified. Indeed, the Hippocratic oath, accepted as a guide to conduct and still recited at graduation ceremonies at many medical schools, prescribes that physicians not only refrain from causing harm but also live exemplary personal and professional lives. If their character turns out to be not quite so meritorious, their deficiencies are readily magnified. Caricaturists and cartoonists have been quick with their censure—from humorous to scathing—whenever physicians fall short of the demands made upon the privileged position they hold. To patients, the doctor often has assumed a dignity hardly warranted by circumstances.

Vanity, greed, indifference, ambition, ignorance, ostentation, corruption, and arrogance have all been pinned on representatives of the medical profession. By turns, physicians have been portrayed as unsympathetic,

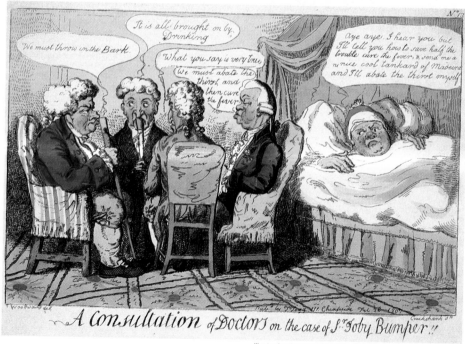

Illustration by Isaac Cruikshank; collection, William H. Helfand

pompous, malicious, evil, lustful, and mercenary; they inspire fear, charge exorbitant fees, fail to provide essential services, make fatal mistakes out of their ignorance, and, if comic valentines can be considered a reputable guide, are repeatedly and thoroughly vile.

Medical manners

Medical consultations, the calling in of colleagues to discuss a case, have long been a popular subject of caricaturists. Hippocrates, traditionally regarded as the father of medicine, in his *Precepts* warned, "Physicians who meet in consultation must never quarrel, or jeer at one another." Sir William Osler (1849–1919), often called the father of bedside medicine, was very dubious about the consultation and wondered, "Can anything be more doleful than a procession of four or five doctors into the sick man's room?" The American physician and man of letters Oliver Wendell Holmes (1809–94) chose the consultation as a theme for a poem:

Now when a doctor's patients are perplexed,
A *consultation* comes in order next—
You know what that is? In a certain place
Meet certain doctors to discuss a case
And other matters, such as weather, crops,
Potatoes, pumpkins, lager-beer, and hops.
For what's the use?—there's little to be said,
Nine times in ten your man's as good as dead;
At best a talk (the secret to disclose)
Where three men guess and *sometimes* one man knows.

—*Rip Van Winkle, M.D., Canto II*

Indeed, such consultations have always been troubling to patients, who could never be sure they were necessary, were almost certain they were a system to raise fees, could not comprehend what was being said, or believed that these "meetings of minds" were, in fact, a conspiracy. The English caricaturist Isaac Cruikshank (1756?–1811) portrayed a frustrated patient's impatience with four physicians who appear to be wasting time in his "A Consultation of Doctors on the Case of Sr Toby Bumper!!" In "The Consultation, or Last Hope," by another well-known English caricaturist, Thomas Rowlandson (1756–1827), who often chose members of the medical profession as the subjects of his pointed attacks, 10 doctors attend a wealthy gout-ridden patient—a look of extreme terror on the sick man's face as he contemplates the inability of the physicians to alleviate his distress.

The doctors hardly are heeding Hippocrates when they not only disagree but come to blows in Isaac Cruikshank's "Doctors Differ and Their Patients Die" or when they resort to out-and-out insulting of one another in the French artist Charles-Emile Jacque's "The Consensus of a Consultation of Doctors." In this 1843 print, one of the doctors says, "I tell you that if this gentleman follows your advice he will not have more than three days to live," and his colleague replies, "If he follows your advice he is a dead man." While a German proverb held that "no doctor is better than three," the caricaturists seem to abide by the Italian proverb that contends, "While the doctors consult, the patient dies."

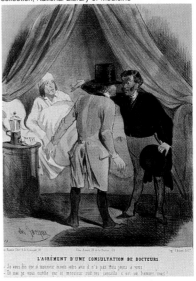

Caricaturists leave little doubt that they question the ability of members of the medical profession to help their patients—the fate of the ailing one being all the more dubious when two or more doctors consult.

25

Caricaturists and cartoonists have been quick with their censure whenever physicians have fallen short of the demands made upon the privileged position they hold. They have been portrayed, among other things, as unsympathetic and incompetent, self-serving and mercenary, impossible to get an appointment with, and, vis-à-vis the female patient, downright lecherous.

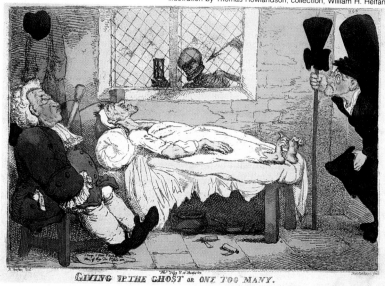

GIVING UP THE GHOST or ONE TOO MANY.

Physicians have also been portrayed in a wide array of situations as utterly unsympathetic, as self-serving, and as capitalizing on their patients' woes. In Rowlandson's engraving "Giving Up the Ghost or One Too Many" (c. 1813), the fat doctor, his gold-headed cane in hand, has fallen asleep as his patient expires; a more alert undertaker, sensing opportunity, has arrived with a coffin. The French artist Honoré Daumier (1808–79) illustrated the exultation of a physician who has his own advancement in mind; he tells a patient, "I'm delighted! You have yellow fever, it's the first time in my life that I will be lucky enough to treat it." In an uncaptioned drawing by the contemporary French cartoonist Claude Serre, there is glee in the eyes of an orthopedic surgeon as he carefully contemplates the bandaged patient before him—the walls of his office already covered with "trophies"

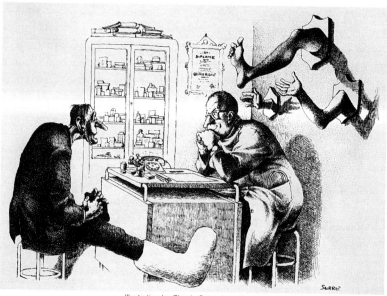

of human hands, arms, and legs. Another Serre cartoon depicts the outright hilarity of a radiologist as he views his disconsolate patient's internal organs on a fluoroscope.

A common theme of contemporary cartoons that are revealing of medical manners is how difficult it is to get to see a doctor when one needs to. The unnecessary and lengthy forms to be filled out, the endlessly long waiting times spent in the physician's office perusing outdated magazines, the requirement for an appointment even in the face of dire emergency, and the impossibility of getting a doctor to make a house call have all been the subjects of cartoons that express the well-warranted indignation of the hapless patient. In one cartoon a nurse asks a patient who appears with an ax stuck in his skull, "Do you have an appointment?" A physician's response to a patient who wants him to make a house call is: "Did Freud make house calls? Did Osler make house calls? Did Sir Alexander Fleming make house calls?" And a woman on the telephone expresses her incredulity: "You mean you *will* make a house call? . . . How can we be sure you're not a quack?"

And largely because male physicians often conduct their examinations in private with female patients, the romantic imagination of the artist has assumed the worst. In a contemporary cartoon by Syd Hoff, the doctor assures his patient he knows best what she needs (as he ravishes her). And cartoonist Whitney Darrow, Jr., presents a doctor who inquires with great interest of his completely disrobed patient's *tonsil!* Dentists, too, are accused of lust, for their female patients are often vulnerable, especially when under anesthesia.

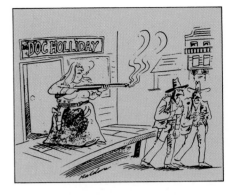

"It's always the same. You can never get past the receptionist."
© *Punch*/Rothco

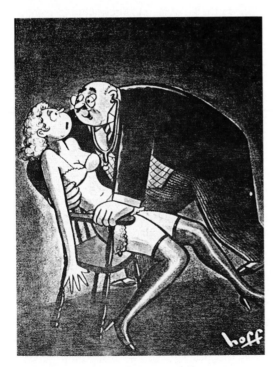

"But I'm your doctor, Miss Faversham, and I know what you need!"
Drawing by Sydney Hoff; © 1938, 1990 The Hearst Corporation

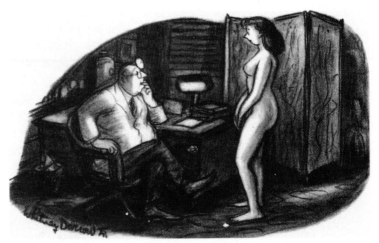

"Now just how long has this tonsil been bothering you, Miss Lorrimer?"
Drawing by Whitney Darrow, Jr.; © 1939, 1967 The New Yorker Magazine, Inc.

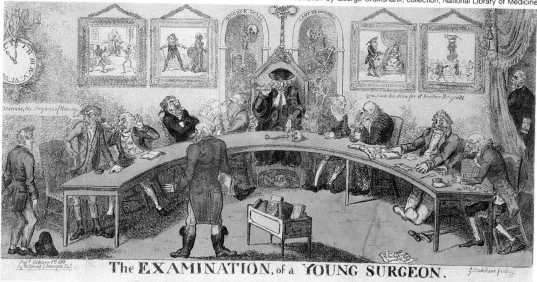

The EXAMINATION, of a YOUNG SURGEON.

George Cruikshank was considered one of the finest caricaturists of his day, surpassing his father, Isaac, with his prolific and dexterous satires on every variety of public event. The follies and failings of members of the medical and surgical professions found ample representation among his spirited etchings. Cruikshank was no respecter of the honored positions of the examiners in the College of Surgeons or of the state of the art of surgery in the early 1800s.

Questionable competence

Professional competence—not to mention professional etiquette—turns up again and again in medical caricatures. Prior to the close of the 19th century and the development of effective therapies, physicians very often could do little or nothing for their patients, but to the satirists that fact was rarely a legitimate justification for their blatant failures. It is not really surprising that with the inadequate state of medicine the skills and knowledge of medical practitioners would be undervalued or despised, but then caricaturists never claimed to be evenhanded.

The French writer Voltaire (1694–1778), a master of satire, wrote: "Doctors are men who prescribe medicine of which they know little to cure diseases of which they know less in human beings of which they know nothing." Caricaturists of Voltaire's day surely reflected that piece of wisdom. In Isaac Cruikshank's "Ghost of the Village Doctor," a physician, on meeting a former patient, inquires, "Any slight returns of the fever?" The patient replies, "No, thank you, doctor—got quite well—been mending ever since you left us—and so has all the village."

Daumier joined those who attributed the death of patients to the artless physician. In his series of satires directed against the greed and immorality that permeated the Second Republic, the physician in the "Clinic of Dr. Robert Macaire" boasts, " . . . gentlemen, you've seen this operation which they said was impossible, performed with complete success." A student then observes, "But, sir, the patient is dead," to which the disdainful reply is, "So what! She would have died even without the operation."

In "The Examination of a Young Surgeon," the British caricaturist George Cruikshank (1792–1878), son of Isaac, ridiculed the lack of medical standards in the early 19th century, suggesting that the deaf, senile, greedy examiners were inadequate to their important task. His attack (dated 1811) was aimed at the recently founded College of Surgeons. While the standards of the surgical profession at the turn of the 18th century may

28

have left a great deal to be desired, it is doubtful that they were quite as deplorable or outrageous as the artist suggested. In caricature, of course, they rarely are.

In addition to criticizing competence and deploring medical standards, caricaturists were quick to direct similar barbs at many of the questionable practices of pre-19th-century "doctors." These included: graverobbers ("Resurrectionists" and "Sack-em-up Men"), who flourished in the early 1800s, especially in Great Britain, guaranteeing a continual supply of cadavers for dissection in anatomy class; transplanters of teeth, who took fresh supplies from poverty-stricken adolescents and attached them to stumps in the mouths of willing adults; and uroscopists, who emerged in the early Middle Ages and held their position well into the Renaissance, purporting to divine patients' illnesses from their urine, and basing their far-reaching conclusions on study of the color, density, content, and clouds that formed in such specimens. Even the artist Albrecht Dürer (1471–1528), not particularly known for his satire, exhibited his contempt for uroscopy in a drawing executed in the margin of a prayer book. The depiction was apparently inspired by a line ("Thou who has healed the sick woman . . . ") from a prayer, "In Recognition of One's Frailty"; his caricature of a pompous doctor examining the contents of his urine flask was hardly flattering.

Quackery in all its forms was (and still is) a frequent subject, with even well-meaning and well-trained physicians depicted as quacks in the caricaturist's zeal to offend. Of course, it was not always a simple matter to identify proper quacks and charlatans, especially in periods before the late 19th century, when the behavior of all health practitioners, from highest to lowest, was not too dissimilar. The English writer Horace Walpole (1717–97) recognized the ambiguity: "By quack I mean imposter, not in opposition to but in common with physicians." So also had the playwright John Ford

From Albrecht Dürer's *Randzeichnungen aus dem Gebetbuche des Kaisers Maximilian I*, Munich

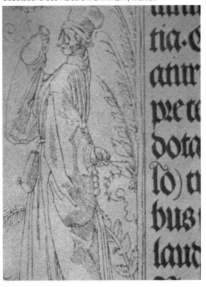

Nearly six centuries ago Albrecht Dürer was one of many artists to show his contempt for uroscopy, a practice that flourished from the Middle Ages into the Renaissance and whose practitioners diagnosed illnesses from the color, density, and clouds that formed in a specimen of urine. But today's practitioners, with all the wondrous advances of medicine at their disposal, are no less frequently ridiculed for their diagnostic methods.

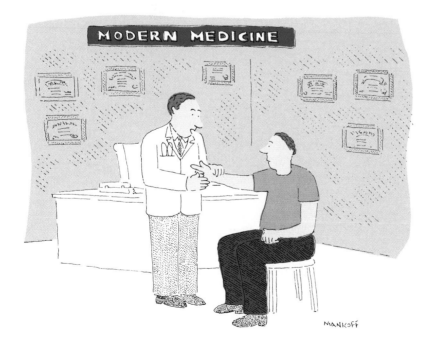

"Well, Bob, it looks like a paper cut, but just to be sure let's do lots of tests."

Illustration by
William Hogarth; collection, William H. Helfand

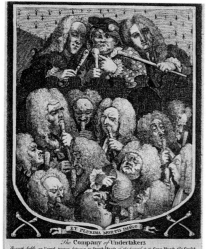

Quackery is an age-old subject for artistic attack, but the distinction between quacks and well-meaning and well-trained doctors is not always so obvious.

a century earlier; in *The Lover's Melancholy* (1628) Ford wrote: "Mountebanks, empirics, quack-salvers, mineralists, wizards, alchemists, cast-apothecaries, old wives and barbers, are all suppositors [supporters] to the right worshipful doctor." In "The Company of Undertakers" the English painter and engraver William Hogarth (1697–1764), who gained his reputation as a supreme moralist and satirist, made this point well in placing three foolish-looking quacks garbed as physicians prominently above 12 rightful and very serious-looking physicians.

Time and again the graphic satirists have challenged not just the competence of the practitioners but their proclivity for botching their treatments or for making fatal "mistakes." A 1910 cartoon from *Punch* shows a girl returning a bottle of medicine to the doctor and saying, "Please, sir, I've brought the remains of the medicine you gave grandfather. He's dead, and mother thought you might like it for somebody else." And despite today's medical expertise, to the cartoonists the competence of practitioners of medicine seems just as questionable as ever. They rely on needless fancy tests or cannot seem to manage the simplest test. (One cartoon shows a patient whose blood has been drawn for a cholesterol test now needing a tetanus shot.) Dentists are forced to make excuses for pulling the wrong tooth, surgeons for removing the wrong limb or not fully accounting for all their instruments, and pharmacists for using the wrong ingredient. The fate of a poor victim in one contemporary cartoon is that "the doctor treated him for jaundice for three months and today learns he is Chinese."

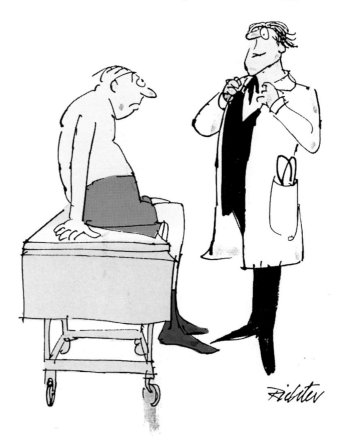

"Orthodox medicine has not found an answer to your complaint. However, luckily for you, I happen to be a quack."

Drawing by Richter; © 1973 The New Yorker, Inc.

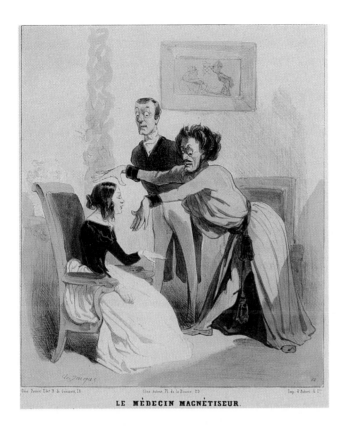

LE MÉDECIN MAGNÉTISEUR.

Systems of treatment: bizarre to brutal

New and unorthodox systems of treatment have always been fair game for caricature. A prime example was Franz Anton Mesmer's animal magnetism; the Austrian physician (1734–1815), having made experiments on the supposed curative power of magnets, came to believe that he possessed a kind of occult force. In Paris he devoted himself to curing diseases, holding hypnotic séances in his magnetic tubs. The tubs contained a weak solution of sulfuric acid. His ailing patients formed a circle in the tub, each of them holding onto iron bars that conducted magnetic currents. With much flourish and artifice, Mesmer then proceeded to "treat" his patients by touching the afflicted parts of their bodies. A commission appointed by the French government denounced him as an impostor, but his treatment gained devoted followers throughout Europe, and many practitioners in his wake used his magnetic principles.

Samuel Hahnemann's homeopathy was another new approach to treatment that was widely ridiculed when it was first introduced in the early 1800s. His system was based on the premise that like cures like (*similia similibus curantur*), that diseases can be cured by giving patients infinitesimally small doses of agents that would in healthy persons produce symptoms of the disease being treated. In Norwich, Connecticut, Elisha Perkins (1741–99) achieved notoriety with his "tractors"—two metallic rods, one blunt and the other sharply pointed, that he claimed could "extract" illnesses by being stroked downward on the affected part of the sick person's body. The English caricaturist James Gillray (1756–1815) expressed his disdain for

31

Perkins' tractors, which could, according to his irreverent depiction, assuage discomfort from "red noses, gouty toes, windy bowels, broken legs, and hump backs." Vinzenz Priessnitz (1799–1851), a Silesian farmer, was the best-known advocate of hydropathy (or hydrotherapy). He proposed that sprays, baths, douches, cold packs, and wet sheets could cure a variety of illnesses. Not surprisingly, the caricaturists found his methods well worth mocking. And the German practitioner Franz Joseph Gall (1758–1828) was among the most acclaimed and attacked scientists of his day when he introduced phrenology. His system suggested that various brain functions as well as an understanding of personality and character could be identified by bumps on the head.

In all of the above cases, caricaturists were quick to take up the invitations offered by the novel approaches—approaches that in most cases proved to be pseudoscientific at best, no matter how firmly their practitioners believed in them. But even scientifically sound methods were condemned by artists when they were new. Shortly after Edward Jenner discovered preventive inoculation in 1796, Gillray's caricature "The Cow Pock—or—the Wonderful Effects of the New Inoculation!" appeared, leaving no doubt of the artist's ridicule, in the face of what has proved to be a valid method.

Above all, it was the so-called heroic medicine, practiced in both Europe and America during the 18th and 19th centuries, that was probably the most bitterly attacked. French caricaturists, most prominently Jacque, savaged the radical bloodletting and drastic counterirritation preached by a leading French physician, François-Joseph-Victor Broussais (1772–1838). Broussais thought that life depends on irritation, in particular on heat, while disease depends on localized irritation of a specific organ such as the stomach; for cure a powerful weakening regime was necessary, and to

Elisha Perkins from Connecticut adamantly believed his treatment—stroking the affected part of the sick person's body with two metallic rods, one blunt and the other pointed—could cure just about anything, but the English caricaturist James Gillray had his doubts. Vinzenz Priessnitz, a Silesian farmer, advocated water treatment (hydropathy or hydrotherapy) as a certain cure for most illness. The French caricaturist Charles-Emile Jacque, however, was more prone to pity the poor patient who was subjected to such dousings.

Illustrations by (left) James Gillray and (right) Charles-Emile Jacque; collection, National Library of Medicine

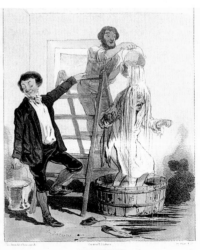

LES HYDROPATHES.

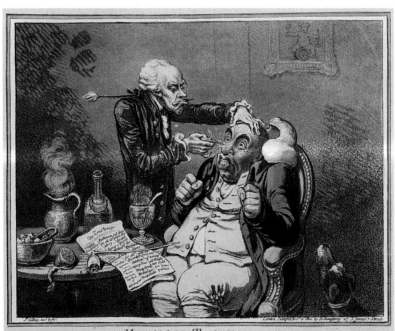

METALLIC-TRACTORS.

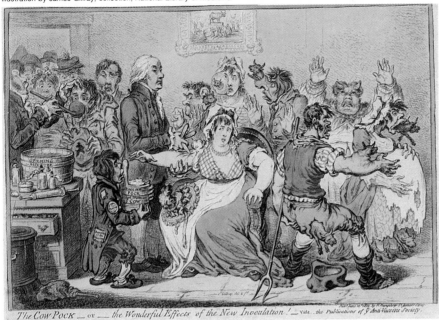

The Cow Pock _ or _ the Wonderful Effects of the New Inoculation! _ vide. the Publications of Y Anti Vaccine Society.

this end leeches, as many as 50 at a time, and fasting were prescribed. In Jacque's lithograph "A Disciple of Broussais," the doctor shows surprise that 40 leeches have not worked and consequently increases the dose to 60. In Jacque's "The System of Magnetic Brushes," a patient is subjected to the fanaticism of the bristle wielder: " . . . since I've been told to make your blood circulate, I'm going to make it circulate throughout the apartment." Bloodletting, in fact, had been around for centuries. In 1545 the eminent French physician, astronomer, and mathematician Jean Fernel noted, "The physician today seems athirst for blood. Blood-letting, like wine-drinking, is

James Gillray was no less skeptical about scientifically sound methods than he was of pseudoscientific ones. His ridicule of Edward Jenner's newly discovered cowpox inoculation to confer immunity against smallpox was just as sharp as his attack on Elisha Perkins' metallic tractors.

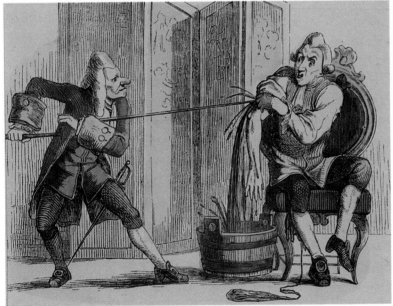

Bloodletting was a means of purging the body of its "fouled fluids." It began with Hippocrates and was practiced well into the 19th century. Of all the so-called heroic forms of medicine, this one probably incited the most vigorous and frequent attacks; artists' depictions inevitably showed the most copious quantities of the precious fluid being let. Reflecting on the practice, Oliver Wendell Holmes wrote: "The lancet was the magician's wand of the dark ages of medicine." Indeed, as a result of such brutal if well-intentioned therapy, many victims were in fact bled to death.

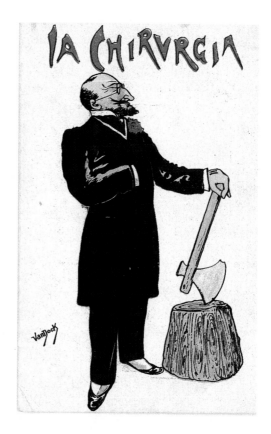

right in moderation, but in excess it leads to disaster." As the caricaturists two and three centuries later made evident, however, Fernel's word was hardly heeded.

Perhaps these criticisms contributed to the decline of at least some of the unorthodox and pseudoscientific systems of treatment. With the advent of modern medicine and its potent therapeutics and complex surgical approaches, the bite of the caricaturist shifted to the modern physician, an awesome and antiseptic figure in a white coat, and *his* systems of

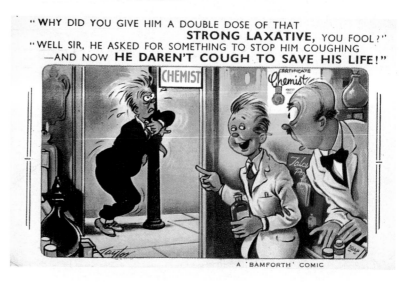

treatment—his armamentarium of diagnostic machinery, probes, powerful drugs, and fear-invoking surgical instruments.

An Italian postcard from the 1920s depicting a "modern" representative of the surgical profession presented a self-important and imposing figure and his instrument: an ax. A British postcard from the mid-1960s showed a grinning pharmacist who has supplied a strong laxative because the client "asked for something to stop him coughing and now he daren't cough to save his life!" These satires are typical in that they exhibit skepticism rather than esteem for the "wonders" of 20th-century medicine; in fact, they portray "modern" medicine as barely short of primitive.

If any single brutal treatment can be said to have shown itself more often than any other in caricature and cartoons, it would probably be that experienced in the dentist's chair. Anticipation of a visit to the dentist inevitably foreshadows pain, and the dentist is the one who delivers it. Daumier captured the situation perfectly in his 1864 lithograph captioned, "Come on . . . open your mouth!" in which a pale, trembling patient anticipates the fateful moment, his eyes pinned on every least movement of the dentist's hand. But countless artists centuries before Daumier did the same, and today dental phobia is as ripe a subject as ever. A classic drawing by the late *New Yorker* cartoonist Charles Addams shows a dentist's office waiting room; the pictures that decorate the walls of this practitioner's office are prominent, and they have a single theme: pain. No caption is needed.

Side effects

The side effects of treatments have always troubled those for whom they are prescribed. Morison's Pills, potent purgatives first marketed by James Morison through his British College of Health in 1825, contained only veg-

Illustration by Honoré Daumier; collection, National Library of Medicine

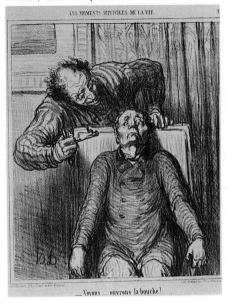

No practitioner, past or present, has inspired more fear—and literally volumes of graphic satires—than the dentist.

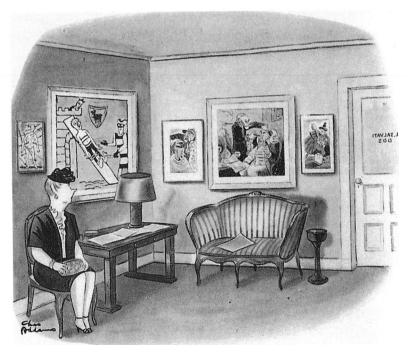

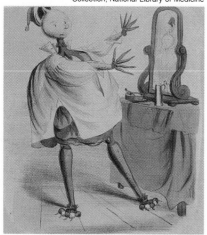

"They told me if I took 1,000 pills at night I should be quite another thing in the morning," exclaimed this believer in the Universal Vegetable Pills promoted by James Morison, a notorious medical man of the early 19th century. His allegedly gentle and side-effect-free all-natural-ingredient remedy for virtually every ill prompted a host of spoofs by cartoonists of the day—spoofs that suggested Morison's famous pills may not have been without side effects after all.

etable ingredients. The cornerstone of their promotion was that they were free of the debilitating effects of calomel and similar harsh preparations so frequently prescribed by the medical profession of his day, or the "faculty," as Morison termed them. Morison's excessive promotion prompted a counterreaction by the cartoonists, who took great pleasure in recording the side effects that could come from his allegedly gentle remedy. In the "Singular Effects of the Universal Vegetable Pills on a Green Grocer," C.J. Grant depicted vegetables sprouting from the body of a grocer who was "order'd to live for the space of one month upon vegetable diet & to take during that time 132 boxes of vegetable pills for the cure of a gangreen & being caught in a shower of rain." Another spoof on Morison's pills showed a man whose nose had turned into a carrot; yet another, a gout victim whose entire body had become covered with grass. A cartoon by George Price that appeared in *The New Yorker* in 1987 could be considered a contemporary variation on the same theme—the side effect of a seemingly benign prescribed treatment; a doctor examines a patient from whose head extend branches of a tree, while his wife asserts, "I *told* him to lay off the high-fibre diet."

Profiting from patients

Medical practitioners have long been seen as mercenary figures, ever anxious to add to their wealth and position. Artists' attacks on doctors' fees date as far back as 1587, when a series of four allegorical engravings from the school of the Dutch engraver Hendrik Goltzius portrayed the physician sequentially as God, angel, man, and devil, each image reflecting the time during the course of the treatment the doctor-patient encounter took place. The devil appeared on the day of financial reckoning.

Adverse effects of treatments continue to trouble patients. With the ever expanding and ever more potent therapeutics of modern medicine, the likelihood of such undesired effects occurring has, in fact, increased.

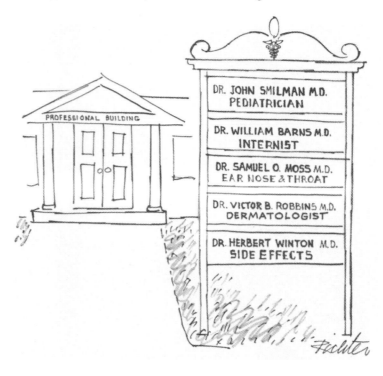

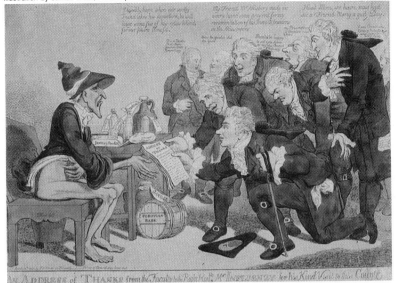

Physicians' notorious greed and ambition and the outrageous fees they charge have been timeless sources of inspiration for satirists. Hence, doctors are likely to be grateful for epidemics—the bigger and longer-lasting the better.

A late 18th-century print by the British artist Robert Dighton of three physicians in a pharmacy included the verse "How merrily we live that doctors be; we humbug the public and pocket the fee!" In an 1803 caricature by the British artist James West, a delegation of physicians, to show their gratitude for increased business, present "An Address of Thanks from the Faculty to the Right Honble Mr. Influenzy for his kind visit to this country." The doctors are clearly reluctant to see the epidemic end.

That physicians can always find novel ways to increase their income has been a source of continual amusement to the cartoonist, a good example being doctors who profited from selling bootleg liquor during Prohibition. A popular song took this as its subject; pictured on the cover of the song sheet is a cartoon of a waiting room full of eager paying patients, each calling out "Oh Doctor" (the song title) as they await their turn to have the winking physician prescribe their suddenly legal drink.

A 1925 *Punch* cartoon by Frank Reynolds has a fashionably dressed doctor and a surgeon in conversation:

Doctor: What did you operate on Jones for?
Surgeon: A hundred pounds.
Doctor: No, I mean what had he got?
Surgeon: A hundred pounds.

Not surprisingly, to the caricaturist doctors' fees are invariably too high. The physician on a postcard published in the 1920s tells his patient, "Here is a prescription to reduce your weight," to which the patient responds, "Never mind doc' your bill will have the same effect." An Italian postcard of about the same time depicts a doctor who is a "specialist in extracting painlessly" as the patient hands over his payment.

Many practitioners emphasize that their services are worthy of their fees, and so do dispensers of drugs. In a cartoon by Alphonse Normandia, an alchemist justifies the cost of his "prescription": "Of course the price

During Prohibition doctors found a new opportunity to increase their incomes: "prescribing" for "liquor mourners." A popular song had this refrain:

> *Oh! Doctor, Oh! Doctor, I'm feeling blue—*
> *Oh! Doctor, Oh! Doctor, it's up to you—*
> *. . .*
> *Write the prescription and please make it say—*
> *"Take with your meals," I eat ten times a day—*

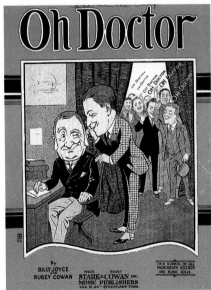

37

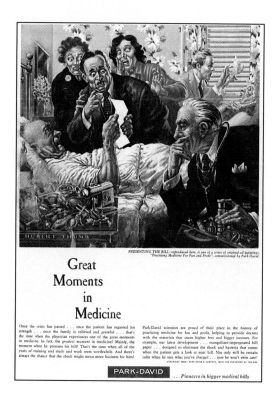

In the 1950s the pharmaceutical company Parke, Davis commissioned the series of paintings "Great Moments in Medicine," depicting many of the heralded discoveries and therapeutic achievements made by physicians through the ages. A takeoff by MAD Magazine *chose as its subject not doctors' ability to conquer disease but their proclivity to charge exorbitant fees.*

Comic valentines, a genre popular in the U.S. and Great Britain at the beginning of the 20th century, were sent anonymously to practitioners of medicine, dentistry, and pharmacy—their verses expressing patients' most heartfelt sentiments toward these not-so-beloved professionals.

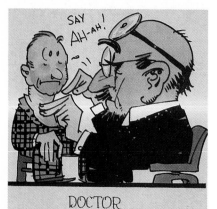

DOCTOR
Powder and pills! Needle and knife!
Cut up the husband, slice up the wife!
Fill up the children with rank castor oil
You just know enough to open a boil.

Collection, William H. Helfand

is high. But ten years ago nobody had ever heard of bats' wings and mandrake roots."

In the 1950s the pharmaceutical firm Parke, Davis sponsored the series "Great Moments in Medicine," a popular collection of paintings by the illustrator Robert Thom, featuring 45 key events in medical history, from medicine in ancient Egypt—a physician treating a sick old man with lockjaw—to crucial therapeutic advances of the 20th century, such as the discovery of the first chemical "bullet" in 1910, which successfully cured syphilis. *MAD Magazine* in its characteristic irreverent fashion parodied the series with an illustration entitled "Presenting the Bill . . . one of a series of original oil paintings 'Practising Medicine for Fun and Profit,' commissioned by Park-David."

Doctors and dentists and druggists: loving to hate them

Finally, there is a special genre of artistic offense that was popular in England and the United States around the turn of the century—the comic valentine. Sent unsigned to those people loved the least, these "penny dreadfuls" attacked all professions and trades equally; pharmacists, dentists, and physicians all certainly came in for their share. Scurrilous caricatures accompanied by acerbic verses summed up a variety of complaints.

To a druggist: Keep on grinding poisonous pills,
See that each cathartic kills.
Strive to play a doctor's art,
Of quack nostrums sell your part;
Never 'tending pharmacy school,
You're a murderer and a fool!

To a dentist: Your patients always greet you
With groans and howls and curses;
For all that you can extract well
Is money from their purses.

To a doctor: Powder and Pills! Needle and knife!
Cut up the husband, slice up the wife!
Fill up the children with rank castor oil
You just know enough to open a boil.

Why all these relentless attacks? Why abuse rather than adulation? Why treat with such contempt those who do so much for preserving and improving human health? Why so many graphic castigators expressing their irreverence toward medicine and so few Norman Rockwells sentimentally honoring the beloved and patient country doctor practicing his gentle bedside manner?

One explanation is that physicians have great power over patients, who need a means to retaliate when excesses demand it. Because illness is unpleasant no matter how one views it, medical satire helps mitigate fears; it is an outlet that provides psychic relief. The French philosopher Henri Bergson (1859–1941) thought that people laugh at what they fear the most. In an article in 1921 discussing the psychology of medical satire, Isador H. Coriat, a leading Boston psychiatrist with an abiding interest in the history of medicine, suggested that satires were "produced at the expense of overcoming deep resistances and repressions concerning illness and death and the constant struggles against these unforeseen and unavoidable accidents of human life." As the late physician, literary critic, and French academician Henri Mondor, writing about Daumier's medical caricatures, argued: "It is in accordance with the oldest literary traditions that doctors should be involved in the endless charges brought by malcontents against established institutions, by the frivolous minded against everything serious, by writers against science, by the ignorant against any subjects they find hard to understand, and finally by the sick and born grumblers against the men who heal them slowly or incompletely or who appear to tend them roughly and automatically rather than with sympathy."

Irreverence, finally, must be viewed positively. Its deformations and exaggerations stress deviations from the high ideals the medical profession claims as its own and, one may hope, in the process, will serve to keep health professionals closer to these lofty standards.

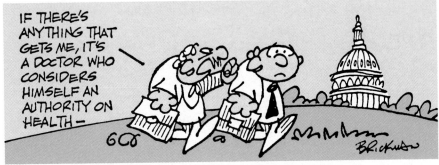

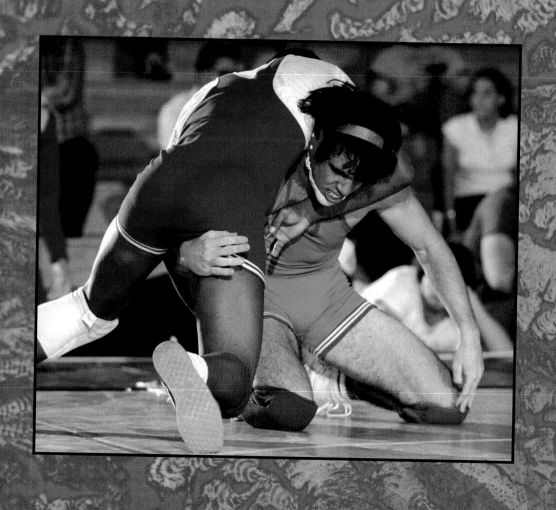
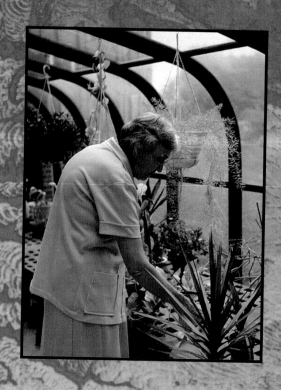

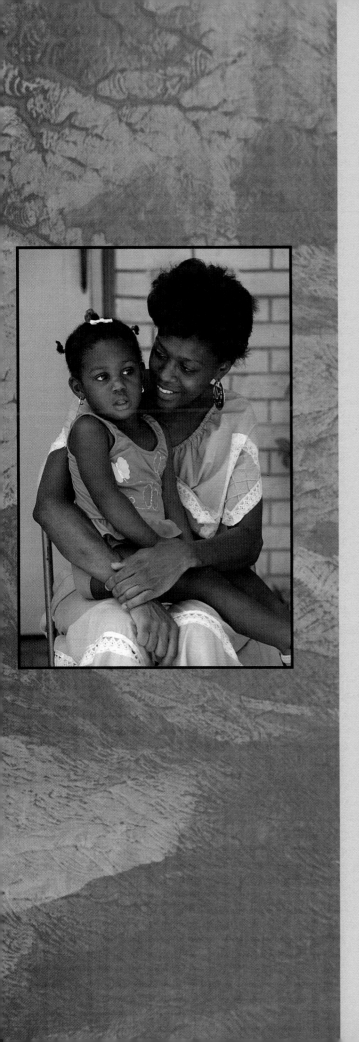

Awash in Hormones:
The New Endocrinology

by Nicholas P. Christy, M.D.

Endocrinology—the study of hormones and the cells and tissues that secrete them—has changed more drastically over the past 30 years than any other field of medicine. Cardiology, for example, which has witnessed spectacular advances during that time in the understanding of the physiology of the heart and circulation, remains a limited, well-defined field. Gastroenterology, which has likewise made brilliant progress, still treats the gut (gastrointestinal tract), the pancreas, and the liver. In endocrinology, however, new developments in many branches of science—genetics, immunology, biochemistry, and molecular biology among them—have so transformed and enlarged the field that its borders have grown indistinct and the definitions of *gland* and *hormone* have had to be radically revised.

Classic endocrinology: hail and farewell

From ancient times to the middle of the 20th century, endocrinology was defined anatomically, in terms of distinct glands exerting specific effects on the body. The relation of the testes to maleness has been known since antiquity: a castrate bull is a steer, a castrate man a eunuch. Other glands had to wait for centuries before their functions became known. It was not until 1855 that the English physician Thomas Addison identified destruction of the adrenal glands, located just above the kidneys, as the cause of the affliction now known as adrenocortical insufficiency, or Addison's disease. The deleterious effects of excessive and deficient function of the thyroid, at the base of the neck, were familiar to British and Irish clinicians by the end

Nicholas P. Christy, M.D., is Writer in Residence and Senior Lecturer in Medicine, Columbia University College of Physicians and Surgeons, New York City, and Attending Physician (Medicine), Presbyterian Hospital, New York City. He has conducted extensive research in adrenal and pituitary endocrinology.

Until the mid-20th century, endocrinology constituted a field clearly defined in terms of distinct glands exerting specific bodily effects. The purpose of such glands as the testes has been comprehended in a general way since ancient times, while the functions of others, like the pancreas, had to await the rise of modern science for clarification. In 1922, in experiments on dogs, Charles Best and Frederick Banting (left and right) showed the ductless portion of the pancreas to be the source of the blood-sugar regulator insulin. By the 1950s researchers and physicians felt confident that most endocrine disorders could be traced to excesses or deficiencies of a small number of hormones secreted by an even smaller number of glands (see Table, opposite page).

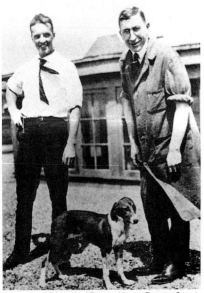

University of Toronto Library, Toronto, Canada

of the 19th century. In the early 1920s the famous experiments of Canadian medical researchers Frederick Banting and Charles Best established the endocrine, or ductless, portion of the pancreas as the source of the blood-sugar-regulating hormone insulin. In 1937 the American P.E. Smith proved that the anterior pituitary, at the base of the brain, is essential for the normal structure and function of at least three other glands: the cortex (outer portion) of the adrenals, the ovaries, and the testes.

By the 1950s clinical endocrinology occupied a well-demarcated anatomic province, consisting of the anterior and posterior portions of the pituitary, the thyroid, the parathyroids (also in the neck), the cortex and medulla (inner portion) of the adrenals, the islets of Langerhans in the pancreas, and the gonads: the testes and ovaries. Physicians and research workers were content to interpret most endocrine disease in terms of excessive and deficient production of the hormones uniquely secreted by those nine glands. The classic idea of a hormone (Greek *hormōn,* meaning "to excite, set in motion, spur on") prevailed: a substance made by one organ, secreted directly into the bloodstream, and transported to a more-or-less distant organ or tissue where it exerted some regulatory action. This model, which predominated during what may be called the descriptive phase of endocrinology, still constitutes a major portion of the practice of clinical endocrinologists today.

Overlapping that descriptive phase, there began in the 1920s the period of chemical purification, identification, and synthesis of most of the hormones. Then, beginning in the 1940s, investigators discovered several hormonal disorders of sexual development resulting from abnormalities in the chromosomes. Such findings opened up increasingly sophisticated genetic studies that continue to influence endocrine research today.

The 1960s and '70s saw the development by Solomon Berson and Rosalyn Yalow, working in an endocrine laboratory at the Bronx (New York) Veterans Administration Hospital, of the technique of radioimmunoassay (RIA), a revolutionary method of measurement that enabled detection of minute quantities of hormones in bodily fluids. It would not be hyperbole to claim that the capacity of RIA to measure picograms of a substance per milliliter of fluid (trillionths of a gram in about 20 drops) is equivalent to detecting a pinch of salt in a fair-sized pond. This ability contrasted sharply with older chemical and biological assay methods, which often took days to perform. One achievement that RIA made possible was the measurement of all the known protein and peptide (small protein) hormones of the anterior pituitary. Because researchers could finally make numerous sequential determinations, they learned that each of those hormones undergoes its own peculiar oscillatory cycle of secretion over a 24-hour period. Hitherto, a single determination a day was all one could reasonably expect.

The past two or three decades have also seen sophisticated studies of the biochemical mode of action of hormones upon cells. New substances with hormonal or hormonelike properties have been discovered; examples are the ubiquitous prostaglandins and many compounds secreted by lymphocytes (specialized white blood cells) and other cells of the immune system. Hormones have now been shown to exert not only classic endocrine activity (*i.e.,* activity at a point distant from the site of the secretion)

Simplified canon of human endocrine diseases, 1950

gland	overfunction	deficiency	damage to gland	hormone involved	clinical disorder
anterior pituitary	X		secretory tumor	growth hormone	acromegaly[1], giantism
		X	nonsecreting tumor, hemorrhage	growth hormone, gonadotropins, thyrotropin, corticotropin	hypopituitarism (deficiency of pituitary secretions)
posterior pituitary		X	destructive, unknown cause	vasopressin[2]	diabetes insipidus[3]
thyroid	X		autoimmune reaction?	thyroxine	Graves' disease (thyrotoxicosis)[4]
		X	autoimmune reaction?	thyroxine	myxedema[5]
parathyroids	X		secretory tumor	parathyroid hormone	high blood calcium, bone disease
		X	destructive, unknown cause	parathyroid hormone	low blood calcium, tetany
adrenal cortex	X		overgrowth[6], secretory tumor	cortisol[7], androgens[8]	Cushing's disease[9], virilism[10]
		X	destructive, tuberculosis	cortisol, aldosterone[11]	adrenal insufficiency (Addison's disease)[12]
adrenal medulla	X		secretory tumor (pheochromo-cytoma)[13]	norepinephrine[14]	episodic hypertension
pancreatic islets	X		secretory tumor	insulin	low blood sugar
		X	destructive, unknown cause	insulin	high blood sugar, diabetes mellitus[15]
testes	X		Leydig cell tumor[16], unknown cause	testosterone	precocious puberty
		X	genetic, pituitary failure	testosterone	failure of sexual development
ovaries	X		secretory tumor[17], unknown cause	estradiol	precocious puberty
		X	genetic, pituitary failure	estradiol	failure of sexual development

[1] enlargement of skeletal extremities and internal organs

[2] or antidiuretic hormone; causes the kidney to retain water

[3] uncontrollable loss of water via the kidneys

[4] generalized increase of metabolic rate, weight loss, fatigue, tremors, prominent eyes

[5] generalized decrease of metabolic rate, loss of energy, pasty complexion, puffy face, hoarseness, hair loss

[6] or hyperplasia; due to excessive corticotropin secretion by the anterior pituitary

[7] or hydrocortisone; its synthetic analogs are used in large doses to treat cancers and allergic and inflammatory diseases

[8] testosterone and weaker androgenic steroids (dehydroepiandrosterone, androsterone, and others)

[9] cortisol excess; round face, thin skin, obesity of the trunk with thin arms and legs, easy bruising, high blood pressure, diabetes mellitus, brittle bones (osteoporosis or osteopenia); identical clinical picture (Cushing's syndrome) may follow treatment with high doses of cortisol analogs over long periods

[10] precocious puberty in boys, masculine features in girls and women

[11] the salt-retaining hormone of the adrenal cortex; causes the kidney to retain salt

[12] weight loss, weakness, bronze skin, low blood pressure, undue susceptibility to minor illnesses; fatal if not treated with cortisol and aldosterone analogs

[13] rare tumors, benign or malignant; they secrete adrenaline-like compounds that cause intermittent or constant rise in blood pressure

[14] or noradrenaline; there is no known deficiency state of this hormone

[15] by far the most common endocrine disease (affects 7% or more of U.S. population)

[16] tumors affect the testosterone-secreting cells of the testis; exceedingly rare; precocious puberty in boys is due usually to unduly early pituitary secretion of gonadotropins; the cause of the premature secretion is unknown

[17] the granulosa cell tumor of the ovary; exceedingly rare

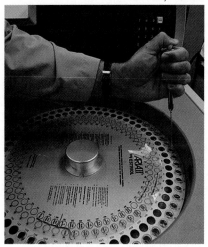

Contributing to the current explosion of knowledge about hormones has been the technique of radioimmunoassay (RIA), a method involving the use of antibodies and radioactive isotopes to measure precise levels of very low concentrations of substances in blood and other bodily fluids. Almost all of what is known about regulation of hormonal secretion and the interactions among hormones has been derived with RIA, beginning in the 1960s.

Near the end of the 20th century, a large part of clinical endocrinology remains concerned with the functions and disorders of the nine traditional glands: the anterior and posterior pituitary, the thyroid, the parathyroids, the cortex and medulla of the adrenals, the pancreatic islets, and the ovaries and testes. During the past three or four decades, however, medical research has discovered hormonal activity for compounds secreted by a bewildering, ever expanding assortment of tissues and organs, among them the hypothalamus and pineal gland in the brain, the heart, the thymus, the lungs, the kidneys, and the gastrointestinal tract. This knowledge has added to an altered, vastly complicated picture of the human endocrine system.

but also activity that is autocrine (acting on the same cell in which the substance is made) and paracrine (acting on cells neighboring the secretory cell). Conventional hormones and substances structurally resembling them have been found to be secreted by some kinds of malignant tumors. Finally, hormones and hormonelike compounds occur in and are secreted by a bewildering array of organs and tissues, differing markedly from the traditional glands. Examples are the brain, the gut, the heart, the thymus, and the kidneys.

This revolutionary phase of endocrinology, in concert with advances in biochemistry and molecular biology, has greatly enlarged the field, intermingling it with many other branches of biological science. Furthermore, this new knowledge has altered and vastly complicated the perception of the endocrine system and hormones. Medical researchers are only now beginning to fathom the full range of what hormones do, where they come from, how they carry local and distant messages, and the myriad ways they govern such aspects of human experience as growth, maturation, defense against infectious organisms, and mental and psychological function. Few would have predicted, for example, the results of a study published in 1990 in which giving synthetic growth hormone to elderly people for six months appeared to turn the clock back by increasing muscle mass and bone density, reducing body fat, and, in certain patients, improving strength and exercise capacity.

Hormonal control: an increasingly complex picture

In recent decades it has become apparent that the body's control of hormone secretion is more complicated than previously supposed. By the 1940s the principle of negative-feedback inhibition of hormone secretion had been firmly established. For example, the parathyroid glands regulate

Nine "classic" endocrine glands and some less conventional sources of hormones

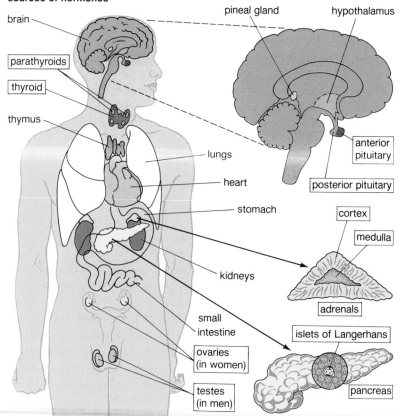

the concentration of calcium in the blood serum by secreting parathyroid hormone (PTH), which raises serum calcium levels. When calcium levels fall, the parathyroids are stimulated to secrete more PTH in order to elevate the calcium concentration to appropriate levels. On the other hand, high serum calcium levels are a signal to the parathyroids to reduce hormone production: negative-feedback inhibition. Similarly, the anterior pituitary makes two so-called gonadotropins—luteinizing hormone (LH) and follicle-stimulating hormone (FSH)—which among other actions regulate the levels in the blood of sex hormones secreted by the gonads. When sex hormone levels are high, the pituitary's secretion of LH and FSH is inhibited. Later work on the hormonal control of reproduction in women uncovered another effect: positive-feedback control. Midway through the menstrual cycle, the ovaries release high amounts of sex hormones called estrogens, an event that is followed by a peak in the pituitary's secretion of LH, which in turn is followed by ovulation, or release of the egg from the ovary. Such new observations have enabled precise identification of the hormonal events surrounding ovulation, greatly simplifying the treatment of menstrual disorders and infertility in women.

The discovery of a new hormone has complicated the picture of how pituitary gonadotropins and the sex hormones testosterone (the predominant androgen, or male hormone) and estradiol (the predominant estrogen in the female) interact. The standard idea had been that testosterone in the male and estradiol in the female suppressed the pituitary's secretion of FSH and LH by negative-feedback inhibition and that such hormonal interplay sufficiently explained the workings of the menstrual cycle. However, the observation in the 1920s of men and women suffering from certain kinds of gonadal lesions accompanied by extraordinarily high levels of FSH suggested the existence of an as yet unidentified gonadal hormone, dubbed inhibin, that was being produced by the gonads and that played an important role, perhaps the chief role, in regulating pituitary FSH secretion.

For almost a half century this hypothetical substance failed to gain a respectable place in the canon of hormones. Finally in the 1970s the World Health Organization, which was seeking a male contraceptive, began funding inhibin research, reasoning that a substance that inhibited FSH would consequently inhibit sperm production. By the 1980s it had been established that both the testes and the ovaries secrete a substance having FSH-inhibiting activity. Subsequently that substance was purified, and by means of modern techniques of molecular biology its structure was completely determined. Today, necessarily accepted as a hormonal reality, inhibin is known to suppress ovulation, and studies are in progress to find out whether it suppresses sperm production. In addition, researchers have produced antibody molecules that specifically recognize and bind to inhibin; when tested in laboratory animals, the antibodies block inhibin action. If the work on inhibin can be applied to human beings, the hormone itself may come to serve as a contraceptive, while inhibin blockers may find a place in treating infertility.

Inhibin may have further significance both within and outside the reproductive system. Through chemical rearrangement of its two component

Negative-feedback control of parathyroid hormone secretion

- high calcium levels block parathyroid hormone secretion
- low calcium levels allow parathyroid hormone secretion

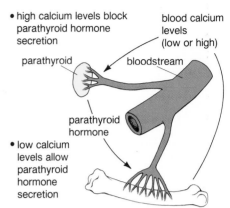

parathyroid hormone releases calcium from storage in bone (and accelerates calcium absorption from gut)

Positive- and negative-feedback control of gonadotropins in women

- high estrogen levels ordinarily block LH and FSH secretion (negative feedback inhibition)
- at mid cycle high estrogen levels stimulate LH surge and consequent release of egg from ovary (positive feedback)
- low estrogen levels allow LH and FSH secretion

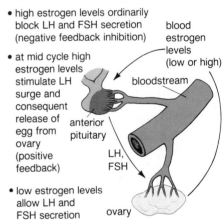

LH and FSH stimulate secretion of estrogens from ovary

The body's control of hormone secretion exploits negative and positive feedback. The former occurs, for example, in the regulation of blood calcium by the parathyroids (top). Low calcium levels stimulate secretion of parathyroid hormone (PTH), which makes calcium more available, whereas high calcium levels block PTH secretion. Negative feedback also operates in women in restraining pituitary secretion of gonadotropins (LH and FSH), which stimulate estrogen release from the ovaries (above). At mid cycle, however, positive feedback occurs: release of high levels of ovarian estrogens elicits a surge of pituitary LH and consequent ovulation.

parts to form a substance called activin, inhibin takes on the capacity to stimulate FSH secretion. Inhibin and activin also affect the synthesis of hemoglobin, the oxygen-carrying pigment of red blood cells, and are thought to influence aspects of the immune response.

The sources of inhibin are the ovaries, the testes, and, during pregnancy, the placenta, which arises from fetal cells. Since it is now possible to measure inhibin in the blood serum, such determinations will probably prove useful in evaluating several types of impaired fertility. Measurements of inhibin levels in the blood are already proving valuable as markers in detecting recurrences of two kinds of cancer: the granulosa-cell tumor of the ovary and a tumor of the placenta known as hydatidiform mole.

Contributions from genetic advances

Between 1940 and 1960 a whole new territory of reproductive endocrinology grew up around the discovery that certain types of ovarian and testicular disease are related to chromosomal abnormalities. The normal man has 44 ordinary paired chromosomes (named autosomes) plus the sex chromosomes X and Y, expressed in shorthand as 46,XY. The Y chromosome carries all the genes that determine maleness. The normal chromosomal constitution of woman is 46,XX. Applying rather simple biological methods, Canadian researcher Murray Barr and others identified chromosomal anomalies in many hitherto inexplicable disorders that are marked by failure of the gonads to develop. For instance, in female-appearing individuals afflicted with Turner's syndrome—characterized by rudimentary ovaries, short stature, high levels of FSH in the blood, and sometimes skeletal and other deformities—it has been established that the chromosomal constitution is 45,XO; that is, one of the X chromosomes is missing. In male-appearing persons having Klinefelter's syndrome—characterized by a body form resembling that of a eunuch, small testes, complete or nearly complete failure of sperm production, and raised FSH values—the chromosomal constitution is shown to be 47,XXY; that is, an extra X chromosome. Individuals with the syndrome who have more extreme degrees of feminization show chromosomal patterns still more abnormal: 48,XXXY and 49,XXXXY. A rare constitution, 47,XYY, has been found in normal-appearing males who, although not excessively virile, often exhibit serious degrees of mental deficiency and behavioral disorders. Such findings and many more like them have shed new light on human sexual development and on how chromosomes affect it. The detection of such anomalies makes possible early counseling of the afflicted and their parents and enables timely treatment of hormonal deficiencies where they exist.

Sophisticated genetic and cellular studies recently have revealed some of the molecular mechanisms underlying three distinctly different endocrine diseases. One, familial pseudohypoparathyroidism, stems from a cellular resistance to the normal actions of parathyroid hormone, which include stimulating calcium release from storage in bone and fostering the absorption of calcium from the gut. Victims of the disease show low levels of calcium in the blood and several kinds of defects of the skeletal structure. The second disease, Albright's hereditary osteodystrophy, is marked by

While excess secretion of pituitary growth hormone in childhood is responsible for the giant stature of the man in the 19th-century illustration below, his disproportionately enlarged hands and jaw, characteristic of the condition called acromegaly, is a result of continued overproduction of the hormone in adulthood. In recent years researchers probing the molecular mechanisms underlying acromegaly have uncovered genetic mutations in some cases that allow the growth-hormone-secreting cells of the pituitary to escape proper regulation by the brain. The result is overgrowth of those cells and overproduction of growth hormone. Conceivably, advances in genetic engineering one day may allow the defective genes to be corrected.

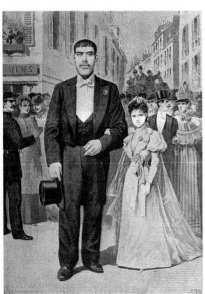

Jean-Loup Charmet

short stature, short fingers and toes, and bony deposits under the skin. It results from a cellular resistance to PTH as well as to several pituitary hormones that stimulate the thyroid and the adrenal cortex and help in regulating water balance and the concentration of dissolved substances in the bodily fluids. The third disease, acromegaly, is characterized by gradual enlargement of the skeletal extremities and internal organs and thickening of the skin and is the result of overproduction of pituitary growth hormone, caused by a pituitary tumor.

In all three diseases researchers have found abnormalities in certain intracellular proteins (G proteins) that act as modulators and transmitters of hormonal and other signals. The protein abnormality in acromegaly releases the growth-hormone-secreting cells of the anterior pituitary from proper regulation by the brain. The result is uncontrolled overgrowth of those cells, the formation of a growth-hormone-secreting tumor, and consequent acromegaly. In pseudohypoparathyroidism, acromegaly, and Albright's syndrome, specific mutations in genes that code for G proteins have been identified. These observations go some distance in explaining the molecular basis of the three disorders. It is conceivable that in the future genetic engineering could be used to correct the defective DNA that encodes the abnormal proteins.

Cellular receptors and endocrine disease

Some hormones work on all cells. Cortisol (hydrocortisone) and related steroid compounds (glucocorticoids) of the adrenal cortex, which are essential for life, have ubiquitous action. The same is true for the major thyroid hormones, thyroxine and triiodothyronine. On the other hand, for the many hormones that act on a few special organs or tissues, it is reasonable to ask how they can "know" their specific targets. Early work in the field showed that in the case of the female hormone estradiol, radioactively labeled estradiol that was injected experimentally concentrated in the uterus, obviously a target tissue for the ovarian estrogen. From such studies grew the identification of a host of hormone receptors—now known to be protein molecules—having great specificity and avidity for molecules of the appropriate hormone. Sex hormone receptors are concentrated chiefly in the cells of androgen- and estrogen-responsive tissues: the breasts, uterus, penis, and skeletal muscle. By contrast, glucocorticoid and thyroid hormone receptors are found in virtually all cells.

Precisely how these receptors affect hormone action is a complex matter. In general, some hormones bind specifically to receptors located within the cell, in the cell sap (cytosol). The resulting hormone-receptor complex then acts, either within the cell nucleus or elsewhere, to affect the translation of genetically coded instructions into protein. Other hormones find their receptors on the surface of the cell, whereupon they begin a cascade of biochemical reactions that carries into the cell and exerts many regulatory effects.

The fields of toxicology and environmental health have been recent beneficiaries of research into hormone receptors. It turns out that the industrial toxins known as dioxins (including the most toxic dioxin, 2,3,7,8-TCDD) act

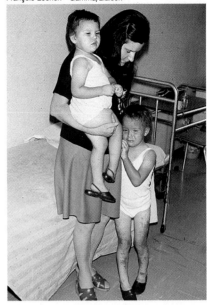

Severe skin rashes afflict two children shortly after their exposure to a dioxin-laden cloud that emanated from a chemical plant explosion near Seveso, Italy, in 1976. Dioxin (specifically 2,3,7,8-TCDD) and its close relatives, the undesirable toxic by-products of industrial chemical synthesis, have been found to act on receptors of human body cells in a way virtually identical to that of the adrenal hormone cortisol and the sex steroid hormones. In fact, much of the detailed knowledge of the effects of these toxins on cells has been derived from research on hormone receptors.

47

on cell receptors in a manner virtually identical to that of cortisol and the sex steroids. Dioxins—environmental contaminants produced in such industrial activities as garbage incineration and automobile and paper manufacturing and known infamously as a contaminant in the defoliant Agent Orange used in Vietnam—bind to intracellular receptors, bind to DNA, and inappropriately affect genetic processes. In experimental animals dioxins disrupt embryological development and damage gonadal function; in humans they have been linked with the skin disease chloracne and possibly with a type of cancer known as non-Hodgkin's lymphoma. Interestingly, the detailed knowledge of how these poisons work has been gained from the unlikely source of endocrinologic research.

Hormone receptors play a significant role in human afflictions. The presence or absence of estrogen receptors in samples of breast cancer tissue has long been used to determine whether removal of the ovaries will effectively deprive the mammary tumor of a growth factor and thereby cause its regression. Clinically, women whose cancers contain estrogen receptors are candidates for ovarian removal; if receptors are lacking, ovarian removal will be ineffective.

Inherited deficiency or absence of receptors characterizes a number of conditions. Pseudohypoparathyroidism, as mentioned above, arises when cells of the target tissues that normally respond to parathyroid hormone resist its action. In some of the several forms of the disease, this resistance is due in part to lack of specific receptors on cell membranes. Consequently, PTH cannot bind to the cell and thereby stimulate calcium release from bone or absorption of calcium from the gut. Another hereditary disorder, testicular feminization, affects people who are genetic males (46,XY) but have ambiguous external sex organs and at puberty develop feminine body form although their gonads are testes. The cause is deficiency, absence, or abnormality of the cellular receptor for testosterone. Neither the individual's own nor administered testosterone has any effect.

French medical researcher Etienne-Emile Baulieu, developer of the compound RU-486, diagrams the mechanism whereby the drug terminates pregnancy by blocking certain receptors (one is depicted as a large crescent) in the uterine lining from binding the ovarian hormone progesterone (P), an event needed to accept and sustain the fetus in the womb during pregnancy. Used in conjunction with prostaglandins to induce uterine contractions, RU-486 has proved to be extremely effective when taken during the fourth to sixth weeks after conception. It is also being investigated as a conventional contraceptive, an aid to ease difficult deliveries, and a cancer treatment.

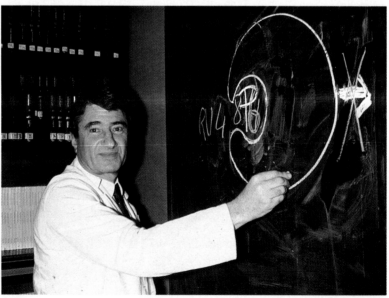

The most common hormone receptor disorder is non-insulin-dependent (adult-onset) diabetes mellitus, associated with obesity and often occurring in middle age. In this case the numbers of insulin receptors are reduced in red blood cells, in white blood cells known as monocytes, and in fat cells. Such diabetes responds only sluggishly to administered insulin, making control of blood sugar levels difficult and highly dependent on diet.

In the field of reproductive endocrinology, hormone receptors are the key to a recent development of great potential significance. RU-486, or mifepristone, a drug marketed by the French pharmaceutical company Groupe Roussel-Uclaf, is a progesterone receptor antagonist; it acts to prevent receptors in the uterine lining from binding the ovarian hormone progesterone, an action essential for implantation of the fertilized egg and maintenance of the fetus during pregnancy. The substance, taken in conjunction with prostaglandins, is extremely effective in terminating pregnancy during the fourth to sixth weeks after conception. RU-486 has been available since 1988 on an experimental basis in France, where thousands of women have chosen it over surgical abortion. As of mid-1990, in part because of resistance by pro-life activists, Roussel-Uclaf had not yet released it for sale in other countries. Investigators have begun exploring other potential uses for the drug; for example, as a conventional contraceptive, a labor inducer, a promoter of wound healing, and a treatment for certain kinds of tumors.

Hormones from improbable organs

One of the most far-reaching changes in the concept of hormones has come from the finding of hormonal substances in organs and tissues that no one had ever considered to be secretory glands. The lungs, seemingly an unlikely source of hormonal influence, have been found to process hormone precursors—activating some, inactivating others, and synthesizing still others (prostaglandins). Certain of these substances may play a role in the lungs' reaction to injury by embolisms, vessel-blocking blood clots that travel from other sites in the body.

The kidneys, plainly not glands in the traditional sense, produce at least one protein, erythropoietin, that acts like a hormone. Erythropoietin stimulates the bone marrow's production of red blood cells in response to lack of oxygen, as is experienced by people living at high altitude or by those with severe lung disease. In rare cases tumors derived from kidney cells synthesize and release enough of the protein to cause excessive red cell production, a condition called polycythemia. In some instances of renal cancer, measurements of erythropoietin values in the blood serum are useful as tumor markers.

The thymus, a lymphoid organ in the upper chest, has been regarded as playing some part, not yet well defined, in the body's immune response to infectious disease. Recent work has disclosed several thymic peptides that help regulate the maturation of primitive lymphocytes into T cells; that is, cells that are immunologically capable of defending against bacterial and viral invasion. Further, the thymus elaborates two other peptides that have found limited therapeutic use. Thymopoietin has shown some beneficial effect against human rheumatoid arthritis. Alpha-1 thymosin has benefited

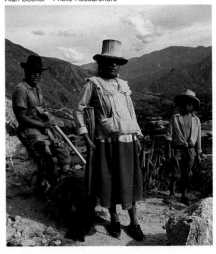

Blood unusually rich in red cells (erythrocytes) is found in people living at high altitude, such as the mountain dwellers of the Bolivian Andes above, and in victims of lung disease severe enough to starve the tissues of oxygen. This compensatory mechanism is mediated by a hormone, erythropoietin, produced by an unlikely endocrine organ, the kidney. Secreted in response to lack of oxygen, erythropoietin stimulates the bone marrow to increase production of red cells. People afflicted with severe kidney disease may experience a deficiency of the hormone and consequent anemia, which has been shown to respond to treatment with erythropoietin. In 1989 a form of the hormone producible in quantity by means of genetic engineering became available in the U.S. for such treatment.

A nursing mother, an emotionally exhausted political candidate, and a first grader who towers over his classmate—the linking thread is that their life experiences are being influenced by pituitary hormones normally controlled by the hypothalamus in the brain. While one hypothalamic hormone governs prolactin, the pituitary hormone that regulates milk production in women after childbirth, another controls pituitary secretion of a hormone that prompts the adrenal cortex to release cortisol, a major player in the body's response to stress. Pituitary growth hormone is ordinarily regulated by hypothalamic releasing and inhibiting hormones, but certain pituitary abnormalities in childhood, particularly tumors, may cause oversecretion of growth hormone and consequent pituitary gigantism.

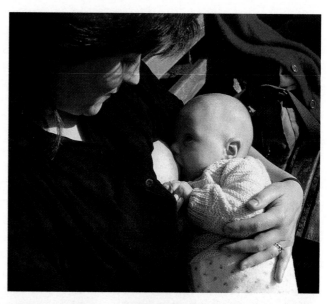

Photographs, (top) Barbara Alper—Stock, Boston; (bottom left) Honl—Gamma/ Liaison; (bottom right) Arthur Grace—Stock, Boston

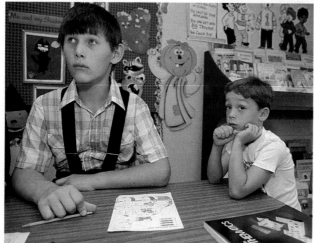

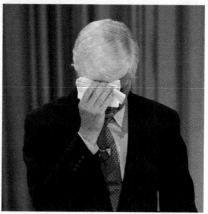

children with genetic immunodeficiency diseases and cancer patients who have suffered dangerous reductions in blood lymphocytes as a result of chemotherapy.

Even the heart turns out to have an endocrine activity, as was unexpectedly discovered in the early 1980s. When the heart begins to fail as a pump and the blood volume consequently rises, the thin-walled upper chambers, or atria, of the heart stretch, causing what earlier had been observed to be a compensatory "reflex" excretion of salt and water via the kidney. The reflex is now known to result from the release from special cells in the atria of a hormone called atrial natriuretic peptide (ANP; also known as auriculin and atriopeptin). This new diuretic substance may well play an important natural role in offsetting the effects of heart failure and in the normal function of the heart and blood vessels. Furthermore, it may have therapeutic applications in patients with heart failure, high blood pressure, some kidney diseases, or other illnesses associated with the retention of fluid.

50

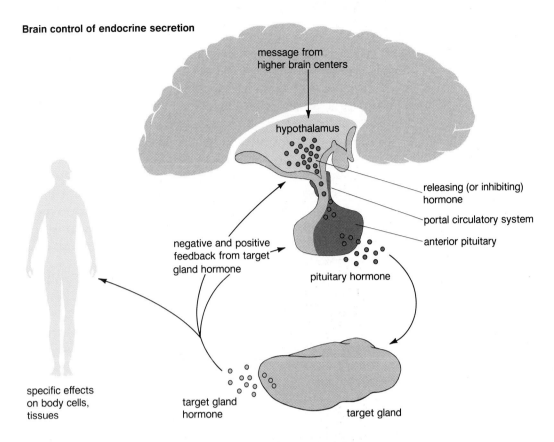

message from
higher brain centers

hypothalamus

releasing (or inhibiting)
hormone

portal circulatory system

anterior pituitary

negative and positive
feedback from target
gland hormone

pituitary hormone

specific effects
on body cells,
tissues

target gland
hormone

target gland

The past two decades of research have shown the gut to be a factory of hormones. More than 35 such peptide hormones are secreted by the so-called APUD cells, which are distributed diffusely throughout the intestinal tract. Within the gut they are thought to regulate gut motility and secretion of digestive fluids. Studies of their actions outside the gut are just starting but promise surprising disclosures. Certain gastrointestinal tumors oversecrete gut hormones—for example, gastrin and somatostatin—and the gross excess of the substances gives rise to disorders having well-defined symptoms. Measurement of the hormones in blood serum affords the opportunity for early diagnosis and treatment.

Brain hormones

The brain and other parts of the central nervous system are now known to produce many hormones and neurotransmitters that have endocrine, autocrine, and paracrine activity. Among the earliest to be discovered were chemicals made by the hypothalamus—a small structure at the base of the brain just above the pituitary—that stimulate the anterior pituitary. From work done in the 1960s and '70s, it is known that this minute volume of brain tissue secretes peptide hormones that travel by way of a special circulatory system to the pituitary gland, where each peptide acts to regulate the synthesis and release of a specific pituitary hormone. Among the hypothalamic peptides are growth-hormone-releasing hormone (GRH) and growth-hormone-inhibiting hormone (somatostatin). Prolactin, the pituitary hormone that regulates milk production in women after they have given birth, is controlled almost entirely by a prolactin-inhibiting hypothalamic hor-

The basic relationships among the brain, anterior pituitary, and the pituitary's dependent glands are diagrammed above. Under the control of higher brain centers, the hypothalamus secretes any of several hormones that travel via a special system of blood vessels (portal system) to the anterior pituitary, inducing that organ to release hormones targeted for specific dependent glands. The hormone released by the dependent gland not only exerts its endocrine effects on the body but also provides negative- and positive-feedback control of the hypothalamus and pituitary. The discovery of the hypothalamic hormones during the 1960s and 1970s deepened understanding of the interworkings of the endocrine system and the brain and shed new light on the causes of endocrine disorders.

51

mone that is not a peptide but an amine, the neurotransmitter dopamine. Gonadotropin-releasing hormone (GnRH) controls the pituitary's secretion of FSH and LH; thyrotropin-releasing hormone (TRH), that of thyrotropin (thyroid-stimulating hormone; TSH); and corticotropin-releasing hormone (CRH), that of corticotropin (adrenocorticotropic hormone; ACTH).

These hypothalamic hormones all can be considered neurotransmitters; secreted by neural tissue, they transmit chemical signals to the pituitary. Their discovery won for the Americans Rosalyn Yalow, Roger Guillemin, and Andrew Schally the Nobel Prize for Physiology or Medicine in 1977. The vast amount of research on these compounds has deepened understanding of the relationships among the brain, the pituitary, and the pituitary's dependent glands, has disclosed new diseases, and has opened doors in reproductive endocrinology.

One recent benefit of this research, coupled with the measurement capabilities of radioimmunoassay, has been the recognition that an elevated level of prolactin in the blood, a condition known as hyperprolactinemia, is the most common neuroendocrine disorder. In addition to causing galactorrhea (inappropriate breast milk production), hyperprolactinemia has been found to be involved in significant numbers of cases of other reproductive disorders, including infertility and amenorrhea (absence of menstrual periods) in women and impotence in men. In most cases the elevated prolactin results from a pituitary tumor, but it has also been associated with an abnormality of hypothalamic secretion or some other cause outside the pituitary itself. Studies have shown that treatment with substances that inhibit prolactin secretion in many cases is preferable to surgical or radiation treatment of the pituitary. In particular, numerous reports have documented the success of bromocriptine, an alkaloid drug that can stimulate dopamine receptors on the prolactin-secreting cells of the pituitary and thereby mimic the natural inhibiting action of dopamine, in reducing prolactin levels and, surprisingly, in reducing the size of pituitary tumors.

Many other hormonal substances, presumably neurotransmitters, are found in the central nervous system. Perhaps the most dramatic are the so-called endogenous opioids (or natural opiates)—the endorphins and enkephalins—which are widely distributed in brain tissue and are found chiefly in cells that have opiate receptors; i.e., specific receptors for the addictive narcotics like morphine. These small peptides have many incompletely understood influences on human experience; they affect sleep, eating and drinking behavior, body temperature, the perception of and response to pain, and, amazingly, memory and learning. They have been offered as explanations for such diverse phenomena as the ability of acupuncture to produce anesthesia and the druglike euphoria reportedly experienced by runners, weight lifters, and other athletes during intense workouts. Investigation of the significance of the endogenous opioids still has a long way to go. Researchers expect to find them involved in the bodily response to stress and suggest that they may operate in the higher central nervous system in ways that today can barely be imagined.

At least 10 other hormonal peptides have been isolated from brain tissue. Among the more interesting is cholecystokinin (CCK), first known as a gut hormone that stimulates the gallbladder. The question of what CCK is doing in the brain may have begun to be answered with recent observations that the substance induces satiety—*i.e.,* it lowers appetite and food intake—in laboratory animals, leading to the hope that the hormone could find a place in the understanding and management of human obesity and in the development of drugs that stimulate or suppress appetite.

As mentioned above, certain cancers secrete hormones and hormonelike substances. Benign, but more commonly malignant, tumors of virtually every organ have been reported as sources for protein hormones: vasopressin (antidiuretic hormone, or ADH, normally a pituitary secretion), gonadotropins, ACTH, insulin-like growth factors, and many others. Overabundances of these inappropriately secreted substances can cause serious disorders of their own. Measurements of their levels in the blood are useful as tumor markers, enabling monitoring and prompt treatment. These observations have led to the realization that almost all cells have the potential for hormone secretion. The nature of the cancerous process that releases this potentiality is the subject of intense study.

Hormones from many sources

A variety of protein substances that influence growth have been and continue to be discovered in numerous tissues. Whether they are hormones may be simply a question of semantics, since they certainly have endocrine, autocrine, and paracrine activity. One, epidermal growth factor (EGF), influences growth, development, and the proliferation of cells in fetal life. EGF has shown promise in clinical trials as a healing agent; it slightly accelerates the healing of superficial incised wounds in the skin. As can be supposed, very active research on this compound is under way.

Other substances in this category are platelet-derived growth factor, which affects blood clotting, and fibroblast growth factor (FGF), which influences the growth of connective tissue. Somatomedin, synthesized in the liver, acts as a mediator that permits the widespread action of pituitary growth hormone. Nerve growth factor (NGF) affects the development of nerve cells and fibers and may be involved in the failure of brain development seen in cretins, infants who are deficient in thyroid hormone in fetal life and early infancy and thus experience major problems in physical and mental development. Clinical trials have been initiated to determine whether NGF is useful in promoting the healing of wounds in peripheral nerves.

Prostaglandins, powerfully active compounds formed from essential fatty acids, are present in most tissues. They and related substances, eicosanoids and leukotrienes, generally act as local regulators (paracrine hormones), and over the past two decades they have been shown to mediate an astonishingly diverse array of functions. Prostaglandins have neuroendocrine actions in the regulation of thyrotropin, corticotropin, prolactin, and gonadotropin secretion by the pituitary. The finding that they stimulate contraction of the uterine muscle has led to the successful treatment of menstrual cramps by administration of prostaglandin inhibitors, such as ibuprofen, and to the use of prostaglandins as labor-inducing agents. Some prostaglandins influence the immune response of lymphocytes and help mediate inflammation; oth-

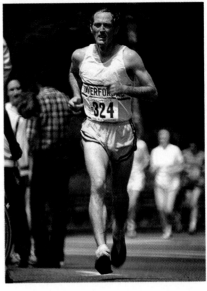

Runners, weight lifters, and other athletes have reported experiencing euphoric "highs" during peak physical activity, an effect that some attribute to the release of hormonelike substances called endogenous opioids. Discovered in the brain and spinal cord in the 1970s, these peptide compounds bind to the same receptors as do the opiate narcotics. They are clearly involved in the body's perception of and response to pain, show strong evidence of being connected with so-called pleasure centers in the brain, and seem to influence a variety of other human experiences, including sleep, eating behavior, and memory and learning.

ers are intimately involved in the process of blood clotting; and still others affect the digestive tract. Prostaglandins are also strong vasodilators, relaxing the muscles in the walls of blood vessels and thereby enlarging the vessel diameter and lowering blood pressure.

Hormones in behavior, aging, and stress

Hormones may play a part in what ranks among the most common of human diseases, depression. First, research suggests that there may be abnormalities of various neurotransmitters in the brain of the depressed person. Second and more certain, some forms of depression are marked by definite and major endocrine disturbances.

The best studied and most obvious is excessive secretion by the adrenal cortex of its major glucocorticoid hormone, cortisol. In some forms of depression, levels of cortisol and abnormalities in its secretory control are as great as those found in Cushing's disease, an illness resulting from overstimulation of the adrenal cortex by an ACTH-producing pituitary tumor. Some researchers postulate that areas of the brain above the hypothalamus stimulate excessive secretion of hypothalamic corticotropin-releasing hormone, a suggestion supported by the discovery of high levels of this hormone in the cerebrospinal fluid of depressed patients. Other support comes from the frequent occurrence of depression in true Cushing's disease. Other neuroendocrine abnormalities—involving somatostatin, vasopressin, growth hormone, and TSH—have also been discovered in depression. Understanding the significance of these endocrine changes should lead to the design of effective therapies.

Hormones are becoming increasingly implicated in the biology of stress and aging. When a person is confronted with prolonged stress—for example, a family tragedy or a high-pressure job—the body may respond with increased secretion of CRH from the hypothalamus, which induces pituitary secretion of ACTH, which in turn stimulates cortisol secretion from

Studies in laboratory animals suggest that in the elderly the hormonal response to stressful situations may remain "switched on" longer than in young individuals. Stress initiates a chain of hormonal secretions beginning in the brain and culminating in the release by the adrenals of cortisol and other hormones, which among their actions raise blood pressure, step up metabolism, and make nutrients more available to cells and tissues; at high levels cortisol also can impair the functioning of the immune system. In the aged, chronically high levels of cortisol may actually damage part of the brain responsible for endocrine control, thus making the brain even less capable of responding appropriately to stress.

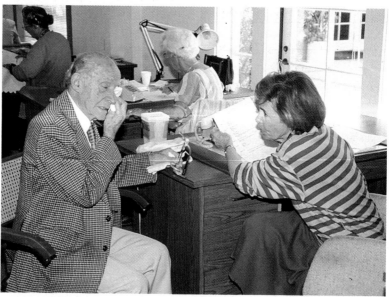

Bill Aron—Photo Researchers

the adrenal cortex. Among other actions, cortisol raises blood sugar and steps up metabolism; there is evidence that it also suppresses the immune system. Laboratory studies of old rats have revealed that the adrenal cortical response to various stress situations does not "turn off" nearly as rapidly as in young animals. Furthermore, experimentally exposing aging rats to a characteristic feature of stress, namely, high blood concentrations of cortisol, actually induces the death of cells in a part of the brain called the hippocampus, located in the limbic system, a part of the brain involved in neuroendocrine control. Put another way, chronic stress may damage the brain and, in a vicious circle, render it less and less capable of mounting appropriate emotional and physical responses to adverse stimuli from the environment. Whether these laboratory observations are true for human beings remains to be shown.

In recent years researchers have reported finding abnormally high cortisol levels and disordered regulation of cortisol secretion associated with other behavior-related problems, ranging from manic-depressive illness to the eating disorder anorexia nervosa to shyness and poor psychological adjustment in teenagers. It falls to future studies to establish whether a cause-and-effect relationship for these associations actually exists and, if it does, whether the hormonal disturbance is the root or a result of the behavior disorder.

The pineal, a small gland located at the center of the brain, secretes a unique hormone, melatonin, whose physiological significance in humans is still largely unknown. The pineal's production of melatonin varies both with the time of day and with age, which has led to the suspicion and some experimental demonstration that it plays a role in the body's responses to cycles of light and dark, in daily biological rhythms, and in bringing on sleep. In the early 1980s psychiatrists recognized a cyclically recurring form of depression, termed seasonal affective disorder (SAD), that afflicts people during the months of shortened daylight hours and that could be relieved by daily exposures to bright artificial light. Because strong light has been shown in experiments to suppress melatonin secretion in humans, some researchers believe the hormone to be involved in the causation of SAD.

The future

Over the past few decades medical research has discovered that hormones help govern virtually every aspect of human experience—from growth and development to metabolism, to reproduction, to responses to physical injury and mental stress, and even to thought processes themselves. Where medicine was once content to define endocrinology in terms of fewer than two dozen chemical substances, it now must deal with hundreds. Even the idea of a hormone itself has broadened to include just about any substance made by a cell that can change what that cell or some other cell in the body is doing. In the future the rapid pace of hormone research will surely uncover even more of the body's biochemical secrets, hastening the day when people no longer will live entirely at the mercy of their hormones but to some degree will control that delicately balanced mix of chemicals to lead longer, healthier, more self-directed lives.

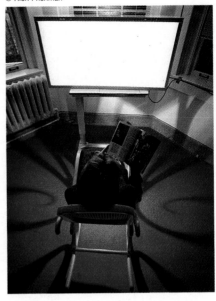

Daily exposure to strong supplemental light for an hour or more, particularly in the morning, has been found therapeutic in relieving a cyclically recurring form of depression called seasonal affective disorder (SAD). Recognized for only about a decade, SAD afflicts its victims during the fall and winter, when hours of daylight are shortest. The pineal, an organ located deep in the brain, secretes the hormone melatonin, whose production follows a daily rhythm that is affected by changes in the day-night cycle and can be suppressed completely by strong light. In large doses melatonin also has been shown to induce sleepiness and slow down reaction time, leading to speculation that the hormone is somehow involved in the causation of SAD.

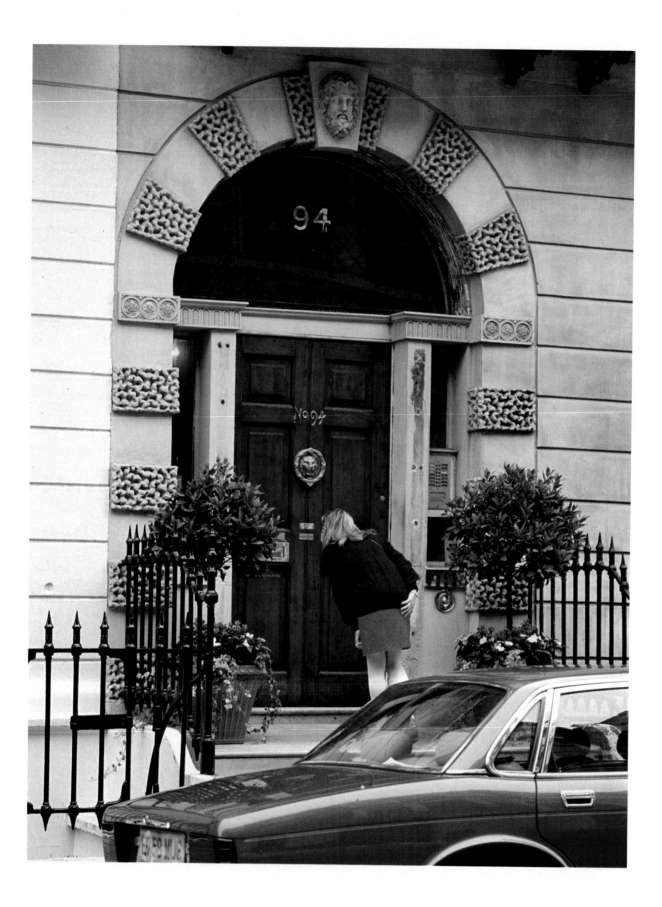

A Practice with Prestige—
DOCTORS OF HARLEY STREET

by Jerry Mason

London has its Harley Street, New York has Park Avenue, and few are immune to the snob value of having consulting-rooms on the chosen street.
—The Principles and Art of Plastic Surgery

Liz still, after all these years, found satisfaction in giving her address. Each time a shop assistant or a clerk or a tradesman wrote down Dr. E. Headleand, Harley Street, the same thrill of self-affirmation, of self-definition would be re-enacted. Liz . . . had become Liz Headleand of Harley Street, London W.1. Nobody could argue with that, nobody could question it. . . . Her largest dreams, her most foolish fantasies had been enacted in bricks and mortar and mantel shelves and tiled floors and plaster ceilings. . . . The Headleands of Harley Street. Resonant, exemplary. Myriad uncertainties and hesitations were buried beneath that solid pile, banished by the invocation of a street name. *—The Radiant Way*

Mention Harley Street, London, and people the world over associate it with doctors—not just any doctors but the most eminent of specialists. Indeed, an address in Harley Street automatically bestows the perception of excellence and exclusiveness upon the doctor who practices there, where the highest fees are routine.

The Harley Street doctor has been lampooned by George Bernard Shaw in *The Doctor's Dilemma* (1906), reviled by the Scottish novelist A.J. Cronin in *The Citadel* (1937), and held up as the epitome of yuppie elegance by the contemporary British novelist Margaret Drabble in *The Radiant Way* (1987). On the one hand, the Harley Street specialists have been castigated for their greed by the government and the press. On the other hand, they owe much of their glamour to newspaper reportage, and the British government sought first to gain *their* cooperation, rather than the general practitioners', in the creation of a National Health Service (NHS) in 1948. The specialists negotiated the right to continue in part-time private practice; therefore, the new system, which pledged medical treatment free at the time of need to all citizens of Great Britain, did not undermine the prestige of Harley Street. Specialists in all fields of medicine are clustered there still, with the overflow of preeminence long established in neighboring Wimpole Street.

Jerry Mason is a London-based free-lance photojournalist.

(Opposite page) London has enjoyed a long history as a major center of medicine. Since the early 19th century, when specialists began to exert their eminence, many of the city's most prosperous and illustrious medical consultants have been clustered in the several blocks of stately Georgian houses that line Harley Street. (Wimpole Street, its parallel neighbor, is also the abode of prominent physicians.) Photograph, Jerry Mason

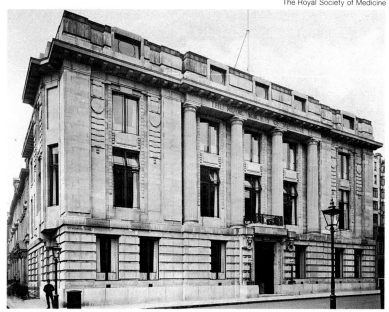

On May 21, 1912, a new building for the Royal Society of Medicine was opened in a formal ceremony by King George V and Queen Mary. The society's president expressed "grateful appreciation" to "Your Majesties, who at all times show very active sympathy in the work of the great hospitals and similar institutions, and in everything that tends to alleviate sickness and relieve suffering." Today the society maintains its position as the bastion of British medicine, and the original Wimpole Street building still serves as its headquarters. Between 1982 and 1986 a major development of the premises expanded and modernized the facilities, which now include meeting halls, lecture theaters, an enlarged library, an academic center, and gracious club facilities with comprehensive amenities.

Number 1 Wimpole Street

Appropriately, 1 Wimpole Street is the address of the Royal Society of Medicine—the bastion of British medicine. Founded in 1805 as the Royal Medical and Chirurgical Society of London, the society had, and still has, as its purpose the advancement of medicine, surgery, and related sciences, and its motto states: *Non est vivere sed valere vita* ("One must enjoy good health to live fully").

The Wimpole Street headquarters were opened in 1912 by King George V and Queen Mary. Designed by John Belcher, with columns of Portland stone on a Cornish granite base, the stately structure was commended by the *Architectural Review* for "a dignity eminently in keeping with the institution housed within its walls," a feature sustained in the later additions to the building as the society has grown.

Today the Royal Society of Medicine has 17,000 members and 34 specialty sections, which ensure the progress of debate, collaboration, and research in each recognized field of medicine. The society's conference rooms are kept busy, and the library is one of the largest medical research collections in Europe. In addition to its monthly *Journal,* the society publishes *Tropical Doctor* and, since 1987, *The AIDS Letter*. There is also a Royal Society of Medicine Foundation, with premises in New York City.

Brass plates: Harley Street emblem

Between them, the five-block stretch of Harley Street and the four blocks of Wimpole Street today accommodate over 1,000 doctors and some 200 dentists in the original Georgian houses and a scattering of newer buildings, amounting to one of the largest concentrations of medical professionals anywhere in the world. Harley Street has long been famous for the shining brass nameplates emblazoned on virtually every address and bearing the names of the eminent consultants within.

58

Photographs, Jerry Mason

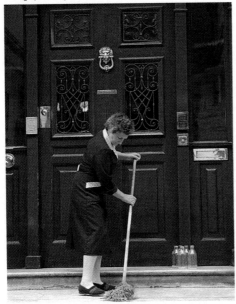

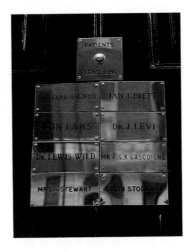

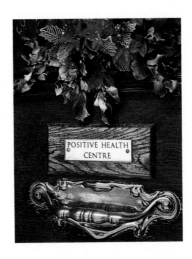

Of Harley Street the Michelin guide to London says, "Seemingly every door, three steps up from the pavement, is emblazoned with consultants' brass plates." (Not all names on the plates begin with "Dr."; in Britain surgeons and dentists usually call themselves "Mr." or "Mrs.")

Several years ago the *British Medical Journal* published a "Survey of Nameplates in a Well Known London Street," the street being, of course, Harley Street. The research was undertaken by an otolaryngologist, Catherine Milton, and a surgeon, Richard Bickerton, to follow up a similar survey that had been done 35 years earlier by another doctor, Scott Stevenson. Stevenson had recorded 798 brass nameplates in Harley Street in 1951, at which time he noted: "I did not realise that the latest snobisme [sic] of Harley Street is to have no door plate at all—a natural reaction to the common spectacle nowadays of a dozen or even (in two instances) twenty name plates on one door." The greatest number of plates Bickerton and Milton counted at any one site was 40. Yet they reported, "Since this last

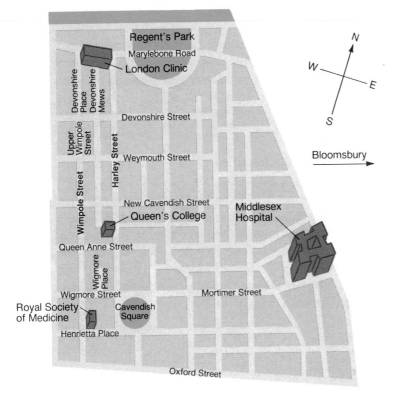

The fashionable physicians' quarter, famed for its private consulting rooms, is situated between Regent's Park to the north and Oxford Street to the south. Many Harley and Wimpole Street specialists hold appointments at the noted Middlesex Hospital, a few blocks to the east in Mortimer Street.

survey was conducted the number [the total number for the entire street] has decreased by 23." This surprising finding is attributed to "the communal entryphone"—the entryphone is next to the nameplates and used for patients to announce their arrival—and to "the emergence of the shoddy plate"—that is, one made of plastic tape. Bickerton and Milton further discovered: "The legal profession occupied several sites, particularly in the south. It came as no surprise to observe the dimensions of their plates, being many times greater than those of the medical profession."

The facetious survey was presented in formal journal format: including abstract, statement of purpose ("In view of the time that has elapsed since the last survey it seemed essential that a further review should be undertaken"), defined units of measure (1 plate [P] = A plaque consisting of any material on the door or doorway bearing one or more names [1KP = 1,000 plates]"), statement of methods ("The survey took place in daylight, early one Sunday morning . . ."), graph, table, and references. The report was hardly subtle in its suggestion that the Harley Street specialist, however venerable a part of the establishment, is a cliché.

This was no less true at the beginning of the century—the "golden age" of Harley Street—when the practitioner lived in his house and one brass plate was the norm for each door, with two indicating a father and son in practice. There was even a doctor Robert Harley (1829–96) of Harley Street, a heroic character who was proud of the coincidence of his name. He exemplified the Victorian faith in the scientific method, living for days on asparagus to induce diabetes, swallowing nitroglycerine to study its effect, and curing himself of morphine addiction by sheer power of will. In his drawing room at Number 25, the first perforated wax gramophone was played, and guests, including novelist Charles Dickens and painter Sir Edwin Landseer, were treated to breakfasts of donkey sausage, Pomeranian goose, and 1,000-year-old eggs from China.

Dickens, however, thought it appropriate in *Little Dorrit* to house the swindler Mr. Merdle (not a doctor) in Harley Street, where "the opposing rows of houses . . . were very grim with one another." Likewise, Benjamin Disraeli called Harley Street and its neighbors "flat, dull, spiritless streets." Both disdained the austere good taste of the houses, built of brown London stock brick, that lined the streets. Shaw reserved his criticism for the physicians living in Harley and Wimpole streets; *The Doctor's Dilemma* is an impassioned attack on their snobbery and wealth and on the complete sham of their profession.

Mountebanks and charlatans

In fact, the first famous medical men to live in Harley Street had been mountebanks and charlatans. The very first doctor to live there (in 1775), Robert Perrean, was publicly hanged before he could set up in practice (convicted of raising money to buy the house on a forged bond). William Rowley (1742–1806) of Number 66 (now Number 4) was a keen collector of degrees, with self-proclaimed expertise in numerous fields. He gave himself the title "Man-Midwife," campaigned vigorously against vaccination, and insisted he had a cure for cancer.

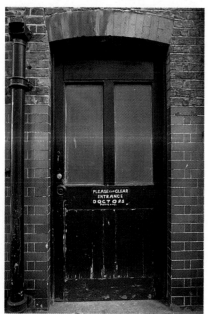

Medical facilities now occupy a site in Devonshire Mews, originally built as stables for horses. In the "golden age" of Harley Street, when the immediate neighborhood was the dwelling place of nobility and gentry, the prominent physicians who lived there went about in horse-drawn carriages, and their standard garb was top hat, astrakhan collar, and spats. Those too were the days when the Royal Horse Guards daily paraded down Harley Street, the ceremonial route from their Regent's Park barracks to Whitehall.

Jerry Mason

60

But the famed street's most sensational practitioner was the infamous and rich John St. John Long (1798–1834), "king of quacks," of Number 41 Harley Street. Although professional skill rather than quackery was to become the abiding reputation of practitioners in the street, no doctor, qualified or not, before or since, has been quite so popular as the empiric Long. "The Pied Piper of Harley Street" lured rich, often titled, lady patients to Number 41 in such numbers that the street was daily jammed with carriages. Inside, a labyrinth of mysterious pink tubing distributed a corrosive inhalant for the communal phase of his treatment that was employed for virtually any female ailment, with whole bevies of ladies "plugged in" at once. The effect was often mass hysteria. Private massage sessions followed, with a lotion so corrosive two patients subsequently died from gangrene.

Long was found guilty on his first charge of manslaughter, but he was spared harsh punishment when, during his trial, one of his devoted lady patients, the Marchioness of Ormonde, whispered in the judge's ear; he was fined but £250. Because he was earning in excess of £10,000 per annum, comparable to any Wall Street raider today, the prosecution must be said to have failed, as it did in a second trial when Long was acquitted on another charge of manslaughter. Commenting on the trials, *The Law Review* noted that a verdict of murder would certainly have been justified. Long was ruined anyway and was to die at age 36 from tuberculosis—one of the ailments he claimed his formula, "The Saviour of Mankind from All Ills and Ailments, the Great Lengthener of Life, the One and Only Distributor of Health," could cure.

Stead of gentry

The original grand plan for the development that became the world-renowned abode of eminent physicians was drawn up by John Holles, Duke of Newcastle, at the beginning of the 18th century to provide "residences for the nobility and gentry." Holles was married to Lady Margaret Cavendish (commemorated in the square of that name at the south end of Harley Street). Their daughter, Henrietta, married Edward Harley, Baron Harley of Wigmore (1689–1741), who, on inheriting the land, proceeded to develop it. He and his titled descendants had the honor of being remembered in the grid of streets that came to be.

The City had always been the favored location for doctors, close to the long-established teaching hospitals of the capital. Appointments as physicians to these hospitals conferred prestige to the practitioners who held them. As London's affluence spread westward, medical men moved first into Bloomsbury and then, with the founding in 1745 of the Middlesex Hospital in Mortimer Street, into the neighborhood of Harley Street. The practical value for a doctor of an address in Harley Street had been assured with the building in 1756 of the New Road—London's first bypass road—which cut through green fields from Islington to Paddington, and which has become the congested Marylebone Road at the north end of Harley Street and Devonshire Place.

Because doctors gained their reputations chiefly in teaching hospitals, which in London were voluntary institutions—*i.e.,* nonpaying—they de-

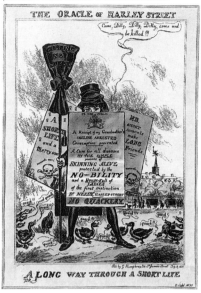

The infamous and rich John St. John Long, "the oracle of Harley Street," lured wealthy ladies to his home with the promise of miraculous cures for every known ailment. In fact, his "treatments" produced mass hysteria, gangrene, and at least two deaths. In 1830 the "king of quacks" was widely pilloried in the press (note the ducks in the cartoon's foreground); subsequently he was publicly denounced as a murderer.

pended on a private income. At first, leading doctors would let it be known that they might be consulted at certain hours in the coffee houses of the area. Then in 1795 Matthew Baillie moved into Cavendish Square and advertised his presence at home to patients. Among the patients who consulted him there was the poet Lord Byron. Baillie was prominent in the founding of the Royal Medical and Chirurgical Society and for 10 years was physician to the mad King George III.

Among the eminent doctors who first lived and practiced in Harley Street was John Latham, who was president of the Royal College of Physicians from 1813 to 1819. His predecessor, Sir Lucas Pepys, had lived in Wimpole Street. Augustin Sayer, physician to the Duke of Kent and prominent advocate of sanitary reform, was a resident of Harley Street. Henry Southey, younger brother of the English poet laureate Robert Southey, could be seen leaving his house in Harley Street to attend King George IV (who died in the same year John St. John Long was twice tried for manslaughter). By 1855 there were 19 doctors living in Harley Street, including Alfred Baring, expert in the disease foremost among the ails of the Victorian upper classes—gout. His high-living neighbors were no doubt among his patients.

The distinction of specialists

The early specialists who made Harley Street what it is had a hard fight to secure recognition within the profession, finding themselves out of favor with medical colleges and often excluded from the hospital appointments that were so important to their status. To exploit his reputation to the fullest among fee-paying patients, a doctor had to specialize. It was not so easy to begin with. The respected teacher at Guy's Hospital, Thomas Addison (1793–1860), made no bones about it; a specialist "savoured of quackery."

Consultant had first been used to refer to physicians and surgeons who had hospital appointments. General practitioners (GPs), represented by the

The widely revered physician Matthew Baillie (below) began to treat patients at his home in 1795. Baillie was prominent in the founding of the Royal Medical and Chirurgical Society (which later became the Royal Society of Medicine). He wrote one of the first textbooks on pathological anatomy, The Morbid Anatomy of Some of the Most Important Parts of the Human Body *(1793), and for 10 years he was physician to King George III (right).*

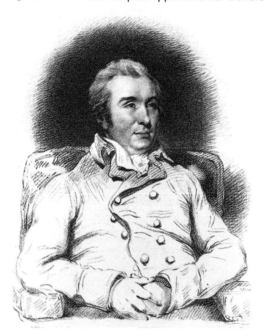

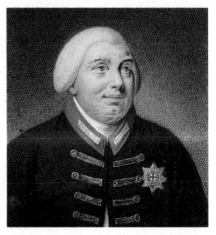

youthful British Medical Association, established in 1832, rebelled against the consultants, competing with them for well-heeled clients. Not long after the Public Health Act was passed in 1848, general practitioners forced an agreement on the specialists: physicians and surgeons who set themselves up as specialists would see private patients only on referral by general practitioners. This suited both sides and added further distinction to the term *consultant*.

Harley Street played a major role in the dissociation of consultants from others in the medical profession. By catering to the rich and famous, Harley Street doctors became celebrities themselves, aided by the interest in royal health of Victorian newspaper readers. Throat specialist Sir Morrell Mackenzie of Number 19 Harley Street, for instance, was made so famous by news coverage of his treatment of the German crown prince, author Lady Duff-Gordon recalled, that "people [stood] on chairs in a hotel restaurant to watch Mackenzie at dinner." The crown prince was seen leaving Mackenzie's "flower filled" consulting rooms "with a look of doom on his face" and died shortly thereafter from cancer of the larynx. Mackenzie published a book on the affair in defense of his treatment, and 100,000 copies were sold in two weeks. Despite the death of the prince, the celebrated doctor continued to thrive in what was surely one of the most lucrative practices in all of Britain. Mackenzie was perhaps being disingenuous when he said in the *Fortnightly Review* of 1885, "The truth is, we are just a little doubtful as to our position in the social scale."

One of the first "bedside baronets" was the urologist Sir Henry Thompson of 35 Wimpole Street, who was in attendance at the deathbed of Napoleon III in 1873. Sir Henry's famous dinner parties, known as Octaves, were attended by the Prince of Wales and the king, among other elite members of society. The parties began at 8 PM and consisted of eight courses, with eight wines, for eight guests. In the 1890s Arthur Conan Doyle could be found there, having walked the short distance from Devonshire Place, where in 1891 he had rented a consulting room for £120 per annum in order, ostensibly, to practice ophthalmology. In fact, Doyle did not see a single patient there, but he did write the first of his Sherlock Holmes stories.

Sir Henry successfully treated King Leopold I of Belgium for stones in the bladder and was paid £5,000 for the job; he justified his fee by remarking afterward that the use of new implements in the operation was significant. Sir Frederick Treves of 6 Wimpole Street, famous for his care of John Merrick (known as the Elephant Man), was also serjeant-surgeon to both King Edward VII and King George V. His removal of Edward's appendix on June 24, 1902, inspired a lasting fashion for the operation. Nevertheless, the operating coat used by Treves in his honorary post at the London Hospital had been, according to the hospital governor, so stiff with congealed blood it would "stand upright on its own when placed on the floor."

Two women of Harley Street

In the latter half of the 19th century, many daughters of Harley Street doctors attended Queen's College at Numbers 43–49, which had been established in 1848 as the first school in the country for the higher education

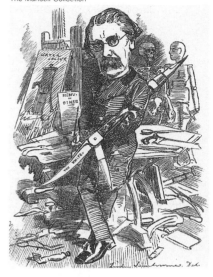

The urologist Sir Henry Thompson (1820–1904) lived at 35 Wimpole Street. He attended Napoleon III at his death and treated King Leopold I of Belgium for bladder stones but perhaps was best known for his dinner parties, known as Octaves—eight courses and eight wines for eight elite guests.

The renowned surgeon Sir Frederick Treves (1853–1923) also enjoyed all the trappings and glamour of a Wimpole Street address (Number 6). Treves, who has been called by a recent biographer "the extra-ordinary Edwardian," served four monarchs but was most famous as the benefactor of the Elephant Man.

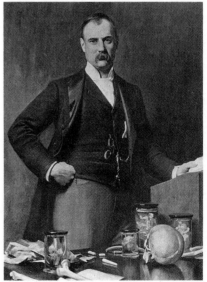

63

Many doctors' daughters attended Queen's College, which was founded in 1848 at 43–49 Harley Street as the first school in England for the higher education of women.

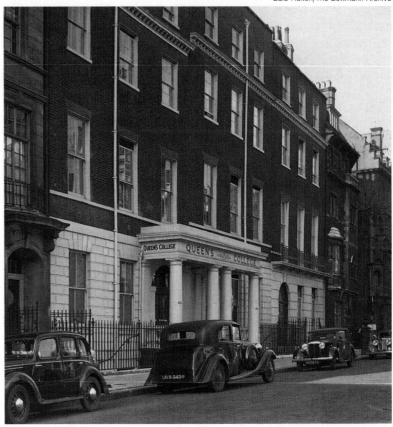

of women. One of these was Sophia Jex-Blake (1840–1912), who became the first qualified woman doctor to practice in Britain and a leader in the movement to open up medical education to women. After graduating from Queen's College, she studied medicine in the United States and Edinburgh and subsequently founded the London School of Medicine for Women and the Edinburgh Hospital for Women and Children.

Perhaps as a child Sophia had seen Florence Nightingale (1820–1910), who had lived at Number 47 Harley Street before the house was incorporated into the college. Nightingale is remembered as well at Number 90 Harley Street (then Number 1 Upper Harley Street), the address to which, as superintendent, she moved the Institution for the Care of Sick Gentlewomen in Distressed Circumstances in 1853. No one was prepared for the zeal the new Lady Superintendent was to show.

Nightingale saw the need for organization at the heart of care for the sick, and there was no detail too small or too obvious to escape her attention. Within her first 10 days she dismissed most of the institution's suppliers, from the coal merchant to the butcher; installed windlasses for delivering hot food to patients, bells with valves to indicate a patient in need, and a new kitchen range; supplied hot water to all the wards; and changed the institution's name to the Institute for Gentlewomen During Illness. Much against the orthodoxy of the day, she stipulated that the institute was to take in all denominations as well as widows and daughters of men in the services. The institute was soon running smoothly, and Nightingale was visiting hospitals in London to collect facts needed for the reform of the nursing profession, for which she ultimately became so famous.

From Number 1 Upper Harley Street, she left for the Crimea in 1854; the miracle of determination she worked in the appalling conditions of the war caught the public imagination. Shortly thereafter, "Nightingale nurses" were being trained by the thousands in Britain, Europe, and the United States; it was the beginning of modern nursing.

Advent of multiple lettering

The golden age of Harley Street, when doctors actually lived there, lasted through World War I. In the early postwar years a venereologist sublet 14 rooms of his residence at Number 88 Harley Street as consulting rooms for other doctors to practice in, charging £300 per annum each. He had feared a sharp drop in patients with the establishment of three national societies dedicated to wiping out venereal disease, but he was perhaps overly hasty. At the end of the war, the National Council for Combating VD, which was established at Number 143 Harley Street, issued a warning that 300,000 servicemen were infected. Another resident, at Number 79, shrewdly followed the example of the venereologist at Number 88 and sublet the rooms his family had occupied. A large portion of the doctors who took up practice in the newly available consulting rooms on Harley Street were venereologists, who maintained highly lucrative practices; some offered discreet cubicles in the waiting room for their patients' privacy, and some paid hospital porters commission for patients received.

Added to the financial incentive to sublet was the difficulty, after the war,

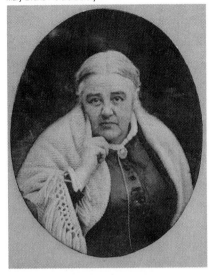

An early pupil of Queen's College was Sophia Jex-Blake, who went on to become a doctor and a leader of the movement to open the medical profession to women in England.

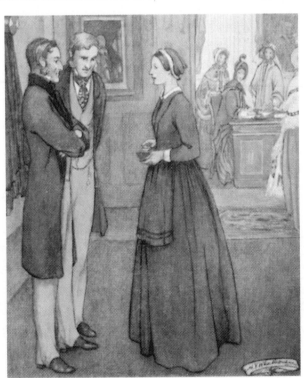

Florence Nightingale lived as a young girl at Number 47 Harley Street in a house that was later incorporated into Queen's College. At age 33, after years of longing for "a profession, a trade, a necessary occupation, something to fill & employ all my faculties," she moved the Institution for the Care of Sick Gentlewomen in Distressed Circumstances to Number 1 Upper Harley Street (left). Despite the fact that her father was firmly against "ladies" accepting paid employment, she served as the institution's zealous Lady Superintendent; it was there that she began to pioneer some of the sanitary reforms for which she later became so famous. In 1909 the facility moved to another part of London and was renamed the Florence Nightingale Hospital for Gentlewomen. Carved in the stone of the building in Harley Street is the tribute: "Florence Nightingale left her hospital on this site for the Crimea—October 21st 1854."

in finding the domestic servants needed to run a large Harley Street house. Single-family residences in the area gradually became scarce and multiple-professional occupancy the norm.

Aggrandized by an address

At its height of glamour, Harley Street had but 200 resident doctors. Ernest Jones of Number 81, the great English interpreter of Sigmund Freud, re-called: "What a closed corporation, like an expensive club, the consulting world of those days was, where everyone gossiped with the other and looked askance at anyone who was not quite the thing!"

Arbuthnot Lane of 21 Cavendish Square, an eminent surgeon at Guy's Hospital, proved himself to be "not quite the thing" when in 1926 he set up the New Health Society for "the prevention of the diseases which are incident to civilization." His missionary approach was deeply offensive to his fellow doctors. When he signed articles propounding the society's cause in the *Daily Mail,* his name was struck from the Medical Register. His student and protégé at Guy's, Sir Heneage Ogilvy, never forgave "the hyenas of Harley Street, the confidence men of medicine who trade on the goodwill and trust established by generations of honest men, who gamble on the magic of an address as able to suggest long training and established posi-tion, who have learned to hand out the patter of a speciality without having the training that patter should represent."

The report of a royal commission on university education in 1915 had criticized Harley Street consultants for being more interested in their bank balances than with advancing medical knowledge. Not many consultants resigned from private practice in order to pursue research, but Wilfred Trotter of Number 101 Harley Street did, despite being serjeant-surgeon to King George V. He chose to dedicate himself to his profession in the less than elegant wards of University College Hospital.

A view of the lower end of Harley Street in the 1920s appeared in the book Wonderful London, *with the caption: "The limousines of those who expensively enjoy bad health are a feature of the street."*

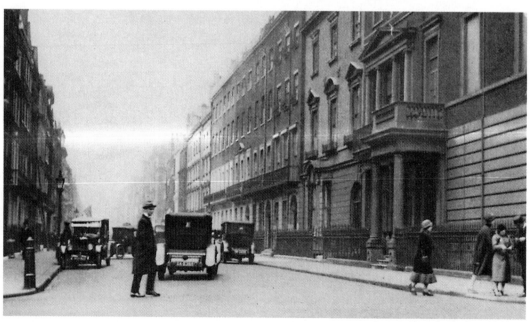

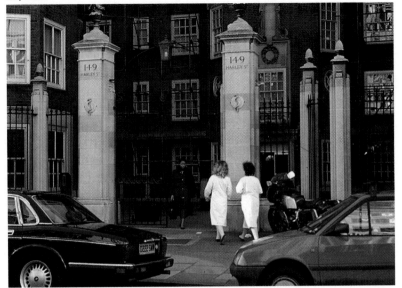

The London Clinic and Nursing Home opened at the north end of Harley Street facing Regent's Park in 1932—a private enterprise offering the most sophisticated hospital care, with luxury accommodations for convalescents, an outpatient clinic, and suites for private practitioners. Five of the physicians attending the present royal family are based there. The list of wealthy and internationally famous people who have been patients at the clinic over the years is a long one. In 1961, during the filming of Cleopatra, *Elizabeth Taylor suffered from complications of pneumonia and needed an emergency tracheotomy. The clinic's resident anesthetist saved the actress's life—and also that of the now-classic movie.*

In 1918 *The Lancet* disparaged specialists as a creation not of the profession but of the public: "The public is obsessed with the glamour of specialization." In 1920 *The Times* reported a "crisis in Harley Street" as specialists struggled to earn the £4,000 a year necessary to sustain a practice there. N. Bishop Harmon of Number 108 Harley Street pointed out that patients required that doctors be "enshrined in suitably substantial elegance."

Elegance and glamour did not satisfy all patients, however. In 1922 the great newspaper baron Lord Northcliffe was treated for infective endocarditis by the world-renowned heart specialist Sir James Mackenzie of Number 133 Harley Street and Sir Thomas (later Lord) Horder of Number 141 Harley Street. They prescribed a "non-specific fresh air regime," for which Northcliffe spent his last days in a hurriedly constructed shelter on the roof of the Duke of Devonshire's house in Pall Mall, pain crazed and threatening his doctors with a revolver.

Hospital for the wealthy

A decade later Lord Northcliffe would perhaps have fared better, despite the continuing craze for the fresh-air regime. The big teaching hospitals, where so many Harley Street doctors practiced their skills part-time on nonpaying patients (the "worthy poor" of the voluntary system), had never been considered suitable for the middle class, let alone the aristocracy. However, the work of Nightingale, Joseph Lister (who was remembered for his pioneering work in antisepsis with the naming of Number 11 Wimpole Street Lister House), and others had so improved conditions that a great many middle-class people were now, for a fee, using the voluntary hospitals themselves (as well as supporting them with donations). In 1932 the London Clinic and Nursing Home was opened at Number 149 Harley Street, a large, fully equipped modern hospital designed for the rich sick, such as the unfortunate Lord Northcliffe. Windows in patients' rooms were designed to fold completely away to create a loggia effect of openness to

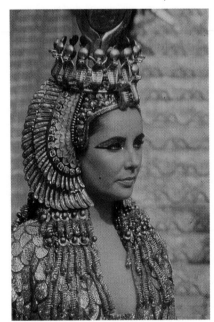

the air from Regent's Park, and an elevator took patients in their beds up to the roof garden.

The London Clinic was the brainchild of a group of Harley Street physicians and surgeons—purpose-built for private patients, a place combining the comforts of a luxurious convalescent home with the facilities for diagnosis and therapy such as normally exist only in the larger teaching hospitals. The Harley Street wing of the clinic houses consulting suites for 50 doctors in all the medical specialties. (Today 5 of the 10 doctors who attend the royal family in London have consulting rooms there.)

Although the enterprise quickly stumbled into financial difficulties caused by the emergent Depression, it weathered hard times by specializing in elective care for the upper echelons. It soon became famous for its expertise in cosmetic plastic surgery (among others, Elizabeth Arden, Helena Rubenstein, and the Duchess of Windsor visited for this purpose). The London Clinic's list of wealthy and internationally famous patients is extremely long. Among those treated there during World War II were Ernest Hemingway and Dwight D. Eisenhower, the former for alcohol dependency. As a young congressman, John F. Kennedy was rushed there during a visit to London for treatment of Addison's disease. In 1961 Elizabeth Taylor, who was suffering from complications of pneumonia and had to have a tracheotomy, had her life—and also the life of the film *Cleopatra*—saved by the clinic's resident anesthetist. Howard Hughes and his entourage took over the entire top floor of the clinic in August 1973, when Hughes had a broken leg. John Paul Getty II convalesced at the London Clinic for 18 months, from October 1984 to March 1986, while he was undergoing treatment for phlebitis. King Hussein of Jordan and Yoko Ono are just two others numbering among the Harley Street hospital's celebrity patients.

A client at the Executive Health Centres undergoes an evaluation using highly sophisticated muscle- and joint-testing equipment. The private establishment opened at 48 Harley Street in 1989 with the purpose of serving London's business community by providing consistent preventive medicine as the basis of maintaining good health. Its resources include a physiotherapy and sports rehabilitation unit as well as a complete gym and health club with personal exercise trainers.

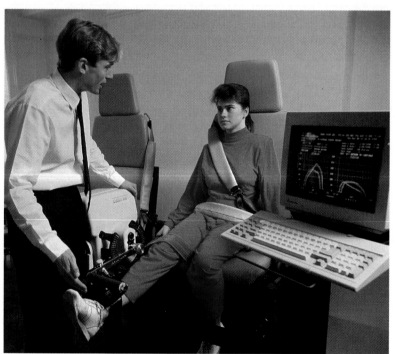

Executive Health Centres PLC

Harley Street today: healthy as ever

The availability of hospital care in Harley Street after 1932 ensured the survival of the street's credibility. Other private hospitals that provide extensive care have sprung up in the neighborhood: the Wellington Day Surgery Centre (a Humana hospital) and the Harley Street Clinic (actually in Weymouth Street), part of the AMI hospital chain. In 1989 Executive Health Centres established itself at Number 48 Harley Street as the first genuine health management organization in the U.K., providing complete specialist health care for the business community. In London it offers "company-specific" programs tailored to the needs of the employees of each company it serves. Its wide-ranging care includes medical screens; health seminars on weight management, stress management, and smoking cessation; and personal exercise training in the private state-of-the-art gym at Harley Street. Executive Health Centres also advertises internationally and offers its exclusive services to foreign visitors.

Harley Street's enduring distinction has not meant that scandals and charlatanism died with Long or Lane, however. In 1989 disquiet was aroused by a Harley Street trade in human kidneys and by an aggressive advertising campaign offering "body sculpture" and "permanent eyeliner" by a cosmetic surgeons' group in Wimpole Street.

The greatest testimony to the stability of the Harley Street medical practice and all that it came to represent was its ability to withstand the creation of the National Health Service, which was launched on July 5, 1948. By the end of World War II, plans for reconstructing a "new Britain" had become widely known. Following the landslide victory of the Labour Party in July 1945, it fell to Aneurin Bevan as the new minister of health to implement a national health service. He swung into action and at once encountered almost overwhelming opposition from doctors to the nationalization of hospitals and the prospect of salaried GPs. Bevan allayed fears by allowing consultants part-time contracts, which protected private practice, and by establishing GPs as independent contractors in the new system. Lavish "merit awards" further reconciled the hospital doctors.

Nowadays all Harley Street specialists are trained by the NHS, and most work at NHS hospitals several days a week, returning between bouts to attend their private patients. In recent years, however, the national system, which treats 30 million Britons a year, has foundered. Long waiting lists for surgery and delays in treatment have caused great dissatisfaction in the populace. On the one hand, polls have repeatedly shown that people still endorse the concept of a publicly financed health system. On the other hand, the policies of the present Conservative government have encouraged the growth of the private sector insurance and, some contend, threaten the future of the NHS. About 5.3 million people out of a population of 57 million are presently covered by private medical insurance, which enables them to obtain faster and better treatment. Private insurance cases now supply approximately 75% of the specialists' business. With increasing pressure on the state medical system, the private sector epitomized by the Harley Street specialist has never been in better health.

Jerry Mason

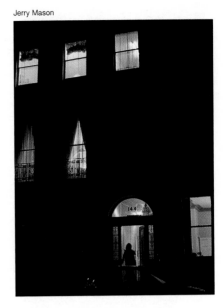

At Number 144 Harley Street, consultants work well into the evening. Most specialists today work at National Health Service hospitals several days a week in addition to seeing their private patients. Although the publicly financed NHS guarantees free medical care to all British citizens, the system has suffered considerably from underfunding, staff shortages, and long waiting lists for surgery. Business in Harley Street consequently has never been better.

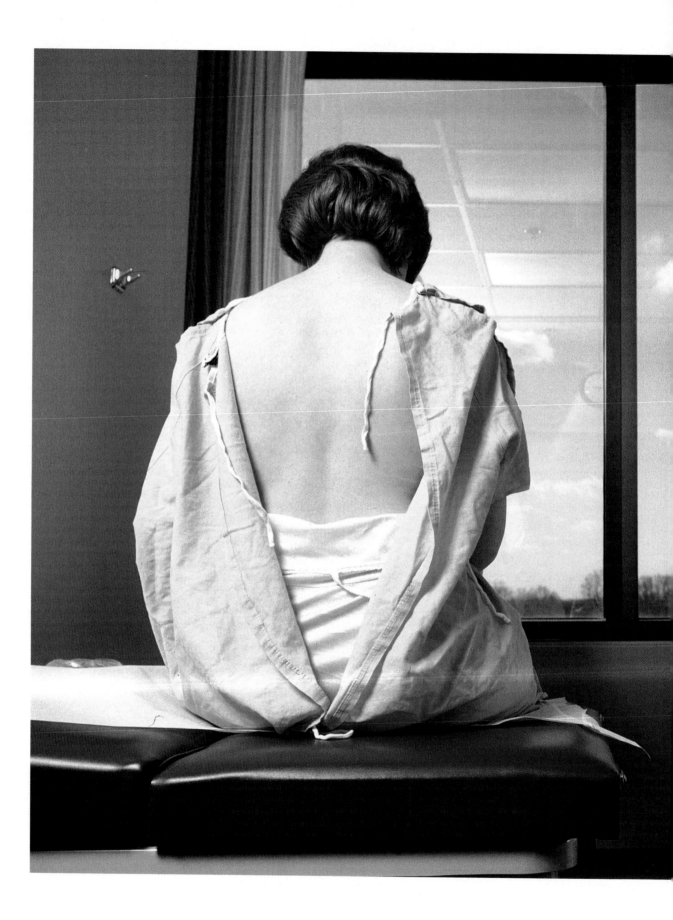

Breast Cancer in Perspective

by Donald J. Ferguson, M.D., Ph.D.

Continuing intensive research has made possible early diagnosis and effective treatment for breast cancer, while the survival rate has remained unchanged or has even slightly decreased over the last several years. This incongruity, implying needless mortality, calls for better education. If the facts about breast cancer were widely perceived, and if women were sufficiently encouraged to act on them, the death rate could probably be halved. Even the more literate public, however, is likely to get its information in scattered snippets that are at times difficult to fit into a whole picture or that appear to be contradictory. What follows aims to provide a convenient framework of common knowledge on the timely subject of breast cancer, as a basis for both appropriate personal care and more critical understanding of advances reported in the news.

Cancer is uncontrolled cell division caused by genes that were altered by inherited or acquired damage. The cellular process of becoming malignant varies; it usually occurs in stages, and a diagnosis is seldom possible until many months or years after the first cell begins unregulated division. In breast cancer, as the disease progresses, the malignant cells continue to change; some of them proliferate more rapidly and become independent of hormonal regulation, and they show a greater tendency to spread (metastasize) outside the original area.

Breast cancer is rare before age 25, but about 10% of women eventually are affected; in the United States the diagnosis is made at an average age of 52. Mortality approaches 50%, so almost everyone has or will have some distressing personal contact with it. The mention of breast cancer probably suggests mutilation and mortality to most women. Among those who treat the disease, there is active controversy because all types of therapy combine uncertain prospects of cure with predictable disadvantages and risks.

Breast development and cancer risk

The human breast begins with a cluster of 15–25 glands derived from the epidermis during embryonic development. Carcinoma, the common type of breast cancer, originates in the epithelial cells of the mammary gland. Many carcinoma cells retain the capacity to form keratin, a protein of skin, by which they can be identified in metastases.

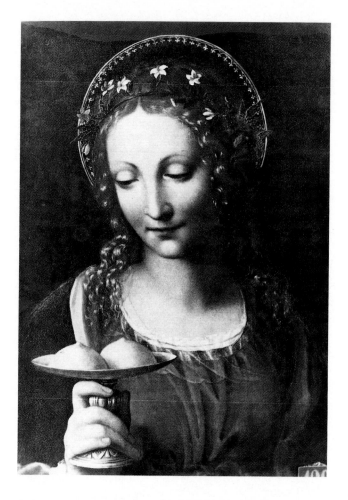

Donald J. Ferguson, M.D., Ph.D., *is Professor of Surgery Emeritus, the University of Chicago.*

(Overleaf) A woman at high risk for breast cancer has regular checkups at the Clinical Center of the National Institutes of Health, Bethesda, Maryland. Photograph, Maggie Steber—JB Pictures

In males the breast remains rudimentary except in relatively rare cases in which there is abnormal growth of breast tissue (gynecomastia). The male incidence of breast cancer is about 0.1%; it is 100 times more common in women. In the female a coordinated increase of hormones (blood-borne secretions of the pituitary, ovaries, and other endocrine organs), associated with puberty, induces permanent mammary enlargement with potential capacity for secretion of milk. This development is associated with increased risk of cancer, further augmented by early onset of menstruation (menarche) and by late menopause. On the other hand, women deprived of essential hormones before age 37, as by removal of the ovaries, have a lower risk.

Mammary glands in humans originally were indispensable for perpetuation of the species, as they continue to be for other mammals. Lactation early in life and multiple pregnancies reduce the incidence of mammary carcinoma, which is, accordingly, more common in women who have never borne children than in parous women. The latter may benefit from the reduction in the total number of menstrual cycles, with their recurrent hormonal stimulation of mammary tissues.

Breast cancer is more frequent in mothers, sisters, and daughters of patients with the disease than in other women, indicating an inheritable cause. The risk in affected families can be high enough to justify early preventive

72

mastectomy and avoidance of pregnancy to prevent passing on bad genes.

The incidence of breast cancer can be compared in those parts of the world where there are cancer registries. Some registries, however, may not accurately reflect the whole population of their area. The wide variation—from 11 women per 100,000 among non-Jews in Israel to 87.5 women per 100,000 among native Hawaiians—is not fully accounted for, but differences in hereditary susceptibility and in diet are suspected. Although Japanese women have a very low incidence of breast cancer in their own country, where the diet consists largely of grains and vegetables, the incidence is higher among Japanese women who have lived many years in the U.S. and adopted a "typical" American diet, in which meat and dairy products and foods that are high in fat content are consumed in much greater quantities. The global pattern of mortality from breast cancer varies roughly with the incidence, but the correspondence is probably affected by local variations in diagnosis and treatment.

There are several known avoidable risks. These include use of hormones for birth control before age 20, exposure of the breast to radiation in small doses at an early age (as from repeated diagnostic X-rays or radiotherapy given to nearby structures), smoking, more than occasional use of alcohol, and probably high fat content in the diet.

Self-examination—the first step in diagnosis

At about age 25 women should begin to examine their own breasts for signs of disease, and they should continue to do it monthly throughout life. Before and during the menstrual cycle, the breasts typically become tender and swollen, sometimes painful, and sometimes more lumpy; a better time to examine is a week or two later. Inspection, aided by a mirror and good lighting, can reveal protuberance, retraction or dimpling, asymmetry, changes in the skin of the nipple, and discharge from the nipple. Drops

Breast cancer incidence: population variations*	
population	rate per 100,000
U.S.: Hawaii (Hawaiian)	87.5
U.S.: Hawaii (Caucasian)	85.6
U.S.: Connecticut	77.9
U.S.: Atlanta, Georgia (white)	76.7
Canada: Ontario	64.6
U.S.: Utah	63.8
U.S.: Atlanta, Georgia (black)	61.9
Israel (American and European Jews)	61.7
U.K.: Southern Thames	58.4
Italy: Varese	57.6
U.S.: Hawaii (Chinese)	55.3
Israel (Israeli Jews)	54.0
U.S.: Hawaii (Japanese)	47.1
Finland	40.1
Poland: Cracow	35.2
Israel (African and Asian Jews)	34.3
U.S.: Hawaii (Filipino)	25.7
India: Bombay	21.2
China: Shanghai	19.6
Japan: Osaka	12.7
Senegal: Dakar	11.8
Israel (non-Jews)	11.0

*Selected international range: availability and reliability of cancer statistics vary widely by location

Adapted from G. Melvyn Howe (ed.), *Global Geocancerology* (Edinburgh: Churchill Livingstone, 1986), p. 29

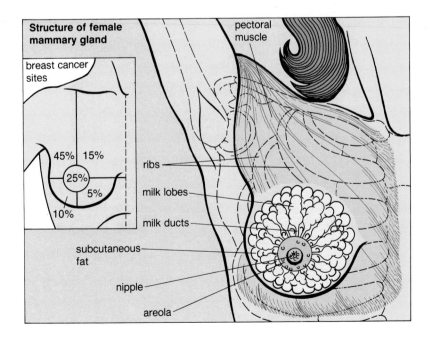

The breast is composed of a mass of glandular tissue that is supported by fibrous tissue and covered with fat and skin. About half of all breast carcinomas, the most common type of breast cancer, fall in the upper outer quadrant, the area containing the largest volume of breast tissue.

Early detection of suspicious changes in the breast, achieved by regular self-examination, annual checkups, and routine use of mammography, could significantly reduce breast cancer mortality. Every woman, beginning in her early twenties, should check her own breasts once a month for unusual lumps or masses under the skin and changes in consistency of breast tissue; initially it is best to receive instruction from an expert to ensure that she masters the proper technique. (Opposite page) Beginning about age 35 to 40, women should have mammograms every few years and on an annual basis after age 50. Breast X-rays using modern equipment and interpreted by experienced radiologists assure optimal results. Mammography today is a safe and indispensable tool for detecting cancers before they can be felt. Nonetheless, findings can be erroneous, and doubtful readings are not uncommon. A biopsy (excision of a tissue sample for microscopic examination by a pathologist) therefore is sometimes necessary. The X-ray (opposite page, top) shows a somewhat suspicious one-centimeter (about one-third of an inch) shadow deep in the breast of a 50-year-old woman who had had no palpable mass or clinical findings for cancer. A biopsy was done; the lesion that is clearly present on the mammogram showed no evidence of cancer. The middle mammogram shows a shadow that is characteristic of cancer in an elderly woman; she, too, had no palpable masses. Biopsy, however, indicated there was an eight-millimeter cancer. Eleven years after a mastectomy she was disease free. The bilateral mammograms (bottom) were read as normal even though a lump could be felt in the left breast. In this case, a six-centimeter tumor not visible in the X-ray was present.

of watery or bloody fluid that appear spontaneously on the nipple may be confirmed by gentle pressure around the full breast circumference, beginning about five centimeters (two inches) from the areola and moving toward the nipple; sites where any discharge is produced should be noted. The breasts should be palpated both in upright and supine positions and any variation in the normal mild to moderate lumpiness of breast tissue and any lumps in the armpit noted. Every woman should initially be instructed by an expert in these methods; she should also be examined annually or more often as needed by a medical professional. None of the signs noted above is specific for cancer, but each should be closely watched for and if found should promptly be called to the attention of a doctor.

Mammography: importance and limitations

It has been estimated that the present mortality of breast cancer could be reduced by as much as one-third by universal attention to early detection. Mammography (or xeromammography), an X-ray study of the breast, is indispensable for this purpose. However, mammograms do not show all cancers, and cancer may develop during the interval between procedures (a year to several years), so monthly self-examination and annual checkups by a physician are equally necessary. Mammography is advisable for every woman, beginning at age 35 to 40 and increasing in frequency to annually after age 50; the associated exposure to radiation is small and is

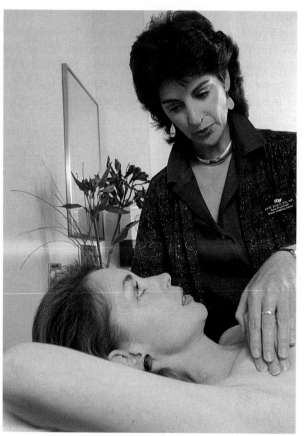

Liane Enkelis

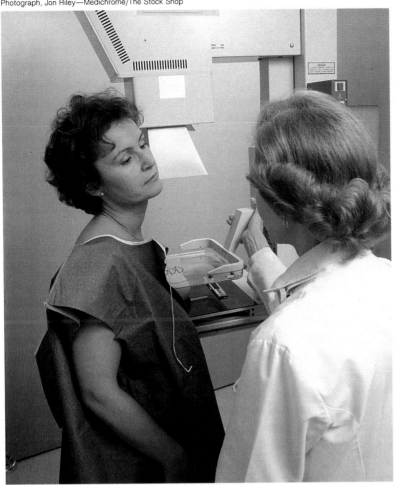

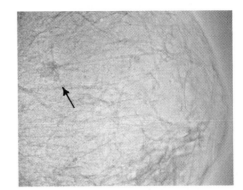

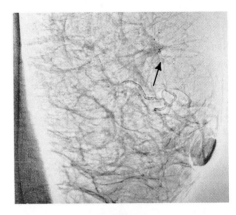

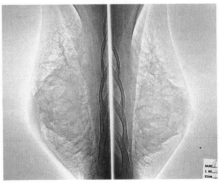

considered safe by authorities who have studied the risk. Mammography is sometimes used earlier and more frequently in patients known to be at high risk because of family history or following results of a biopsy showing changes considered premalignant.

Mammograms can reveal early signs of carcinoma before they can be detected by any other currently available method. Moreover, a cancer that is too small to be felt is highly curable. A mammogram is also needed whenever any possibly cancerous sign is detected in the breast. The mammogram can sometimes confirm or alter a clinical diagnosis, or it can reveal additional disease that is otherwise not suspected in the same breast or in the opposite one.

Optimal results from mammography require modern equipment and an experienced radiologist. It is preferable that the mammographer examine the patient before the X-ray picture is taken so that any lumps or scars can be tagged with radiopaque markers to aid interpretation. At best, some cancers are invisible by X-ray. Therefore, a palpable mass or discharge from the nipple may require biopsy even though the mammogram is negative. Findings suggesting cancer on the mammogram may also be erroneous in a proportion of patients. In fact, doubtful readings are not uncommon; if they are not resolved on prompt reexamination, a biopsy is safer than waiting to see what happens.

Biopsy and needle localization

A biopsy consists of removal of part or all of a lump and microscopic examination of the processed and sectioned tissue by a pathologist. Excision of the tissue can be safely and painlessly accomplished under local anesthesia in an outpatient procedure. By freezing a portion of the excised tissue, the pathologist can complete the examination in a matter of a few minutes, although some lesions require more elaborate techniques that need more time for evaluation. The scar left after the biopsy incision usually is scarcely detectable.

Alternatively, a diagnosis of cancer can sometimes be made by examination of cells aspirated through a fine needle or a small core cut with a larger needle, depending on the expertise of the pathologist, but negative findings by these techniques have not been proved to be completely reliable, and the lesion in such cases, whether palpable or mammographic, should be excised for more adequate scrutiny. Even if it is not cancer, it may show signs of precancerous change, and in any case it is better removed than left to provoke continuing diagnostic uncertainty.

Benign lumps

The commonest tumor (lump) in premenopausal women is a benign cyst, which is more likely to be painful than cancer is. These cysts can be recognized by ultrasound examination but are more quickly and certainly found by removal of the fluid with a needle and syringe. Another common lump in young women that is nearly always benign is the fibroadenoma, a smooth firm mass. A biopsy is often needed to confirm the diagnosis.

Pathological diagnosis

The pathologist will report whether cancer is present, whether it is invasive or noninvasive, the type of growth, the grade or apparent degree of malignancy, and whether hormonal receptors are present—information essential for planning treatment. The important question of whether lymph nodes are involved (by metastases) can be answered only after their surgical removal and the pathologist's examination, since enlargement may occur in the absence of cancer, and nonpalpable nodes may contain cancer.

Staging of invasive cancer is based on the apparent size of the mass in the breast, apparent attachment to or ulceration of skin, swelling, redness of the skin, attachment of the mass to muscle, presence of axillary nodes larger or harder than those felt in normal persons, attachment of these nodes to each other, palpable nodes in the neck, and any signs or symptoms of disseminated cancer. After biopsies and surgical specimens have been interpreted, the much more accurate pathological stage can be given. The involvement of lymph nodes is the most useful single indicator; tumor size is less important. A simple version of both types of staging is as follows: stage 1, invasive cancer confined to the breast (clinically a lump may or may not be felt within the breast); stage 2, confined to breast tissue and axillary lymph nodes; stage 3, spread to adjacent regional tissues, *e.g.,* adjacent skin or tissue between involved lymph nodes, causing them to be clumped; and stage 4, generalized spread, *e.g.,* to bones, lungs, liver, or brain.

After the workup has been completed, the patient should receive a sympathetic but objective assessment of her status, usually from the referring physician in consultation with the surgeon who did the biopsy. It is important that the woman with a breast cancer diagnosis have available to her professional guidance toward establishing her priorities and corresponding options in the choice of treatment; *e.g.,* from experts in radiotherapy and plastic surgery (the latter can inform her about the possibility of breast reconstruction following mastectomy).

Nodal involvement

The breast, like most other body tissues, is drained by a system of tiny vessels, the lymphatics, which carry tissue fluids to groups of lymph nodes, normally ranging in size from about that of a pinhead to that of a lima bean, where particulate matter such as bacteria or cancer cells is filtered out before the fluid reenters the bloodstream. The nodes contain cells (lymphocytes and macrophages) that attack bacteria and perhaps some tumor cells. The nodal groups draining the breast are mainly in the armpit (axillary) and behind the ribs near the breastbone (internal mammary).

Spread of cancer to axillary lymph nodes eventually causes their enlargement, which can be felt, but metastases to the internal mammary nodes are not palpable because they are behind the chest wall. Palpable cancers that appear to be confined to the breast tissues have spread to the axillary nodes in about half of all patients and to the internal mammary nodes in about one-fifth. These are usually the first sites of metastases, which are present in 37% of patients whose cancers are up to one centimeter (the size of an aspirin pill) in diameter. Metastases are uncommon when the disease is noninvasive or only microscopic in size. Reported incidences of nodal metastases are affected by the thoroughness of the surgical dissection and the care with which the resected tissues are examined. Nodes free of cancer, in the one or two sections of each that are routinely studied under the pathologist's microscope, will show small metastases in 20 to 30% of patients if several hundred more sections are made. However, this is not practical for regular use. Nevertheless, it is clear that regional spread of breast cancer into lymph nodes must usually be considered in planning treatment even if the nodes are reported to be negative.

Breast cancer in pregnancy

Occasionally, a cancer may be discovered during pregnancy. The attending physician should follow the same diagnostic procedures as usual, except for the use of mammography, which is better avoided. There is probably no risk to the fetus in the use of local anesthesia for biopsy. At any stage of the pregnancy, the treatment of cancer should be that used for any other patient, with no delay. The available data are compatible with the supposition that survival can be essentially the same as in nonpregnant women. Difficulty with diagnosis of small lumps in the enlarging breast, a

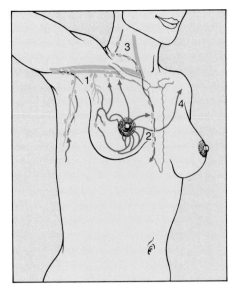

The lymph node chains are the routes by which primary breast cancers metastasize. Assessment of the nodes at the time of initial diagnosis is important for both treatment and prognosis. The diagram shows the lymphatic drainage of the breast to regional node groups: (1) the main underarm (axillary) nodes, (2) the internal mammary nodes, (3) nodes over the collarbone (supraclavicular), and (4) the lymphatic channels leading to the opposite underarm nodes. The axillary and internal mammary nodes are usually the first sites of metastases.

Today the probability of disease-free survival with adequate treatment is routinely possible for the woman with a diagnosis of breast cancer. After the complete workup, every patient should have an objective assessment of her status. She will need to discuss her options for treatment with her physician. Psychological guidance may be helpful in establishing priorities.

reluctance to biopsy, a timid approach to treatment, and a policy of delay until pregnancy has been completed have probably increased mortality in the past. During the first trimester, abortion may be considered if cancer is proved, because during that period the fetus is most susceptible to injury by general anesthesia, radiation, and drugs used for the mother's treatment.

Treatment

The treatments for breast cancer that are used today include surgery, radiation, endocrine treatment, and chemotherapy. Before attempting to evaluate these methods and their combinations, one should understand the principal modern tool that has been and continues to be used to test and assess breast cancer treatments—the controlled clinical trial.

Clinical trials (and their tribulations). By the process known as randomization, a group of patients with a similar disease is divided into two or more subgroups of nearly equal size, which are selected purely by chance. The aims (which can be assured only by this method) are to avoid bias in selecting patients for a comparison of management strategies and to equalize unrecognized variables that might affect the results. The conditions of such controlled trials are as follows. First, the investigators must believe that both of the alternatives to be studied represent management as good as is available and that they are equivalent with respect to the welfare of patients to be enrolled. This requirement means that if any difference is found it is likely to be small, and it can then be established only if hundreds of patients are enrolled in the trial and expert statistical advice is retained from the beginning. Second, logically there should be only one known variable for any comparison of two subgroups. And third, every patient must, at least in the United States, sign an instructive document indicating her informed consent to participation and her awareness of possible harmful consequences. This document stipulates that she has the option to withdraw from a trial at will.

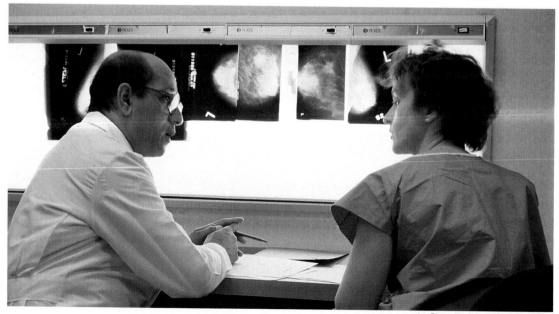

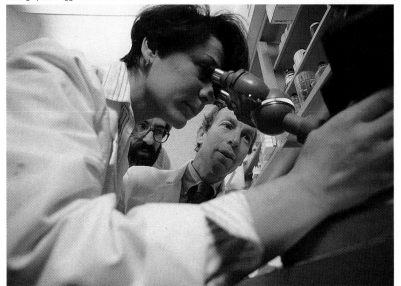

Physicians at the Warren Grant Magnuson Clinical Center in Bethesda, Maryland, examine breast cancer cells under the microscope. The Clinical Center is a unique facility where physicians from each of the National Institutes of Health work in close cooperation to apply research findings to new therapies. The breast cancer patient below has a checkup at the center, where she is a participant in a clinical trial. All patients who are accepted into research protocols at the Clinical Center must give their informed consent to participate after being fully instructed about possible risks. Trial subjects pay no fee, and they have the option of withdrawing from the study at any time.

This is a legal protection of patients' rights, which was not observed in the past and still is not practiced worldwide.

The first and third requirements have slowed or even prevented enrollment in such trials. Some investigators have not participated in a given trial because they did not agree that the alternatives were equivalent or because they did not accept either of them as the best management.

Patients, too, have had strong objections; they have objected to being "guinea pigs," and many lose faith in a practitioner who says he or she does not know which treatment is better. This latter difficulty has been alleviated to some extent by randomization of patients before (instead of, as is usual, after) they have been informed about the alternative treatments and have given their consent. The success of this strategy must be due to the fact that although the patient is still informed, the practitioner can now recommend the allotted treatment. This procedure of prior randomization has been questioned and defended on scientific and moral grounds.

Definition of cure and other distinctions. Cure of breast cancer means that patients live a normal lifetime after treatment, with no evidence of recurrent disease. Recurrences are rare after 15 years.

What is termed *locally recurrent cancer* is usually persistent cancer; *disseminated recurrence* may also be persistent but unrecognized at the time of first treatment, or the cancer may have spread later from a local recurrence. A local recurrence is most realistically defined, especially from the patient's point of view, as the presence of cancer in the locally treatable area of the original cancer—*i.e.,* in the operative scar, regional nodes, or residual breast tissue after incomplete mastectomy.

Evolution of surgical treatment. Effective treatment of breast cancer is only about 100 years old. Throughout earlier history, cure of any type of cancer was rare. Diagnosis depended on clinical observation and was based on rudimentary knowledge, which meant that it was seldom made at an early stage. Up until the late 1920s, surgeons not uncommonly did

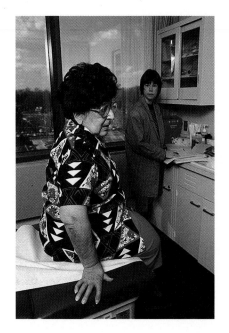

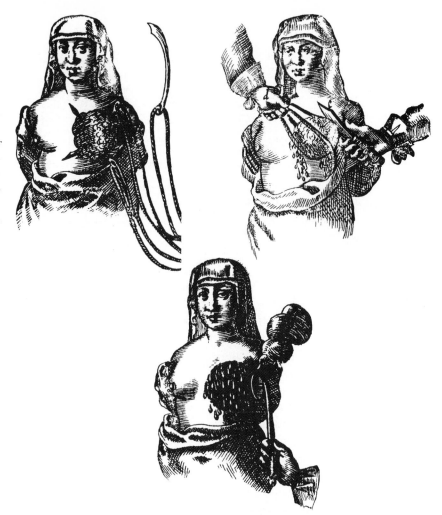

Effective treatment of breast cancer is only about 100 years old. Until the 1840s mastectomies were crude, usually done as a last resort when cancers were very advanced, and mortality rates from the operations undoubtedly were high. The 17th-century German surgeon Johann Schultes illustrated a method of amputation that first tied off the breast with cords; the breast was severed with a sharp knife; cautery was then used to stop the bleeding.

mastectomies without a preoperative tissue diagnosis, so obvious was the grossly advanced lesion; the usual patient, because of fear or ignorance, had not promptly sought help.

Until the advent of general anesthesia in the 1840s, careful surgical removal of tumors of the breast was not feasible, and partial or near total mastectomies, done only as a last resort, were quick, crude, and rarely helpful; moreover, they probably carried a high mortality rate. The only effective alternative for relief from an ulcerated mass was cauterization with a hot iron or chemicals. Asepsis and antisepsis were not effectively practiced before 1890. Blood banks, for the most part, did not exist until the 1940s, and at about that time the development of safe anesthesia for open chest operations came into general use. These were the final steps that allowed the most advanced surgical techniques to be used safely in the treatment of breast cancer.

Radical mastectomy. William S. Halsted, who was the first surgeon in chief at Johns Hopkins Hospital, Baltimore, Maryland, where he established a world-renowned school of surgery, remarked in 1894 that none of his teachers had seen a patient cured of breast cancer. He advocated a general principle of cancer surgery, based on the consensus among the most progressive surgeons at that time, that the local and regional cancer must be

80

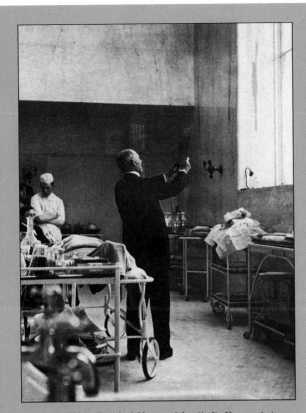

Case XXIX. (Surgical No. 1718.)—C. B. K., aged sixty-two ; widowed ; one child. Abscesses in both breasts during lactation, thirty years ago. Four months ago noticed soreness in left nipple, and a few days later a lump above the nipple. Cancer, now the size of a duck's egg, chiefly below but embracing nipple. Movable on muscle. Nipple retracted and fissured. Bleeds easily. A large mass of glands in the axilla. July 16, 1892, complete operation. Prognosis favorable as to local recurrence. Died in ten months from internal metastases. No local nor regionary recurrence.

William S. Halsted, who revolutionized surgery, emphasizing skill and technique, established his world-renowned school of surgery at Johns Hopkins just before the turn of the century. He was the innovator of many operations, including the radical mastectomy, which required complete removal of the breast along with wide excision of skin, pectoral muscles, and other tissues without cutting through any tissue that might contain cancer cells. In 1894 Halsted reported on 50 radical mastectomies that he had performed in five years; case number 29 was one of these. Because the majority of his patients had advanced disease, most died from metastases to internal organs. His operation did, however, prevent high rates of local and regional recurrence, something that had never been achieved previously, and a few of his patients were cured.

Photograph, The Bettmann Archive; case, from William S. Halsted, "Operations for Cure of Cancer of the Breast," *Annals of Surgery*, vol. XX (July–December 1894), p. 522

completely removed with wide margins—en bloc—that is, without cutting through any tissues that might contain cancer cells, either growing or in transit. His mastectomy was called radical because of wide excision of skin and other tissues, including the pectoral muscles, carried out in pursuit of this important principle. At least partial removal of muscle was considered necessary because some cancers rest on or near it, lymphatic vessels traverse it from the cancer to the lymph nodes, and there are nodes between the two pectoral muscles. Removal of muscle also facilitates the dissection of axillary nodes, which is otherwise less likely to be complete or en bloc.

Halsted himself obtained a few long survivals, but his patients were at a late stage of disease—all with cancer spread to the axillary nodes—and most of them died of recurrence. His operation remained the standard treatment until the 1970s, eventually achieving, as diagnoses were made earlier and operations were facilitated by advances in anesthesia and availability of blood banks, a survival rate at 10 years of about 75% for patients with

Table 1: **Radical versus extended radical mastectomy** (in patients with medially and centrally located cancers at clinical stages 1 and 2)		
A. 286 patients, 52% node+		
	% local recurrence (10 years)	% survival (10 years)
extended radical mastectomy (in-complete: not Urban type)	9	56
radical mastectomy	9	62
probability that observed difference occurred by chance		not significant
Compiled from Umberto Veronesi *et al.*, *Cancer* 47:170 (1981)		
B. 70 patients, 50% node+		
extended radical mastectomy (Urban type)	0	86
radical mastectomy	0	60
probability that observed difference occurred by chance		<0.03
Compiled from Paul Meier *et al.*, *Cancer* 63:188 (1989)		

negative lymph nodes, about 50% for those with positive nodes at stage 2, and about 25% for those at stage 3.

Radical mastectomy has achieved nearly as high a survival rate as any treatment subsequently devised. At about 15 years after radical mastectomy, the survival of patients free of recurrence is the same as that of women at the same ages who have not had breast cancer. Both groups, however, may have a continuing incidence of new cancers.

Extended radical mastectomy. Metastases in internal mammary nodes have been successfully treated by surgical removal from patients whose cancers are in the central or medial parts of the breast—a group that comprises 60% of total patients. Radiotherapy (*see* below) added to radical mastectomy does not increase survival, which indicates that it probably does not eliminate metastases in internal mammary nodes. The extended radical operation, described most adequately in 1952 by New York surgeon Jerome Urban, is a mastectomy that is performed so as to remove the internal mammary nodes en bloc with the rest of the removed tissues. This is a difficult operation and has been performed as Urban described it by only a few surgeons. The more commonly used incomplete versions of the extended operation appear to have provided no advantage over radical mastectomy. Comparative results of both complete and incomplete types versus radical mastectomy are shown in Table 1.

Radical surgery need not be disabling. The principal objection to it by patients is loss of the breast. By modern surgical techniques the lost tissues, including muscle, can be replaced starting at the time of the original operation, resulting in appearance and function that most patients so treated, whose priority was the maximum probability of survival, have found very acceptable.

Modified operations. As indicated above, radical mastectomy should include most of the axillary nodes as well as removal of the underlying muscles, and extended radical mastectomy includes the same plus the internal

Although radical mastectomy has acquired a reputation for being mutilating, the operation as performed today can achieve the maximum probability for survival, resulting in both function and appearance that many patients find quite acceptable.

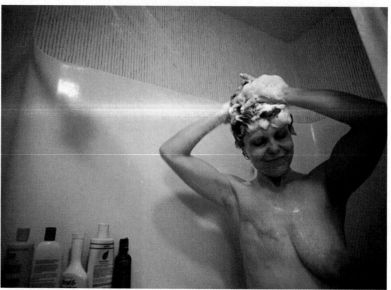

Lynn Johnson—Black Star

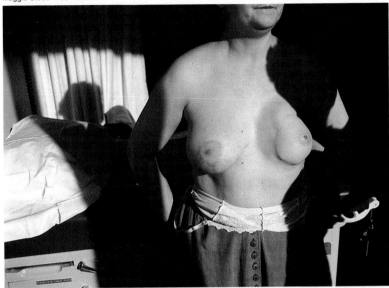

An option that thousands of women who have mastectomies are choosing today is to have breast reconstruction. For some women this is done at the same time as the cancer surgery. The decision about the advisability and timing of reconstruction should be made by the woman in consultation with her cancer surgeon, a plastic surgeon, and other physicians involved in her treatment. The methods commonly used involve silicone implants or transfer of tissue (known as a musculocutaneous flap) that is taken from the underlying muscle of the woman's back or abdomen. A few months later a new nipple can be formed from skin of the chest overlying the implant or from the skin of the flap. A new areola is simulated by an additional graft of skin or in some cases by tattoo. These techniques produce an excellent resemblance of a breast, which for many women helps restore feelings of confidence and well-being after the trauma of breast cancer.

mammary nodes. Removal of the part of the breast containing a cancer or other tumor is termed *partial mastectomy* or, sometimes, *lumpectomy. Total (or simple) mastectomy* refers to removal of all mammary tissue and some skin including the nipple and areola but no other tissue. The term *modified radical mastectomy* refers to a variety of procedures including removal of the breast and at least some of the axillary nodes.

Surgery for noninvasive cancers. There have been no randomized clinical trials with long-term follow-up of patients treated for noninvasive breast cancers. There are two main varieties of treatment, with different implications for management. Because multicentricity (several sites of disease within the breast) is common with these cancers, the safest treatment is total mastectomy, which is nearly 100% curative. Noninvasive cancers are relatively benign, however, and many patients have survived 10 years or more after only a biopsy or partial mastectomy. As many as one-third of those so treated eventually develop invasive cancer, which is assumed to have arisen from a site of noninvasive disease and affords the same survival probability as other invasive lesions. Most of the multiple foci of noninvasive cancer are unlikely to progress, but there is no way to predict which will do so.

Comparing surgical outcomes. As of 1990 there had been a total of nine randomized clinical trials carried to 10 years comparing radical or extended radical mastectomy with smaller operations (partial or total mastectomies), with or without radiation. Some end results of four of them are given in Tables 1–3, comprising two of the four studies that found no significant difference in survival (part A of Table 1 and Table 3) and two of the five that found statistically significant increases of survival following the larger operation (part B of Table 1 and Table 2).

These data have supported a variety of interpretations. In comparing survival data with the extent of mastectomy, completeness of the resections should not be taken for granted. In multi-institutional trials it is probably impossible to assure that first-rate surgery or radiotherapy have been given to patients accepted for study from many different sources. Hence the conclusions of such studies apply to the named treatment as commonly given but not necessarily to its full curative potential.

Radiotherapy. Shortly after the German physicist Wilhelm Röntgen of Würzburg reported his discovery of X-rays in 1895, X-radiation began to be used in the treatment of breast cancer. In some cases inoperable lesions were effectively reduced. A widespread policy of supplementing radical mastectomies with postoperative radiation was gradually adopted, although no evidence existed then or has been found since that it increased survival.

In 1948 Robert McWhirter, a radiotherapist in Edinburgh, while accepting the view that breast cancer is curable by adequate local treatment, proposed that radiation could be a more effective therapy than surgery for involved lymph nodes, especially for the internal mammary chain, which few surgeons at that time had ever attempted to remove. He presented data on total mastectomy supplemented with radiation to the regional nodes. Survival appeared comparable to that previously obtained with radical mastectomy. Although these data were not altogether persuasive because they did not compare carefully matched groups of patients, they initiated a revolution in treatment that has proved very acceptable to women, who naturally favor operations that are less radical if they seem equally curative.

Increasing use of radiotherapy as a substitute for surgery and as justification for not observing the surgical principle discussed above—*i.e.,* performing a thorough operation to remove the cancer and adequate numbers of lymph nodes in order to increase the chance of survival and prevent recurrence—has led to the present popularity of partial mastectomy, with partial removal of axillary nodes often included in order to improve the accuracy of the staging. The purpose, of course, is to preserve most of the breast and adjacent tissue and, it is hoped, to achieve high rates of survival.

It has become apparent that radiation of cancers larger than three or four centimeters (between 1 and 1.5 inches) in diameter and radiation of

---

Table 2: **Partial mastectomy versus radical mastectomy, both with postoperative radiation**
(randomized 10-year comparison from Guy's Hospital, London)

A. 376 patients age 50+ (excluding medial cancers)

	% local recurrence		% survival	
	stage 1	stage 2	stage 1	stage 2
partial mastectomy	30	56	57	35
radical mastectomy	13	21	51	50
probability that observed difference occurred by chance	< 0.003	< 0.001	—	< 0.05

B. 252 patients, all ages (including medial cancers) at clinical stage 1

	% local recurrence	% survival
partial mastectomy	29	58
radical mastectomy	6	68
probability that observed difference occurred by chance	< 0.001	< 0.002

Compiled from J.L. Hayward in *Conservative Management of Breast Cancer,* edited by J.R. Harris *et al.* (Philadelphia: Lippincott, 1983), p. 77

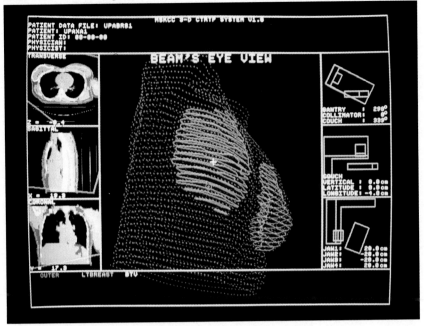

the axilla are likely to be followed, sometimes many years later, by severe tissue damage. Therefore, when radiation is to play a major role in breast cancer treatment, the surgeon is asked to remove such tumors and many of the axillary nodes, especially any that are palpable.

As in the case of the varied extent of surgical procedures, the most objective evaluation of radiation is based on randomized clinical trials comparing treatments and following up the patients treated for prolonged periods of time. A 10-year comparison of results of radical mastectomy and total mastectomy with or without radiation is given in Table 3.

Hormonal treatment. Estrogen and progesterone, secreted mainly by the ovaries, have powerful effects on the breast and on breast cancer. It was first observed by George T. Beatson of Edinburgh in 1896, before the concept of hormones was established, that patients with advanced breast cancer sometimes demonstrated remarkable improvement after removal of the ovaries, a treatment still sometimes useful. The concept of hormonal control of some types of cancer was more fully explored by Charles B. Huggins at the University of Chicago, who received a Nobel Prize for Physiology or Medicine for his work in 1966.

It has been shown that suppression of hormonal secretion can be used for the treatment of disseminated cancer. A response of cancer to hormonal treatment is much more likely if the cells contain hormonal receptors. These structures allow the cell to bind and then use specific hormones, including estrogen and progesterone. Hormonal receptors, accordingly, are routinely measured in biopsied breast cancer. Modern endocrine treatment and prophylaxis depend mainly on the drug tamoxifen, which appears to act, at least in part, by blocking hormone receptors in the cancer cells, thereby preventing a stimulus to cell division. Tamoxifen is given as two pills a day and has only a few, usually mild, side effects.

Radiation began to be used in the treatment of breast cancer shortly after the discovery of X-rays in 1895. Today radiation therapy is considerably more refined than it was originally and is most often used as an adjuvant treatment with a modified form of surgery; e.g., a lumpectomy, which essentially removes just the tumor, leaving most of the breast intact. The sophisticated procedure known as BEAMS Eye View uses dozens of computed tomography scans to pinpoint the exact location of the tumor and serves as a treatment guide for the radiation therapist. At the left of the screen are various anatomic views. The center screen is a view as seen from the source of radiation. The right three views indicate the positioning of the radiation equipment. This kind of precision targeting of the tumor helps to minimize radiation damage to noncancerous tissues.

85

Table 3: Surgery and radiation: three treatment approaches (1,665 women up to age 70)	% local recurrence (10 years)		% survival (10 years)	
	stage 1	stage 2	stage 1	stage 2
radical mastectomy	6	8	58	38
total mastectomy and radiation	4	14	59	39
total mastectomy	9		54	
probability that observed difference occurred by chance	—	—	0.5	0.7

Compiled from Bernard Fisher et al., "Ten-Year Results of a Randomized Clinical Trial Comparing Radical Mastectomy and Total Mastectomy with or Without Radiation," New England Journal of Medicine, vol. 312, no. 11 (March 14, 1985), pp. 674–681.

Two relatively simple but representative and instructive randomizations concerning the effects of tamoxifen as an adjuvant to surgery are summarized in Tables 4 and 5. It should be noted that six controllable variables that might affect results—stages, ages, presence or absence of estrogen receptors, extent of surgery, duration of treatment, and use of a placebo (inert substance made to look like the drug)—vary within one or the other of the studies or between the studies. Planned but uncontrolled variables within studies interfere with a scientific evaluation of the results and also may reduce their significance by hindering plausible comparisons between projects. Further, the follow-up times were less than the 10-year minimum desirable for assessment of breast cancer treatments. These shortcomings, of uncertain significance, some of which are difficult to avoid, are not unusual; they are cited to indicate the critical attention that must be applied before the conclusions of such reports can be fully accepted.

Nonetheless, the two sets of data on tamoxifen suggest that for the short term this drug reduces recurrent cancer when given after total or partial mastectomy, whether estrogen receptors are present or not. In both pre- and postmenopausal women, it may or may not affect survival at about four years. Other endocrine agents that can suppress breast cancer in some patients include the ovarian hormone progesterone, the antiprogesterone RU-486 (a contraceptive), and the male hormone testosterone. Some remissions have been achieved with these agents and have endured for several years.

Chemotherapy. A number of chemicals have been discovered that are particularly lethal to dividing cells and so affect cancer more than they do most normal tissues. Different parts of the cell-division cycle are affected by different drugs, so rational combinations can be used. Unfortunately, these drugs also poison the rapidly dividing normal cells in the bone marrow, the lining of the gastrointestinal tract, and the hair follicles. Their use therefore requires careful attention to dosage and to these and other side effects, some of which can be lethal. Long-term toxicity has rarely included drug-induced cancers.

Multiple drugs given as adjuvants to primary treatment in patients with stage 1 and 2 breast cancer have shown up to 7% increases in five-year survival. Disease-free survival has been improved in several groups of premenopausal patients who had one to three positive axillary nodes. Many other randomizations of adjuvant chemotherapy have been done, although very few are followed to 10 years. Numerous variations in the trials make concise summarization unfeasible, but none so far has established a more distinct success.

Recently it has been proposed that adjuvant chemotherapy be given to all patients at stage 1 whose cancers lack hormone receptors even though the 10-year survival of such patients should be 70% or more without the drug. A reduction in four-year recurrence rates by use of the drugs in a randomized comparison of such patients was cited as the reason for the recommendation. Survival, however, was not altered. Objections have been raised that the benefit to a few might be countered by injury to the 70% who did not need the drugs. The issue remains a controversial one and is unlikely to be settled until more data and longer follow-up are available or until an accurate method of recognizing persistent cancer is discovered so that only those patients who need such treatment would receive it.

Ongoing research

Because breast cancer is not yet always a curable disease, medical science continues to seek better explanations, better diagnostic potential, and better treatments. Research is active on many fronts.

Diagnostic refinements. The problem of selecting the minority of patients with apparently early breast cancer who need adjuvant chemotherapy may be eased by analysis of particular genes, proteins, or nucleic acids found more abundantly in cancers that are most likely to have spread. For the same purpose a sensitive technique is under development for early detection of cancer in the bone marrow, a common site of metastasis. It is based on the fact, already mentioned, that breast cancer cells commonly form keratin, a protein that is not normally present in the marrow. A test

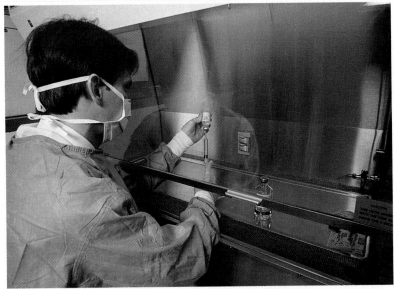

C.C. Duncan—Medical Images, Inc.

Table 4: Postoperative tamoxifen for five years versus placebo (2,644 patients up to age 70, with mammary cancer containing estrogen receptors and negative axillary nodes, following total or partial mastectomy)

	% with no recurrence (at 4 years)	% surviving (at 4 years)
tamoxifen	83	93
placebo	77	92
probability that observed difference occurred by chance	<0.001	0.3

Compiled from Bernard Fisher et al., "A Randomized Clinical Trial Evaluating Tamoxifen in the Treatment of Patients with Node-Negative Breast Cancer Who Have Estrogen-Receptor–Negative Tumors," New England Journal of Medicine, vol. 320, no. 8 (Feb. 23, 1989), pp. 479–484

Table 5: Tamoxifen for two years versus no postoperative treatment (1,129 patients up to age 75, with mammary carcinoma at stages 1 or 2, with or without estrogen receptors, after total mastectomy with node dissection or sampling)

	% with no recurrence (at 45 months)	% surviving (at 45 months)
tamoxifen	73	80
no tamoxifen	61	72
probability that observed difference occurred by chance	<0.001	<0.002

Compiled from M. Baum et al., "Controlled Trial of Tamoxifen as Single Adjuvant Agent in Management of Early Breast Cancer," The Lancet, vol. I, no. 8433 (April 13, 1985), pp. 836–839

Adjuvant chemotherapy involves giving multiple drugs in conjunction with local therapy—either surgery or radiation. In patients who have stages 1 or 2 carcinoma, five-year survival has been increased up to 7%. The drugs used are cytotoxic agents that destroy cancerous cells shed into the bloodstream and the lymph system by the original tumor. Combinations, schedules, and dosages vary. Because all anticancer drugs have potentially serious side effects, they must be administered by professionals experienced in their use.

New York City artist Nancy Fried had a mastectomy for breast cancer in 1986 at age 40. After her operation she produced a series of terra-cotta sculptures that helped her come to terms with the loss of her breast.

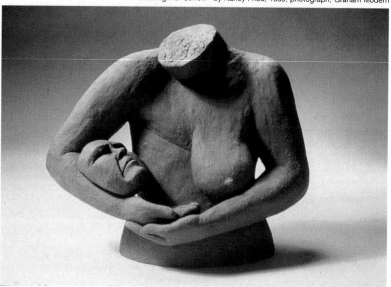

for keratin can be used to recognize tumor cells in marrow that has been removed from the patient by needle aspiration. It is probable that many such cells are not capable of growing as metastases, but tests for this or other markers can give evidence of spread outside the breast and suggest the need for systemic treatment.

Several recent reports have associated the enzyme cathepsin D, secreted by breast cancer cells, with poor prognosis. A test measuring cathepsin D may prove useful in identifying women at high risk of metastatic disease.

Understanding metastasis. Most cancers that remain localized are relatively easy to cure. It is the spread of the disease that makes cancer fatal. Studies of the metastatic process have identified potentially treatable elements. First is the secretion by the cancer cell of enzymes that enable it to bore through tissue and capillary walls, into or out of the bloodstream. Second is the component of the cancer cell surface that sticks to the wall of a capillary blood vessel at the potential site of metastasis, after which the cell penetrates the wall and enters the tissue. And third is release of a blood-vessel-producing (angiogenesis) factor that is needed for growth at the new site. The steadily growing comprehension of the process of metastasis could lead to methods of prevention based on the probability that, lacking any one of these three capacities, the cancer cell would be rendered relatively harmless.

Seeking the basic mechanism of cancer. Knowledge of the molecular basis of cancer is a long-range research goal. Its achievement seems likely to provide a rational basis for prevention or medicinal cure. Clues concerning the process of cancerous growth have arisen from a rapidly increasing knowledge of molecular genetics. An example is the elucidation of function for many normal genes, known as proto-oncogenes (capable of becoming cancer-causing genes), which, through the proteins they encode, regulate cellular division and differentiation. When these genes are activated or altered to become oncogenes, their products contribute to the induction of cancer. Activation may be due to an external agent such as radiation, hormones, or chemicals or to translocation within the chromosome, perhaps a result of misalignment during cell division. Genes are made of thousands of pairs of nucleic acids arranged in specific sequences that code for the structure of proteins. Every human being (except for identical twins) has a unique set estimated to contain from 50,000 to 100,000 genes, arranged for the most part unvaryingly in the 46 chromosomes of each cell.

The function of most of the genes is yet to be determined. Usually several of them are involved in a series of steps before a cell becomes cancerous. Although particular oncogenes have been shown to be unusually active in some breast cancers, they also become active in normal cells dividing in culture. Their role is not yet clear, nor is that of the suppressor genes, which have been shown to control other gene activity. Loss or inactivation of a suppressor can thus result in activation of an oncogene.

A new process that can speed genetic research is the polymerase chain reaction. By converting messenger nucleic acid molecules (mRNA) associated with oncogenes into complementary DNA sequences, which can be greatly amplified by this reaction, it can be determined in a very small sample of cells which genes are active or inactive. Progression of this work has potential application to diagnosis and treatment of any type of cancer.

Causes of altered gene function that have been associated with human breast cancer include hereditary defects, hormones, radiation, and cancer-causing chemicals in the environment. Certain foods, tobacco, and alcohol have all been implicated as altering gene function and thereby increasing the risk of breast cancer.

Gene therapy. Replacement, correction, and augmentation of particular genes have been accomplished in mammalian cells, then introduced into mouse embryos. With greater understanding of genetics and the cancer process, it is not unreasonable to anticipate that such gene therapy may eventually be applied in curing human cancer.

Today's outlook: justifiably optimistic

After any type of treatment for breast cancer, a lifetime of follow-up is important, though it need be not different in kind from the routine screening recommended for all women. Early discovery of local recurrence requires more frequent than annual checking during the first five years. Frequent repetitions of X-rays and scans looking for systemic spread in asymptomatic women, on the other hand, cause unnecessary anxiety and expense and are without demonstrable effect on survival.

The earliest practicable diagnosis of breast cancer can be achieved by monthly self-examination, annual checkups by a doctor, and routine use of mammography. Needless mortality can in this way be significantly reduced.

Current treatment involves surgery of variably appropriate extent, supplemented in suitable cases by adjuvant radiotherapy, hormonal treatment, or chemotherapy. The probability of 10-year survival exceeds 75% after adequate treatment of breast cancer discovered as early as is now routinely possible. Rapid and wide-ranging progress of biological research suggests that prevention and medical cure of breast cancer are rational prospects.

Because breast cancer strikes one in 10 women and is not always curable, medical science continues to seek better treatments and ways to prevent the disease. Even today, however, there is much needless mortality. If women knew the facts and were encouraged to act on them, the death rate from breast cancer probably could be cut in half.

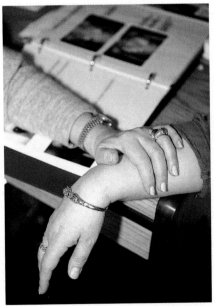

Maggie Steber—JB Pictures

Children with Cancer:
Odds in Their Favor

by Anna T. Meadows, M.D., and
Beverly J. Lange, M.D.

At some time in life, one in six people develops cancer. Most often that time is old age; in rare cases it is childhood. One in 600 children develops cancer by age 15, a figure that has not changed substantially in 40 years. What has changed is the outlook for children with cancer: 40 years ago most children with cancer died—usually within weeks or months; today over 60% of these children survive more than five years, and many are cured. Still, in 1990 in the developed nations of the world, only accidents cause more childhood deaths than cancer.

Cancers of children differ from those of adults. Carcinomas of the lung, colon and digestive tract, breast, prostate, uterus, and ovaries make up 80% of the cancers in adults. Leukemias, brain tumors, Hodgkin's and non-Hodgkin's lymphomas (tumors of lymph nodes), sarcomas (tumors of muscle and bone), Wilms' tumor of the kidney, and neuroblastoma (a tumor of adrenal glands or other glandular nerves) make up 80% of the tumors in children. Most childhood tumors arise in embryonal cells; that is, precursor cells present in the developing embryo. In the last months of pregnancy or the first months of life, embryonal cells are normally programmed to mature to form the blood, brain, bone, muscle, kidney, liver cells, and adrenal and other glands. What causes an embryonal cell to become a malignant cancer cell, which then multiplies and divides, is not known. Without knowledge of the cause of these cancers, prevention is impossible. However, it is possible to treat them.

Childhood cancer is generally not treated at community hospitals; it is treated by specialists in a small number of pediatric units and cancer centers. Treatment entails long hospitalizations. It requires donated blood and potent medication. It involves uprooting families over weeks or months, which often means loss of time from work for parents. Socioeconomic support is essential to reduce the emotional burden on the child and family.

The cure of childhood cancer is one of the medical miracles of this century. Physics, chemistry, biology, and statistics have all contributed to the miracle. Millions of dollars and volumes of blood donated by concerned citizens have helped bring it about. Perhaps, above all, it is the triumph of the children and their families who have agreed to participate in daring human experimentation.

90

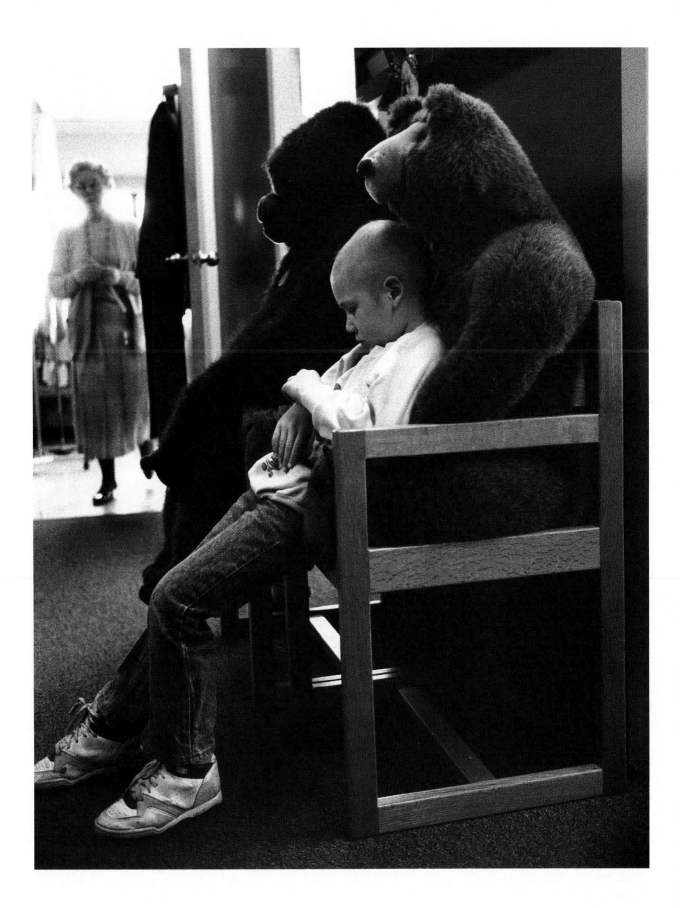

Anna T. Meadows, M.D., is *Professor of Pediatrics, University of Pennsylvania School of Medicine, and Director of the Division of Oncology, Children's Hospital of Philadelphia.*
Beverly J. Lange, M.D., is *Professor of Pediatrics, University of Pennsylvania School of Medicine, and Associate Director of the Division of Oncology, Children's Hospital of Philadelphia.*

(Overleaf) Six-year-old John Mackenzie, who has been in treatment for leukemia for five years, awaits his chemotherapy in the pediatric oncology department of Boston's Massachusetts General Hospital. Photograph, Eddie Adams—Sygma

Evolution of a cure

Acute lymphoblastic leukemia is the most common childhood cancer. It is called acute because without treatment it is fatal in a matter of weeks. It is called lymphoblastic because it is a cancer of immature bone marrow cells called lymphoblasts. Normal lymphoblasts (sometimes referred to simply as "blasts") mature to form the immune defense system. In leukemia abnormal lymphoblasts overgrow the normal cells of the marrow—*i.e.,* the other white blood cells that fight infection, red blood cells that carry oxygen to the rest of the body, and platelets that clot the blood. Without any treatment, children with leukemia succumb to anemia, bleeding, or infection. By the 1940s red blood transfusion could treat anemia, and sulfa and penicillin antibiotics could treat infection and postpone death by weeks or months, but neither transfusions nor antibiotics actually cured anyone.

Step one: discovery of chemotherapy. After the discovery of sulfa antibiotics to kill bacteria, chemists developed similar drugs, called chemotherapy, to kill cancer cells. The first of these was aminopterin. In 1948 Sidney Farber, who was pathologist in chief at the Children's Medical Center in Boston, gave aminopterin to 16 children with leukemia. The drug temporarily eradicated the leukemia of 10 of these children—that is to say, it caused a remission. Unfortunately, in all of the children, the leukemia reappeared, and none was cured.

The experiment with aminopterin identified two problems: (1) resistance: the leukemia, which had apparently been eliminated, came back, presumably because aminopterin failed to kill all the cells and those that remained were

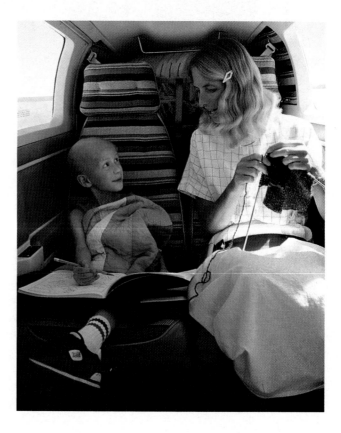

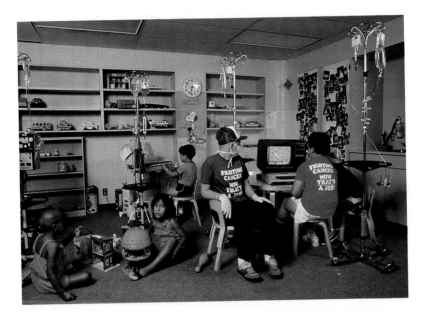

Childhood cancer is treated by oncology specialists at select pediatric cancer centers. Aggressive treatments frequently require families to be uprooted for weeks or months. The young patient and his mother (opposite page) are being flown home to Oakland, California, after his hospitalization for treatment in Los Angeles by Air Life Line, an association of private pilots who offer their services on "errands of mercy." The cure of childhood cancer is one of the greatest achievements of modern medicine, but the battle itself can be arduous, painful, and long. It is the children who undergo the tough treatment regimens who know this best; the brave cancer fighters at left are patients at Texas Children's Hospital in Houston.

Photographs, (left) J.P. Laffont—Sygma;
(opposite page) Karen R. Preuss—The Image Works

resistant to it; and (2) toxicity: aminopterin led to many severe, potentially life-threatening side effects. Not only did aminopterin kill leukemic cells, it also killed normal cells—especially those of the marrow and those lining the mouth or intestines—and it damaged the liver. Despite the progress that has been made, these two problems, toxic side effects and emergence of resistant cells, remain impediments to total cure.

Step two: combination chemotherapy. The partial success of aminopterin in the treatment of childhood leukemia inspired the search for other chemicals to treat cancer. Between 1950 and 1990 thousands of compounds were tested. Only about 50 turned out to be appropriate in cancer treatment. Many of the drugs used to treat lymphoblastic leukemia today were available by 1960: methotrexate (a less toxic form of aminopterin), vincristine (made from periwinkle plants), 6-mercaptopurine, prednisone (a form of cortisone, or steroid hormone), and l-asparaginase (a substance in guinea pig serum). Through a series of comparisons of combinations of different drugs using different schedules, it became apparent that some drugs such as vincristine, prednisone, and l-asparaginase were most useful in the first weeks of treatment to eliminate the majority of the leukemia cells, whereas others such as methotrexate and 6-mercaptopurine were more useful afterward to eliminate the few remaining cells. The comparisons, called clinical trials, often take years, and new trials are now under way.

Step three: prevention of leukemic meningitis. In 1960, even with combinations and sequences of drugs, few children were cured. Sooner or later the leukemia recurred; about half the time it recurred in the brain or in the lining around the brain and spinal cord as leukemic meningitis. Leukemic meningitis could be treated with radiation to the brain and spinal cord, methotrexate injected into the spinal canal, or both; however, control was usually temporary, and the leukemia would soon reappear in the marrow. Then there was a breakthrough; investigators decided to prevent the leukemic meningitis by giving radiation treatments to the brain

Acute lymphoblastic leukemia is the most common form of pediatric cancer. Fifty years ago virtually no children survived. Today nearly 80% are cured. The bone marrow (magnified 1,000 times) from a seven-year-old boy with this form of cancer is shown below: a monotonous population of leukemic lymphoblasts is evident. The photomicrograph of the same patient's marrow (at bottom) was taken after 28 days of treatment with cancer-fighting drugs; here normal red blood cells and normal white cell precursors have returned. Although there are no longer any visible leukemia cells, experience has shown that if treatment were stopped at this stage, the leukemia would reappear within weeks or months.

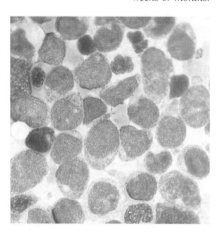

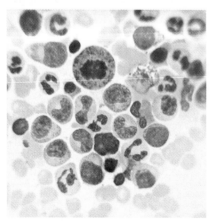

or methotrexate by spinal tap *before* the disease showed itself as meningitis. By the end of the 1960s, Joseph Simone and Donald Pinkel at St. Jude Children's Research Hospital in Memphis, Tennessee, had devised and tested a treatment plan called "total therapy." Total therapy involved (1) three or more drugs in the first month to reduce the leukemia to an undetectable level, (2) addition of at least two other drugs for years to treat the undetectable leukemia, and (3) prevention of leukemic meningitis with radiation, chemotherapy, or both. The total therapy of the late 1960s cured about one-third of children with this disease. The basic strategy of total therapy underlies treatment in 1990.

Step four: recognizing more than one disease. Once cure was possible for some children, the obvious question was, "Why not for all?" In the 1970s and 1980s, research in cellular and molecular biology provided the answer: not all children have the same disease. In most children the lymphoblastic leukemia is a disease of an immature precursor of the B-lymphocyte, the antibody-making cell of the immune system; in about 20% of children it is a disease of the T-lymphocyte—the memory cell of the immune system. The T-cell leukemias often divide and multiply more rapidly than the early B-cell leukemias and require different treatment. Infants under one year of age have yet another form of lymphoblastic leukemia, in which the leukemic blasts are less mature than those of older children. Infant leukemia requires a treatment different from that used in other forms of lymphoblastic leukemia. Again, stepwise comparisons of standard treatment to treatment with new drugs and higher doses of traditional drugs have made it possible to cure over 75% of children with acute lymphoblastic leukemia.

Step five: preventing death from treatment side effects. The addition of more drugs and higher doses of drugs increases the risk of death from side effects. One way to reduce side effects of treatment is to reduce treatment in children who may need less. For two decades the Children's Cancer Study Group (CCSG) conducted a series of randomized trials to determine what treatments could be safely eliminated. CCSG is the world's largest organization conducting research on the cancers of infants, children, and adolescents and developing new treatments and cures for these diseases. Over 20,000 children have been treated in CCSG studies, and more than 2,000 physicians and research scientists at 100 member institutions are a part of the group. Together, CCSG, the Pediatric Oncology Group in the U.S., and several collaborative pediatric groups in Europe have made possible research on large numbers of children with rare diseases.

In a randomized trial, patients agree—or in the case of children, their parents give consent for them—to accept either a standard treatment or an experimental one, not knowing which they will receive. In 1970 total therapy with five years of chemotherapy and radiation to the brain was the standard treatment for acute lymphoblastic leukemia. Comparison of three years with five years of treatment showed that three years was as good as five, and a comparison of two with three years showed that for girls two years was as good as three. Similarly, it was shown that in many children injections of methotrexate into the spinal cord could prevent leukemic meningitis as effectively as radiation, with fewer serious side effects.

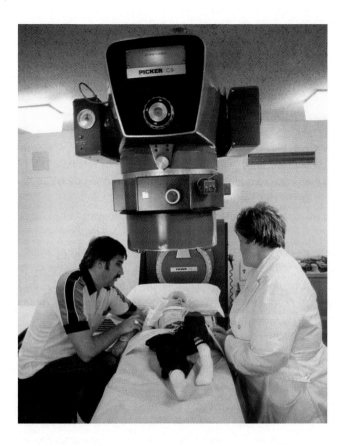

A child is prepared for radiation treatment. Therapy for lymphoblastic leukemia often includes radiation of the brain and spinal cord region to prevent leukemic meningitis; these treatments are given after a series of drugs has effectively rid the marrow of abnormal lymphoblasts.

Photograph, Tom Tracy—MediChrome

Infection is the most common cause of death in children with leukemia. Infections that are a particular problem for children with lymphoblastic leukemia are a form of pneumonia, *Pneumocystis carinii* pneumonitis, and chickenpox. Walter Hughes and co-workers at St. Jude Children's Research Hospital proved that giving an antibiotic called trimethoprim-sulfamethoxazole to children receiving chemotherapy could prevent pneumocystis pneumonitis. Chickenpox can be prevented with a special hyperimmune gamma globulin, and today it can be treated with antiviral drugs. Also, Japanese investigators have developed a vaccine to prevent chickenpox, which has been used investigationally in the U.S. in children with leukemia. However, because it is a live vaccine and has the potential to give a modified form of chickenpox, the children need to discontinue chemotherapy one week before and after the vaccine is given, and a booster immunization is necessary. Moreover, because antiviral drugs are so effective, use of the vaccine is likely to remain quite limited.

The next step. Curing 75% of children with lymphoblastic leukemia is not enough. The main impediment to a 100% cure rate remains the inability of available treatments to eradicate all the leukemic cells, which means leukemia, although inapparent for years, may recur. When it comes back, it can be treated and retreated sometimes for months, sometimes for years, but if it recurs in the bone marrow, usually it is fatal. Ways to deal with recurrent lymphoblastic leukemia such as bone marrow transplant have been borrowed from approaches that have worked in other forms of leukemia.

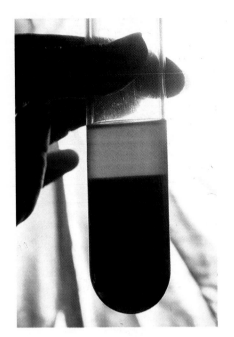

Bone marrow transplants are curative for about 50% of children with the myeloid form of leukemia. The idea behind bone marrow transplantation is to destroy both the blast and the normal cells in the patient's marrow, then to transfuse carefully matched donor marrow (usually from a sibling or parent) into the child with leukemia. The photograph above shows centrifuged blood in which lighter blood cells and marrow are separated. The diagrams below are from a book that helps children with leukemia understand what their treatment will involve.

Treatment of less common leukemias

About 20% of children with leukemia do not have acute lymphoblastic leukemia. Most of these have either acute nonlymphoblastic leukemia or acute myeloid leukemia; a small number have chronic myeloid leukemia. Drugs that kill the leukemic lymphoblasts fail to kill myeloid leukemic cells. Other drugs may make the leukemia go away temporarily, but in the majority of children myeloid leukemia returns in months or years. In the 1970s physicians at the Fred Hutchinson Cancer Research Center in Seattle, Washington, used bone marrow transplantation to eliminate the disease in children with recurrent leukemia. This novel approach cures some children whose leukemia has recurred.

Bone marrow transplantation involves huge doses of chemotherapy and radiation to eliminate from the blood all the leukemic cells as well as normal bone marrow and immune cells. Then normal marrow removed from a brother or sister with the identical white blood cell type is transfused into the child with leukemia. Bone marrow transplantation is used early in treatment of children with myeloid leukemia to bring about a cure rate of about 50%. However, only one in four children has a suitable donor for marrow transplantation. Other ways to carry out transplantation are being investigated, particularly that of removing the child's own marrow at a time when the leukemia is inapparent and purging the marrow of residual leukemic cells with drugs or antibodies.

It is clear that other forms of chemotherapy need to be tried and that other treatment approaches to the various forms of childhood leukemia need to be developed. A whole new class of drugs called growth factors is being tested. Growth factors are hormones made by normal blood and tissue cells. Recombinant DNA technology has made it possible to produce massive quantities of these growth factors. In some cases growth factors can increase the killing effects of chemotherapy, and in others they can reduce the side effects of chemotherapy, hastening the return of the patient's own normal white blood cells and increasing the ability of these cells to fight infection.

Wilms' tumor: model for treating solid tumors

The cure of acute lymphoblastic leukemia is one model of the stepwise approach to childhood cancer; Wilms' tumor offers a second model. This

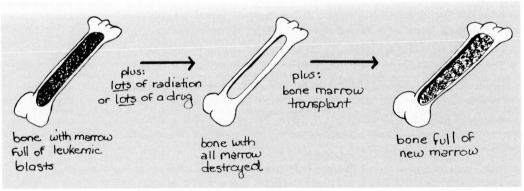

bone with marrow full of leukemic blasts

plus: lots of radiation or lots of a drug

bone with all marrow destroyed

plus: bone marrow transplant

bone full of new marrow

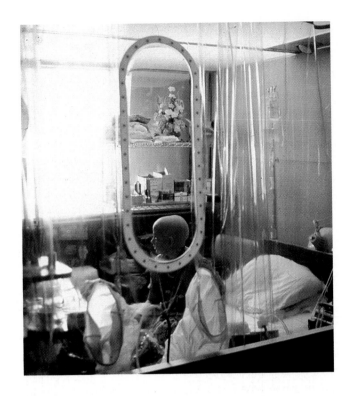

tumor occurs as a solid mass or a solid tumor in the kidneys in children who are usually between the ages of two and four years. Removal of the involved kidney by surgery cures about 30–40% of children with Wilms' tumor. Radiation to the abdomen may cure another 10%. However, without further treatment half the children who have no visible tumor in their lungs will develop disease there months after the kidney tumor is removed. This implies that tumor cells were always in the lung but were too few in number to be detected by a chest X-ray. Furthermore, in some children chest X-rays show that the tumor has already spread (metastasized) to the lungs; in others the tumor may involve both kidneys. In these situations surgery does not suffice.

In the 1950s Farber discovered that a new chemotherapeutic drug called actinomycin-D could treat children with Wilms' tumor. The same logic that led to prevention of leukemic meningitis in children with leukemia (*i.e.,* prevention of predictable disease rather than treatment of obvious disease) was applied to prevent the growth of Wilms' tumor in the lungs. Farber showed that when actinomycin-D and abdominal irradiation were given to children right after surgery, before the tumor could be seen on chest X-rays, the cure rate rose from 40% to over 80%. The National Wilms' Tumor Study group, headed by Philadelphia pediatrician and radiation therapist Giulio D'Angio, used the clinical trial approach throughout the United States and was able to show that a two-drug combination, actinomycin-D and vincristine, could cure over 90% of children with stage I and II Wilms' tumor and that radiation was unnecessary when the tumor had been completely removed. In a later study by the same method, the length of treatment was reduced from 15 months to 6 months for most children. Cutting back treat-

97

Wilms' tumor occurs as a solid mass in one or both kidneys of children who are usually between the ages of two and four years. After many years of evolution of progressively better treatments, it was found that surgery to remove the entire tumor followed by the two-drug combination of actinomycin-D and vincristine given over a six-month period could cure the majority of patients. This highly effective approach spares children from the side effects and ordeal of radiotherapy and a longer regime of chemotherapy.

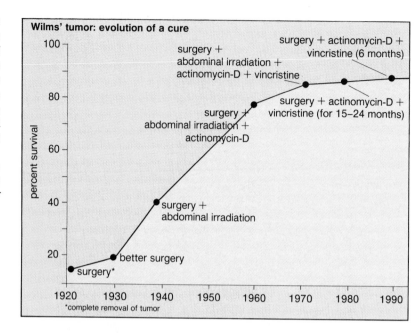

Wilms' tumor: evolution of a cure

Osteogenic sarcoma, the most common bone tumor in children, most often occurring during the adolescent growth spurt, is also one of the most difficult to treat. The X-ray shows an osteogenic tumor in a patient's right knee, which has caused the leg to swell and has destroyed the normal structures of the tibia (shin bone). The tumor causes pain, and the fragile leg is vulnerable to fractures.

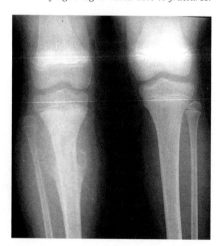

ment for some children took great courage in the face of excellent survival in a formerly fatal disease. Furthermore, combinations of chemotherapy and radiation have made it possible for children with Wilms' tumor in both kidneys to survive with ample normal kidney function.

The strategy used for Wilms' tumor was applied to treatment of other solid tumors such as those of the liver, the testes, and the ovaries and sarcomas of muscle and bone. Success in these diseases is good, but not quite as good as in Wilms' tumor.

Osteogenic sarcoma. The most common tumor of bone is called osteogenic sarcoma. Osteogenic sarcoma (or osteosarcoma) has proved more difficult to treat than other childhood solid tumors. Most osteogenic sarcomas occur around the knee, and most occur in adolescence during the growth spurt. In the past the standard treatment was the amputation of the affected leg or arm. However, even with amputation 80% of the patients had metastatic tumors in their lungs within one year and 80% had died by two years. Through the 1950s and 1960s and in the early 1970s, the drugs used in other childhood tumors failed to have any effect on these tumors. In the 1970s Gerald Rosen at Memorial Sloan-Kettering Cancer Center in New York City and Norman Jaffe at Children's Hospital in Boston showed that extraordinarily high doses of methotrexate could make some of the tumors in the lungs shrink and that high-dose methotrexate, given early in this disease, before tumors were apparent on chest X-ray, could cure 50% of the patients. Other drugs such as cis-platinum and adriamycin were also found to be effective treatment for this disease.

Today chemotherapy has made it possible to avoid amputation in some patients; if chemotherapy is given before amputation and shrinks the tumor so that it can be removed with the bone, an artificial (prosthetic) bone can be inserted and the surrounding muscles can be spared. This kind of prosthesis generally cannot be used in young children but is appropriate for some teenagers, thus avoiding amputation of the leg. Sometimes it is possible to preserve the hands of children who have osteosarcoma of the arm, regardless of age.

Neuroblastoma. Neuroblastoma, like Wilms' tumor, occurs in infancy and early childhood, but unlike Wilms' tumor, which usually occurs in only one kidney, most neuroblastomas have already spread to the bones and bone marrow when they are first diagnosed. These tumors are resistant to combinations of 3 and 6 and as many as 10 drugs, and few such children are cured even with aggressive treatment followed by bone marrow transplantation.

Sometimes neuroblastoma occurs as an isolated solid tumor; in this case it can be cured by surgery. Some babies with neuroblastoma may have a tumor in the adrenal gland and multiple tumors in liver, bone marrow, and skin, but their disease does not behave at all like cancer. This disease, designated stage IVS (S for *special*), was first defined by the former U.S. surgeon general C. Everett Koop and Audrey Evans at the Children's Hospital of Philadelphia. The children appear healthy despite the widespread cancer, and in most the tumor goes away over weeks or months without treatment. The reasons for this disappearance remain one of the most challenging mysteries of pediatric cancer.

In about 70% of the children with neuroblastoma, the tumor makes hormone substances that can be detected in the urine. Japanese and some American investigators are screening millions of samples of urine from babies to determine whether early detection of a tumor prevents widespread disease later in childhood. It is not yet clear that these screening programs will be either practical or successful.

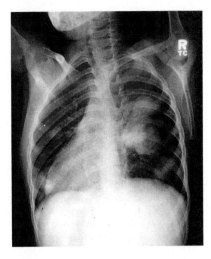

Tumors that metastasize to the lungs are frequent in children with osteogenic sarcoma. This chest X-ray shows tumors in both lungs of a 13-year-old whose leg was amputated 10 months earlier. The metastases had not been present when the bone cancer was first diagnosed. Because the tumors are too close to the heart and major blood vessels, they cannot be removed surgically. Today all children with sarcomas are given chemotherapy at the time the tumor is discovered in the bone so as to prevent the subsequent development of such malignant growths in the lungs.

Brain tumors

Brain tumors are the most common solid tumors in children. Some brain tumors are benign; that is, they do not invade the surrounding normal brain and do not spread outside the brain. Many of these can be cured by surgery, if surgery is possible. However, over half of pediatric brain tumors invade and spread. Progress in curing the majority of malignant brain tumors has been relatively slow. The first impediment to cure in childhood brain tumors was the difficulty in diagnosing them. Before 1975 there were no X-ray studies capable of showing any but the largest brain tumors. The development of computed tomography (CT) scanning and more recently magnetic resonance imaging (MRI) have made it possible to see the brain through the skull and identify tumors, infections, or blood clots.

The second problem in curing brain tumors has been, and still is, that many of them cannot be removed by surgery. Often they are located in areas that control breathing or heartbeat or swallowing—areas essential for life—or they may be located in areas necessary for normal coordination. Newer instruments and techniques now allow neurosurgeons to carry out delicate surgery in these areas; complete surgical removal is now possible more often. Among these surgical innovations is the cavitron, an ultrasonic nebulizer that aerosolizes the tumor and sucks out the aerosolized particles; it eliminates the need for dissecting out some areas of the tumor

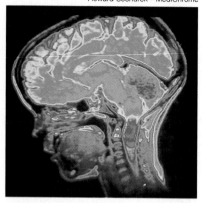

Highly refined imaging techniques have made it possible to identify children's brain tumors before they have grown to a size that makes them inoperable. Magnetic resonance imaging produced the picture above, in which a tumor in the child's brain stem is evident (the large red area). Using newly available instruments and innovative surgical methods, neurosurgeons are now able to perform extremely delicate operations to remove brain tumors in many young patients.

with the usual surgical equipment. The dissecting microscope, which has two lenses that give a 5- or 10-fold magnification to the area where the neurosurgeon is operating, allows more precise and delicate dissection of nerves and arteries in areas of the brain. A technique known as stereotactic surgery involves attaching a grid to the head of the patient; a computer simultaneously correlates the grid on the patient's head with a grid on a CT scan, which shows where the tumor is located in the brain. Then the neurosurgeon uses the computerized image and the two grids to guide a needle to biopsy a mass in an area that is considered unreachable by standard neurosurgical techniques.

The third problem has been the difficulty of treating incompletely removed tumors. The doses of radiation necessary to eradicate these tumors can cause serious and even fatal injury to the normal brain cells. Only in the past decade has it been shown that chemotherapy for some brain tumors increases the cure rate. Giving chemotherapy before radiation in very young children, thereby postponing radiation until children are older, may also permit larger, more curative, and less toxic doses of radiation to be given.

Defining "cure"

In the 1970s it was clear that many children treated with combinations of surgery, radiation therapy, and chemotherapy were living for 5 and even 10 years from the time their cancer was discovered. Nevertheless, no one dared to use the word *cure*. Today the accumulated observations of 20 years allow pediatric oncologists to say with confidence that when a child has received no treatment for two years and is free of disease for five years, that child is "cured." Recurrence of leukemia more than four years after discontinuation of therapy happens occasionally, and sometimes brain

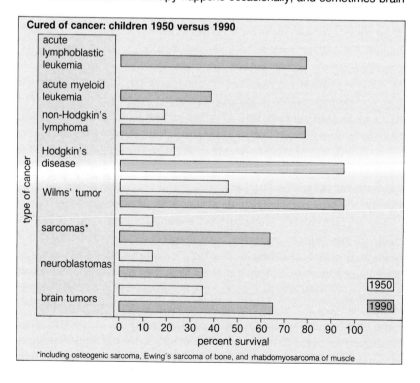

Cured of cancer: children 1950 versus 1990

*including osteogenic sarcoma, Ewing's sarcoma of bone, and rhabdomyosarcoma of muscle

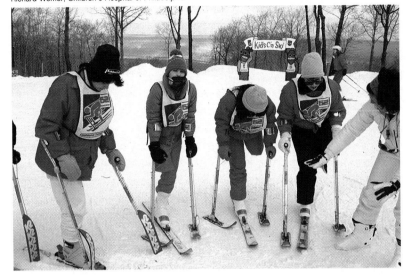

Many surgical treatments that effectively cure childhood cancers leave obvious physical defects that survivors must learn to live with. It is important that these young people have appropriate psychological support and that they discover ways to overcome their disfigurements. A group of former bone cancer patients from Children's Hospital of Philadelphia take an annual ski trip with one of their physicians. These youngsters clearly have not let their limb amputations limit their participation in demanding physical activities.

tumors, Hodgkin's disease, or neuroblastoma reappear years after treatment. However, except for these rare cases, cure has become a realistic expectation for the majority of long-term survivors of childhood cancer.

A crude estimate of the actual number of cured patients is based on the following calculations: if one in every 600 children develops cancer by age 15, and if approximately 60% of them have been cured since 1970, by the year 2,000, one in every 1,000 young adults will be a survivor of childhood cancer. This is a formidable population of potentially productive citizens—provided the disease or its treatment has not left them with debilitating or lethal late effects.

Treatment-related complications: new insights

Although the benefits of treatment have been obvious for years, only recently have the complications become apparent. All three types of cancer treatment—surgery, radiation therapy, and chemotherapy—injure other, noncancerous cells in ways that are permanent. Most often these injuries are minor, sometimes they are serious, and occasionally they are fatal. Children cured of cancer are expected to survive many more years than cured adults. Many treatment-related complications are especially damaging to children; children are often more susceptible than adults to the undesirable effects of surgery, radiation, and chemotherapy.

Problems after surgery. Solid tumors require a biopsy for making the diagnosis and surgery for removing tumor masses. Because it is necessary for the edges of the mass to be absolutely free of tumor, some normal tissue is removed along with the tumor. Some surgical procedures cause only subtle defects, apparent only to an astute observer; others, such as amputation of a limb or removal of an eye, produce obvious defects. Sometimes the results are disfiguring or may be cosmetically unacceptable. In these cases every effort is made to provide appropriate psychological support to the children and their families and to work closely with plastic surgeons, who often are able to perform reconstructive "miracles."

101

Many children with cancer have abdominal surgery either to diagnose the tumor or to remove it. These children run the risk of intestinal obstruction and need to be aware that they must consult a physician whenever sudden, severe, or prolonged abdominal pain develops—even years following surgery.

The removal of the spleen in a young child places the child at risk of overwhelming infection from certain bacteria. Today immunization with pneumococcal and *Haemophilus influenzae* vaccines and daily penicillin offer these children some protection, but they still need special medical attention when they develop fevers. A child who has had a kidney removed for Wilms' tumor may never have any problems unless he or she injures the remaining kidney.

Radiation effects. Radiation therapy is aimed at tumor masses or potential tumor masses, as in the case of prevention of leukemic meningitis. Only those tissues or organs in the field of radiation therapy are susceptible to damage; the bulk of this tissue usually is the tumor, but surrounding normal tissues also are affected.

Chemotherapy damage. Chemotherapy taken by mouth or injected in a vein goes everywhere, and thus every cell in the body is at risk of damage caused by chemotherapy. Cells that are especially susceptible to the effects of chemotherapy are those that are dividing each day, such as the cells that make hair and the cells of the bone marrow and the intestine. Fortunately, the ability of these cells to repair damage and to renew themselves is so great that the damage caused by chemotherapy is usually temporary. Occasionally, however, it is fatal.

Chemotherapy uses special drugs that destroy cancer cells, but healthy cells may be harmed as well. The drugs are usually given intravenously over several months. Hair loss, fatigue, nausea, vomiting, and painful mouth sores are all common side effects. Fortunately, most of these problems are temporary; nonetheless, children need to be taught that these difficult regimens are worthwhile because the drugs are likely to make them well. The youngster below has the support of his mother and a younger sibling while he receives his chemotherapy at the Cancer Treatment Center in Bethesda, Maryland. At Children's Hospital of Philadelphia, dolls help instruct patients about chemotherapy; the children can play doctor, administering the injections to the toy patients.

Photographs, (left) Randy Taylor—Sygma; (right) Donna Ferrato—Black Star

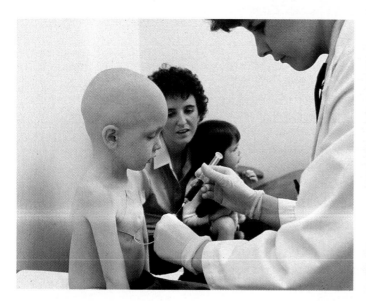

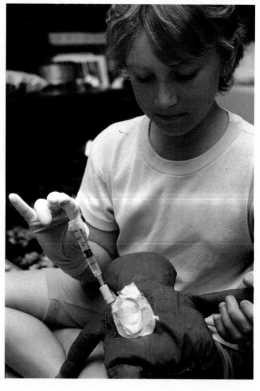

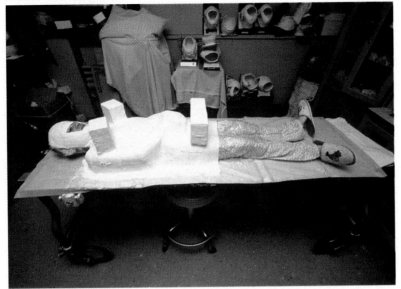

Radiotherapy attempts to target cancerous tissue only, but if a patient moves even a single millimeter during treatment, vital surrounding tissues and essential organs may be damaged. Impenetrable casts that expose only certain areas and that prevent the patient from moving have been specially designed to minimize the chance of healthy tissues being irradiated.

Many chemotherapeutic agents used to treat children's cancers have few, if any, long-term sequelae. Drugs such as methotrexate, 6-mercaptopurine, vincristine, cytosine arabinoside, l-asparaginase, 6-thioguanine, actino-mycin-D, and the corticosteroids have been in regular use for 25 years or more and do not appear to have delayed toxicities, except in rare cases and, perhaps, in conjunction with other predisposing factors. It may be too early to detect damage resulting from newer drugs because frequently effects do not become manifest until decades after these drugs are given.

Essential organs affected. When radiation treatment of tumors encompasses surrounding normal tissue such as the heart, lungs, or kidneys, the radiotherapist tries to limit the radiation dose to one that will not damage these organs. Sometimes it is necessary to use doses less than necessary for eradicating the tumor cells in order to spare normal organs. However, there are situations in which damage occurs in spite of precautions. For example, even modern treatment to both lungs or both kidneys can cause serious long-term disabilities. Certain prophylactic measures such as re-fraining from smoking, avoiding exposures to fumes or dust if the lungs have been irradiated, and monitoring blood pressure and urine for early signs of problems if the kidneys have been irradiated can delay or prevent these problems.

A class of chemotherapeutic agents called anthracyclines (especially adri-amycin and daunomycin) can cause the heart to fail as late as 14 years after treatment. Awareness of this risk facilitates early diagnosis of the problem, and proper care may keep it dormant for long periods. Today physicians test children's hearts before, during, and after cancer treatment to detect abnormalities and prevent irreversible damage.

A relatively newer drug called ifosphamide, used extensively to treat sarcomas, can damage the kidney such that essential salts, sugars, and proteins leak out of the body into the urine. The long-term effects on children who suffer from this complication are being studied now.

103

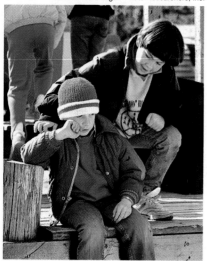

Chemotherapy is never easy. A little comfort afterward can make all the difference.

Growth impairment. Children do not grow during periods of very intensive cancer therapy—usually during the first year after diagnosis. After that, however, they usually recover a normal growth rate, even when they continue treatment. Nevertheless, there are some childhood cancer patients who fail to "catch up" completely, and their height as adults is somewhat less than expected.

As radiation retards the growth of malignant cells, so can it retard growth of bone and muscle in the surrounding normal tissues. The smaller the fraction of potential growth attained at the time of irradiation, the greater the growth impairment. Young children are, therefore, most vulnerable; their expected loss will depend on the dose of radiation, the size of the area treated, and whether critical growth centers such as the hips or knees received radiation.

Hormones also are important in determining whether the child's full growth potential will be achieved, especially thyroid hormone and growth hormone. When the neck receives high doses of radiation therapy, children can develop thyroid deficiency. This condition can be managed easily, if detected, by the taking of daily thyroid hormone in pill form. Growth hormone is produced by the pituitary gland, and radiation to the brain in doses that children with many types of brain tumors receive can abolish the production of growth hormone. Now recombinant DNA technology has made it possible to replace growth hormone. Theoretically, recombinant growth hormone could encourage growth of the original cancer or the development of a new one; however, there is no evidence that growth hormone favors tumor growth.

Effects on sexual development and fertility. Normal sexual development does not occur in some children with cancer. In girls the normal function of ovaries to make eggs and produce sex hormones may be affected by cancer treatment. Girls whose ovaries have been removed or have been irradiated fail to produce the hormones necessary for puberty, and thus they never ovulate or menstruate. Today synthetic hormone replacements can induce puberty in these girls, and if the uterus is normal, pregnancies may be possible with *in vitro* fertilization of donated eggs and careful hormonal management. Women who have had abdominal irradiation who become pregnant have been reported to have small babies and high rates of fetal loss. These women need expert prenatal care.

In boys the ability of the testes to make male sex hormones and sperm may be reduced. Irradiation of the testes causes relatively less hormonal damage than irradiation of the ovaries, but the sperm are more easily killed than eggs by irradiation. Sterility often is a consequence of relatively little testicular irradiation, while testosterone production continues in boys treated with higher doses. Storage of frozen sperm specimens in "sperm banks" prior to treatment may enable postpubertal boys to preserve fertility.

The class of drugs known as alkylating agents can damage both male and female sex hormones and lead to infertility. Younger children appear to tolerate larger doses of these drugs better than older children, especially when the latter have already entered puberty. Total dosage and age effects have not been established well enough for useful estimates of risk to be

104

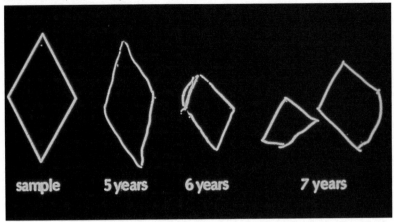

sample 5 years 6 years 7 years

As part of a study to determine whether radiation to the brain to prevent leukemic meningitis had any deleterious effects, a five-year-old boy was asked to copy the diamond on the left. His first diamond was drawn about a month after he developed leukemia—before radiation. One and two years later he was asked to draw the same diamond. It is apparent that he had lost considerable facility. This awareness of treatment-related learning problems has led physicians to seek therapies that cause the least amount of damage without compromising the cure.

made, and surprise pregnancies have resulted after an erroneous prediction of male or female infertility.

Studies of the offspring of former child cancer patients have not shown them to have an excess of birth defects or cancer compared with a non-cancer population. Because of the young ages of most survivors treated with modern chemotherapy, it may be too early to be certain that problems in offspring will not arise as they grow up. Continued monitoring of former patients and their offspring is therefore necessary.

Learning deficits. Once treatment is complete and its immediate side effects have resolved, most long-term survivors function normally. Until large numbers of survivors with leukemia or with brain tumors were able to return to the normal activities of daily living, especially to school, where demands were made to perform, problems with learning were not appreciated by parents or physicians. Then, in the late 1970s and early 1980s, these authors and colleagues at the Children's Hospital of Philadelphia found the first evidence of reduction in IQ in children treated with brain irradiation to prevent leukemic meningitis. Children less than six years old at the time of such brain irradiation appear most affected. Although these children can learn and function in adult life, it has become clear that they benefit from individual tutoring or special classes to achieve their maximum potential.

The clinical trial process has now permitted investigators to determine, first, that lower doses of radiation can still prevent leukemic meningitis while resulting in fewer learning problems and, later, that many children can be successfully treated without any radiation at all. Most children with brain tumors and some with leukemia continue to require brain irradiation; studies are under way to determine whether individualized teaching methods can help these childhood cancer patients overcome their learning problems.

Psychological problems. The initial adjustments of a child with cancer often depend more on the psychological health and coping skills that the child and the family bring to the situation than on the severity of the disease. At most treatment centers professionals and volunteers work with the children and their families to guide them in dealing with stress and grief, to help them organize their resources and reorganize their lives, and to assist the children and the school system with the children's school reentry. For most

School is an essential part of life for most children with cancer, and they overextend themselves to attend. If they are in classes during the rigors of therapy, they may have a hard time coping with temporary physical impairments such as hair loss, unsightly scars, or weight gain, and they may have problems concentrating or keeping up with their work. It is important that they receive psychological support, and some children may need special tutoring so they do not fall behind.

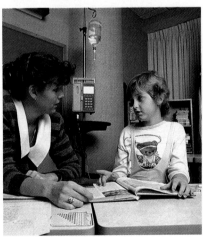

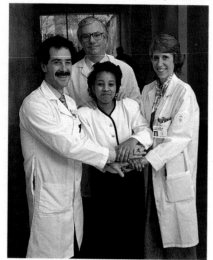

At age 10 Stacey Males was diagnosed with leukemia. Despite aggressive chemotherapy and radiation treatments, she suffered two relapses. She then had a bone marrow transplant at New York's Memorial Sloan-Kettering Cancer Center, which cured her. In November 1989, at age 19, she had a reunion with the transplant team that saved her life.

Michael Italiano had bone cancer in his leg. Rather than amputate, his doctors replaced much of the bone with titanium. Because this is a new treatment, potential long-term effects are not known. Nevertheless, Michael feels triumphant. He has embarked on a career as a securities trader, and he recently married another victorious cancer survivor, Maura Donohue. Maura, a 26-year-old graduate student in art history, was cured of childhood non-Hodgkin's lymphoma.

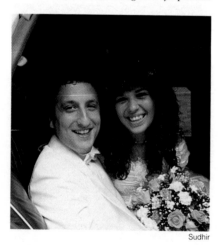

children with cancer, school is an essential part of life, and they overextend themselves to attend.

The children also must cope with physical debilities during treatment, such as weight gain with the drug prednisone, hair loss with chemotherapy, and eating problems and severe nausea with chemotherapy. Most children deal remarkably well with the changes in appearance, which they know are usually temporary. Hair loss can be dealt with by wigs, but an increasing number of children seem to be willing to go bald or wear scarves or hats. The hair loss is almost always temporary. Chronic nausea is a vexing problem; attempts are made to alleviate it with antinausea drugs, but they do not always work. Weight loss can be handled by various kinds of hyperalimentation—that is, feeding children, usually at night, either by means of a tube passed down through the nose to their stomachs or with intravenous administration of nutrients.

Some children feel guilty about the time and expense of their treatment and its impact on their families. Some protect their parents and help them deal with the pain of diagnosis and treatment, even with the process of their own death. The impact of these illnesses can cause siblings to feel guilty for being well or resentful of the sick child for requiring so much attention; in the U.S. there are numerous sibling support groups that enable them to talk about the problems.

Because developing childhood cancer is always devastating, it is not unexpected to observe a host of emotional problems. Nonetheless, surprisingly few graduates of cancer treatment have been found to carry a disabling psychological burden throughout their lives. In fact, many seem to have acquired an appreciation of life and an emotional maturity that are quite special.

Second cancers. Perhaps the most unacceptable side effect of cancer treatment is that it can cause other cancers. Thus, a child cured of one cancer many years later may develop a second, unrelated malignant tumor. When the second cancer is in some way associated with treatment for the first, there are understandably mixed emotions. On the one hand, without the proper treatment the years of extra life—ideally, well lived—would not have been possible. On the other hand, one must question: was it worth it?

Early reports of second cancers were limited to children with retinoblastoma, a tumor occurring often in both eyes and requiring radiation for cure and for sight. Some children with retinoblastoma carry a gene that also predisposes them to bone and muscle sarcomas around the eye and in the leg—where bone sarcomas often occur in children without the gene. The risk of bone cancer in these children is estimated to be approximately 10%. Medical attention is essential for these youngsters at the earliest sign of abnormality. There may be susceptible children with other cancers, and one of the great challenges is to determine who they are when they receive their initial treatment so that they can be more closely monitored and appropriately educated.

High doses of radiation can cause new cancers of bone and soft tissue in the area irradiated; the higher the dose, the greater the risk. The addition of certain chemotherapies, notably adriamycin and cyclophosphamide, often-

106

used drugs in pediatric oncology, increases the risk. Radiation and some drugs in the alkylating agent class cause leukemia. When leukemia occurs, it usually is after a substantial dose of chemotherapy. The risk of leukemia can be lessened by a reduction in the amount of alkylating agent and replacement with another equally effective drug, if such an alternative exists.

Much still to be learned

Concern for the health and well-being of childhood cancer survivors has led to a major effort to study and follow up on the consequences of successful therapy. As the average child with cancer is only five years old, present knowledge of the effects of disease and treatment is limited to mostly school-aged children, adolescents, and young adults; it is too soon to be able to predict the full range and depth of problems likely to be encountered as they age. For example, reliable data about marriage and divorce patterns of cured cancer patients are limited owing to lack of appropriate control subjects, and the data about the divorce rate of their parents are conflicting. The two major problems that long-term survivors do face are employment discrimination and difficulty in obtaining insurance. Support groups often can provide former cancer patients with guidelines about insurability and employability.

Those children with poor cancer prognosis currently are being exposed to an even greater range of medications at ever higher doses with currently unknown but perhaps more serious consequences. Fear of these unknown effects cannot deter attempts to improve upon present results but should provide a strong impetus for continued observation and assessment of potential toxicity to provide the best balance between cure and complications.

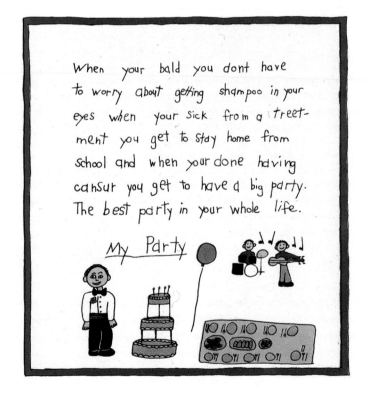

When your bald you dont have to worry about getting shampoo in your eyes when your sick from a treetment you get to stay home from school and when your done having cahsur you get to have a big party. The best party in your whole life.

My Party

At age six Jason Gaes was diagnosed with Burkitt's lymphoma, a rare form of pediatric cancer. For two years he endured a series of difficult treatments, including operations, radiation, and experimental drugs, from which he emerged cured. To let others know that kids with cancer "don't always die," he wrote a book. He wanted to encourage young cancer patients to be brave because the painful process of treatment will probably be worth it in the end. Jason is right. Not only are most children survivors but they emerge from their struggle with cancer having acquired a unique appreciation of life and an emotional maturity that are quite special.

Illustration from *My Book for Kids with Cansur* by Jason Gaes; © 1987 Melius Publishing. Reprinted by permission of the publisher

Healing POOCH and PUSS— from ANGST to ULCERS

by Edward Boden, M.R.Pharm.S.

The therapies used by veterinarians to treat sick animals are, in most cases, adapted from those employed in treating human patients. Consequently, developments in veterinary medicine tend to follow closely those in human medicine. Sometimes the process is virtually cyclical—a technique first tried and perfected in experimental animals becomes a standard treatment for human patients and then, in turn, is widely used in veterinary practice. Both humans and animals ultimately benefit, and increasingly sophisticated types of procedures make their way from human medicine to veterinary medicine. It comes as no surprise, therefore, that some of the current interest in treating certain human ailments by means of "alternative" therapies is now making itself felt in veterinary clinics around the world. Furthermore, clinical psychology, which had until recently been considered an exclusively human province, is being applied increasingly in the treatment of domestic pets whose behavior is causing problems.

Acupuncture: an ancient practice in modern times

Despite the availability and widespread use of advanced diagnostic, medical, and surgical techniques in veterinary practice, there is today an unprecedented interest in acupuncture in the veterinary world. One practitioner of this science is John Nicol, a vet with a busy and successful practice in the pleasant town of Guildford in Surrey, England. Nicol's clinic is equipped with the latest facilities and instrumentation. Every form of up-to-date medicine and the most current surgical techniques are available to the animals taken to him for treatment. Yet the chances are that his clients will ask Nicol to forgo these modern therapies and use instead a system of treatment established thousands of years ago in China. Nicol is one of the growing number of veterinarians throughout the world who have discovered the uses of acupuncture in the care of sick animals. His patients are as likely to have a course of treatment by needles as by drugs.

Across the Atlantic in the United States, Gloria Weintrob, a New Jersey veterinarian, is presented with a four-year-old poodle suffering from a long-standing problem of regurgitation. As a puppy, the animal had been diagnosed as having a congenital malfunction of the esophagus. In her examination Weintrob finds that the dog's esophagus is abnormally enlarged. A

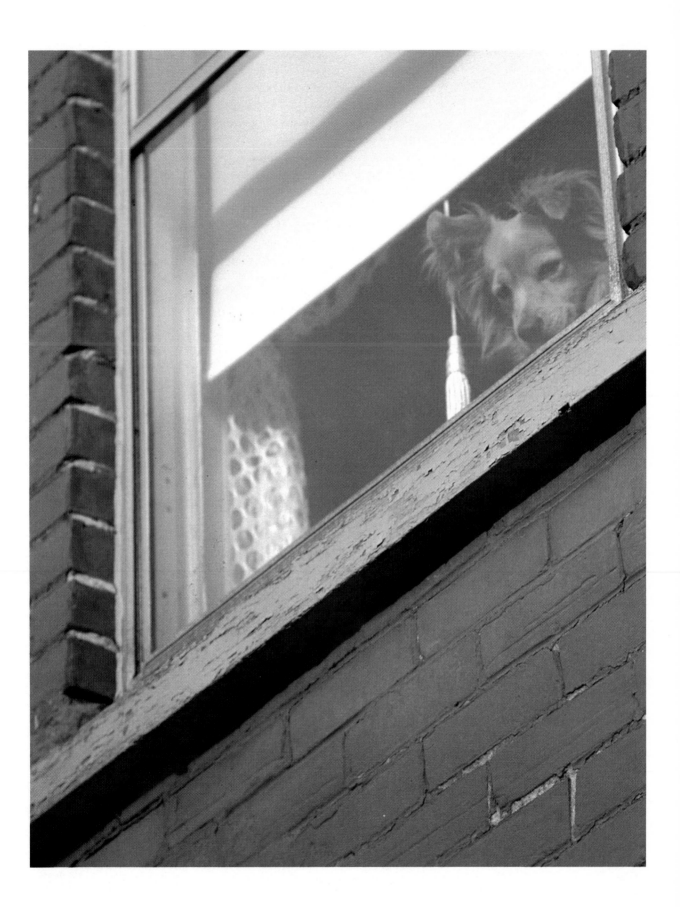

Edward Boden, M.R.Pharm.S., is Editor of The Veterinary Record *and Executive Editor of* Research in Veterinary Science, *publications of the British Veterinary Association, London.*

(Overleaf) Portrait of "animal angst"— a lonely pet awaits the return of its owner; photograph, Owen Franken— Stock, Boston

course of five acupuncture treatments over a three-month period produces progressive improvement resulting in a complete cure; the dog is able to eat normally and has no problem keeping its food down.

William H. McCormick, a veterinarian practicing in Middleburg, Virginia, used acupuncture successfully in the treatment of ulcers that developed on the cornea of a horse's eye. The condition had not been helped by conventional therapy. McCormick injected vitamin B_{12} at the acupuncture points governing the eye and those governing what Oriental medical terminology calls "wind," to which Chinese acupuncturists attribute the problem of ulceration. The treatment was given every third day. McCormick found that after three treatments the animal's eyes had improved, and after the fifth the ulcers were completely healed.

Balancing energy, restoring health. In acupuncture extremely fine needles—not much thicker than a hair—usually of stainless steel, are inserted a few millimeters into the skin at specific points in a network of invisible pathways, called meridians. Each point is related to a particular part of the body. Points on the wrists, for example, may relate to sensations felt in the neck. The notion that a sensitive point can be some distance from the cause of a bodily sensation is not unique to Oriental medicine—it has long been accepted in Western doctrine, under the term *referred pain.* In a human patient a heart condition, for example, may produce pain in the arm. In acupuncture, stimulation of the sensitive point by rotation of a needle, or more often nowadays by mild electrical current or even a laser, delivered via the needle, induces a therapeutic effect in the related part. Often the very thin needles are bent backward so that they are parallel to the skin; they are then taped in position and connected to an electrical stimulator. Sometimes the technique is varied so that an injection, perhaps of a vitamin, is given at the acupuncture point.

The Chinese theory behind acupuncture is that disease is caused by a disturbance of energy flow in the body. The balance of yin (the feminine, negative force) and yang (masculine, positive) energies is upset. Acupunc-

Although doctors of veterinary medicine have at their disposal virtually every "modern" therapy known to medical science, a growing number of vets are becoming interested in the ancient Chinese practice of acupuncture, in which very fine needles are used to stimulate sensitive points on the body. Today the technique may be augmented by the delivery of mild electrical stimulation, as shown at right in the treatment of a bulldog suffering from the painful and potentially disabling condition of hip dysplasia. In veterinary as in human medicine, acupuncture may be used to cure a specific ailment or to provide relief from pain.

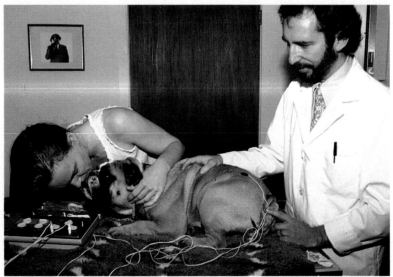

Jim Metzger—The Stock Shop

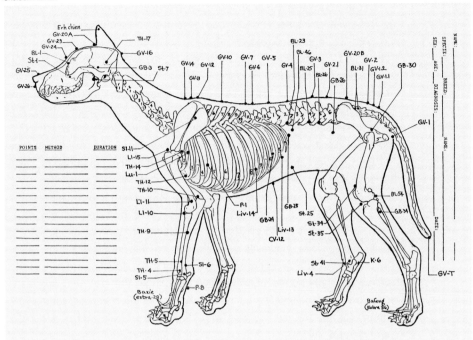

POINTS	METHOD	DURATION
_____	_____	_____
_____	_____	_____
_____	_____	_____
_____	_____	_____
_____	_____	_____
_____	_____	_____
_____	_____	_____
_____	_____	_____
_____	_____	_____
_____	_____	_____
_____	_____	_____
_____	_____	_____
_____	_____	_____
_____	_____	_____

ture can bring it back into balance—and restore the body to health—by judicious stimulation or depression of the flow of energy in the various meridians by needling the appropriate points.

In China the practice is as old as civilization itself. Before there were needles, the acupuncture points were stimulated by sharp stones, fingertip pressure, or heat. Although cruder, these methods followed the same principles as the electrical and laser-beam stimulation now used. Over the centuries, maps showing the acupuncture points have been drawn up. A skilled practitioner can identify these points by touch.

Overcoming Western skepticism. The current Western interest in acupuncture dates back some 25 years, when visitors to China reported seeing complicated surgical operations being performed on human patients who had received no conventional anesthetic. The patients were conscious throughout their operations yet felt no pain. Postoperative recovery was rapid and complete. Western surgeons were initially skeptical, but many became believers when they were able to observe the technique being applied in Chinese hospitals. Veterinarians in China had already begun experimenting with acupuncture in animals, and it was not long before their interest in the process spread to their colleagues in other countries.

Today there is a well-established International Veterinary Acupuncture Society with some 250 members—and many more nonmember vets also practice acupuncture. More than 20 national societies or contact groups exist in various countries, and in the United States alone there are a dozen recognized educational institutions providing courses in veterinary acupuncture. Veterinarians use it to treat a variety of conditions—as already indicated—from eye disease to gastrointestinal complaints. The greatest documented success, however, is in the alleviation of pain-related disorders.

The Chinese theory behind acupuncture is that disease is caused by an imbalance of energy flow along invisible pathways in the body known as meridians. The flow can be affected by inserting needles at sensitive points on the skin that lie along these meridians. The diagram above showing the acupuncture points of a dog was developed by a California veterinarian. Because pain that originates in one part of the body may be "referred" to another part, the sensitive point may be some distance from the underlying cause of the problem. In one study, for example, veterinary researchers demonstrated that stimulating a point on a dog's knee decreased the animal's stomach acidity. Some points are more closely related to the parts they affect—stimulating point GB-30 (at the top of the hip) is said to help relieve hip dysplasia.

111

Chronic lameness cured. In a not untypical case reported by McCormick, a three-year-old steeplechaser had developed a painful chronic lameness in both its forelegs so severe that it was unable to race or train. After identifying the location of the lesion causing the pain, McCormick noted the corresponding acupuncture points—one on the animal's scapula (shoulder blade) and several on either side of the spine in the thoracic region. Into these points he injected vitamin B_{12} enhanced with ammonium sulfate. After two such treatments the horse improved enough to win a race at odds of 24 to 1. A relapse was resolved after McCormick implanted minute quantities of gold, for long-term activation of the most effective acupuncture points. The horse was eventually able to return to a full training program.

How animals—and people—experience pain. The intriguing question is, how can sticking a needle into an animal—or a person—actually relieve pain? It was at first thought that in humans suggestion or hypnosis might play a part. It is, however, unlikely that animals are susceptible to the suggestion that they do not feel pain; in any case, double-blind clinical trials in human acupuncture patients have discounted the idea that suggestion or hypnosis is behind the beneficial effect. The effectiveness seems to be bound up in a fascinating way with the nature of pain and how humans, and animals, feel it.

The question was explored recently by three veterinarians from three different countries—A.M. Schoen (U.S.), L.A.A. Janssens (Belgium), and P.A.M. Rogers (Ireland). They reviewed evidence showing that acupuncture analgesia (relief of pain) works by stimulating nerve fibers at the acupuncture points, from which the stimulus is transmitted to the spinal cord and higher centers in the brain. Their report, published in *The Veterinary Record,* explained that the ascending pain impulses are blocked by a complex interaction involving endorphins—naturally occurring painkilling substances—and certain other substances produced by the body. While the mechanism

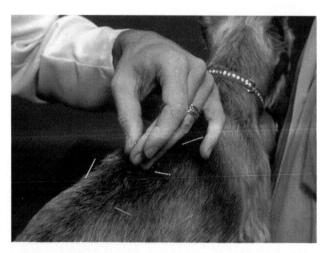

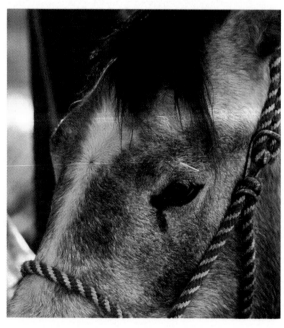

A schnauzer receives therapy for painful spinal arthritis; for pain relief acupuncture may be used instead of or in addition to analgesic drugs. A horse, being treated for an eye inflammation, has a single needle placed in the point known as Ching-shu.

is not entirely understood, a genuine analgesic effect is produced. The fact that it can be reversed by a substance (naloxone) known to combat analgesic effect confirms this theory.

Still, while acupuncture has been shown to work, it is by no means a panacea. Patients must be chosen with care, for although it can be used to relieve pain, acupuncture is not an anesthetic—that is, it does not produce a state of unconsciousness. Thus, a nervous or restless animal is not normally a suitable subject, as it can still move—and bite or scratch—while being treated. Also, there is a marked variation in the effectiveness of analgesia in different individuals and species. Some veterinarians do not think acupuncture works well in cats, for instance.

In veterinary as in human medicine, acupuncture now seems to be finding its place as a technique used along with many others. In combination with conventional drugs, for example, acupuncture may be used to reduce the doses of anesthetics in surgical procedures, thus speeding recovery and healing. In the treatment of painful conditions such as arthritis, it may supplement or supplant medications for pain.

Homeopathy: a therapeutic revival

The practice of homeopathy has a long and not undistinguished history in human medicine and has had veterinary adherents for many years. Recently, however, interest has mushroomed. There are thriving societies for the study and practice of veterinary homeopathy in the United States and Europe. The *International Journal for Veterinary Homeopathy* exists to further knowledge of the subject and circulates to more than 1,500 practitioners throughout the world. Many veterinarians, often in response to client demand, use homeopathic remedies as well as forms of conventional (allopathic) medicine.

Homeopathy and allopathy are two systems of medicine based on two different theoretical concepts. Allopathy, strictly speaking, is the treatment of symptoms by medication that produces an effect different from that produced by the disease the patient suffers from. Homeopathy is designed to work in the opposite way—by using minute doses of a substance that produces symptoms similar to those affecting the patient. For example, minute doses of quinine might be used to treat fever, not because of quinine's antimalarial effect but because an overdose of the drug causes tremor and other signs typically seen in feverishness.

Obtaining an animal's medical history. Homeopathic practitioners also contend that the holistic principle applies in deciding what treatment will be used. In holistic medicine the emphasis is on treating the "whole" patient rather than on viewing each body part or system as separate and amenable to separate treatment. Before prescribing any course of therapy, the homeopathic physician first seeks to obtain as detailed a case history as possible. Obviously, this is harder with an animal than with a human patient. Apart from a thorough examination of the animal, the veterinarian must rely on what the animal's owner can relate about the signs and symptoms of illness. It is on the basis of this information, then, that the appropriate remedy is selected.

113

Deducing the correct treatment for subtly different problems is not always easy; the owner's descriptions may not be accurate. Irmgard Elsholz, a veterinarian from Bonn, West Germany, recounts how, following a detailed examination, she administered a particular homeopathic preparation—a combination of podophyllum, arsenicum album, and rheum—for a cat suffering from severe diarrhea and vomiting. The treatment did not work. Elsholz later discovered that another homeopath had prescribed a different remedy—nux vomica—with successful results. Going back over her case records, she was able to deduce that her own prescription was ineffective because the treatment had been drawn up on the basis of what proved to be an incomplete case history. The cat's owner had told the second homeopath that in addition to the other symptoms, the cat had been waking up at about 4 AM and showing extreme restlessness. This additional clinical sign led to an alternative diagnosis and a different remedy. Skeptics would say that the cat in this particular case would have recovered anyway, regardless of treatment, and that the second treatment simply coincided with a natural improvement.

The "doctrine of similars." The system of homeopathic medicine was formulated by a German physician, Samuel Hahnemann, who was born in Meissen, Saxony, in 1755. After training conventionally as a doctor, he became especially interested in the study of poisons and their effects. Gradually he developed the so-called doctrine of similars, sometimes expressed by the phrase "like cures like"; according to this principle, a disease should be treated with medicines that have been shown to produce in healthy persons symptoms similar to those from which the sick person is suffering. The medicaments he used included plant extracts such as digitalis and nux vomica and chemical substances, for example, arsenic and mercuric sulfide, all diluted hundreds or thousands of times and administered in the form of pills or solutions. Hahnemann made his system public, to a mixed reception from the medical establishment, in 1796.

With time, however, homeopathy attracted more and more adherents, eventually becoming popular and, indeed, fashionable. The success of Hahnemann's system of therapeutics was due at least in part to the crude ineffectualness of much of the contemporary conventional medical treatment. Bloodletting, accompanied by violent purging, was a routine practice in the 18th century. Such treatments were undoubtedly responsible for the early demise of many a delicate, and not-so-delicate, invalid. Hahnemann's therapy, by contrast, involved the gentler administration of medicines that had no adverse side effects; he also emphasized the importance of rest, attentive nursing, and appropriate diet. It is not surprising that, compared with the rigors of conventional treatments, the regime employed by the homeopaths was popular and, in many cases, efficacious.

While there could be no dispute about the popularity of the homeopathic system, though, argument as to why it should work has continued ever since it was introduced. The theory behind the choosing of a given homeopathic remedy is that the more the active therapeutic substance is diluted, the greater is the effect of the remedy. In fact, dilution may be such that a dose of a homeopathic preparation in some cases does not contain a

The practice of homeopathy, which now has a growing number of veterinary adherents, was founded in the late 18th century by a German physician, Samuel Hahnemann. Hahnemann's system of therapeutics was based on the doctrine "like cures like"—thus, treatment consists of the administration of substances capable of producing symptoms similar to those the patient suffers from. Hahnemann's approach was holistic, emphasizing in addition to minute doses of medication the importance of rest, proper nutrition, and good nursing care— a notably gentle regimen, especially when compared with conventional medical practice of his day that relied on bloodletting and violent purging.

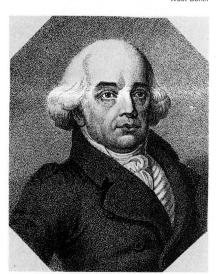

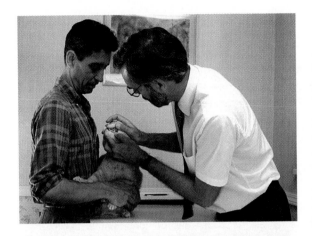

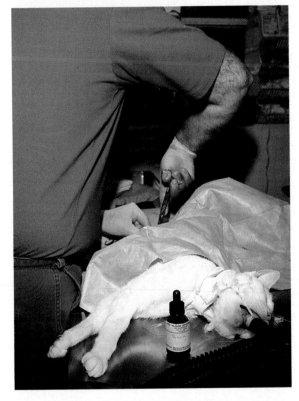

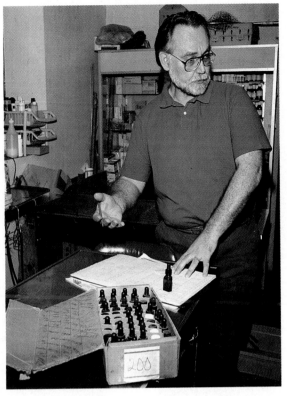

The art of homeopathy lies in learning to identify the remedy—from an armamentarium of more than 1,500 substances—that best matches the overall pattern of physical, mental, and emotional symptoms. (Above left) To aid in the selection of the appropriate remedy, the homeopathic veterinarian relies on a thorough examination of the patient along with close questioning of the owner about the animal's behavior and medical history. Before performing surgery on an injured cat, the vet shown above chooses arnica, a botanical extract used in the treatment of traumatic shock, which is administered to the animal during and after the operation.

Photographs, (top left) Susan H. Pitcairn; (above and bottom left) Jim Metzger—The Stock Shop

single molecule of active substance! Homeopathic practitioners maintain that the special processes of preparation—"trituration" or "attenuation," for solid or liquid dose forms, respectively—themselves confer special qualities on the medicines.

Placebo effect—in animals? The principles used in homeopathic medicine are the same in both human and animal patients: diagnose the symptoms and then administer the remedy indicated by the "doctrine of similars." Opponents of homeopathy maintain that the doses given are much too small to have any effect whatsoever. They argue that the beneficial results of homeopathic medications are due to what is called the placebo effect—that is, the patient's firm conviction that the substance or treatment being given

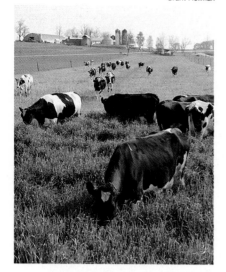

Homeopathic treatment has proved successful for a number of disorders that afflict such economically important animals as dairy cattle. In view of the growing consumer concerns about potent drugs entering the food supply, some farmers now favor the homeopathic approach because it does not involve the administration of antibiotics or synthetic hormones.

will, indeed, be effective. (*Placebo* is Latin for "I please.") In other words, its opponents contend that homeopathic treatment occupies and satisfies the mind of the patient while nature effects a cure.

The placebo effect is, of course, demonstrable in human patients. In fact, it is taken into account in clinical trials of new medicines, which are routinely conducted under a protocol known as a double blind. What this means is that neither the patients nor the researchers know who is receiving the experimental drug and who is receiving a placebo (an inert substance with no therapeutic effect). But can the placebo effect work in animals? Can any animal be said to "believe" that a medicine is curing it? Many a pet owner may think that this is the case, but finding evidence that would convince a scientist, or a skeptic, is another matter. This is the stumbling block that is insuperable as far as the opponents of homeopathic treatment in animals are concerned.

Veterinary homeopaths simply shrug their shoulders and dismiss conventional pharmacological trials as irrelevant to homeopathy. "Homeopathy is not confined to physical parameters," according to H.G. Wolff, whose handbook of homeopathic medicine for dogs has run into three editions since its publication in 1964.

Although few articles on homeopathic treatments are accepted by "conventional" veterinary clinical publications, anecdotal evidence of their success abounds. Often it relates to the type of case in which, the grateful owner testifies, "Everything had been tried, but my pet recovered only after homeopathy."

Benefits of the holistic approach. There are those, too, who have demonstrated the effectiveness of homeopathic treatment in farm animals. English veterinarian Chris Day, a former president of the International Association for Veterinary Homeopathy, uses both conventional and alternative medicine in his busy practice in rural Faringdon, Oxfordshire. Particularly since the enthusiasm for organically grown farm produce has become so widespread—leading to a premium price in the market—Day has found that some of his farmer clients are keen to use homeopathic remedies rather than conventional ones such as antibiotics and synthetic hormones. Day employs homeopathic remedies in treating certain reproductive disorders and mastitis (inflammation of the udder) in dairy cattle and in treating common disorders in sheep, such as mouth ulcers. A homeopathic regime Day instituted for a client who raises pigs proved successful in reducing the incidence of stillbirths, which had been causing severe losses among the farmer's sows; a report of the case resulted in one of the few homeopathic papers to be accepted by a peer-reviewed clinical journal, *The Veterinary Record.*

Day, like German veterinarian Elsholz, attributes a large part of the success of his alternative treatments to the painstaking examination of each case, which includes an evaluation of the temperament and species of the animal being treated as well as the nature of the medical condition. This holistic approach is integral to the successful application of most alternative therapies. And there can be little doubt that the care that goes along with a holistic regime is beneficial.

116

Pet behaviorists to the rescue

Two young professionals say good-bye to their dog, close the door of their smart apartment, and go off to their respective offices. Eight hours later they return—to chaos. Their previously well-behaved canine companion has wrecked the apartment, chewed the furniture, pulled down the drapes, and generally created mayhem. What do the owners do? Chances are, they will punish the dog and hope it is an isolated incidence of misbehavior. If the problem recurs, however, they are in trouble.

An emerging specialty. Until recently, the only answer might have been to have a persistently misbehaving dog put to sleep. Now, however, owners may well call on the services of an animal behaviorist specializing in the treatment of pets. The behaviorist will likely tell the distressed couple in the example above that the dog is suffering from separation anxiety and that the worst thing they can do is to punish it. A diagnosis like this one usually involves a house call. After a period spent watching and noting how the animal behaves, both with and without its owners, and a discussion of their own daily routine, the behaviorist will advise a course of action to relieve the dog's anxiety—and thus remove the cause of the destructive behavior.

It is a measure of the increasingly sophisticated care that is available today to the pet owner that such services can be provided. It is also, perhaps, a comment on contemporary urban life that such services should be needed. But it is a fact that a great many pets are being left home on their own for long periods of time. Just as people can develop psychological problems when isolated for long periods, so can animals, particularly if they are, by nature, social animals. Apartment living can also be hard on animals bred to enjoy an open-air environment where they can get plenty of exercise.

Animal behaviorists who treat pets tend to have taken up their specialty in one of two ways. From working as behavioral scientists or psychologists in research, they may have developed a particular interest in pet-related problems, or they may be veterinarians who, having become interested in animal behavior, have studied it in depth. Many behaviorists remain in the academic environment, concentrating on research, sometimes combining it with an appointment in the clinical department of a veterinary school. Increasingly, however, animal behaviorists are making their skills available in veterinary practice.

Whichever route they follow to this vocation, pet behaviorists are quick to make it clear that they are *not* trainers. Peter Borchelt, a pet behavior consultant working in New York City, points out that, unlike obedience trainers, behaviorists do not use punishment-related techniques or leash training. Whereas obedience trainers concentrate on compliance with basic commands—sit, stay, heel, and so on—behaviorists work to modify undesirable traits that a dog or cat has acquired.

Alleviating animal angst. The separation anxiety described above, which manifests itself as destructive behavior when a dog is left alone, is very common. It arises because dogs, social animals that live in packs in the wild, do not take naturally to the solitary condition. The dog's "pack leader" is its owner. Some puppies quickly get used to being left on their own;

A pup waits anxiously by the window for its human companions to return. Often when owners go off to work or are away for long periods, the dog left at home on its own may experience acute separation anxiety, which it expresses in a variety of undesirable behaviors—destroying furniture, howling endlessly, urinating and defecating indoors. Most such behavior problems can be successfully overcome, often with the aid of a behavior specialist. Patience and persistence in following through with prescribed treatments will be required on the part of the owner, however.

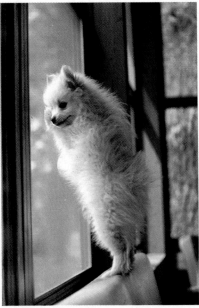

Horst Schäder—Globe Photos

117

others do not adapt and remain anxious. Even when a dog for years has seemed happy enough alone in the house for a while, its anxiety can be triggered by an unexpected or unusual noise or event—a particularly violent thunderstorm, perhaps.

Then the previously well-behaved companion animal becomes destructive and messy. The "displacement behavior" it shows can include wrecking furniture and clothes, howling and whining, urinating and defecating indoors, or perhaps all of these. Nevertheless, if the dog is of basically stable temperament and the owners are prepared to go to some lengths in assisting in the treatment, the behaviorist will usually be optimistic that the problem can be cured.

Peter Neville, a pet psychologist in Britain, sees many such cases during the sessions he holds as a guest consultant to numerous veterinary practices. Neville has found a number of basic guidelines effective in helping to eliminate displacement activity. One step is to provide the dog with a comfortable place of its own—a den—in one room, with its favorite playthings, in which the animal can feel secure. Before the owner leaves the house or apartment, he or she should take the dog for a walk and then feed it. This way, the dog should be ready to go to sleep before the owner departs. Another tactic is for owners to vary their departure habits and periods of absence so that the animal does not become conditioned to a specific routine that triggers its anxiety. In some cases getting another dog, or perhaps a cat, as a companion may help. The wrong choice, however, could make the problem twice as bad, so professional advice is essential. Although response to treatment will take time, as it does in cases of human behavior problems, Neville says that persistence and consistent application of the behaviorist's advice by all who are in contact with the dog will usually resolve the problem.

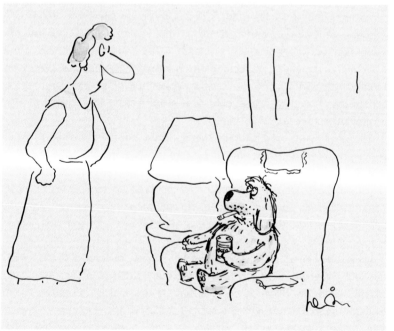

"Bad dog!"

Photographs, Jeanne Carlson

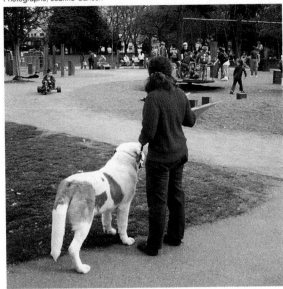 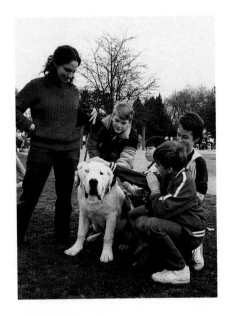

When a dog is aggressive. Separation anxiety, although common, is by no means the only canine problem for which behaviorists are consulted. Dominance and aggression—toward other dogs or toward people—can be not only troublesome but dangerous. One situation that is particularly worrisome is when a dog displays aggression toward a child in the owner's family. The animal may be defensive of its own situation in the household or just plain afraid of an unpredictable toddler. With care, this problem can be overcome. Treatment may involve introducing an infant to the pet dog in carefully controlled conditions, so that neither party acts threateningly toward the other. Gradually the two are brought together, and ultimately the relationship becomes friendly.

The very real risks of canine aggression in uncontrolled situations were brought home in England in 1990 when a series of attacks by Rottweilers left several children dead or seriously injured. Such incidents—involving various breeds in different countries—are unfortunately becoming regular occurrences. According to Borchelt, where the problem of aggression is caused by the dog's sheer dominant nature, a satisfactory resolution of the problem may not be likely; the dog may simply have to go.

Dominance can cause other problems. A not uncommon one often develops when a dog is bought by a couple for protection, perhaps because the husband is frequently away or works a night shift. The dog can become excessively attached to one party to the extent that it will not allow the other near without growling and other aggressive behavior. A classic situation in such cases occurs where a woman keeps the dog in the bedroom at night when the husband is away. A dominant animal may treat the husband as an interloper and attack him, particularly if he returns unexpectedly.

More common is aggression toward other animals. A dominant dog, which may accept a human as overall pack leader, may nevertheless attempt to assert dominance over every other dog. It can be very difficult to exercise a "boss dog" in areas where other dogs are to be found. Neville

Aggressive behavior in dogs—toward other animals or toward people—is a common problem treated by pet behaviorists. Aggression toward children can be particularly troubling. Because fear is often at the root of an animal's aggression, one way to eliminate this kind of undesirable behavior is to progressively socialize a puppy around youngsters. In these photographs a therapist guided an exuberant five-month-old St. Bernard through his initial encounter with children. This practitioner routinely uses massage to calm an animal before introducing it to new, potentially frightening situations. Her next step in this case was to spend some time with the dog observing children at play from a distance. Finally, when the dog and youngsters came together, she stayed close by to make sure that the animal was handled gently and showed no signs of anxiety.

tells of the case of a pair of bull mastiffs that scrapped incessantly. The owner, who had bought the pair as company for each other, found them uncontrollable and sought professional advice. After observing the dogs, Neville noted that the aggressive behavior disappeared when the two were separated. When another home was found for one, both the dogs became docile and well-behaved.

Problem behavior is not confined to commoners' canines. Queen Elizabeth II of England is fond of Welsh corgis, of which she keeps several. Corgis are a notably snappy breed and, although such information is not officially made public, it is understood that Roger Mugford, one of Britain's longest-established pet behaviorists, has been consulted about unspecified misbehavior among the royal corgis. Whether he succeeded in his treatment has not been revealed.

Coping with feline misbehavior. Cats, too, can require behavioral treatment. Although the domestic cat is by nature normally well behaved, persistent problems, such as an animal's marking its territory by "spraying" urine or sharpening claws on furniture, can be infuriating. Spraying is a problem with a complicated etiology. It is a sexual aggression-related behavior; in male cats it can sometimes be successfully treated by neutering. Sharpening claws, as on furniture, is often cured by provision of an alternative, such as a scratching post or a piece of cork, near the cat's favorite claw-sharpening place.

Although aggression is more rarely a problem in cats than in dogs, dealing with a ferocious cat can be a frightening and potentially dangerous experience. Again, fear or phobia on the part of the animal is often the root cause; as in the case of aggressive canines, introduction of the fearful stimulus in a controlled situation is often the solution.

Sometimes, though, a cat's natural territorial defenses can be misdirected against people. Neville relates a case in which a neutered male tabby would sit by the window keeping watch over "his" garden. Whenever he spied another cat on his patch of ground, he growled, his coat bristled, and his tail swished from side to side. When his owner tried to comfort him, the cat attacked her, on one occasion requiring her to be hospitalized. The suggested treatment was that the owner employ distraction techniques such as rolling a ball past the cat or showing him a favorite play object. It might also help to keep the window drapes closed and to place the cat's bed away from an outside view. Another alternative would be to open the door and let him out to protect his anxiously guarded territory. On no account, however, should an owner attempt direct physical contact with the cat in such a situation!

Another common problem in cats is a predisposition to chewing fabric, particularly wool. Many a favorite wooly garment has ended up inside a cat's stomach, to the distress and annoyance of the owner although usually with no harm to the cat. Prevention is the first step—making sure that all tempting items of clothing are put away out of reach. Another ploy is to dose a piece of the cat's favorite fabric with a deterrent substance such as oil of eucalyptus, which cats find offensive but which will not make them ill. Sometimes, however, it seems that nothing will cure this bizarre taste for

This six-month-old puppy, adopted from an animal shelter, was fearful of being held and tried to bite her owner whenever he attempted to brush her. The behavior therapist showed the owner how to gently restrain the dog without arousing her fear of being harmed; as soon as the pup stopped struggling, she was rewarded with stroking and gentle massage. It did not take long for the animal to understand that being gently held was not a threat. Eventually she began to enjoy being groomed and even to look forward to it.

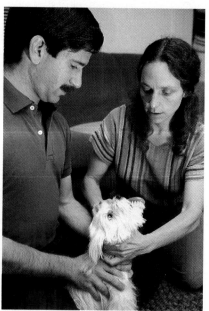

Jeanne Carlson

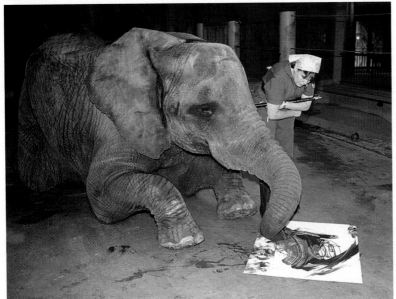

Although offered a brush, Suti, an elephant at the Lincoln Park Zoo in Chicago, prefers to paint with her trunk. Chimps also participate in the zoo's "art classes." As well as being enjoyable, painting serves as a form of therapy for animals who live in restricted environments and are unable to engage in behaviors such as foraging for food, which in the wild would occupy much of their time and energy. Behavioral consultants typically advise zookeepers about how to keep captive animals contented.

fabric. Why do some cats have this proclivity? Behaviorists speculate that it is a retention of infantile behavior patterns. A study being conducted in England at the Bristol University veterinary school is seeking to establish breed and feeding patterns in cloth-eating cats, which may offer a more decisive answer to this poorly understood phenomenon. British interest in feline behavior problems is such that the Bristol veterinary school holds regular clinics to evaluate and treat them.

Creatures small and great. As well as pets kept in the home, zoo animals occasionally require behavior therapy. They are often restricted in their environments and deprived of the opportunity for certain natural activity. Therapists can help by providing the captive animals with activities that help to replace behaviors common in the wild. A Dutch veterinarian, for example, at the marine park at Harderiwijk, The Netherlands, observed that the walruses were displaying a stereotypical behavior in which they endlessly repeated purposeless actions. His solution was to have the animals' meals of fish and mollusks hidden in a trough of stones, from which they could forage as they would in their natural habitat.

Chimpanzees are well known for their enjoyment of play activity. The chimps' "tea parties" held at many zoos are an amusing example of structured play that entertains both the animals and their audiences. Chicago's Lincoln Park Zoo is one of several that provides "art classes" as a source of both therapy and exercise for some animals. Chimps, in particular, hugely enjoy working with paints and crayons. June, a 23-year-old chimp, is one of several Chicago apes that have actually had their work exhibited. The Lincoln Park Zoo's classes are open to elephants as well. The animals set to enthusiastically, using their trunks to make giant "finger" paintings. Animal keeper Dan Krawitz claims he can easily tell by looking at a canvas which of his charges painted it. Such activities can play an important part in creating an environment that keeps the animals content.

Consultants and a caveat. For the present, animal behaviorists practice in only a few Western industrial countries and are virtually restricted, as organized groups, to the United States and the United Kingdom. In the U.S., behavioral consultants have formed an informal group known as the Animal Behavior Society. In the U.K. there is an Association of Pet Behavior Consultants, made up variously of psychologists, behaviorists, biologists, and veterinarians. In other countries behavioral consultants, where they exist, are often veterinarians with a particular interest in the subject or trainers who have shown a special aptitude for dealing with difficult pets.

Because there are so few practicing behavioral consultants, it is not at all unusual for them to hold clinical sessions at local veterinary practices. A vet with patients requiring behavior therapy may arrange for a consultant to visit the practice on a regular basis. Much useful advice, too, can be given in a telephone consultation. In some cases, however, a "house call" is necessary before the problem can be analyzed and a course of action agreed upon. Consultant behaviorist's fees vary considerably, but home visits can be expensive. A house call might cost $200 or more, plus travel and expenses.

A novel approach to pet behavior therapy has, therefore, been introduced by Mugford, the "royal behaviorist," who has organized "puppy playgroups." Attended by young dogs and their owners, the play groups, says Mugford, aim to teach pups the positive behaviors expected of a pet dog. "Play and early socialization of puppies have long been regarded as vital in the development of the happy, well-adjusted adult dog," according to Mugford, who feels that traditional dog-training classes usually accept their pupils too late, when undesirable behaviors may already be well established.

Perhaps the most common mistake owners make in dealing with their pets is in ascribing to them human motives, thoughts, and aspirations. To do this is to negate one of the greatest benefits people derive from interacting with their pets—that is, simply, that they *are* animals, not other human beings.

As well as creating problems of temperament, generations of inbreeding have resulted in physical changes that are not always in the animals' best interests. Nowhere has this been more true than in the breeding of pedigreed dogs for show. The British bulldog is a case in point. Through selective breeding the bulldog of 1820 (below) has evolved into the present-day example of the breed (right), with its characteristically large head, foreshortened muzzle, and narrow hips. While prized by breeders, these traits have contributed to respiratory and reproductive problems for the animals. In the U.S. and the U.K., concerned dog breeders are now moving to revise breed standards in order to eliminate those that are detrimental to the animals' health and well-being.

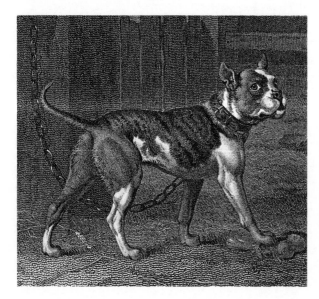 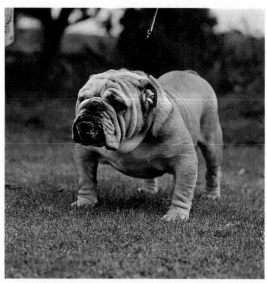

(Left) The Bettmann Archive; (right) Sally Anne Thompson—EB Inc.

Untreatable problems: legacy of inbreeding

Not every case can be treated effectively by a behaviorist. Some problems—for example, those created by maladaptive conditioning or poor handling—can be dealt with; some others cannot. The latter are those problems arising from congenital factors, the intrinsic flaws of temperament in an animal that are not amenable to treatment by any means.

Such congenital defects can occur by chance, but in quite a few instances, unfortunately, they arise from injudicious breeding. Pedigree-dog-showing is nowadays a high-powered business. Prizewinning dogs are much in demand for producing offspring, which in turn will reproduce their winning characteristics. Through inbreeding these traits can become exaggerated. The British bulldog, for example, is bred to have a particular "look" that calls for a large head, a flat face, an undershot jaw, and narrow hips. These traits can be so exaggerated that pups may have to be delivered by cesarean section. Pekingese, bred to have facial characteristics similar to those of the bulldog, often have breathing problems caused by the highly valued flat nose, which results in a compressed upper respiratory tract. Many German shepherd dogs are prone to hip dysplasia, a condition leading to painful lameness. The reason for this is that they are bred from lines of animals that are pleasing in appearance but carry a gene predisposing to hip dysplasia.

Along with such undesirable inbred physical characteristics are to be found, in some breeds, mental traits that cause problems of temperament. The cocker spaniel, traditionally a delightfully friendly dog, can exhibit a rage syndrome in which it goes berserk and may attack its owner. West Highland terriers (Scotties) may also show a tendency to bite. Some German shepherds are temperamentally unsound, becoming nervous, aggressive in guarding their territory, and overly dependent on their owners.

The remedy here is much more difficult. As the problems have been bred in, so must they be bred out. This process requires, first, the development of new breed standards—possibly including specifications for temperament—and then gradual improvement over, perhaps, many generations of breeding. Even so, all behaviorists are faced with dogs having problems of temperament that are, unfortunately, untreatable.

In England, at least, a start has been made in the long process of changing some breed standards. Mike Stockman, a veterinarian and a breeder, is working to revise the present breed standards of the British Kennel Club, most of which were set many years ago, to eliminate any characteristics judged to be against the best interests of the dogs themselves. A similar movement to revise breed standards is also under way in the U.S., the object being the welfare of the animals.

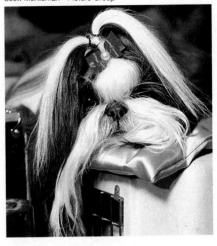

It is an all too common tendency of pet owners to ascribe to their animals human thoughts, motives, and desires. To do this, however, negates one of the greatest benefits people derive from the companionship of animals—quite simply, that they are animals.

Nowhere a Promised Land:

The Plight of the World's Refugees

by Michael J. Toole, M.D., and Ronald J. Waldman, M.D.

There are more than 14 million refugees in the world today. These are people who have fled war, civil violence, and political persecution and who are dependent upon external assistance for their survival. They are Afghan farmers, Vietnamese fishers, Somali camel herders, Ethiopian teachers, Salvadoran doctors, Mozambican mothers of small children, Soviet Jewish merchants, East German students, and Bulgarian bakers. By definition, a refugee is an individual who has crossed from one country into another. But, in addition, there are another approximately 16 million people who have been abruptly displaced from their homes and have fled to other, more secure regions within their own countries. These "internally displaced" persons do not qualify for international refugee assistance. With no access to relief and without legal rights to the protection accorded refugees by international law, these people are frequently in a particularly desperate situation.

History is replete with examples of mass population movements resulting from war and persecution. Moses is said to have led the Jews from persecution in Egypt in the 13th century BC. The journey covered very desolate country, and the refugees had to rely on external sources for sustenance. They are said to have complained bitterly about the lack of food and water. Most of the great wars of the Middle Ages were followed by major population movements in Europe. Later, persecution of the Jews in Spain and of the Huguenots in France precipitated the flight of hundreds of thousands. But the social disruption that followed World War II was a turning point in refugee history. For the first time, the international community took steps to protect the rights of refugees.

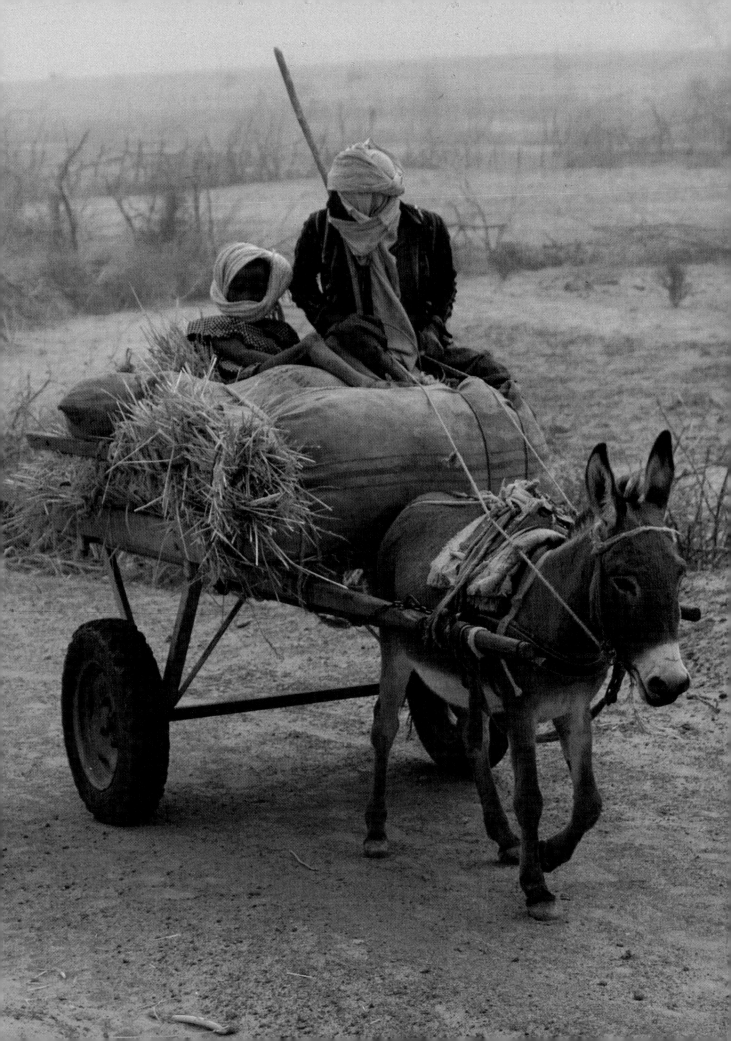

Michael J. Toole, M.D., is a Medical Epidemiologist with the International Health Program Office, Centers for Disease Control (CDC), and Assistant Professor, Emory University, Atlanta, Georgia.
Ronald J. Waldman, M.D., is Director of the Technical Support Division of the CDC's International Health Program Office.

(Overleaf) Photograph, Cynthia Johnson—Gamma/Liaison

In 1951 the Office of the United Nations High Commissioner for Refugees (UNHCR), headquartered in Geneva, was created, and the United Nations Convention Relating to the Status of Refugees (1951) and its 1967 Protocol guaranteed the rights of refugees. According to these agreements, a refugee is defined as "a person who owing to a well-founded fear of being persecuted for reasons of race, religion, nationality, membership [in] a particular social group, or political opinion . . . is outside the country of his nationality."

In some cases the solutions for the settling of refugees have caused new problems. The creation of the State of Israel in 1948, for example, led to the displacement of vast numbers of Palestinians, who were confined to huge camps in Jordan, Syria, and Lebanon. A new UN agency, the United Nations Relief and Works Agency for Palestine Refugees in the Near East (UNRWA), began operations in 1950 to care for these refugees, many of whom now reside in camps in the occupied West Bank and Gaza Strip. Today, with a registered refugee population numbering more than 2.2 million (about half the estimated total number of Palestinians), this group constitutes one of the largest unresolved refugee problems in the world.

Third World refugees

A new chapter in the history of refugees opened in the late 1960s and '70s when colonial powers began to grant independence to new African and Asian nations, frequently without regard to the level of social disruption that might be caused by the arbitrary boundaries created. Sudden population movements of people seeking to rejoin their own tribal, ethnic, or religious groups accompanied ensuing wars and civil insurrections. The wars following Algerian, Indian, Nigerian, and Indochinese independence all generated great numbers of refugees. One of the most dramatic population shifts occurred in 1971, during the war for independence in Bangladesh, when more than eight million refugees fled to neighboring India.

More recently, large refugee movements have occurred with unfortunate frequency in the less developed world. Some of the more publicized include the Vietnamese who fled the Communist victory in 1975, the Cambodians who fled from Pol Pot's murderous Khmer Rouge into Thailand (1975–79), the Ethiopians (largely of Somali ethnicity) who fled into Somalia between 1978 and 1981 and those who escaped into The Sudan (1984–85), and the Afghans who sought refuge in Pakistan from their own civil war as well as the Soviet invasion (1979–80). Today approximately 65% of the world's dependent refugees are in Asia and the Middle East. Afghanistan has generated the largest number of refugees (currently nearly six million). The rest (about 30%) are in Africa; the countries of Mozambique and Ethiopia have each seen more than one million citizens flee to neighboring countries during the past 10 years.

In 1969 the United Nations' definition of refugee status was expanded by the Organization of African Unity to include persons fleeing from war, civil disturbance, or violence of any kind. This latter definition has been ratified by most African governments, such that African nations have become among the most hospitable toward present-day refugees.

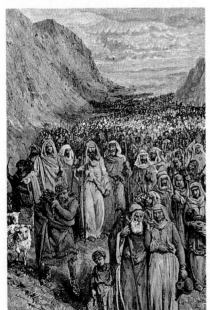

The Bible recounts the mass exodus of the Hebrews from Egyptian oppression in the 13th century BC under the leadership of Moses—perhaps the most widely known example of mass refugee movement in the Western world. The fleeing people traversed desolate country while facing severe shortages of food and water.

Historical Pictures Service, Chicago

126

It is in the Third World that the adverse health consequences of mass population displacements have been the greatest. Refugees in the Third World find refuge in neighboring countries that frequently are already dependent upon external sources in order to meet the subsistence needs of their indigenous populations. They simply cannot afford to provide the assistance necessary to sustain the lives of large numbers of unexpected refugees. Many of the countries currently acting as hosts to large refugee populations (Pakistan, Somalia, The Sudan, Ethiopia, and Malawi) have annual per capita gross national products of less than $400 and infant mortality rates greater than 100 per 1,000 live births per year. Thus, the fate of refugees arriving in these countries depends largely on the quantity and quality of assistance provided by the international community.

Most necessary commodities are donated by individual governments. The current role of UNHCR is to coordinate the collection, delivery, and distribution of relief supplies and other assistance. The procurement and transport of food—the most expensive and probably the single most important commodity—is usually handled by the World Food Program, another UN agency, in collaboration with UNHCR. The U.S. is the leading donor in terms of the overall monetary value of its contributions. The most generous donors on a per capita basis have been the Scandinavian countries, Canada, The Netherlands, and Switzerland.

Many private voluntary organizations offer more direct assistance, often in the form of field personnel. The more experienced of these agencies include Oxfam and Save the Children Fund of the United Kingdom, the French Médecins sans Frontières (Doctors Without Borders), the U.S.-based International Rescue Committee, and the international League of Red Cross and Red Crescent Societies. The number of private voluntary organizations has grown greatly over the past 20 years, reflecting the humanitarian concerns of people of all nations who have become increasingly knowledgeable about

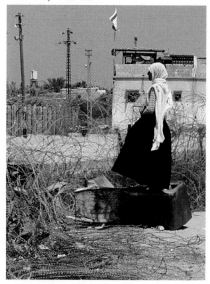

Barbed wire defines the border of a Palestinian refugee camp in the Israeli-occupied Gaza Strip (above). Creation of the State of Israel in 1948 resulted in the displacement of vast numbers of Arabs to camps in the Strip and West Bank territories. (Below) Afghan children gather before a "home" in a bleak refugee camp in Pakistan. Afghanistan's civil war and invasion by the U.S.S.R. in 1979–80 generated what is currently the largest population of refugees from one country—almost six million.

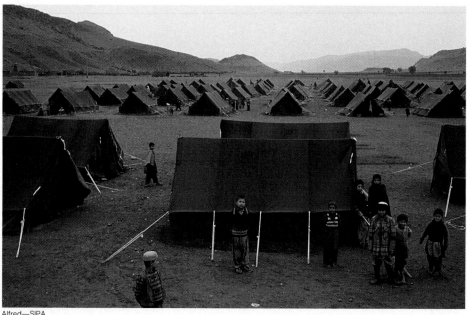

the plight of refugees, largely through the publicity generated by the mass media. Another agency, the Intergovernmental Committee for Migration, organizes the resettlement of refugees in Western countries. When refugees are situated in a zone of continuing armed conflict, the Geneva-based International Committee of the Red Cross (ICRC) frequently attempts to mount a relief effort in the area. This agency has a unique mandate and was created as a result of the Geneva Convention Relative to the Protection of Civilian Persons in Time of War (1949).

The refugee experience: first, the violence

Amnesty International has estimated that more than one-third of the world's governments routinely employ torture as part of their security system. This practice has been particularly common in certain Central and South American nations; in some African countries such as Ethiopia, Somalia, and The Sudan; and in Afghanistan—all of which have generated large numbers of refugees. Beyond the immediate physical trauma, chronic psychological and physical disabilities have been described.

Other refugees have experienced harassment in the form of armed attacks on their homes and villages simply because they were located in areas in which rival armed forces were operating. Refugees in Malawi in

Selected refugee and internally displaced populations in the world today			
source country	refugees	main countries of asylum	internally displaced (range of estimates)
Afghanistan	5,927,000	Iran, Pakistan	2 million
Angola	396,000	Zaire, Zambia	450,000–1.5 million
Burundi	187,000	Tanzania, Rwanda	
Cambodia	354,000	Thailand	
El Salvador*	153,000	Mexico, Honduras	150,000–500,000
Ethiopia	1.1 million	Somalia, The Sudan	700,000–1.5 million
Guatemala	43,000	Mexico	120,000–500,000
Iran	349,000	Iraq, Pakistan	1 million
Iraq	508,000	Iran	500,000–1 million
Lebanon			500,000–800,000
Mozambique	1,147,000	Malawi, Zimbabwe	1.5 million–2 million
Namibia	81,000	Angola, Zambia	
Nicaragua	55,000	Honduras	200,000–350,000
Palestine†	2,273,000	Jordan, Syria, Lebanon, West Bank, Gaza Strip	
Rwanda	218,000	Uganda, Burundi	
Somalia	350,000	Ethiopia	600,000
South Africa	25,000	Angola, Lesotho, Swaziland, Zambia	3.6 million
Sri Lanka	92,000	India	400,000–500,000
Sudan, The	355,000	Ethiopia	2 million–3 million
Uganda	9,000	Kenya, The Sudan	100,000–350,000
U.S.S.R.			156,000
Vietnam	74,000	Malaysia, Hong Kong	
Western Sahara	165,000	Algeria	
Zaire	53,000	Angola, Burundi	

*As of early 1990, all refugees from the three main camps in Honduras had voluntarily repatriated, and the camps were closed.
†The creation of the State of Israel in 1948 led to the displacement of vast numbers of Palestinians.

Source: *World Refugee Survey—1988 in Review.* U.S. Committee for Refugees, Washington, D.C., 1989

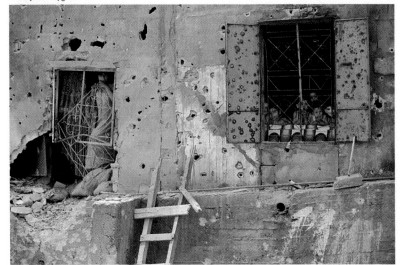

Bullet-sprayed walls frame the countenances of Lebanese civilians who are being driven from their homes to another part of Lebanon by continuing religious strife and civil war. Truly refugees in their own land, they are among the world's 16 million internally displaced people, who by an irony of definition do not qualify for international refugee assistance. Such people often live in crowded camps having little food and virtually no medical facilities.

1988 described in great detail to a U.S. State Department investigator raids on their villages in Mozambique by antigovernment rebels, known as Renamo. Villagers were beaten, mutilated, and raped, and a conservative estimate of 100,000 were murdered for no reason other than their lack of enthusiasm for the rebel cause. More recently, in early 1990, up to 100,000 Liberians fled Nimba county into the neighboring countries of Guinea and Côte d'Ivoire. Refugees reported that Liberian soldiers had brutally and wantonly attacked unarmed civilians following rebel activity in the area. At least 500 civilians were reported to have been killed.

Occasionally, a less developed country's army has invaded a neighbor and imposed its rule by force, creating terror in the general population. This happened when Indonesia illegally annexed the former Portuguese colony of East Timor in 1975. Since then, a protracted guerrilla war, together with famine and disease, has caused an estimated 150,000 deaths and generated thousands of refugees. Even the ICRC has had difficulty in providing medical relief or any other form of assistance to civilians trapped in zones of conflict such as East Timor, where it was denied access entirely for several years. The agency first attempted to gain access to southern Sudan in November 1987; not until December 1988 did both The Sudan's government and the Sudan People's Liberation Army agree to a Red Cross airlift of food into the region. In the meantime, an estimated 250,000 civilians died of starvation. Despite their dire circumstances, refugees are frequently the *fortunate* survivors of organized violence.

The internally displaced

Of the 30 million people today who have been forced from their homes by civil conflict, more than half remain in their own countries. The list of countries with sizable internally displaced populations includes Afghanistan, Angola, El Salvador, Ethiopia, Guatemala, Iran, Iraq, Lebanon, Mozambique, Nicaragua, Somalia, Sri Lanka, The Sudan, Uganda, and the U.S.S.R. Once displaced, these populations often continue to be the targets of violence.

129

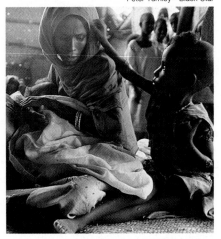

Days of fleeing on foot from an intense clash between Eritrean rebels and the Ethiopian government have left their mark on this gaunt Eritrean mother and daughter. Lack of proper nutrition during the often long and torturous escape from hostilities and then at ill-supplied camps is largely responsible for the extremely high illness and death rates reported among the displaced.

Internally displaced Sudanese, driven to seek refuge in the capital city of Khartoum by civil war in the south, endure the interminable days in communities of makeshift shelters having no clean drinking water, proper sanitation, or organized food-distribution system. Estimates of malnutrition rates in these communities have run as high as 45%. In addition to causing general physical wasting, malnutrition increases vulnerability to common communicable diseases, particularly in children.

For example, the *New York Times* reported that on the night of March 26–27, 1987, a train full of displaced southern Sudanese was attacked at the Ed Da'ein station by hostile militia, who set the train on fire and massacred more than 1,000 people.

Relief programs for the displaced victims of war are often themselves the targets of violence. In southern Sudan a U.S. convoy of food was attacked near the city of Juba in 1987; further attacks occurred throughout 1988. In December 1989 an aircraft flying relief personnel and supplies into southern Sudan was shot down, killing the pilot and three French medical relief workers. During the past five years, relief workers have been kidnapped by government or rebel forces in Afghanistan, Mozambique, Somalia, The Sudan, and Ethiopia.

The internally displaced often congregate in crowded, ill-supplied camps, where food is scarce and health care almost nonexistent. Where mortality rates among the displaced have been documented, they have been found to be much higher than the death rates for the nondisplaced in those countries. For example, the U.S. Centers for Disease Control (CDC) reported a death rate of 120 per 1,000 population per month in a camp in the Southern Kordofan province of The Sudan during July 1988, compared with the usual death rate for nondisplaced Sudanese of 1.6 per 1,000, as reported by UNICEF. This rate was the highest reported for any civilian camp population in the past 20 years and, if it had been sustained for even less than a year, would have resulted in the extinction of the affected population. Average monthly death rates of 12 per 1,000 were sustained in seven other displaced persons camps in the Southern Darfur province of The Sudan during the first half of 1988.

Other displaced populations, such as Ethiopians in Koram in 1985 and Mozambicans in Gaza province, have experienced abnormally high death rates: 70 per 1,000 and 8 per 1,000 per month, respectively. The most common causes of death reported in these camps have been measles, diarrhea, pneumonia, and meningitis. In each of these populations, the

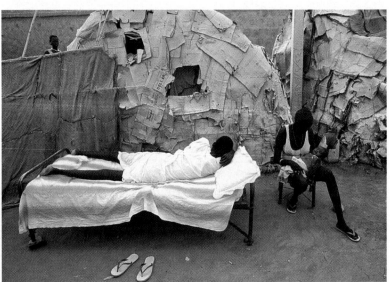

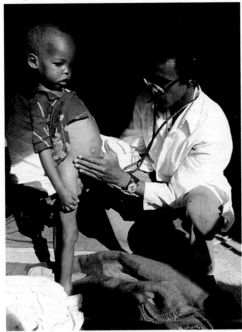

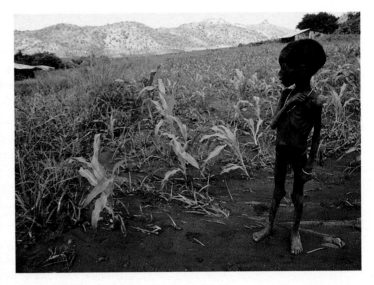

The protein-energy malnutrition (PEM) so common among the displaced can take on various appearances. Certain high-starch, low-protein diets produce wasting plus abdominal bloating, called kwashiorkor (left). The major form of PEM in young children, however, is marasmus (above).

underlying cause of most deaths was most likely malnutrition. The prevalence rates of acute malnutrition measured in children one to five years old in the Sudanese camps already mentioned ranged between 25 and 43%. Malnutrition rates among displaced persons in Mozambique and Ethiopia have ranged between 20 and 70%.

Malnutrition: the root of most health problems. When deprived of food, humans develop protein-energy malnutrition (PEM), or starvation. Malnourished individuals generally show signs of weight loss, weakness, apathy, and depression. Symptoms may progress to cachexia (general physical wasting), diarrhea, anorexia (loss of appetite), immobility, and finally death. Edema (severe bloating caused by fluid retention) is rarely seen in association with total starvation but is commonly seen with semistarvation. While the predominant form of PEM affecting young children is marasmus (wasting only), there are circumstances that can produce kwashiorkor (wasting plus edema), such as was seen so commonly in Biafra in 1969 among young children, whose major energy source was cassava, a starchy food that provides virtually no protein.

PEM affects persons with the highest energy and protein requirements—infants, young children, pregnant and lactating women, the chronically ill, and the elderly. Nutritional status is measured in young children by certain indexes, or combinations of measurements, which are compared with those of a reference population that has been established by the World Health Organization (WHO). A weight-for-height index is the one that most sensitively detects recent PEM (or wasting) in children and is most often used in overall surveys of the nutritional status of populations. Only children under five years of age or less than 115 centimeters (46 inches) in height are included in samples because genetic factors affect height after age five.

Displaced infants, young children, and pregnant and lactating women are among those hit hardest by PEM because of their high protein and energy requirements. Symptoms begin with weight loss, weakness, and apathy and then progress to general wasting, diarrhea, and immobility—until death finally comes.

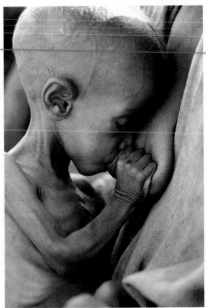

131

The prevalence of acute PEM in nondisplaced, non-famine-affected children in the Third World is usually between 2 and 3%, a rate that is not much different from the prevalence of acute malnutrition in developed countries. In displaced populations in the Third World, however, the prevalence of acute PEM is often very high.

Where less developed countries differ greatly from industrial societies is in the prevalence of "chronic" PEM, or long-standing failure of growth (sometimes known as stunting), which is assessed by an index that measures height-for-age. The prevalence of chronic PEM in developed countries is about 2–3%; in nonrefugee Third World countries, chronic malnutrition affects between 20 and 30% of the populations. Not surprisingly, when Third World chronic PEM victims suddenly become refugees, the rate of chronic PEM soars, and so too do death rates.

Malnutrition among displaced persons is not confined to camps. More than one million Sudanese displaced by the war in the south found their way to the capital city of Khartoum, where they lived in makeshift dwellings without clean drinking water or proper sanitation. No organized food-distribution system was established. Malnutrition rates in these communities were as high as 45%, and it is presumed that mortality was high, although death rates could not be reliably documented. Malnutrition increases the vulnerability of children to common communicable diseases like measles, diarrhea, pneumonia, and malaria; it also increases the fatality rate in these diseases. Because in most cases the root cause of the health problems of displaced persons is lack of food, the challenge to the international community is to find ways of getting adequate food to and other basic needs met for people trapped in zones of conflict, where existing mechanisms for relief and protection are sorely inadequate.

Flight to freedom

The sometimes long and dangerous flight of the refugee takes many forms. Perhaps the most familiar to Western observers have been the dramatic leaps across barbed wire and massive stone walls. Who can forget the images of an East German jumping to freedom in the early days of the Berlin Wall? Or the terrible flight from Pol Pot's Cambodia portrayed in the acclaimed film *The Killing Fields*?

Much less visible have been the escape routes of millions of other refugees. The mountain-dwelling Hmong of northern Laos, for example, walked for days across mountain ranges and through valleys riddled with land mines and infested by malaria-carrying mosquitoes to eventual "haven" in Thailand. Both Hmong and Cambodian refugees arriving in Thailand suffered from exceedingly high rates of malaria. During the first 10 days of their stay in the Sakaeo camp, approximately 1% of the Cambodian refugees died, most from malaria contracted during their escape.

Many of the Tigre who fled war and famine in their northern Ethiopian province in 1985 walked for up to 30 days, mostly at night in order to avoid aerial bombing raids, to reach the camps of eastern Sudan. An indigenous agency, the Relief Society of Tigrai, attempted to distribute food to the fleeing refugees; however, these food supplies were inadequate. Upon arrival

Health workers measure a young displaced child against a weight-for-height index chart in order to evaluate nutritional state. In children under five years of age, this type of index has proved to be the most sensitive indicator of recent PEM. Acute PEM, defined as weight-for-height that is less than 80% of the median of a reference population, is often very high in displaced populations in the Third World compared with nondisplaced Third World children not affected by famine.

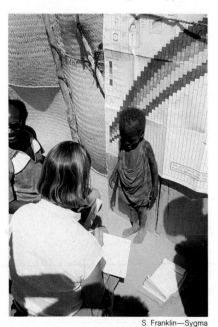

S. Franklin—Sygma

in The Sudan, over 30% of the refugees had acute PEM. Their weakened physical state undoubtedly contributed to the high death rates among these refugees in Sudanese camps.

One of the worst experiences of flight in recent history was that of some 513,000 Vietnamese boat people, who suffered repeated attacks by pirates en route to Malaysia, Thailand, Indonesia, and other Southeast Asian nations. In addition, the refugees had to contend with unpredictable storms in the South China Sea, which often caused flimsy boats to be swamped and overturned. It will probably never be known how many perished at sea during these voyages. Like the internally displaced, the refugee in flight is largely inaccessible to relief assistance. A few heroic agencies hired boats and roamed the seas looking for Vietnamese refugees in danger; however, such interventions have been rare.

Survival in country of first asylum

It is in the refugee camps established by international agencies in the so-called countries of first asylum that the conditions of refugees have been best documented. These camps are largely open to relief workers and are often visited by journalists, international bureaucrats, and elected officials. Nevertheless, few reports on the health problems of refugees had been published until recently. Most health care in refugee camps has been provided by individuals—motivated by humanitarianism—who have worked for a few months as volunteers. While many volunteer relief workers have been skilled and dedicated, their relative inexperience and their short stays have resulted in rapid turnovers with relatively little documentation of their experiences. Given the lack of systematic studies and of published medical reports, what was learned by medical relief workers often needed to be relearned by successors.

During the past five years, the situation has changed somewhat. Several agencies have made the study of refugee health problems a priority, including the CDC, the Refugee Policy Group based in Washington, D.C., the Refugee Studies Program of the University of Oxford, the London School

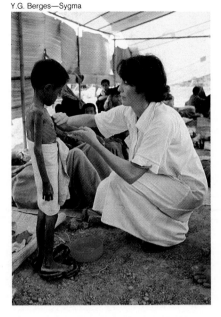

Most health care in refugee camps in countries of first asylum is given by humanitarian volunteers who spend a few months as relief workers before returning to their regular jobs. Until recently this rapid turnover, together with a lack of systematic studies and reports, had resulted in poor documentation of refugee health problems and worker experiences. Since the mid-1980s several agencies based in the U.S. and Europe have given the study of refugee health care priority attention.

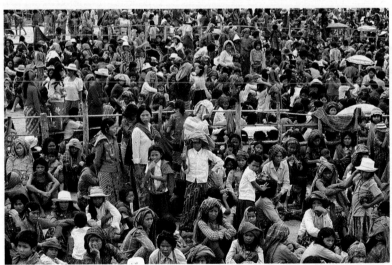

Because the majority of the world's refugees have been granted asylum by poor, less developed nations, exceedingly large and crowded refugee camps, such as this one in Thailand, have become more common. Many camps are located in remote regions of the host countries, far from permanent water supplies and served by inadequate road systems.

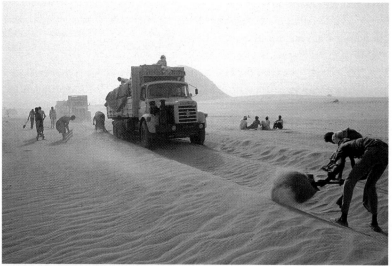

Workers struggle with The Sudan's blowing desert sands to clear a path for food-laden trucks destined for a distant refugee camp. Even when food supplies are forthcoming from the international community, delivering them when and where they are needed is often hindered by such obstacles as poor roads, shortages of trucks and fuel, and inadequate motor maintenance support.

of Tropical Medicine and Hygiene, and the Paris-based Epicentre. In addition, UNHCR, which had been concerned primarily with protection issues related to refugees, has created a Technical Support Services unit in order to reinforce its ability to provide high-quality medical care and nutritional rehabilitation to these populations in need.

Camp conditions. During the last two decades, because the majority of the world's refugees have been granted first asylum by poor, less developed countries, the environmental conditions of most refugee camps have worsened. Many camps are located in remote, arid regions of host countries, where permanent and abundant water supplies cannot be ensured, where roads are poor, and where a reliable political and logistic infrastructure is frequently absent. Some refugee camps have been exceedingly large and difficult to manage. In Thailand (1980), The Sudan (1985), and Ethiopia (1988), camps had populations of more than 100,000. Camps of more than 20,000 people are quite common.

Food and water. The two basic needs of dependent refugees—food and water—have become increasingly difficult to provide in adequate quantity and quality. In 1988, for example, the Ethiopian government placed more than 200,000 Somali refugees in the Hartisheik camp, more than 50 kilometers (30 miles) from the nearest natural water source. Water had to be transported daily by a fleet of donated, unsuitable trucks over rough dirt roads. For much of 1989, refugees were forced to subsist on an average of three to four liters (one liter is roughly equal to one quart) of water per person per day—about one-quarter of the minimum UN standard.

When refugee camps are located many kilometers from the nearest natural water source, simply providing water to these remote sites can become an overwhelming task. In some camps refugees are forced to survive on a fraction of the minimum standard set by the UN.

Even if the international community pledges sufficient quantities of food and fluids for refugees, the obstacles to regular and timely delivery of sustenance supplies to these remote camps are awesome. Pledges do not always materialize in a timely fashion; cargo ships are not always available; ports are often ill-equipped to handle large food shipments; and customs clearance can be delayed by bureaucratic red tape. Beyond the port, there is usually a shortage of both suitable trucks and fuel for delivering the food—

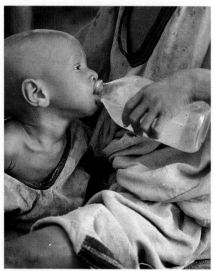

134

usually over very poor roads—to remote camps. The resultant frequent breakdowns overload the poorly trained mechanics, who have no access to spare parts. Unfortunately, this desperate situation is often exacerbated by governments that insist on donating surplus food that is either nutritionally or culturally unsuitable for the needs of the refugees.

The quality and quantity of food supplied to refugees vary with the location and natural resources of the host country and the perceived strategic significance of that country to Western donors. For example, in eastern Thailand in 1979, an adequate food ration was promptly supplied to Cambodian refugees both because Thailand is rich in locally grown food and because donors came quickly to the aid of this country, which was thought to be on the front line of defense against Communism in Southeast Asia. In contrast, inadequate food rations were supplied for the first eight months of the relief operations for Ethiopian refugees in the impoverished African countries of Somalia (1980) and The Sudan (1985), whose public profile and strategic importance on the global scale were deemed much lower. Of the major refugee emergencies of the past decade, the early response in terms of food supply was satisfactory in Pakistan (1979–80), Thailand (1979), Honduras (1980), and Malawi (1987); it was quite inadequate in Somalia (1979–80), eastern and western Sudan (1985), and Ethiopia (1987–88). Six months after the relief program was launched in Somalia in 1980, refugees received general rations containing between 1,000 and 1,200 kilocalories per person per day. The minimum daily refugee ration should contain at least 1,900 kilocalories, as well as adequate protein and micronutrients such as vitamins A, B, and C, iron, folic acid, and iodine.

Death rates. Considering the inadequate food and water and the crowded conditions in many of the world's refugee camps, it is little wonder that death rates have sometimes been unusually high. Refugee camps in Thailand (1979), Somalia (1980), and The Sudan (1985) have recorded death rates during the first month of operation that were more than 20 times the rates reported for the population in the host country. In Bangladesh (1978), Pakistan (1979), Honduras (1980), and Ethiopia (1988–89), death rates have been two to three times the expected death rates for nonrefugees. In the past 12 years, only in Malawi have refugee death rates been comparable to those of the rest of the region.

The highest death toll has occurred in refugee camps where acute malnutrition rates have been high. Data from camps in Ethiopia, Somalia, and The Sudan indicate that the highest death rates were in children less than five years of age—the segment of the population that is most vulnerable to insufficient nutrition. Although sex-specific death rates have rarely been recorded in these camps, there is anecdotal evidence that among adults, women suffer disproportionately high mortality from causes such as anemia and pregnancy-related problems.

Diseases. Although malnutrition is often the underlying cause, the immediate cause of death in refugee camps is usually a common communicable disease. Most lethal among these are measles and diarrhea. During the emergency phase of refugee relief operations in Thailand, Somalia, and The Sudan, between 50 and 80% of all deaths were caused by either measles,

Death rates in refugee populations (per 1,000 per month)		
	refugee deaths	nonrefugee deaths (host country)
Burmese in Bangladesh (1978)	6.3	1.7
Cambodians in Thailand (1979)	31.9	0.7
Ethiopians in Somalia (1980)	30.4	1.8
Ethiopians in The Sudan (1985)	16.2 (8 camps)	1.7
Chadians in The Sudan (1985)	24.0	1.7
Mozambicans in Malawi* (1987)	10.0	16.0

*rate for children under age five

Compiled by Michael J. Toole and Ronald J. Waldman, Centers for Disease Control, Atlanta, Ga.

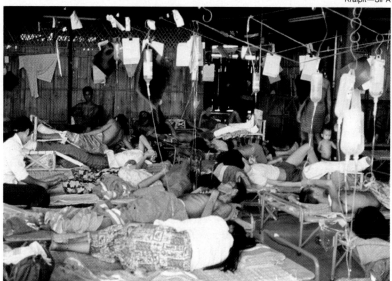

Crowding and malnutrition combine to transform common communicable diseases such as measles, diarrhea, pneumonia, and malaria into devastating epidemics and to make them the usual immediate cause of death in refugee camps. Outbreaks of less common diseases including cholera, meningitis, hepatitis, and relapsing fever also add to the burden of the camps' already overstrained medical facilities.

diarrhea, pneumonia, or malaria. These diseases are already common in the less developed world; it is the high fatality rate suffered by nutritionally compromised refugee populations that renders them unique.

Measles is an especially lethal disease in refugee camps. In Wad Kowli, a camp in The Sudan with a population of approximately 85,000 refugees, an estimated 2,800 children died during a three-month period in early 1985; almost 2,000 of these deaths were reported due to measles.

There have also been reports of epidemics of less common communicable diseases such as cholera, meningitis, hepatitis, and relapsing fever in refugee camps. An outbreak of cholera in one refugee camp in Somalia in 1985 caused more than 1,000 deaths, killing one-quarter of those who experienced clinical symptoms. Enterically transmitted non-A, non-B hepatitis, also called hepatitis C—a viral disease—made its first appearance in Africa among refugees in Ethiopia and Somalia. This variety of hepatitis has a selectively high fatality rate in pregnant women.

Another rare disease that has made a significant appearance in some refugee camps is the ancient scourge of sailors—scurvy—caused by a deficiency of vitamin C in the diet. Not seen in large numbers since World War I, scurvy appeared in Somali refugee camps in 1982 when refugees were deprived of their traditional source of vitamin C, camel's milk. Initially, they exchanged part of their rations for fruits and vegetables in the local market. When the market was suddenly closed for political reasons, however, thousands developed symptoms of scurvy (*e.g.,* spongy gums, loosening of teeth, and bleeding into the skin and mucous membranes). Since then, further outbreaks of scurvy have occurred in other camps in Somalia (1983), The Sudan (1985), and Ethiopia (1989).

"Compassion fatigue." Following the emergency period (which may last from a month to a year, depending on the adequacy of relief efforts), mortality rates begin to approach normal rates for the region. Nevertheless, refugees continue to be vulnerable to disruptions of the relief system.

Floods may cut access to roads for weeks at a time; wells may dry up; and medical supplies may run out. It is after the emergency phase, when the initial publicity fades, that "compassion fatigue" may set in. Volunteers return to their jobs; voluntary organizations find it difficult to raise money; and governments face new crises in other parts of the world. One report from Somalia described high malnutrition rates of between 20 and 25% in five Somali refugee camps in 1988—eight years after they had been opened. Epidemics may still occur in established camps since they may remain densely populated and sanitation facilities may still be minimal. The previously mentioned outbreak of cholera in Somalia in 1985 occurred five years after the initial influx of refugees.

A unique relief effort. Relief programs for refugees have, at times, been based on expediency and the easy availability of resources to the donors, not always on the real needs of the refugee population. Some relief programs have been dominated by the establishment of hospitals and clinics (with sophisticated equipment) staffed by expatriate specialists. Simple, inexpensive lifesaving measures directed at the more common causes of refugee mortality—such as measles immunization, treatment of diarrhea with oral rehydration salts, and the control of other common communicable diseases such as malaria—have not been aggressively implemented.

One successful health program for 700,000 refugees in Somalia achieved sustained improvement in health status by emphasizing preventive interventions, standardizing treatment protocols, implementing an essential drugs policy, and training more than 3,000 refugees as community health workers. Although death rates had been high during the emergency phase of this program (1979–80), the formation of a specialized refugee health unit within the Somali Ministry of Health toward the end of 1980 promoted a united approach to health care in the camps by the 20 or more foreign, voluntary agencies operating in the country. Priorities were established on the basis of regularly collected data on nutrition, mortality, and morbidity. The mark of this program's success was that good health parameters were sustained in this refugee population long after most expatriate relief workers had withdrawn. The program operated successfully until 1988, when it was seriously disrupted by a civil war in the north of Somalia.

The following measures are the very minimum that should be required of relief agencies to ensure prevention of excess mortality in refugee populations: the provision of adequate food and clean water, sanitation, and measles immunization; prompt prevention of dehydration with oral rehydration salts; and effective treatment of malaria and pneumonia where these are epidemiologically indicated. Supplementary feeding for malnourished children, adequate shelter, a health information system, and an effective outreach program that provides access to vital health services all will increase the effectiveness of these interventions. The provision of an adequate family food ration, as described above, is probably the single most important intervention to sustain the good health of refugees. Supplementary feeding for malnourished children is not intended to replace this ration; the goal of this procedure is to provide children who are identified as malnourished with an extra daily supplement of food in order that they might regain their

Major causes of death in refugee camps

Somalia: seven camps in Gedo region
(January 1980)

The Sudan: Wad Kowli camp
(February 1985)

Somalia: Hartisheik camp hospital, children under age five
(January–November 1989)

- measles
- diarrhea
- pneumonia
- malnutrition
- malaria
- fever of unknown origin
- tuberculosis
- hepatitis
- other

Sources: (Top and center) International Rescue Committee/ Centers for Disease Control; (bottom) Administration for Refugee Affairs/Ministry of Health, Government of Ethiopia

137

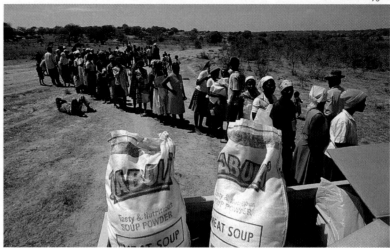

Refugees in Mozambique line up at a food-distribution site. Provision of an adequate family food ration—i.e., food suitable nutritionally and culturally as well as in sufficient quantity—is probably the single most important measure that relief agencies can undertake to sustain the good health of refugees.

normal weight. Supplementary food is usually cooked and served on the spot at a special center; it consists of high-energy and high-protein mixtures of corn-soya porridge, milk, cooking oil, and vitamin supplements.

"Trapped" for years. After the acute emergency phase, when survival is the priority, there may be severe psychological problems as refugees become more aware of the hopelessness of the situation. Several authors have described patterns of apathy, dependence, and depression among refugees who are trapped in camps for many years. Prolonged stays in camps are not unusual; most Afghan refugees have been in camps in Pakistan or Iran for 10 years, and hundreds of thousands of Ethiopian refugees have been in Sudanese or Somali camps for 13 years. A whole generation of Palestinians has been born in the camps of the Middle East.

"Durable solutions"

The three so-called durable solutions to the plight of refugees that are sought by the international community, led by UNHCR, are local settlement, voluntary repatriation, or resettlement in third countries. Unlike the refugees from Eastern Europe, those in Africa and Asia have very little hope of being resettled in another country or of attaining a durable solution. In 1987 only 1.5% of the world's refugees were voluntarily repatriated, 12% successfully settled in the country of first asylum, and 1% resettled in a third country.

Forced repatriation: an illegal "solution." Despite the guarantees outlined by international conventions, a fourth, illegal solution is sometimes enacted by the governments of countries where refugees have sought asylum. This is forced repatriation, termed *refoulement* under international law.

Unfortunately, this desperate measure was taken as recently as December 1989 by the British government when 51 Vietnamese refugees were removed by force from makeshift camps in Hong Kong and flown back to Vietnam against the will of both the refugees and the Vietnamese government. An earlier example of *refoulement* was the large numbers of Cambodians forced back by Thai authorities between 1975 and 1980. Thailand was also accused of forcibly repatriating Burmese students who

138

had fled the violent suppression of the democracy movement in Burma (now Myanmar) in 1988. In Africa an estimated 2,000 Mozambican refugees were sent back monthly to Mozambique by South African authorities in 1987. In Central America the Honduran government reportedly forced 300 Nicaraguan asylum seekers to return across the border in 1988 in an area said to be littered with land mines.

An even more severe form of *refoulement* has been practiced by some Southeast Asian nations—the practice of turning back refugees as they arrive in the country of asylum. This was a common practice during the early 1980s, when countries like Malaysia prevented Vietnamese refugees from landing their boats on beaches. Although the consequences of this practice have not been well documented, it is likely that many of these boats succumbed to further attacks by pirates and that many lives were lost as a result. The international community has been creative in its attempts to avoid these problems, mainly through what has been termed the Orderly Departure Program (ODP), by which Western nations—with the cooperation of the Vietnamese government—have agreed to accept immigrants directly from Vietnam. Since its inception in June 1979, the ODP has enabled 150,000 Vietnamese to migrate safely and avoid the dangers of clandestine flight, piracy on the high seas, and possible rejection by countries in the region. More than 68,000 of these have gone to the United States, with the rest divided among 30 other countries.

More common than the *refoulement* of large groups of refugees, however, is the denial of asylum to individual refugees and their consequent deportation. This became increasingly common in Western Europe and the United States during the 1980s. The United States, for example, approved only 25% of asylum requests between 1980 and 1989. Swiss authorities granted asylum to a mere 4.3% of applicants during the first four months of 1989, less than one-half of the 9% approval rate in 1988. Selective application of refugee status to different nationalities is often based on political biases that override humanitarian considerations. Thus, despite the dismal

To the three internationally acceptable long-term solutions to the plight of refugees—local resettlement, voluntary repatriation, and resettlement in third countries—is sometimes added a fourth, illegal measure: forced repatriation, or refoulement. *Recently the British government in Hong Kong was accused of* refoulement *when it forcibly returned to Vietnam 51 of more than 40,000 boat people who, because they had arrived in Hong Kong after a mid-1988 cutoff date, were being treated as illegal immigrants until they could prove they had fled political or religious persecution. In early 1990 Hong Kong housed about 55,000 Vietnamese who had sailed from their homeland across the South China Sea in flimsy open boats (below left). At a Hong Kong detention center (below), refugees protest government intentions for more forced repatriations.*

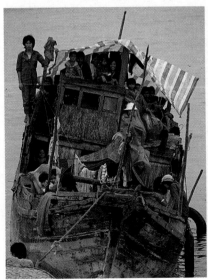

Christopher Morris—Black Star

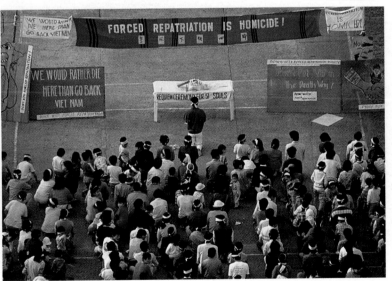

Marc Fallander—SIPA

United Nations High
Commissioner for Refugees; photograph, A. Billard

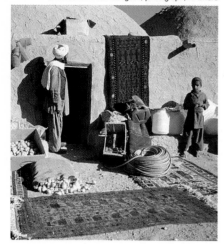

Most Afghans who have sought refuge in Iran have been there more than a decade. Although today many are at least housed in permanent villages (above), they share the fate of the great majority of the world's refugees in not having been given rights to settle locally in the country of first asylum.

human rights record of successive Haitian governments, the United States refuses to grant refugee status to Haitians who flee in large numbers, often risking their lives in dangerous sea voyages.

Local settlement. Although many of the Afghan refugees in Iran and Mozambican refugees in Malawi are at least temporarily housed in villages, very few of the world's refugees have been granted permanent rights to settle in the country of first asylum. Most of those who have settled locally are in Africa. An estimated 200,000 African refugees are now self-sufficient in the country in which they first sought refuge. Most of these are in Burundi, Rwanda, Uganda, Zaire, and Tanzania.

Voluntary repatriation. Most of the successful voluntary repatriations have also taken place in Africa, including the massive repatriation of Zimbabwean refugees from Mozambique following the end of the war for independence in Zimbabwe in 1980. In 1987 and 1988, 86,000 Ugandan refugees were repatriated from The Sudan, and 5,000 Ethiopian refugees returned home from Djibouti. In 1988 successful voluntary repatriations included 53,400 refugees from Rwanda to Burundi only months after their arrival in Rwanda. During 1989, in a widely praised operation, 41,000 Namibian refugees were repatriated from 41 different countries (the majority from Angola and Zambia) prior to a UN-supervised plebiscite in Namibia. Currently, the Somali and Ethiopian governments, together with UNHCR, are planning the repatriation of up to 400,000 refugees from the Ogaden region of Ethiopia, who are residing in 35 camps in Somalia.

In Central America, however, the repatriation of Guatemalan refugees from Mexico initiated in 1986 has been only partially successful because most refugees fear forced relocation into so-called model villages created for security reasons by the Guatemalan government. These villages resemble the "strategic hamlets" created in other countries faced with guerrilla war, such as Vietnam and preindependence Zimbabwe; inhabitants face

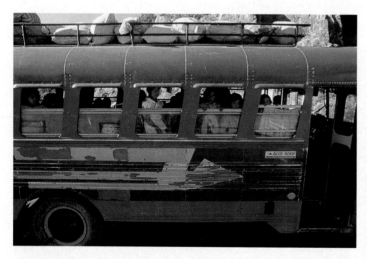

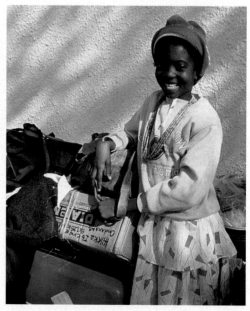

A busload of Guatemalan refugees who have spent years in Mexico (above) and an obviously happy Namibian returnee to Ovamboland (right) begin the process of voluntary repatriation in their homelands.

United Nations High Commissioner for Refugees; photographs, (left) D. Bregnard; (right) L. Aström

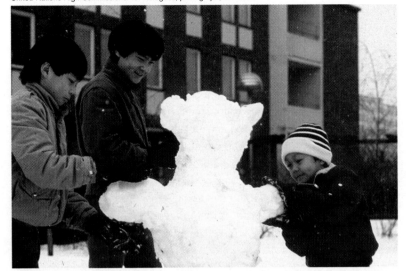

Vietnamese refugee children experience snow for the first time in their new home in Sweden. Fewer than 1% of the world's refugees, the majority from camps in Southeast Asia, are granted permanent residence in a third country each year. On a per capita basis, Sweden ranks near the top among Western nations willing to accept refugees for resettlement.

severe restriction of movement and constant, intrusive surveillance by police—clearly not a climate conducive to leaving the safe haven of Mexico's refugee camps. In Asia small numbers of Laotian refugees have returned home voluntarily from Thailand (3,200 between 1980 and 1989), and approximately 2,000 refugees in Papua New Guinea have returned home to the Irian Jaya province of Indonesia since 1986.

Third-country resettlement. Third-country resettlement is offered to fewer than 1% of the world's refugees each year. The majority of those who successfully apply for resettlement have been in camps in Southeast Asia. For example, between 1975 and 1986 a total of 1,508,500 Indochinese refugees were resettled, the majority in various Western countries. Smaller numbers of refugees from Afghanistan, Ethiopia, Central America, and the Middle East have been accepted for resettlement. The U.S. has accepted approximately one-half of those refugees resettled during the past decade, while on a per capita basis Australia has absorbed the highest number of refugees, followed by Canada, Sweden, and Denmark.

Health of resettled refugees. There is an extensive literature describing the health problems of resettled refugees. Most reports, however, describe exotic illnesses in individual refugees, focusing on the occurrence of diseases that are endemic in the refugee's country of origin but are generally quite rare in the country of resettlement (including various intestinal parasites, leprosy, malaria, hepatitis B, and certain nutritional deficiencies such as beri beri). A high prevalence of dental and gingival problems has been reported among refugees in Australia. While newly diagnosed tuberculosis is more common in resettled refugees than in other population groups, most countries now screen incoming refugees for tuberculosis and usually administer treatment to those who are infected prior to their departure from the country of first asylum.

The U.S. and Australia now screen refugees for the AIDS virus, with the former refusing to admit those who test positive. By the beginning of 1990, only one refugee accepted for settlement in the U.S. had been found

Demonstrators in New York City protest against U.S. government actions that appear to imply that the spread of AIDS is associated with entire ethnic groups rather than with the behavior of individuals. Despite blatant human rights violations by successive Haitian governments, the U.S. has continued to refuse refugee status to Haitians who flee in large numbers, a policy that some blame on prejudiced views that Haitians as a whole are illiterate, promiscuous AIDS carriers. The U.S. has also pursued a policy of mandatory screening of all refugees for AIDS and of refusing those who test positive, causing concern that the discriminatory nature of such screening will encourage even greater restrictions on refugee movement and settlement.

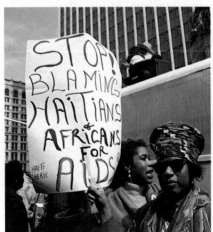

to be positive for this virus. There is increasing concern that the inherently discriminatory nature of such screening will result in the development of more formidable obstacles to the free movement of refugees.

One mysterious medical condition that seems to affect primarily young, male Southeast Asian refugees, in particular the Hmong from Laos, has been described in the U.S. This fatal condition, called sudden unexplained death syndrome (SUDS), strikes apparently healthy men during sleep. Death is preceded by a telltale gurgling and labored breathing; it is suspected that an irregular heartbeat affects the blood supply to the brain. Death, as the name indicates, is sudden, and no traces of drugs or signs of abnormal organs have been found at autopsy. Since 1980 some 120 cases have been reported. The cause of the syndrome remains a mystery.

There have been, in addition, numerous reports of various psychological problems related to the act of resettlement encountered by refugees. For example, a Danish psychiatric journal reported on a study that found the incidence and prevalence of paranoid disorders among Hmong in Minnesota to be high compared with other groups. Although most of the 100 refugees followed had no or mild paranoid symptoms (suspiciousness and mistrust), a few had severe symptoms (so-called ideas of reference—*i.e.,* assuming words and actions of others refer to oneself) and paranoid delusions and hallucinations. Although paranoia has been recognized as a special problem among refugees, it is not known if this vulnerability to paranoia is a premigration or postmigration phenomenon or if it is caused by genetic or organic factors.

An American study found that delusions of contagion (an obsessive fear of repeated infection by contagious diseases) were common, particularly in Hmong psychiatric patients. Two other American studies have linked the high incidence of depressive illness and psychosomatic disorders in refugees with exposure to violence and trauma. One of these studies found that 30% of 404 Southeast Asian refugees seeking psychiatric help reported specific traumatic experiences either in their homeland or during their escape. The frequent reference to Hmong refugees in U.S. reports may

A headstone marks the grave of a 48-year-old male Southeast Asian refugee whose unexpected death from an undetermined cause occurred as he slept. Called sudden unexplained death syndrome (SUDS), the condition that killed him has plagued Southeast Asian immigrants to the U.S. since at least the late 1970s, claiming some 120 victims— primarily young Laotian men of the Hmong ethnic group. Though the nature of SUDS remains a mystery, investigators have suggested that latent, possibly hereditary heart abnormalities coupled with the stressful "culture shock" of resettlement may be responsible.

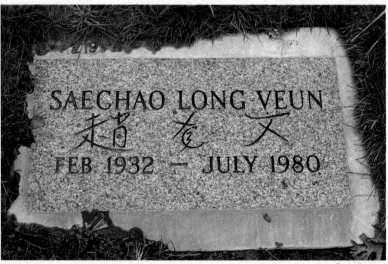

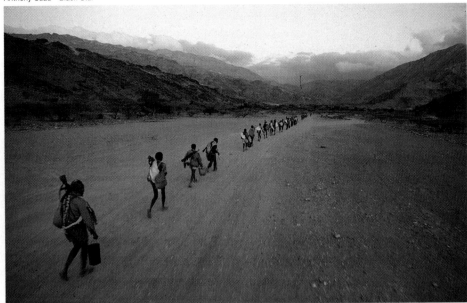

reflect the difficulty that this Laotian ethnic group has had in adjusting to life in the modern, urban United States. Several authors have described the isolation, language problems, unemployment, and cultural misunderstandings that the Hmong have encountered in their resettlement in the U.S.

Unacceptable suffering

Movements of large populations from their homes to areas where they become dependent upon external assistance have become a fact of modern existence. During the past 20 years, several refugee movements managed to catch the eye of the public for a few months, resulting in the provision, at least temporarily, of basic commodities and services. Still, experience has taught that caring for people who are displaced by violence or by environmental factors, regardless of their place of origin, should become a planned activity for governments and multinational agencies, not one that depends on the serendipitous presence of aggressive (and perhaps sympathetic) journalists. The health risks to which refugees are exposed have by now been identified and described. They result in levels of suffering and mortality that far surpass those that should be tolerated by the global community. Interventions can and should be designed to meet the needs of these populations. Contingency plans should be developed to allow relief experts to respond rapidly, providing adequate food and water and appropriate medical care to refugee populations. It is especially urgent that the same protection be provided to internally displaced persons as is already guaranteed to refugees who cross international borders.

It would be naive to think that the global conflicts that create refugees will end tomorrow. One of the few remaining uncertainties in the field of refugee health is when and where the next major crisis will occur; one of the certainties is that a next crisis, unfortunately, will occur. With hope, the world will be equipped to meet it.

That populations will continue to be forced from their homes is a virtual certainty. In recent decades numerous acute refugee problems have caught the public eye for a few months, resulting in initial outpourings of supplies, medicine, and services. All too often, however, "compassion fatigue" has set in after the emergency period, and volunteers and money have faded away while the needs of the refugees have remained. Such experience shows that ensuring the future survival of the world's displaced people— those both within and outside their home country's borders—cannot be left to the whims of sympathy and publicity but must become an anticipated, planned activity for national governments and international bodies.

143

SPIN-OFFS FROM SPACE:
Health on Earth

by Doris J. Rouse, Ph.D.

The stunning successes of the United States space program, scarcely imagined three decades ago, could have been achieved only through major technological developments. Teaming up with industry and the scientific community, the National Aeronautics and Space Administration (NASA) has sent men to the Moon and safely returned them, placed automated laboratories on Mars, begun a systematic exploration of the solar system utilizing planetary probes, and, through the space shuttle program, promised access to realms once only imagined in science fiction. The shuttle has made possible the current capability to launch, retrieve, and service sophisticated payloads and—in its unique microgravity environment—to conduct commercial research that is important to industry and medicine. During the next decade, the shuttle will afford construction of the *Freedom* space station, gateway to planetary exploration and a permanent platform for research.

The diverse and abundant new technologies that have been required for these mission successes—which began on Jan. 31, 1958, when the U.S. sent up its first Earth satellite, Explorer I—continue to be put to use on Earth. The unprecedented pace of technological change has paid dividends in many fields; medicine is one of the beneficiaries.

". . . for the benefit of all mankind"

With these words from the chartering legislation for NASA, the Space Act of 1958 mandated the transfer of technology from the space program to the nonaerospace community. In response to this mandate, NASA established the Technology Utilization Program, with offices at NASA headquarters in Washington, D.C., and each of the NASA field centers located throughout the country. Recognizing the importance of direct contact with potential users of the technology, the Technology Utilization Program established a nationwide network to assist industry and public-sector organizations in accessing and effectively adapting aerospace technology to meet their requirements.

To promote the secondary application of aerospace technology in medicine, NASA works with universities and medical schools, hospitals and medical centers, pharmaceutical manufacturers and companies that

Doris J. Rouse, Ph.D., is Director of the National Aeronautics and Space Administration's Technology Application Team and Director of the Center for Technology Applications, Research Triangle Institute, Research Triangle Park, North Carolina.

Illustration by Kathryn Diffley

144

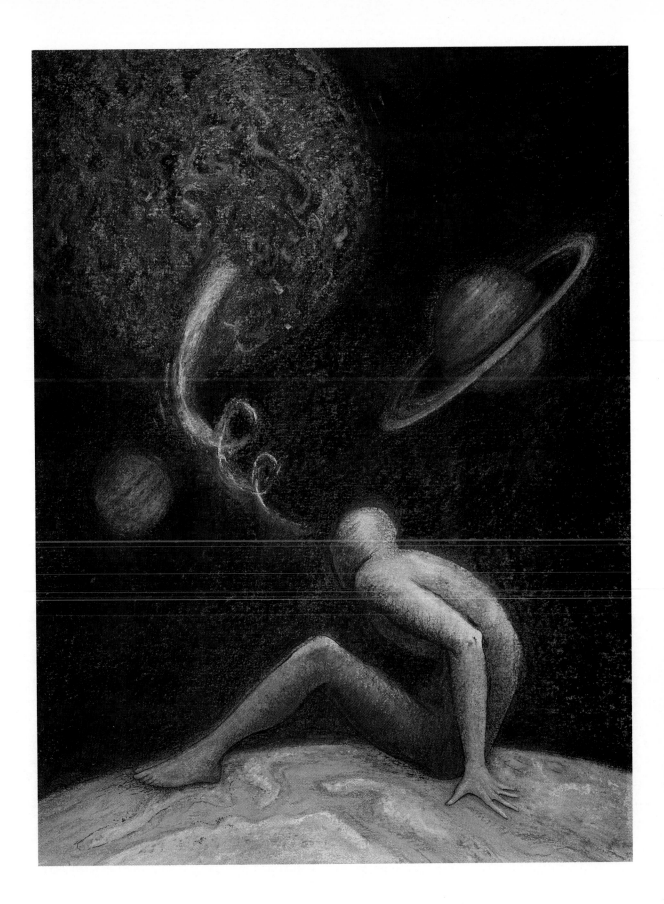

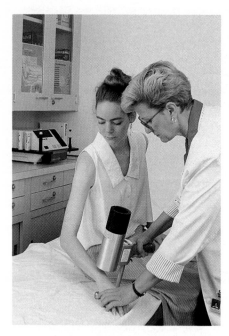

After NASA scientists discovered that some galaxies and stars emit X-rays, they were able to enhance the relatively low levels of radiation from these faraway celestial bodies and develop imaging techniques with wide applicability. One direct spin-off is the LIXI Imaging Scope, a battery-powered, hand-held, portable X-ray device, here being used to examine a patient's injured wrist. With less than 1% of the radiation of conventional medical X-ray machines, the instrument produces a sharp, instant image, making it a remarkably handy tool for immediate assessment of sprained or fractured limbs.

LIXI Imaging Scope provided by Lixi, Inc.;
photograph, Cathy Melloan

produce medical devices, and federal agencies such as the National Institutes of Health and the Veterans Administration. The Technology Utilization Program identifies important technology needs, then matches those needs with technologies and expertise available at the various NASA field centers. Many technologies can be transferred directly; others require adaptive engineering to rechannel them from their aerospace use to an appropriate application in medicine.

Accomplishments of this program in its mission to transfer aerospace technology compare admirably with NASA's successful exploration of space. More than 30,000 secondary applications—or spin-offs—have been developed to improve the quality of health care in the United States and throughout the world. Spin-offs have ranged from complex diagnostic systems to consumer health products that are used every day around the globe. Collectively, these spin-offs represent a significant return on the national investment in aerospace research and development in terms of human health gains. Indeed, the down-to-earth dividends reaped from the Apollo missions alone were characterized by one news magazine as "the best return on an investment since Leonardo da Vinci bought himself a sketch pad."

Windows into the body: innovations in diagnostics

Technologies originally developed to monitor orbiting spacecraft or scan distant planets take on new significance in their application to the improvement of noninvasive medical diagnostics.

Emergency medicine benefits. One such technology, developed and employed first to detect X-rays from distant stars, has been used to build a portable X-ray imaging scope for use in emergency medicine. Researchers at NASA's Goddard Space Flight Center in Greenbelt, Maryland, developed a highly efficient image-intensifying device to enhance the reception of low-level X-ray images from celestial bodies. This image intensifier is equally well suited to use in medical applications because the energy range of X-rays from celestial bodies is similar to that of X-rays used in medical diagnosis. Known as the Lixi Imaging Scope and manufactured by Lixi, Inc., in Downers Grove, Illinois, this device is a self-contained, battery-powered fluoroscope that produces an instant X-ray image. Because the system is portable, it is particularly useful in medical emergencies that demand on-the-spot care; it is also a valuable tool that is used in the homes of bedridden and disabled patients. In addition, the unit is designed to use less than 1% of the radiation required by conventional X-ray devices, thus reducing the potential dosage exposure to both patient and radiologist.

Genetic diseases better understood. Using digital image-processing technologies that have been employed to relay images to Earth from missions to Mars, Jupiter, and Saturn, scientists at NASA's Jet Propulsion Laboratory (JPL) in Pasadena, California, have improved the diagnosis of human genetic abnormalities. Hereditary characteristics are carried in genes contained in the threadlike chromosomes found in the nucleus of a living cell. By studying the arrangement and appearance of these chromosomes, clinicians can diagnose genetic abnormalities. Such information is most useful when presented in a structured form called a karyotype, an arrangement

146

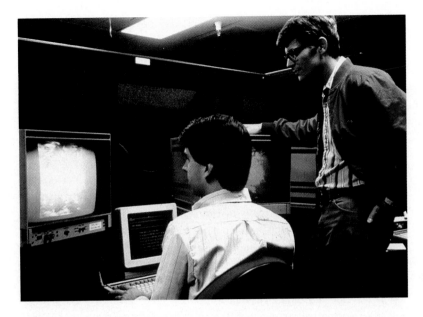

At the Jet Propulsion Laboratory (left), scientists employ digital image processing to relay high-resolution pictures from planets to Earth. The technology was first used in the U.S. space program on the unmanned Ranger missions to the Moon. Since then, image-enhancing methods have opened many new windows onto the human body. The diagnostic body-scanning process known as magnetic resonance imaging (MRI) is just one example. An MRI brain scan produced the computer-processed color composite picture (below left), in which a clearly visible tumor (the white area) has been highlighted. Digital image processing has also made it possible for medical geneticists to scan, assemble, measure, and classify human chromosomes, which, in turn, enables them to diagnose hereditary abnormalities rapidly and accurately. And NASA, of course, continues to reap the bounties of the technology in its ongoing planetary explorations. The image below is one of the dramatic pictures of Neptune that Voyager 2 sent back in August 1989; the intense blue in the image revealed methane gas in the planet's atmosphere.

Photographs, (above and below left) NASA; (below right) JPL/NASA

of chromosomes by type that facilitates the diagnosis of diseases caused by extra, missing, or abnormal chromosomes. The standard method of constructing a karyotype from a photograph of chromosomes within a cell is a labor-intensive endeavor, requiring up to several days. Through the use of digital image-processing technology, NASA scientists and engineers developed an automated light microscope system that automatically scans, assembles, measures, and classifies the chromosomes present in 7 to 16 minutes. This system, subsequently marketed by Perceptive Systems, Inc., of Houston, Texas, will also have a "spin-back" application; NASA plans to use this technology in the future to monitor any effects of increased exposure to radiation in space on astronauts' chromosomes.

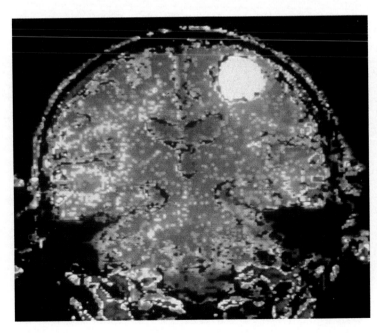

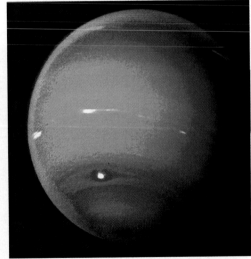

A "temperature pill." Technologies originally developed for transmitting data from orbiting satellites to Earth are being applied to the transmission of physiological data from the interior of a patient's body to the attending physician. In the management of emergency conditions such as hypothermia (dangerously low body temperature) or hyperthermia (dangerously high body temperature), it is crucial to monitor core body temperature accurately. Scientists at NASA's Goddard Space Flight Center and the Johns Hopkins Applied Physics Laboratory of John Hopkins University, Baltimore, Maryland, developed an ingestible thermal monitoring system, better known as the "temperature pill," through the use of several aerospace technologies—integrated circuit miniaturization, telemetry, and sensors. This temperature pill, now produced commercially by Human Technologies in St. Petersburg, Florida, is a highly sensitive thermometer that measures internal body temperature and transmits this information to a computer outside the body. The 1.9-centimeter (0.75-inch) silicone capsule can be swallowed as a pill or inserted vaginally or rectally. When swallowed, the pill makes its way safely through the digestive tract in one to three days. The accuracy of the temperature pill far exceeds that of other thermometers—most thermometers are accurate to one-tenth of 1° C (0.18° F); the temperature pill is accurate to one one-hundredth of 1° C (0.018° F). More important, the

Scientists from NASA's Goddard Space Flight Center have collaborated with scientists from the Johns Hopkins Applied Physics Laboratory in the development of the ingestible thermal monitoring system shown here. A number of aerospace technologies were incorporated into a process that provides extremely precise measurements of internal human body temperatures—readings that are accurate to one one-hundredth of 1° C (most thermometers for recording body temperature are accurate only to one-tenth of 1° C). The capsule-size silicone "temperature pill" is designed to be taken orally or inserted rectally or vaginally. For one to three days it monitors internal temperatures continuously, relaying the vital information to a computer. Such accurate readings are a great boon to doctors in the treatment of patients with hypothermia and hyperthermia, life-threatening conditions in which body temperature is either dangerously low or dangerously high. Physicians foresee using the same technology in other, similar systems, such as fertility monitoring and assessing vital signs in frail elderly patients.

Photograph, NASA

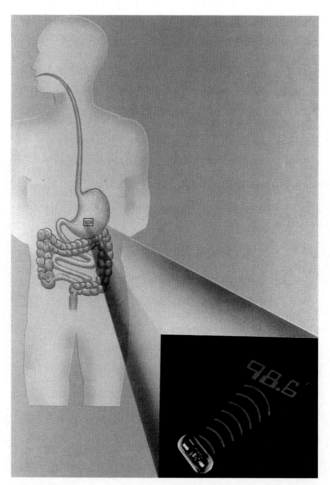

temperature pill is the only means for obtaining deep body temperature that does not require wires and connections to an external temperature monitor. Additional applications envisioned for the temperature pill include monitoring of body temperatures and other sensitive internal vital signs during surgery, in geriatric patients, and in fertility monitoring.

Combating dizziness and instability. It has been well established that prolonged exposure to weightlessness in long-duration spaceflight may result in alterations of the body's mechanisms for maintaining balance and posture. Scientists at NASA's Ames Research Center, Moffett Field, California, developed a sensitive balance system to monitor this phenomenon in astronauts. Recognizing the potential of this system as a clinical diagnostic tool, TherEx, Inc., of Woodside, California, manufactured the device, known as the AT-1 Computerized Ataxiameter, for use in the identification and treatment of balance disturbances and dizziness associated with neurological and musculoskeletal disorders. Capable of measuring visually imperceptible body movements, the system enables the clinician to monitor and precisely quantitate the patient's stability during initial assessment, treatment, and rehabilitation. For example, the AT-1 can be used to evaluate the effects of surgery, medications, physical therapy, or prosthetic devices. In a typical test, the patient stands on footplates fitted with four independent force-measuring transducers for measuring the pressure on the ball and heel of each foot. The transducers quantitate the weight displacements that reflect the direction and amount the patient sways in forward-backward or left-right movements. The patient stands on a stable base, first with eyes open, then with eyes closed; the same measurements taken with eyes open and closed are then taken on a tilted base. All data are processed, displayed, and archived by the computer to facilitate assessment of progress at various stages during the course of a treatment regimen.

Saving the eyes of children. Although all youngsters should be screened for amblyopia (a progressive dimming of vision) and other eye defects, a widespread screening program has not been initiated for want of a simple, reliable system that could be used with infants and preschool children. Image-processing and optics technologies from NASA's George C. Marshall Space Flight Center in Alabama have led to the development of a portable system, the VisiScreen-100, for the detection of eye problems through analysis of the retinal reflex. Because the system can be used with infants and preschool children who otherwise might not be tested until school age, it permits the early detection of ocular alignment problems such as "lazy eye," one form of amblyopia that is a potential cause of limited vision or blindness later in life. It has been estimated that as much as 20% of blindness that develops after birth is the result of the late detection of lazy eye combined with loss of vision in the healthy eye caused by trauma or diabetes. In addition, the system can test the human eye for refractive error and obstruction in the cornea or lens. The VisiScreen's photorefractor camera system sends light into the child's eyes, and the light is reflected back to the camera for recording on color film. The retinal reflex generated by the retina's response to the light is analyzed for defects. If any abnormalities are detected, the child is referred to an ophthalmologist for verification

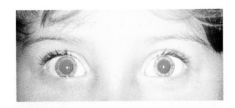
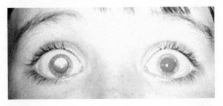
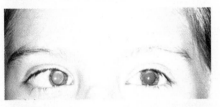
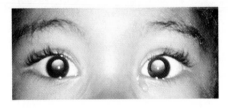

Image-processing and optics technologies have produced a handy, portable device for screening eye problems in children at very young ages. The VisiScreen-100 photorefractor ocular screening system utilizes a camera with an electronic flash that sends light into a youngster's eyes; the response to the flash produces a color image in which the pupils are variously colored and focused. A trained observer can identify the nature of a defect from the image, and the youngster can then be referred to an ophthalmologist for verification. The VisiScreen picture at top shows a child whose eyes are normal (indicated by the two red disks). The second child has hyperopia (farsightedness) in the right eye (indicated by the yellow crescent at the top of the eye). The third youngster's "crossed" right eye indicates the condition strabismus, an imbalance of the muscles of the eyeball. The child at bottom has a slight hyperopia in both eyes (evident from the small yellow crescents).

Photographs, NASA

149

and treatment. The VisiScreen-100 manufacturer, Vision Research Corp., Birmingham, Alabama, has entered into an agreement with Kinder-Care Learning Centers, Inc., to establish this vision-screening program in 1,025 of the company's preschool programs in the U.S. and Canada.

Patients in the hospital: preventing infections and cutting costs. Any innovation that can reduce the length of a hospital stay offers tremendous savings in health care costs. Aerospace technology developed to aid in the identification of microorganisms in space has led to an automated system used by hospital laboratories that detects and identifies infection-causing bacteria in a fraction of the time it once took. Detecting potentially harmful microorganisms has always been necessary in the space program for protecting critical life-support elements such as water-reclamation and air-revitalization systems and for minimizing the risk of crew-member disease due to microbial infection. As more is learned about the effects of long-term spaceflight on the human immune system, microbial detection may become more critical in future missions. To be effective in the spacecraft environment, the microbial diagnostic system must be rapid, accurate, comprehensive, and automated—characteristics shared by the demands on hospital laboratories. For the Voyager space missions, McDonnell Douglas Corp. worked with scientists at the Lyndon B. Johnson Space Center in Houston to develop a system to detect bacterial contamination on the spacecraft. This Voyager/Mars mission technology is now commercially available through Vitek Systems, Inc., of St. Louis, Missouri, a McDonnell Douglas subsidiary. The traditional method for detecting and identifying harmful organisms and determining an effective treatment requires several steps and two to four days. The AutoMicrobic System does the same job in virtually half the time. Advantages of the system include minimized human error, reduced technician time, and increased laboratory output as a result of the system's ability to handle up to 240 patient specimens at one time. More important to the patient is the shorter hospital stay that results from faster analysis of the infecting organisms and earlier treatment. In another "spin-back" to the space program, Vitek is once again working with scientists at Johnson Space Center to adapt the system for use on the *Freedom* space station (AutoMicrobic System II).

Assessing burn injuries and saving lives. Of the approximately two million Americans suffering serious burns each year, more than 10,000 die and at least 70,000 require intensive care and long hospital stays. Early identification and surgical removal of dead tissue is essential to minimizing bacterial infection, a primary cause of death in burn victims. The key to the early differentiation between dead tissue and tissue that will heal naturally is the ability to measure the depth of the burn injury. A partial-thickness burn that involves only the surface epidermis and a portion of the underlying dermis will regenerate new skin and does not need to be removed. A full-thickness burn, however, involves the epidermis, the full thickness of the dermis, and the underlying tissue. In these deep burn injuries, the skin cannot regenerate; therefore, skin must be removed and skin grafts applied. Unfortunately, the depth of a burn injury is difficult to determine. To meet the need for precise diagnosis of burn depth, NASA applied ultrasound technology origi-

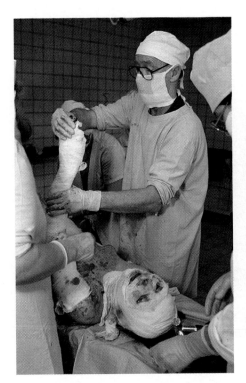

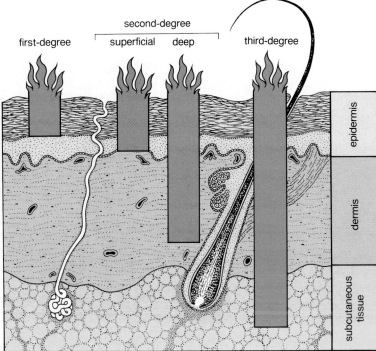

nally used to detect flaws in spacecraft materials. An instrument developed jointly by scientists at NASA's Langley Research Center in Hampton, Virginia, and burn surgeons at the Virginia Commonwealth University Medical College of Virginia directs ultrasound waves at the burn area; the difference in tissue density between the damaged tissue and the healthy tissue causes a reflection at the interface that can be analyzed to determine burn depth to an accuracy within 0.1 millimeter. Clinical studies have indicated that the system accurately measures depths of flame, scald, and chemical burns in humans, providing burn surgeons with an enormously valuable tool for noninvasive assessment of burn injuries.

Once-unthinkable treatments

Countless people who suffer from a wide variety of medical problems are already the beneficiaries of remarkable new therapies derived directly from NASA accomplishments of the past three decades.

Lasers for the heart. Nearly a quarter of a million patients in the United States may be spared the trauma and expense of coronary bypass surgery through the use of a new technique derived from NASA research for space-based lasers. Approximately 225,000 Americans undergo coronary artery bypass surgery annually at a cost of $25,000 to $40,000 per operation. One alternative to surgery has been balloon angioplasty, a procedure in which a catheter is threaded through an artery to the blockage and a balloon in the catheter is then inflated, compressing the arterial plaque against the walls and creating a larger opening for blood flow. Although this technique is less expensive ($7,000 to $9,000 per procedure) and less traumatic than bypass surgery, it serves only to compress the plaque and

The severity of a burn is classified according to the depth of the injury. A superficial (first-degree) burn involves only the epidermis. A partial-thickness (second-degree) burn involves varying depths of the dermis. But a full-thickness (third-degree) burn that involves the full depth of the dermis and underlying subcutaneous tissue must be treated as an open wound because new epidermal tissue will not regenerate. As surface assessments may not reflect the true depth of a burn, it has been difficult to determine when aggressive treatment is required. Now, however, ultrasound technology first used by NASA to detect flaws in spacecraft—internal cracks, for example—will reveal to an accuracy of within 0.1 millimeter the point below the skin surface that viable tissue interfaces with tissue that has been destroyed. This ability to obtain precise and immediate depth measurements means surgeons can hasten the treatment of burn-injured patients—minimizing the risk of infection, fostering healing, and in many cases saving lives.

Photograph, Robert Tonsing—Picture Group

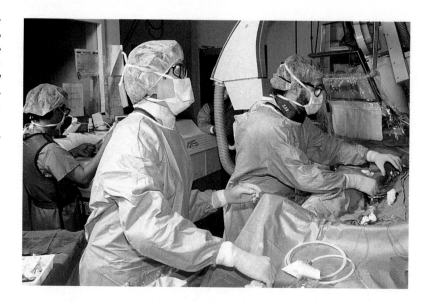

At Cedars-Sinai Medical Center, Los Angeles, surgeons use excimer lasers to vaporize plaque in obstructed coronary arteries. This promising new approach offers an alternative to costly and traumatic coronary bypass surgery. The excimer laser uses pulses of ultraviolet light to break up the chemical bonds in plaque without causing damage to artery walls, as heat lasers can. The precision control afforded by the lasers comes from a magnetic switching element that was designed by NASA scientists at the Jet Propulsion Laboratory and subsequently adapted for surgical use.

Photograph, Cedars-Sinai Medical Center, Los Angeles

does not remove it. As a consequence, one-third of all balloon angioplasty patients must undergo a repeat procedure or subsequently have open-heart surgery. A promising approach to removing plaque involves use of a laser threaded through a 1.5-millimeter catheter to the blocked coronary artery. This innovation was developed by physicians at Los Angeles' Cedars-Sinai Medical Center working with scientists from JPL. The laser vaporizes the plaque to remove it from the artery, thus greatly reducing the possibility of reobstruction. A concern of surgeons was that the heat from most lasers might damage the artery wall and result in the formation of a clot or new plaque buildup. One solution to this problem, the vaporization of the plaque without the use of heat, has been made possible by the use of excimer laser technology. The excimer laser uses pulses of ultraviolet light rather than thermal energy to break the chemical bonds in the plaque. Precise control of the laser pulse width is made possible by NASA magnetic switching technology. The excimer laser angioplasty system, manufactured by Advanced Interventional Systems, Inc., of Costa Mesa, California, has been used successfully on humans since November 1988. As this technique becomes more widely available, an increasing number of patients may realize permanent relief from coronary artery obstruction without the trauma and expense of bypass surgery.

Conquering incontinence. A device currently under development may provide relief to some of the estimated five million persons in the U.S. suffering from urinary incontinence, an inability to control emptying of the bladder. In the elderly, incontinence is a major health care problem, affecting one in 10 persons over age 65, often resulting in the affected person's exclusion from recreational and social activities and increased need for nursing care. In addition to the geriatric population, approximately 150,000 mentally retarded persons in the U.S. are incontinent, which presents a significant barrier to their being mainstreamed into society. In many cases incontinence can be managed by behavioral training; however, the limited success of this approach may be improved by the addition of a signal to indicate bladder

152

fullness. Such a device would provide a way of translating the sensation of a full bladder into the instruction to void.

NASA has teamed with the Association for Retarded Citizens (ARC) and the National Institute on Disability and Rehabilitation Research to develop an assistive device that can unobtrusively monitor the fullness of the bladder and provide a signal to the wearer or the care giver. Ultrasound and signal analysis technologies originally developed for the nondestructive testing of aerospace materials at NASA's Langley Research Center have been adapted to facilitate this wearable bladder-fullness monitor. Rather than having it use distance measurements to compute volume, Langley scientists found a characteristic ultrasound "signature" that relates the power content of the signal from the back wall of the bladder to the extent of bladder fullness. The device, currently being clinically tested by ARC, should afford those who suffer from incontinence vastly improved or full control of the debilitating problem and, therefore, much greater access to educational, social, and employment opportunities.

Transcending disabilities

A very important application of NASA technology has been the rehabilitation of those with physical disabilities so that they might live barrier-free, more productive, and happier lives.

A comfortable wheelchair. A program to develop materials for improved crash protection for airplane passengers has led to a technology with widespread benefits for the disabled. An open-cell polymeric foam material was found to have better impact protection and enhanced passenger comfort on long flights because it distributed body weight and pressure evenly over the entire contact area of the airplane seat. This slow-springback foam, developed by NASA's Ames Research Center, adapts to match the contour of the body pressing against it; it returns to its original shape once the pressure has been removed. Originally marketed as Temper Foam®,

In the 1960s scientists at Ames Research Center in California conducted a research program that led to the development of a new material for aircraft seats that offered protection from impact as well as comfort for long flights. This open-cell polymeric foam is now widely used in spin-offs for rehabilitation medicine. (Below left) The liquid foam material is mixed, poured, and contour-molded for a custom-made wheelchair for a paraplegic patient. The seat (below) will provide support and comfort and, by distributing body weight and pressure evenly, will reduce the potential for developing painful pressure sores.

Photographs, NASA

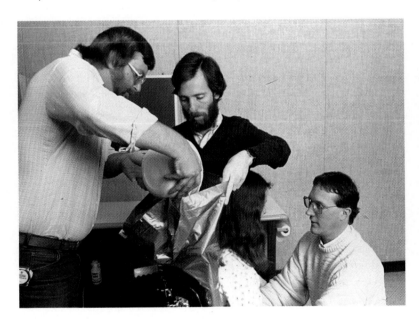

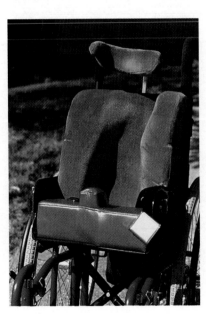

this material has been widely used in wheelchair seating to relieve soreness and fatigue and to help prevent the costly and serious problem of pressure sores. Recently, seating specialists have been able to custom mold the foam seats to achieve the most therapeutic body position for an individual. In addition, this aerospace foam has proved to be remarkably useful in numerous other medical applications—including cervical collars, operating table pads, padding for splints and braces, a hand exerciser, and a strap for "tennis elbow" designed to support forearm muscles and relieve pain. Other uses of the foam include padding for automobiles, football helmets, body pads, and chest protectors.

Friendlier skies. A joint effort between NASA, the University of Virginia, and the airline industry resulted in a product that will make the skies friendlier to the wheelchair-bound. Narrow aisles and small lavatories preclude the use of standard wheelchairs on most airplanes, making long airline flights difficult or impossible for the approximately 700,000 persons in the U.S. who rely on wheelchairs for mobility. The University of Virginia Rehabilitation Engineering Center asked NASA's Langley Research Center for assistance in designing a wheelchair that could be kept on the airplane to provide mobility for the in-flight passenger. Challenging aspects of this design effort were many; the chair had to be strong enough for the safe support of a 90-kilogram (200-pound) person yet weigh very little so as to keep airline fuel costs down, narrow enough to be maneuverable in airplane aisles, and collapsible for easy storage in an overhead compartment or behind the last row of the airplane's seats. Difficult size and weight constraints such as these were nothing new to the engineers at the Langley Research Center, however. To optimize spacecraft strength while minimizing weight, these engineers developed structural design and analysis techniques as well as new materials that could be used in the construction of an airline wheelchair. Wheelchair users and the airline industry were important contributors to the NASA and University of Virginia development effort. The result of this collaboration was a chair that met all of the size, weight, and strength requirements; however, the final obstacle of access to the cramped airplane washroom remained. In response to this problem, the Boeing 767 was designed with an option for a door at the side of the toilet so that a disabled person could move the wheelchair into the washroom and more easily transfer from it to the toilet seat. United Airlines is now using this NASA-University of Virginia chair, called the Stowaway, on some of its Boeing 767s. Use of the Stowaway is not limited to airplanes; hotels and buses are also finding that travel for the disabled can be made safer and more convenient with such a specially designed chair.

Keeping cool. Some of the same technologies that made it possible for astronauts to work outside their environmentally controlled spacecraft have provided many disabled persons the freedom to leave their controlled home environment to pursue educational, career, and recreational opportunities. Maintenance of astronaut body temperature during extravehicular activity presented special challenges to NASA engineers; in Earth orbit, temperatures can climb as high as 136° C (277° F) in the sunlight. A solution was found in a portable cooling system developed by engineers at NASA's

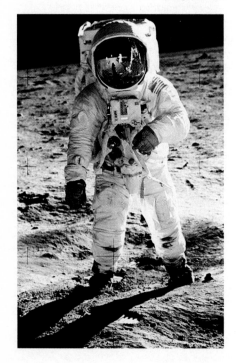

Edwin ("Buzz") Aldrin, who was a member of the first crew to land on the Moon, joined fellow astronaut Neil Armstrong outside the Apollo 11 spacecraft on July 20, 1969; he spent one hour and 44 minutes on the Moon's surface, conducting experiments and collecting rocks and soil samples. The space suit worn by Aldrin took many years to design. It required a special cooling system because the temperature outside the controlled environment of the spacecraft could reach 136° C (277° F); it also needed to provide ample flexibility for movement. (The historic photograph below was taken by Armstrong.)

Photograph, NASA

154

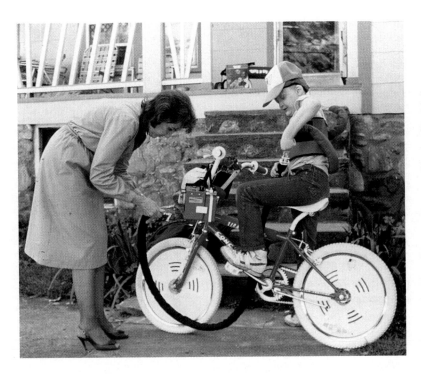

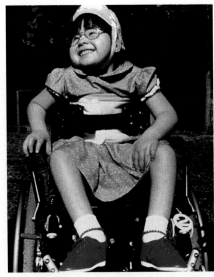

Stevie Roper of Waynesville, North Carolina, and Lynette Bowers of Myrtle Beach, South Carolina, are both beneficiaries of the space-suit technology that enabled Buzz Aldrin, Neil Armstrong, and many subsequent astronauts to make forays outside their spacecrafts and perform their extravehicular feats. Roper was born without sweat glands, which meant any kind of activity would cause his body temperature to rise precipitously; he faced the constant threat of heat exhaustion. Thanks to NASA technology, he can now play almost as actively as his peers. His personal "cool suit" was specially designed for him in 1987, when he was nine, by Life Support Systems, Inc. (LSSI), of Mountain View, California. LSSI is an aerospace spin-off company that mainly manufactures protective garments for workers whose jobs subject them to heat stress. Roper's easily portable system circulates coolant through tubes to a vest he wears on his torso and a head covering (worn under his cap). The suit eliminates 40–60% of his body heat and keeps his heart rate low enough to prevent fatigue. Before he takes off on a bike ride, his mother connects the suit's hose to a pack that stores and pumps the coolant. Bowers also suffers from a life-threatening disorder that makes her vulnerable to overheating. Her new lavender cool suit, which she models above, was designed by LSSI to meet her special needs.

Photographs, NASA

Ames Research and Johnson Space Centers. Used by the astronauts while they work outside the spacecraft, the self-contained system consists of·a space-suit undergarment with a network of tubes through which a cooling fluid is circulated. The fluid is cooled by a heat exchanger and delivered by a battery-powered minipump. Like the astronauts, individuals with certain medical conditions that make them vulnerable to heat stress even in moderate temperatures are unable to work outside a controlled environment. Quadriplegics, for example, generally are unable to perspire below the level of their spinal cord injury; their bodies therefore have limited cooling capabilities. Individuals with a congenital condition known as hypohidrotic ectodermal dysplasia are born without sweat glands, critical elements in the body's natural cooling system. Individuals with these and other conditions affecting the control of body temperature are often unable to leave their homes without the risk of life-threatening overheating. Thanks to the adaptation of NASA's space-suit technology by Life Support Systems, Inc., of Mountain View, California, many disabled persons are now enjoying newfound freedoms.

In another adaptation of the astronauts' cool-suit technology, Composite Consultation Concepts, Inc., of Houston has developed a scalp cooler for use during chemotherapy. Many drugs used in the treatment of cancer have the side effect of inducing hair loss. Use of this CHEMO-COOLER℗™ cap during chemotherapy delivery has been found to lower the scalp temperature and reduce the amount of drug absorbed by hair follicles, thus preventing hair loss in many patients without affecting the anticancer effect of the drugs. Other exciting commercial applications of the cool-suit technology include protection for miners, race-car drivers, and other workers in occupations where exposure to elevated temperatures can be dangerous.

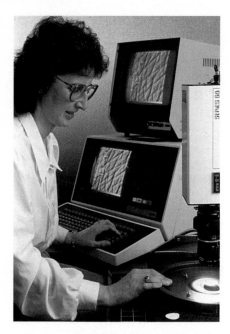

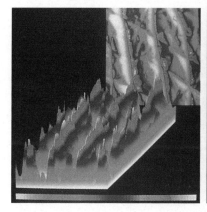

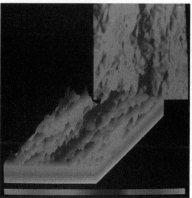

At the Skin Study Center, an independent testing laboratory near Philadelphia, Ortho Pharmaceuticals' product Retin-A was tested as a topically applied antiwrinkling formula. (Above) An image-processing specialist examines the wrinkling patterns in a skin sample by means of a digital image analyzer, a spin-off of NASA image-processing techniques developed for analyzing images of the lunar surface. She rotates the specimen, taking measurements at several different angles. The process is repeated at various times during a course of Retin-A therapy. The computer-processed color images (center and right) highlight peaks and valleys of wrinkles in a cross-section of skin before and after Retin-A treatment; noticeably fewer peaks and depressions are evident in the latter picture—a clear indication of the skin-smoothing potential of the preparation.

Photographs, NASA

Consumer products: enhancing life-styles

Twice-used NASA technologies have had numerous payoffs in a very wide range of products that make life on Earth not only healthier but also safer, happier, and simply more livable.

Cosmetics from the Moon. Exciting pictures of other planets transmitted to Earth by imaging satellites are processed by the previously described procedure known as digital image processing. This NASA technology has inspired numerous spin-off applications not only in medicine but in industrial quality control and consumer-health products. Processing techniques for the analysis of images of the lunar surface are being applied to the research, evaluation, and demonstration of skin-care products. Among the companies using this digital analyzer technique are the cosmetics manufacturer Estée Lauder Inc., of Melville, New York, and pharmaceutical firms such as Ortho Pharmaceuticals and Hoffman-LaRoche.

Strange as it may sound, the Moon's topography and human skin have a lot in common. Dermatological researchers found that the normal skin surface has folds and ridges that can be measured most accurately by computerized image processing; to analyze this skin topography, they adapted NASA technology originally used to determine accurately the topography of other planets and the Moon from satellite imaging transmissions. First, techniques to convert the analog imaging signals from the spacecraft to digital signals were developed. Computer enhancement techniques were then devised to adjust the image to correct for changes in contrast or variations in sensors and to emphasize critical topographic elements. In the same way, the topography of the skin can be translated into numerical descriptions, making possible the quantitative and qualitative assessment and comparison of the effects of cosmetics and medicinal preparations. Changes in the skin surface as a result of cosmetics were previously assessed through skin examinations and comparisons by a panel of experts, an approach that was costly, time-consuming, and imprecise. According to an Estée Lauder spokesperson, the adaptation of NASA technology to cosmetics manufacturing has been immensely valuable: "The use of the digital analyzer technique allows us to perform these examinations at lower cost, with more flexibility, much more frequently and with greater assurance of reproducibility of results. It aids us in developing, screening, and marketing

156

new products that might otherwise not be made available, because the benefits of the product are not readily apparent to visual inspection or touch."

In the past, changes in the skin due to aging or excessive exposure to the sun could only be repaired by surgery or concealed by makeup. Recent research, however, has shown that the use of retinoid preparations may result in a smoother, less wrinkled skin. Understandably, this dramatic development has generated a great deal of public excitement and a concomitant need for scientific assessment. Using the digital imaging technique, researchers are comparing changes in the degrees of roughness and wrinkling of skin over time in subjects using Ortho Pharmaceuticals' product Retin-A and in similar age subjects using a placebo preparation.

Survival in the elements. Materials used to protect astronauts are now being used in lightweight blankets for cold weather emergencies as well as in outdoor wear and sleeping bags. Metallized materials, a plastic film coated with a fine film of vacuum-vaporized aluminum to create a foil-like reflective surface, have found a variety of space applications and are used on almost every spaceflight—manned or unmanned. This material has been used in flight as a reflecting insulator or thermal barrier to protect astronauts and their sensitive equipment from temperature extremes and solar radiation. Metallized Products of Winchester, Massachusetts, worked with NASA to develop the early applications of this material and has since commercialized a broad line of spin-off products for industry and the consumer.

One product evolved from a requirement for ocean survival of the astronauts. In all manned U.S. spaceflights prior to the space shuttle, the spacecraft returned to Earth by parachuting into the ocean. Upon landing, the astronauts would leave their spacecraft and board a raft to await helicopters from the recovery fleet. This wait could be a long one; in some cases spacecraft splashed down as far away as 400 kilometers (250 miles) from the recovery fleet. To protect the astronauts and assist in the recovery mission, NASA asked Metallized Products to develop a raft canopy with a mirrorlike reflective surface that could be more easily detected by radar or seen from a distance. In addition, it would protect the astronauts from the heat, cold, and rain. Subsequently, Winslow Company Marine Products of Osprey, Florida, licensed the technology for this material, called TXG, and is marketing it in its line of survival rafts.

Another product made from this material is the blanket carried by many emergency medical teams for use in ski accidents or cold weather automobile accidents. The blanket is reflective, retaining up to 80% of the user's body heat. Another advantage is its light weight and small storage size; a 0.9 × 2.1-meter (3 × 7-foot) blanket weighs only 85 grams (3 ounces) and folds into a package the size of a deck of playing cards. Other metallized materials used in the interlining of space suits to provide a reflective barrier to the escape of radiant energy are used by manufacturers of outdoor wear, such as gloves, pants, and jackets, and sleeping bags for climbers, campers, and skiers.

For eyes only. The excellent visual acuity of eagles, hawks, and other birds of prey can be attributed in part to their built-in eye filters, which absorb near ultraviolet and blue light. Humans do not have these filters, and

A score of spin-offs have emanated from a material developed by NASA to protect astronauts and their equipment from the elements and used on space missions both as a reflecting insulator and as a thermal barrier. Here an emergency ski patrol covers an injured skier with a metallized blanket that will retain up to 80% of his body heat, thus helping to prevent postaccident chill and shock. The lightweight, large blanket, which folds to the size of a pack of cards, is easily carried by emergency teams and rescue squads of all types.

Photograph, NASA

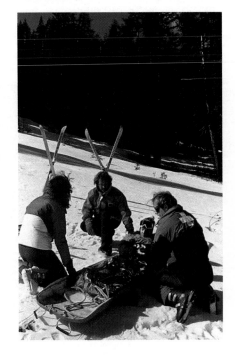

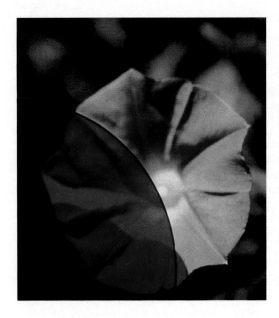 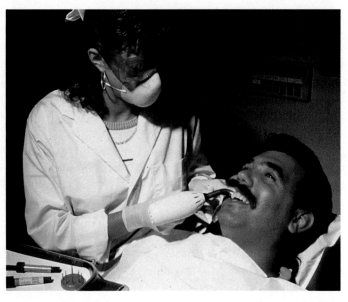

Physicists and engineers from the Jet Propulsion Laboratory worked with the manufacturer Suntiger™ to produce unique filters for eyeglass lenses, known as Polarized Selective Transmission (PST™) lenses. Suntiger markets eyeglasses that are specially fashioned for workers and recreationists who are in contact with light sources that are potentially hazardous to eyes. PST lenses not only eliminate 99% of harmful light wavelengths but also reduce glare, increase visual acuity, improve night vision, and brighten the intensity of colors.

In the photograph above, a morning glory is shown in natural view and, at its most vivid, as seen through a Suntiger lens. At right a dentist using a special ultraviolet treatment method wears protective eyeglasses designed to filter out harmful wavelengths while maximizing nonhazardous light so that she can see more clearly the teeth on which she is concentrating.

Photographs, NASA

occupational safety research has shown that exposure to blue, violet, and ultraviolet rays can contribute to the development of human eye disorders, including cataracts and age-related macular degeneration, the two principal causes of vision loss in Western nations. Researchers at JPL developed a dye formulation capable of filtering out harmful blue and ultraviolet rays produced during welding operations. This dye formula was then adapted for use in protective eyeglasses for welders and others who work in occupational environments that may be hazardous to eye health. These lenses, which were derived from the NASA technology and commercialized by Suntiger™ of LaCrescenta, California, eliminate 99% of the harmful light wavelengths. Visual acuity is also improved, with reduction of glare and the effects of haze. Other products that have been based on this technology are goggles for skiers, who are exposed to very bright and damaging sun rays reflected by snow at high altitudes, and protective lenses for dentists who use ultraviolet curing systems, which can produce harmful blue and ultraviolet light.

In another spin-off, the scratch resistance of sunglass lenses made of plastic has been dramatically improved. Advantages of plastic lenses are that they weigh only half as much as glass lenses and that they can be more easily shaped to facial contours. The primary disadvantage of most plastic lenses is that they are easily scratched. Researchers for a major sunglass manufacturer, Foster Grant Corp. of Leominster, Massachusetts, spent several years in search of a coating that would protect plastic lenses from scratching without interfering with their other positive properties. A solution was ultimately found in an abrasion-resistant coating developed at NASA's Ames Research Center for protecting the plastic surfaces of spacecraft and aerospace equipment in harsh environments. Utilizing this technology, Foster Grant manufactured a new product, called the SPACE TECH Lens, that is five times more resistant to scratching than conventional plastic lenses.

158

Agenda for tomorrow

Two human imperatives—exploration and improving the condition of humankind—have found common ground in the space program. Technologies developed to meet the awesome challenges of exploring realms *beyond* the planet Earth in the past three decades have paid extra dividends in improving the quality of life *on* Earth. Just a few of the medical innovations derived from space technology that will likely be seen in the next decade are a technique for noninvasive measurement of intracranial pressure, a critical parameter in the treatment of head injury; a device to aid in the management of dangerous wandering behavior in patients with Alzheimer's disease; improved heart valves made possible by computational fluid dynamics, an analytic technology developed for aerospace applications; and an adjustable shunt for improved control of cerebrospinal fluid pressure in children born with the condition hydrocephalus.

Furthermore, during the next decade NASA's earth sciences program initiative, Mission to Planet Earth, will create an integrated system for global monitoring of Earth's biosphere, the life-support system that includes the atmosphere, water, and land surface. This scientific mission will lead to a better understanding of global changes in the environment such as ozone depletion, global warming, and acid rain—all of which have important ramifications for human health.

The vast resource of technologies that can be adapted to improve health care and the quality of everyday life will not end there. In the new century, missions to explore other planets and to expand the human presence beyond Earth's orbital space will require many novel technologies—ones very likely to result in spin-offs that will further enhance global human health in ways yet undreamed of.

During the next decade, the gateway to future planetary exploration will be constructed. There is little doubt that the permanently manned, 150-meter (500-foot)-long, 290-ton space station Freedom *will yield a vast resource of new technologies. Many will be adaptable to novel spin-offs that will further enhance the quality of everyday life and health on Earth.*

An artist's conception of the *Freedom* space station; photograph, NASA

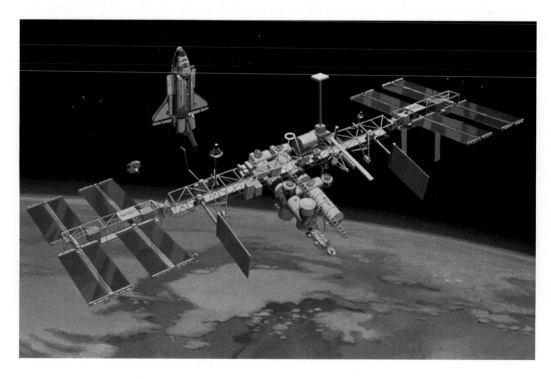

WOMEN
in the
MIDDLE

by Elaine M. Brody, M.S.W.

Elaine M. Brody, M.S.W., is Senior
Research Consultant, Philadelphia
Geriatric Center; Clinical Professor
of Psychiatry, the Medical College of
Pennsylvania; and Adjunct Associate
Professor of Social Work in Psychiatry,
University of Pennsylvania School
of Medicine.

(Opposite page) Jaci Joseph (right),
age 35, epitomizes the contemporary
American "woman in the middle." The
women in Jaci's four-generation family
are her mother, who lives independently
and works full time; her grandmother,
who, since being diagnosed with
Alzheimer's disease, has lived with the
Josephs; and her daughter, eight-year-old
Jillian. The males in the Joseph
household are her husband, Ron, and son,
Jeremy. Photograph, Mark Seliger

In a situation that is unprecedented in history, millions of women today find themselves occupying a unique position in society. They are the "women in the middle": they are usually in their middle years; they are, in the main, a middle generation in three- or four-generation families; and they are caught between the competing requirements of the various roles they are expected to fill. Many are now confronted with the responsibility of caring for their disabled elderly parents, parents-in-law, or other elderly relatives. As a consequence, these women also occupy an uneasy middle ground between two sets of competing values: a powerful, deeply rooted traditional value—that the care of older people in the family is *their* responsibility—and the newly emerging value that says it is acceptable—even necessary—for women to work outside the home.

These women are experiencing the stunning impact of a variety of demographic and socioeconomic trends that have converged to make "elder care" the norm, a typical life experience. In trying to respond to the many demands on their time and energy and to determine some sort of reasonable priorities, many of them are experiencing severe emotional stress.

True, spouses, sons, grandchildren, and at times even other, further-removed relatives become care givers to older people. Daughters, however, form the largest group of helpers for the greatest number of disabled elderly individuals. Daughters outnumber sons in a ratio of about four to one as primary care givers to severely disabled parents and in sharing their homes with those who can no longer manage alone. And, although their contribution is generally underrated, daughters-in-law often provide the actual care in families where sons are named as the main care givers.

Focusing on women care givers, and specifically on daughters and daughters-in-law, is not meant to deprecate the commitment or efforts of other family members. Elderly spouses, in particular, are usually enormously loyal to each other when one of them becomes disabled. But because of the discrepancy in life expectancy, the greatest number of care-giving spouses are women rather than men.

160

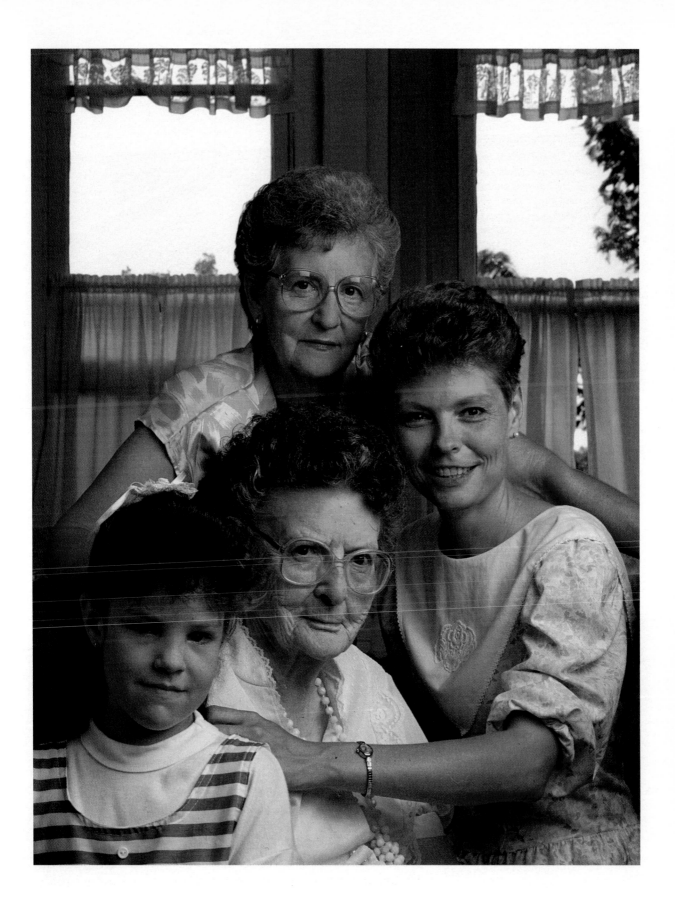

Women who have the responsibility of caring for their elderly parents vary widely in age and stage of life. At right, a woman in her middle years cares for her mother at home. The women in the rose garden (opposite page) are mother and daughter, in their eighties and sixties, respectively. Many such daughters, already past retirement age, find they are called upon to provide care at a time of life when they themselves had expected to be "taken care of."

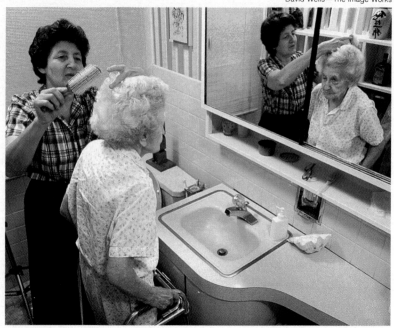

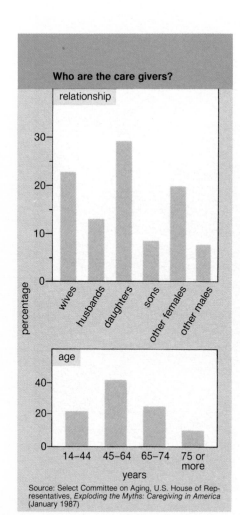

Who are the care givers?

relationship

percentage

wives · husbands · daughters · sons · other females · other males

age

14–44 · 45–64 · 65–74 · 75 or more

years

Source: Select Committee on Aging, U.S. House of Representatives, *Exploding the Myths: Caregiving in America* (January 1987)

Facts and figures

Women vary widely in age and stage of life during their parent-care years. In 1982 a U.S. government long-term-care survey found that almost two-thirds of daughter care givers were between the ages of 45 and 64, 25% were under age 45, and 13% were 65 or over. Almost one-fourth still had children under 18 living at home, while others had reached the theoretical "empty nest" stage. Those over the age of 65, however, exemplify an increasingly common situation—one generation of older people, the "young" old, taking care of members of a still older generation.

Women care givers are extremely diverse in other ways, too—in their socioeconomic and ethnic backgrounds, marital status, personalities, adaptive capacities, and the quality of their relationships with their parents. Some have lived "traditional" lives as homemakers, but most are now in the labor force. Some who worked when they were young gave up their jobs for marriage and motherhood; others have worked all of their adult lives. Still others move in and out of the labor force as their own and their families' needs dictate.

Contrary to popular belief . . .

Research shows definitively that ties between the generations continue to be strong and viable. Intergenerational exchanges of services are the rule rather than the exception: the elderly give as well as receive help from other family members. In short, the notion that the extended family has been replaced by the isolated nuclear family is wrong, and there is good evidence refuting it.

Another common misconception is that dependent elderly people are unceremoniously "dumped" into nursing homes by families unwilling to care for them at home. In the overwhelming majority of situations, the perma-

162

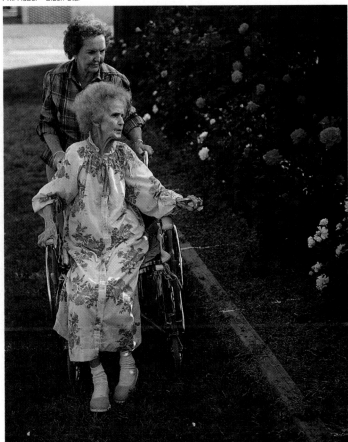

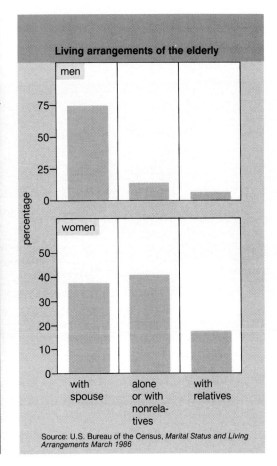

Living arrangements of the elderly

men

women

with spouse

alone or with nonrelatives

with relatives

percentage

Source: U.S. Bureau of the Census, *Marital Status and Living Arrangements March 1986*

nent placement of an individual in a nursing home occurs only after families have endured unrelenting strains for many years. The fact is that in the U.S. only about 5% of the elderly are in nursing homes at any given time. Furthermore, the institutionalized elderly have fewer family members than their noninstitutionalized counterparts—most are widowed or have never married; many are childless; and those with children have fewer children and fewer daughters.

Finally, the majority of older people are *not* dependent. Of all people 65 and older, 76% need no help whatsoever to function in their daily lives. Only about 5% are so disabled that they require help in five or six essential activities such as dressing, bathing, or going to the toilet.

Demographic trends: reshaping family and society

The steady growth in the number and proportion of older people in the population—particularly in the industrialized countries—has been one of the most dramatic and influential developments of the 20th century. In the U.S., for example, at the turn of the century, there were 3.1 million people who were 65 or over, representing 4% of the population. By 1987 there were about 30 million—12.2% of the population, or nearly one in eight of all Americans. That number is projected to increase to 39.4 million (14%) by the year 2010 and to 65.6 million (21%) by 2030.

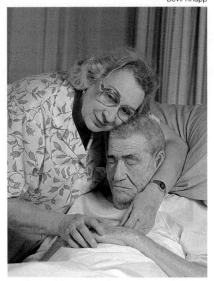

Not all disabled elderly people are dependent on their children. Those who have a surviving spouse will probably be well cared for should they become incapacitated. But because women on the whole are healthier in their late years and live longer than men, it is most often the wife who cares for an ailing husband.

Affecting filial care even more directly is that in the U.S. the number and proportion of *very* old people, those 75 or over, have increased more rapidly than the total older population. At present, about 40% of all older people in the country are 75 and over, and that proportion is on the increase.

At the same time, the declining birthrate has made even more pronounced the alteration in the ratio of old to young. In 1900 the average U.S. family had four children; today that average is less than two. Thus, older women today tend to have fewer children than their own mothers had. Having a smaller number of children also means having fewer daughters. And since many women are daughters-in-law as well as daughters, they have greatly increased chances of being called upon to provide care for more than one set of elderly people.

Another trend that will be accentuated in the future is more people caring for very old persons after they themselves have reached retirement age. Between 1900 and 1967 the number of middle-aged couples with two or more living parents increased from 10 to 47%. By 1980 there were about 9 persons 85 and over for every 100 persons aged 60–74, a ratio that is predicted to reach 33 per 100 by 2050, when the majority of the baby boom generation reach 85 and over. At that time, every third person 60 to 74 years old could have at least one surviving parent!

In addition, rates of widowhood soar as the population moves toward advanced old age, so fewer of the very old have a surviving spouse on whom to depend. When spouses *are* present, they are also likely to be in advanced old age and to have health problems that make them less able to provide care and therefore more likely to rely on adult children.

Finally, while more care-giving adult children will be old or approaching old age in the 21st century, the tendency of women to postpone childbearing until their late thirties and even early forties means that more of the women providing elder care will also have young children at home. With more families having two generations in the aging phase of life, some adults already find themselves helping both parents and grandparents.

The steady growth in the proportion of people aged 65 and over has been one of the most dramatic demographic trends of the past 50 years and has equally portentious implications for the next 50. Affecting the issue of care giving even more directly, perhaps, is that as more people survive into their eighties and nineties (graph, opposite page), increasingly, older people will themselves have at least one surviving parent. Some adult children are likely to find themselves caring for two generations of aging relatives.

year	percentage of population						
	under 18	18–24	25–34	35–44	45–54	55–64	65+
1960	35.8	8.7	12.7	13.4	11.4	8.7	9.2
1990	25.6	10.4	17.5	15.1	10.2	8.5	12.6
2020	21.4	8.5	13.3	12.8	12.4	14.0	17.7

An aging population

Sources: U.S. Bureau of the Census, *1960 Census of Population,* and *Projections of the Population of the United States, by Age, Sex, and Race: 1988–2080*

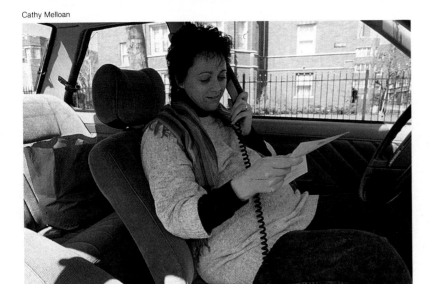

Cathy Melloan

Today more women work outside the home, and couples tend to postpone childbearing; these women in or approaching middle age often find themselves taking care of small children and elderly parents—in addition to holding down a job. Many feel torn by the requirements of these competing responsibilities and the attendant demands on their time and energy.

Remarkable changes in women's life-styles

As already stated, another striking change that has had widespread socio-economic reverberations throughout the Western world is the enormous increase in the number of women who are employed either part or full time. In the United States the proportion of women of all ages who work outside the home has increased vastly over the past several decades. In 1930, 10 million women, or 24% of all working-age women, were in the labor force, and these women made up 22% of the total work force. By 1985, 7 of every 10 women 25–54 years old were working (44% of the members of that age group in the work force). By 1995 the proportion of those working will rise to 8 of 10 women—60 million strong—and women will make up 46% of the work force. This situation is not unique to the United States but is similar to that in the United Kingdom, Denmark, and other industrial countries. Furthermore, middle-aged women—those who are most likely to

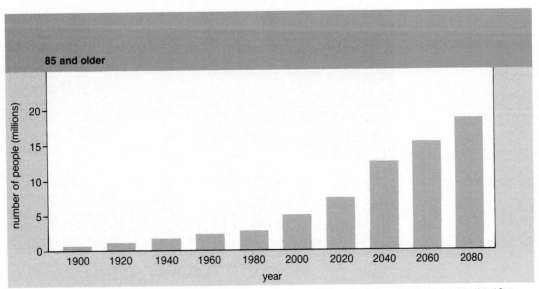

Sources: U.S. Bureau of the Census, *America in Transition: An Aging Society* (September 1983), and *Projections of the Population of the United States, by Age, Sex, and Race: 1983 to 2080*

be in the parent-care years—have been entering the labor force much more rapidly than women of any other age group.

Women's lives have been taking increasingly diverse paths in other ways, too. Patterns of marriage, divorce and remarriage, and childbearing have been changing rapidly. The rise to 44% in the proportion of women in the U.S. population who are not married during the parent-care years is undoubtedly a result of the increase in the number of women who do not marry or who are divorced or widowed in middle age. There is, of course, a tendency for an elderly parent to rely on the adult child who has the fewest competing responsibilities.

Parent care: satisfactions and stresses

Typically, a woman may begin by spending only a few hours a week helping a minimally disabled parent or parent-in-law; ultimately she may find herself providing around-the-clock care when the older person becomes severely disabled. Almost half of care-giving daughters have been providing care for one to four years; one out of five has been doing so for more than five years; and for some, more years are spent in parent care than in raising their own children. Data from this author's research show that caring for an older person often is not a one-time event; many women have care-giving "careers" in that they help more than one elderly person either simultaneously or sequentially.

Nonetheless, the vast majority of women *want* to care for their elderly parents—and do so willingly. They derive many positive benefits: fulfilling what they see as their filial responsibilities, adhering to religious and cultural values, expressing feelings of affection, seeing to it that the parent is well cared for, reciprocating help the parent gave them in the past, and serving

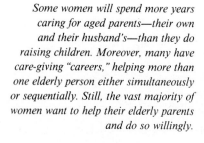

Some women will spend more years caring for aged parents—their own and their husband's—than they do raising children. Moreover, many have care-giving "careers," helping more than one elderly person either simultaneously or sequentially. Still, the vast majority of women want to help their elderly parents and do so willingly.

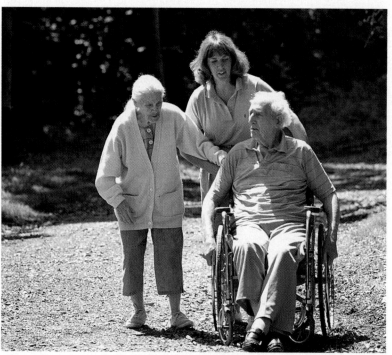

Caroline Pallat

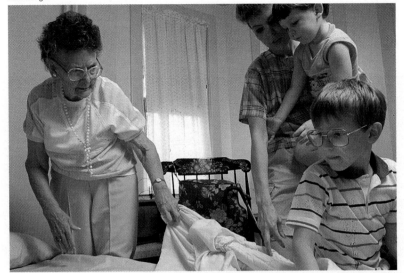
Mark Seliger

Taking responsibility for the care of an elderly person is stressful even when the help is gladly and willingly given. A number of factors may combine to make the situation particularly trying. One of these is caring for an individual who is mentally incapacitated. Another is sharing one's household with a disabled elderly person, especially when more than two generations are involved. Lack of privacy and conflict between family members can create a high level of tension; the woman who is quite literally "in the middle" must keep peace between the generations.

as good role models for their own children. At the same time, more than half of the women providing elder care experience significant degrees of stress and are often overwhelmed by feelings of depression, anger, anxiety, frustration, guilt, demoralization, conflict from competing demands, help-lessness, and irritability. Women who are older, who have been providing care for long periods of time, and who cannot afford to pay for help are especially vulnerable to emotional stress.

Many also report detrimental effects on their own physical health. Interestingly, there has as yet been very little research on the physical health effects of care giving. In a few studies to date, the care givers of Alzheimer's patients have been reported to use more health care resources and prescription medicines and to have generally poorer health than comparable women who were not care givers.

Caring for the elderly person who is mentally disabled—as compared with the physically debilitated—creates the greatest emotional stress. The marked behavior changes associated with Alzheimer's disease and other dementias stand out in this respect and are particularly important because of the increase in the number of elderly people with such ailments. Taking care of such people can be extremely trying—they require considerable personal care and may be forgetful, incontinent, combative, and unable to communicate their needs or to provide appreciative feedback. Adult children, feeling that they may have a genetic stake in the matter, are particularly frightened and anxious. "Will this happen to me?" they wonder.

High on the list of factors associated with emotional stress is sharing a household with a disabled elderly parent. Compared with those who live alone, older people who live with their children tend to be much more disabled (which is why they moved in to begin with) and need more intensive care. Along with overcrowding and loss of privacy, enforced close contact among family members creates fertile ground for conflict. And when the care giver's "nest" also contains her own children, the strain on her is intensified. Some tensions may be relieved when the parent is ultimately

Caring for a parent who lives far away has its own set of anxieties. When Charlas Rhodes, 51, was told that her 71-year-old mother, Arena Whytus, needed to be put into a nursing home, Rhodes chose to relocate even though it involved a long-distance move. Now the two share a house; the daughter managed to find a new job and is satisfied with the care her mother receives during the day at an adult day-care center. Where there are strong intergenerational ties, this kind of selflessness is not unusual.

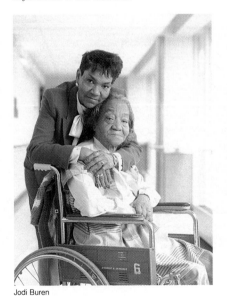
Jodi Buren

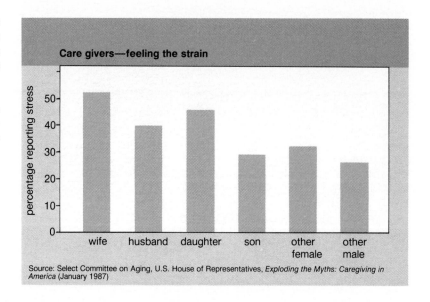

Care givers—feeling the strain

Source: Select Committee on Aging, U.S. House of Representatives, *Exploding the Myths: Caregiving in America* (January 1987)

placed in a nursing home, but new stresses appear, such as worry about the quality of care the parent is receiving in the institution.

Adult children who live far away from a disabled elderly parent also feel anxiety about the parent's decline and experience emotional stress, though to a lesser extent than children who are nearby. Distance presents its own problems, however, such as needing to make frequent, and sometimes costly, trips to visit; being unable to respond quickly to parents' needs; and feeling guilty about not being able to do more to help.

Juggling job and care giving

Recently, information has begun to emerge about a previously little-noticed effect of being responsible for parent care: disruption of the care giver's work or career. In a study funded by the National Institutes of Health that this author conducted in Philadelphia in 1981, 150 women care givers, working and nonworking, were interviewed. Twelve percent of them (28% of the nonworking women) had left their jobs in order to care for a parent. In addition, 13% of those interviewed (26% of the women who were working) were considering quitting or had already reduced their work schedules. Figures from the aforementioned 1982 long-term-care survey were strikingly similar to the Philadelphia findings—11.6% of care-giving daughters surveyed had left their jobs for parent care; 23% had reduced their work hours; and 35% had rearranged their work schedules.

In the Philadelphia study, the women who were still working cited as a problem their anxiety about what was happening to the parent while they were at work. Despite these acknowledged pressures, the women's parents were not receiving less care than the parents of the nonworking women.

Similar reports about the problems of balancing work responsibilities and parent care come from British research and studies conducted by U.S. businesses. In one such study the Travelers Corp., an American insurance company, found that 20% of its employees over the age of 30 were providing elder care. A majority of this group were women.

Subjective experiences

It is notable that women rather than men typically take on the job of parent and parent-in-law care. It has also been found that when men do become care givers, they experience less stress than their female counterparts. Further, sisters of women care givers, whether they live nearby or at some distance, experience more stress than their brothers do, and daughters continue to feel more stress than sons even after a parent has been institutionalized. Nonetheless, many daughters go on to provide care for long years—often beyond what appear to be the limits of human endurance. In the stories these women tell about their experiences of parent care, several subjective themes recur that cast some light on these differences between male and female, son and daughter.

Who assumes responsibility—and why? An overarching theme is that parent care *is* a woman's role—a tenet that is fundamentally accepted by both sexes. Though men too can be nurturing, there is no doubt that women are nearly always the ones who become the care givers whenever anyone in the family needs help. One reason may be that the sexes are socialized so differently in early life; girls learn early on that they will look after the needs of others, while boys are reared to be wage earners. These roles are so deeply ingrained that it does not even occur to most daughters that their brothers could be the ones to provide parent care. Daughters-in-law tend to accept the same assignment of roles by gender. Even women whose life-styles reflect the newer "enlightened" views of women's roles often behave in accordance with these "traditional" values.

One reason that care-giving daughters experience more stress than their male counterparts is that daughters provide both more help and more "hands-on" help. Furthermore, women tend to feel responsible not only for performing needed tasks but also for providing for the emotional well-being of the older person. Sons, on the other hand, are more likely to give their parents emotional support—and to provide financial help when need be—but they tend to become the primary care givers only when they have no sisters. It is then that their wives—the daughters-in-law—often assume the role of care giver.

Expectations, guilt, and a struggle for control. Women's expectations of themselves as care givers increase their emotional strain. They feel, in effect, "I have to do it all, do it well, and see to it that they are happy." Since making people happy can be a basically unrealistic goal, its pursuit is often doomed to failure. A woman's guilt about this "failure" is intensified whenever meeting her own needs conflicts with making the older person happy. Another source of guilt that is virtually built into the parent-care situation is that negative feelings exist side by side with positive ones—dislike and compassion, for example, or resentment and sense of obligation.

The expectation that role reversal will take place when a parent becomes disabled also contributes to emotional stress. Daughters (in particular, when caring for mothers) often say, "She took care of me; now it's my turn to take care of her." Certainly some of the tasks of caring for an elderly parent are similar to those that the parent once performed for the child—feeding, bathing, or changing diapers, for example—but there the resemblance

Women care givers usually expect more from themselves than men in this role. Women feel responsible not only for providing help with the tasks of everyday living but also for making the elderly person "happy"—a basically unrealistic goal and one that may be doomed to frustration. Further, whereas men are called upon to furnish emotional and financial support for their elderly parents, women provide most of the "hands-on" care, a task that can be physically exhausting as well as emotionally draining.

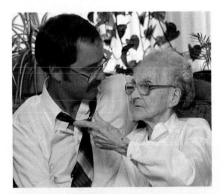

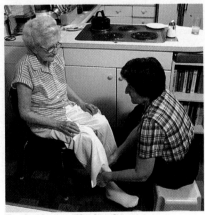

(Top) Paul Damien—TSW-Click/Chicago; (bottom) David Wells—The Image Works

169

ends. A mother's feelings about her baby's wet diapers are not the same as an adult child's feelings about incontinence in an elderly parent. The future holds the promise of a gradual reduction in an infant's dependency—caring for an older person presages only increasing dependency. By the very nature of the parent-child emotional relationship, the parent cannot truly become "the child" in the new relationship.

An especially difficult aspect of parent care, then, is the need for parent and adult child to rebalance their relative dependency and independence and the struggle for control that may ensue. It was the parent, of course, who once had power over the child. But when the parent becomes disabled, does the child have the right to exercise control? The difficulty of the situation is compounded because the ailing parent often is struggling to retain autonomy over his or her own life.

"Empty nests" refilled. Still another theme in women's subjective experiences derives from their stage of life at the time they are called upon to provide care. Since parent care may be needed when a woman is in her thirties or in her seventies, it cannot be said to be a "developmental" event, one normally to be expected in young adulthood, say, or in late middle age. Rather, it may be what has been called an "off time"—and therefore more stressful—event. Women in their thirties, for example, often feel too young for the parent-care stage; they may also have young children at home. Women in their middle years, the theoretical "empty nest" stage, say, "I thought I would be free at this time of my life." Instead, their "nests" are refilled. Finally, women who are older—and often themselves experiencing the decrements of aging—say, "I am too old for this; I'm old myself."

Family dynamics

Inevitably, parent care affects relationships throughout the family. Though what happens at this stage of family life depends on the historical quality of those relationships, the new pressures can exacerbate preexisting problems. The quality of the relationship between an elderly parent and a caregiving daughter is important in easing or increasing the latter's stress. It

Two sisters, themselves both well past middle age, help to pack their aging mother's belongings in preparation for her move into a nursing home. Despite the prevailing belief that the dependent elderly are unceremoniously "dumped" into nursing homes by family members unwilling to care for them, the fact is that the decision to place a parent in an institution is always an agonizing one, usually made only after families have endured long years of unrelenting strain and have no other options. In the U.S. only about 5% of the elderly population reside in nursing homes.

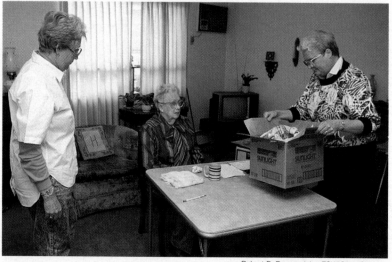

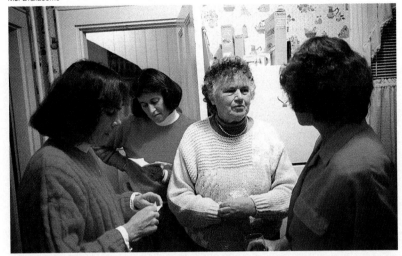

Mel DiGiacomo

A woman who has Alzheimer's disease visits in her kitchen with three of her daughters. Long before the disease was actually diagnosed, her children had noticed that their widowed mother was often confused and forgetful. At a family conference they decided that she could no longer live alone, but they were determined to help her to be as independent as possible. The solution: her son and daughter-in-law moved into her house; her daughters, all of whom work full time but live nearby, agreed to provide respite care on weekends and to take time off from their jobs when necessary to accompany their mother to doctor's appointments and on other outings. Caring for a parent inevitably affects relationships throughout a family; the quality of interaction among siblings in this situation may range from bitter refusal to loving cooperation—or anywhere in between. Not every family manages as well as this one.

is less of a strain to help a dearly loved parent than to care for a parent who has been cold or indifferent. The strain is intensified if the elderly person is critical of the care giver and other family members. Nevertheless, most adult children feel a strong sense of responsibility, and most provide the care even when relationships are poor. In fact, children often go on providing high levels of care even where considerable tension exists.

In most cases, one adult daughter becomes the principal care giver and provides the bulk of help. Her "election" to the role may be due to her sex, geographic proximity, or being an only child. Beyond those straightforward factors, women who are principal care givers attribute their assumption of the role to having fewer competing responsibilities (husbands and children or work) than their siblings, having always been the family "burden bearer," or being the favorite (or least favored) child. The amount of help and support they receive from siblings is variable. Sibling interactions regarding parent care can range from extreme bitterness to amicable cooperation or anywhere in between.

Interestingly, sons-in-law are often unsung heroes in these situations, helping their parents-in-law and providing considerable emotional support to their wives. Most married couples agree that parent care does not affect their basic relationship. Moreover, marital partners often see helping each other's parents as an unspoken part of the marriage contract.

Included among the family supports of daughters-in-law are, of course, their husbands—the sons of the elderly people being cared for. These women may even feel grateful to the men for helping with care of the latter's own parents! Such is the depth of women's socialization to the caring role and the force of social, cultural, and religious values that define and keep them in that role, this despite the fact that helping an elderly in-law has its own unique set of stresses because there is no biological link to provide the powerful motive of reciprocity and the deep emotional bonds. In households where an elderly person lives with an adult child, daughters-in-law experience more severe stress than any other category of relative, including sons-in-law.

The care givers' children—and sometimes grandchildren—are a significant competing responsibility. Women report more symptoms of mental and emotional distress when three generations live under the same roof than when the elderly person does not live with the adult child or the third generation has already left the "nest." Living concurrently with one's parents and one's children is especially turbulent when the children are adolescent. Then the care giver is in the middle in still another sense—that is, in her position as mediator of conflicts among family members. There can be a positive side to this picture; mature teens and young adults often act as a backup system of care, providing emotional support to their parents and coming to the fore when special help is needed.

Women with many relatives can be fortunate in that they often receive much emotional and instrumental support. Studies show that although the actual amount of help the care giver receives may not be significant, she reports feeling less burdened when she knows she has the emotional support of other family members and feels that they can be depended on in times of need. There are, however, some women who quite literally have no one—who are not married, who are childless, and who are "only" children. While they may not experience the sensation of being torn by conflicting loyalties and competing responsibilities, they often feel lonely and alone in the task of providing parent care and worry about what might happen if they get sick or if they predecease their elderly parent. Women who are childless, and therefore have no potential care givers for themselves, have still another worry: "Who will take care of me when I am old?"

Singleness and "double dependency"

In the U.S., at least, high rates of divorce and lower marriage rates mean that in the future more women will be single during their parent-care years. Singleness among women (being divorced, widowed, or never married) has increased by almost 75% over the past two decades. Beset by problems of limited income and single parenthood, such women may be less available to their aging parents. At the same time, the trend toward more remarriages

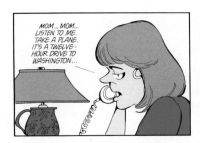
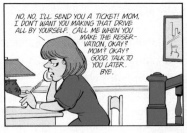
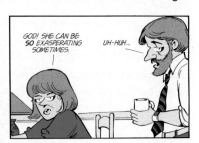
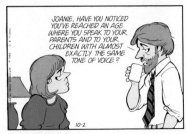
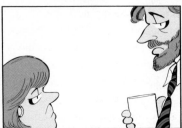
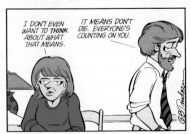

Doonesbury © 1988 G.B. Trudeau. Reprinted with permission of Universal Press Syndicate; all rights reserved

may present adult children of the future with a new dilemma; when one—or both—parents are remarried, to which set of parents is filial responsibility owed? The problems of disabled elderly women without husbands will be compounded; such women already constitute the bulk of the disabled population because of the differential between life expectancy for men and women. Not only will more women enter old age unmarried but as divorce late in life is becoming more common, more women who were married during most of their adult lives will find themselves unmarried in old age.

Because developmentally disabled people—for example, those with Down syndrome—are living longer, more care givers will experience "double dependency," caring simultaneously for their elderly parents and their disabled adult children. Another form of double dependency, caring for young children and elderly parents at the same time, is also increasing, as many women are having their first babies later in life. "Nests" of women in their middle years not only are remaining filled with offspring for longer periods of time but are being refilled to a greater extent by young adults who return home. Currently, 19 million single adults 18 to 34 years old live with their parents, an increase of one-third since 1974. Still another trend is the increase in geographic mobility, which separates parents and children.

Sorely lacking resources

Social policy has made some progress during the past few decades in relieving families of the crushing financial strains of caring for the elderly. Medicare and Medicaid came into being in the 1960s, and an income floor was established in 1974 with the enactment of supplemental security income (SSI) for the aged. Medicaid and SSI together eliminated compulsory financial support of the old by their adult children. With the original Social Security legislation (1935) to provide a baseline of support, the proportion of older people who were wholly dependent on family for economic support dropped from about 50% in 1937 to 1.5% in 1979. All of these programs, together with individual savings and private pensions, enable an increasing proportion of the elderly to maintain their own households and to realize their wish not to depend on their children for either income or the costs of catastrophic illness.

It is generally agreed, however, that the resources of families for providing long-term care have been exceeded. There is a need for both social policy that will create and fund a continuum of long-term care services—including services and facilities for those with chronic mental as well as physical disabilities—and federally funded long-term-care insurance. A recent report by the Brookings Institution, Washington, D.C., concluded that most people could not afford to purchase such insurance privately.

Tapping existing resources

In the U.S. formal services, as they currently exist, are uneven regionally, in short supply, fragmented, and fiscally inaccessible. Care givers are often both confused and frustrated in their attempts to gain access to an array of services delivered by a variety of different organizations, each of which has different funding and eligibility criteria.

173

Still, many sources of help do exist, and more are being developed. Each of the 50 states has an area agency on aging (AAA) in its capital, and there are additional county and regional offices. There are now 700 such AAA offices. (Local offices may be listed in the state government or community service listings of the phone book.) They provide information about the help available locally and make referrals to appropriate agencies and facilities. They may also provide some services.

Among the existing resources that may be available to care givers are adult day-care centers, respite care programs, in-home services (home-makers and home health aides), senior housing and other residential facilities, evaluation and assessment services, counseling services, family service agencies, and hospital departments of social work, which assist in discharge planning when an elderly person has been hospitalized. A network of private professional geriatric care managers has sprung up, a form of help particularly useful to family members who live far away from the older person. Information is available from the National Association of Private Geriatric Care Managers, 1315 Talbott Tower, Dayton, OH 45402. Support groups, notably those connected with the advocacy organization for Alzheimer's patients and their families, can be helpful to many troubled care givers and also provide information about techniques of care and local sources of services. More information can be obtained from The Alzheimer's Association, Inc., 70 E. Lake Street, Suite 600, Chicago, IL 60601 (phone: 1-800-621-0379 [in Illinois: 1-800-572-6037]).

One newly emerging source of help comes from business and industry. As companies have become aware that the responsibilities of parent care can negatively affect employees' productivity, they have become more willing to help their employees cope with these responsibilities. Some firms are even considering the inclusion of elder day care as an employee benefit option. Others have established referral programs for employees trying to negotiate the maze of available services. There has been virtually no discussion, however, about forms of relief similar to those requested by workers with small children—flextime, sabbaticals, job sharing, and the like.

Youngsters in the intergenerational day-care center at the Stride Rite Corp. get help with their construction project from newfound friend Eva DaRosa. DaRosa, 79, was among the first of the seniors to join the pioneering program that extends day-care services to the aging relatives as well as the children of employees. The Cambridge, Massachusetts, shoe manufacturer invested in the generation-bridging facility after a company survey found that approximately 25% of the company's workers had responsibility for an aging parent and at least 13% expected to find themselves in such care-giving roles in the years ahead. Stride Rite has long been a leader among U.S. corporations in providing family-oriented employee benefits; in 1971 it opened one of the country's first on-site child-care centers.

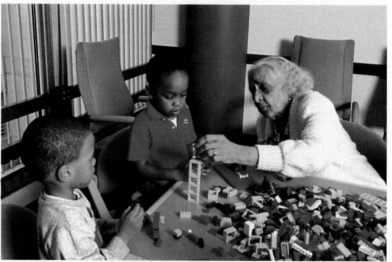

Models for the U.S.: how other countries cope

Almost all industrialized nations except the U.S. and Canada give economic supplements, such as attendance allowances or social security credits, to care-giving families. Among the policy options that have been proposed in the U.S. are direct payments for care giving, Social Security benefits for those who leave jobs for care giving, and tax relief for care givers.

While no country has developed a complete system of supportive services for family care givers, many have moved beyond the U.S. in doing so. Nearly all industrialized nations except the U.S. and Canada provide a "constant attendance allowance" or similar substitute to help the disabled elderly receive care at home. In-home services (home nursing and home-maker services) are vastly more available in European countries. Housing assistance (such as low-interest loans and specially designed housing units) is offered to encourage multigenerational living in the U.K., Japan, and Sweden. Apartments or annexes structurally modified to suit the needs of the elderly ("granny flats") are constructed as a form of public housing in the U.K. and Australia.

What tomorrow will bring

While some human needs change with age or alterations in social circumstances, certain needs remain constant. What elderly people need today from their children is what aging parents have always needed and wanted—affection, contact, and emotional support. Evidence is strong that parents will continue to receive these kinds of caring. Increasingly, however, it is becoming evident that care givers, in order to keep from exceeding the limits of their endurance, will need more help than they are now getting with the tangible services they themselves cannot provide. There is, of course, no single or enduring solution to these dilemmas—change is the only constant. The characteristics and needs of the elderly change as each successive cohort ages, as new scientific and social developments occur, and as the social and economic climate changes and evolves.

In the meantime, certain trends continue: the vulnerable, very old population continues to grow; the falling birthrate continues to reduce the supply of filial care givers; and the proportion of women in the labor force continues to rise. In looking to the future, however, one must be careful not to predict ever increasing needs and neediness of the elderly. Biomedical advances and improved life-styles could reduce dependency among the aged by preventing or ameliorating age-related ailments. Already, many people remain healthier and more productive well into old age.

A major imponderable is how the tension between changing and constant values will be resolved—that is, between the new values surrounding women's roles and the "enduring" values that label care of the elderly a woman's responsibility. It remains to be seen whether men will participate more actively as care givers, but with a majority of women working outside the home and more families than ever before providing parent care, couples will inevitably have a larger package of *shared* responsibilities.

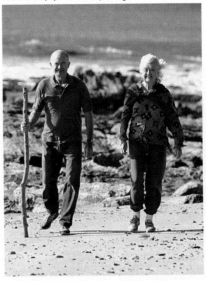

Although the elder-care "crisis" is a very real one, the present situation should not be viewed in an entirely gloomy light. Indeed, there are many men and women who remain healthy and productive well into old age. Moreover, with improved life-styles and biomedical advances, there is every likelihood that the number of active, independent seniors will increase in years to come.

Do Frescoes Make You Faint?
Warning for the Impressionable Tourist

by Graziella Magherini, M.D.

The day before yesterday, descending the Appenines on the way to Florence, my heart was beating fast. What childishness. . . . Memories crowded into my heart, and I felt in no condition to reason, so I abandoned myself to my folly as one does beside the woman one loves.

So wrote the French novelist Stendhal (Marie-Henri Beyle) in his diary on Jan. 22, 1817, as he traveled southward through Italy on his way to the celebrated city of Florence. Italy became Stendhal's adopted home, where he served as a diplomat but chiefly devoted himself to studying and writing about Italian art and planning his novel *The Red and the Black*.

In Florence Stendhal visited the Franciscan church of Santa Croce, where so many famous Italian artists, writers, and men of learning are buried or memorialized. Upon seeing the tombs and funeral monuments of great men such as the poet Vittorio Alfieri, Michelangelo, and Galileo, Stendhal was deeply moved. Of this experience he wrote:

What men! What a stupendous collection! My emotion is so profound that it almost becomes pitiful. The gloomy religiousness of this church, its vault of simple wood, its unfinished facade, all this sent powerful messages to my soul.

A monk then guided him to the Niccolini chapel in the north transept of the church, where Stendhal was to see the frescoes by the 17th-century Florentine painter Volterrano that decorate the cupola. These works of art could not have had a more profound effect on the already overwhelmed Frenchman:

He accompanies me there and then leaves me by myself. And there, sitting on a step of a kneeling place, my head abandoned on the pulpit, in order to look up at the ceiling, Volterrano's "Sibyls" gave me what was perhaps the greatest pleasure I have ever had from a painting. . . . I had reached that emotional point where one meets those celestial sensations given by the beauties of art and by passionate feelings. Coming out of Santa Croce my heart was beating strongly, what in Berlin is called nerves: the life in me had run out, I walked along afraid I would fall down.

In recent years more than a few unwary travelers in Florence, on encountering its art works for the first time, have had unexpectedly intense emotional reactions and have gone for treatment to the department of

Graziella Magherini, M.D., is Chief of Psychiatry and Director of Mental Health Services at Santa Maria Nuova Hospital, Florence, Italy; Professor of Psychopathology in the School of Psychiatry, University of Florence; and a member of the Italian Psychoanalytic Society. She is the author of La Sindrome di Stendhal, *published in Florence in 1989.*

(Opposite page) Michelangelo's "David"; photograph, Charles-Pierre Remy

176

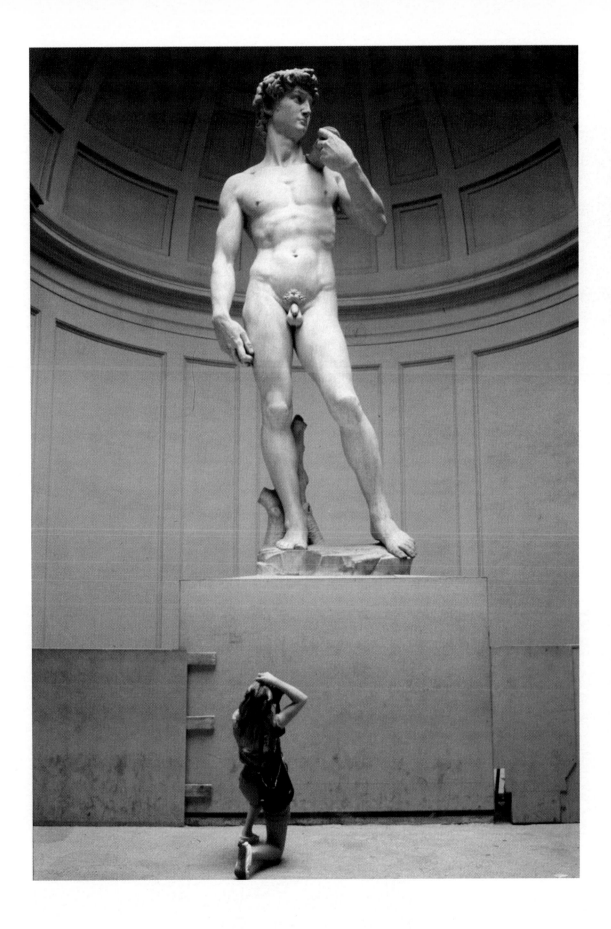

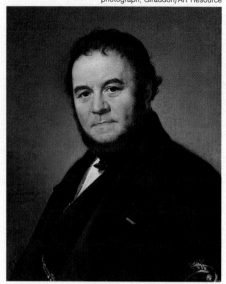

In 1817 the French writer Stendhal visited Florence and was profoundly affected by the city's rich history and its wealth of great works of art and architecture. The frescoes by Volterrano in the church of Santa Croce gave him "perhaps the greatest pleasure I have ever had from a painting" and aroused within him "those celestial sensations given by the beauties of art." Stendhal was so staggered by the experience that upon emerging from the "gloomy religiousness" of the church, he "walked along afraid I would fall down." Such turbulent feelings in travelers confronting the sumptuous art of Florence have captured the interest of Italian psychiatrist Graziella Magherini.

Along with her colleagues at Santa Maria Nuova Hospital, she has treated over 100 overwrought tourists who have had reactions remarkably similar to Stendhal's; hence, she has named the condition "Stendhal syndrome."

psychiatry at the hospital of Santa Maria Nuova in Florence. The emotional disorientation that this author and her colleagues at the hospital have observed and treated is strongly reminiscent of the mental state that Stendhal described upon leaving Santa Croce. Consequently, the name "Stendhal syndrome" has been given to the often overpowering experiences—sometimes accompanied by physical symptoms—that occur in some visitors on holiday in cities of great art. These tourists are suffering more than the common rigors of travel; their overwrought reactions to art go beyond ordinary "museum fatigue." The intention here is to describe the turbulent feelings that may be aroused in extremely sensitive individuals when, in strange surroundings far from home, they confront powerful and deeply moving works of art.

It should perhaps be noted that Stendhal was not the only well-known writer to experience strong emotions upon encountering Florence's aesthetic magnificence. Henry James, in *Italian Hours* (1909), wrote: " 'Lovely, lovely, but it makes me "blue," ' the sensitive stranger couldn't but murmur to himself as, in the later afternoon, he looked at the landscape from over one of the low parapets." And Mary McCarthy, in *The Stones of Florence* (1959), had this to say: "All great Florentine art, from Giotto through the *quattrocento,* has the faculty of amazing with its unexpected and absolute truthfulness. . . . The immediate effect of a great Giotto or a Masaccio is to strike the beholder dumb. Coming into the first room [actually Room 2] of the Uffizi or the Brancacci Chapel of the Carmine, he is conscious of a sensation he may not even associate with what is today called beauty . . .

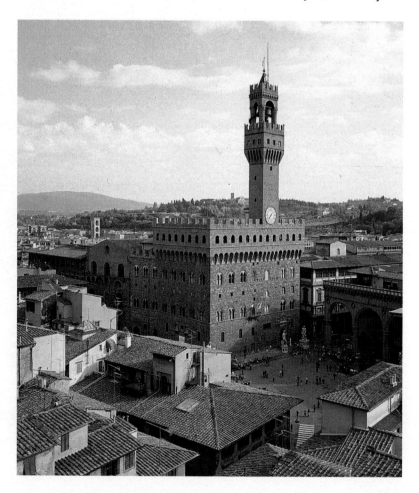

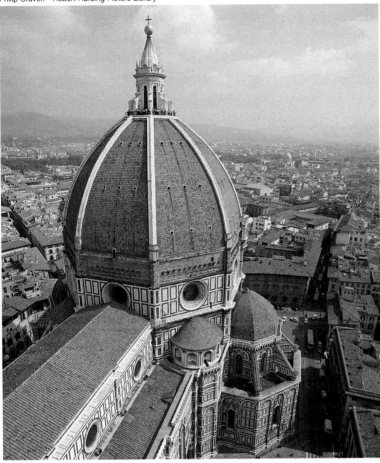

these paintings are, as it were, already coated with legend and literature so that they play on the fancy like fairy-tales . . . an event still so untoward and brusque that it results in a loss of speech, like the announcement of the conception of the Baptist to the old priest Zachary that deprived him of the use of his tongue."

Florence—the city and its treasures

Florence, the cradle of the Renaissance, is a city abounding with palaces and piazzas, churches and cloisters, domes and towers, sunlit public gardens and winding, shadowed byways. It is a city with perhaps the densest concentration of works of art in the whole of Italy—enormous artistic wealth crowded into a tiny area. The city's splendors are stamped by the personalities of the great artists who created them. The historic center of the city consists of the Duomo, or cathedral of Santa Maria del Fiore, with its delicate multicolored marble exterior; the Baptistery, known especially for its monumental bronze doors by the sculptor Lorenzo Ghiberti; and the Piazza della Signoria, a public square dominated by the majestic Palazzo Vecchio, the center of Florentine government from the Middle Ages to the present day. In the piazza Michelangelo's "David" once stood in the open. (The original has since been removed to the safety of the Accademia, but a

The Duomo, or cathedral, shown above in a view from the adjacent campanile, is the center of both traffic and tourism in Florence. The massive structure, with its delicate multicolored marble tracery exterior and majestic red-tiled cupola, dominates every panoramic view of the city. Nearby, also in the historic heart of the city, is the Palazzo Vecchio (opposite page), a fortresslike palace that has served as the seat of the municipal government since the Middle Ages. In front of this imposing medieval building lies the city's major public square, the Piazza della Signoria. In spring and summer months, Florence's resident population of 460,000 more than doubles with international sightseers basking in the city's rich atmosphere of art and culture.

(Opposite page) Photograph, Scala/Art Resource

179

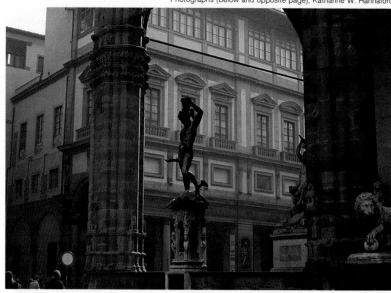

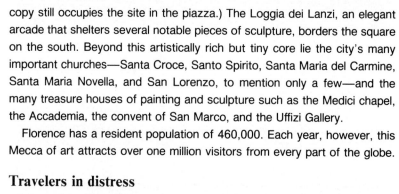

The Loggia dei Lanzi, its graceful arches framing the south side of the Piazza della Signoria, was built in the 14th century to shelter dignitaries during public ceremonies. Over the centuries the loggia became an open-air art gallery, housing many notable pieces of sculpture, including Benvenuto Cellini's "Perseus" (1554). The building in the background is the Uffizi Gallery.

Visitors to the Uffizi Gallery view Giotto's "Madonna in Glory," or "Maestà" (c. 1305–10). In her book The Stones of Florence, *Mary McCarthy wrote: "The immediate effect of a great Giotto . . . is to strike the beholder dumb. Coming into the first room [Room 2] of the Uffizi . . . he is conscious of a sensation he may not even associate with . . . beauty . . . these paintings . . . play on the fancy like fairy-tales."*

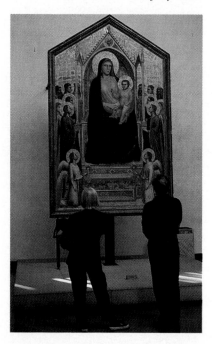

copy still occupies the site in the piazza.) The Loggia dei Lanzi, an elegant arcade that shelters several notable pieces of sculpture, borders the square on the south. Beyond this artistically rich but tiny core lie the city's many important churches—Santa Croce, Santo Spirito, Santa Maria del Carmine, Santa Maria Novella, and San Lorenzo, to mention only a few—and the many treasure houses of painting and sculpture such as the Medici chapel, the Accademia, the convent of San Marco, and the Uffizi Gallery.

Florence has a resident population of 460,000. Each year, however, this Mecca of art attracts over one million visitors from every part of the globe.

Travelers in distress

In the heart of the city, slightly to the east of the Duomo, is Florence's oldest hospital, Santa Maria Nuova, established in 1288. The foreign visitors whom the psychiatrists at Santa Maria Nuova have had occasion to treat mostly have been suffering from acute psychic disturbances lasting from a few days to eight or more days. The disturbances are characterized by clinical manifestations of two kinds: mental and psychosomatic. The former take the form of disturbances of the sense of reality, variously described as feelings of strangeness or alienation; altered perception of sounds and colors; anxiety or euphoria, sometimes intermingled in a disconcerting way; and a sense of persecution by the immediate environment. The psychosomatic symptoms that have been reported include rapid heartbeat, chest pain, faintness, sweating, and, in some cases, stomach pains, all of these often accompanied by anxiety and confusion.

Some tourists who have presented themselves at the hospital have been treated only briefly as outpatients. Over the 10-year period from 1977 to 1986, however, 106 travelers, male and female, were briefly admitted to the hospital. Of this group, most were unmarried and under 40 years of age; there was a particularly high percentage of unmarried women between the ages of 26 and 40. Interestingly, although about one-third of the tourists who visit Florence are native Italians, no Italians were to be found among these patients. Another noteworthy observation is that a majority of them—and particularly the female patients—came from countries in Western Europe. The proportion of visitors to Florence from Western Europe, however, is smaller than that from other parts of the world—North America, for example. Further, while 37% of visitors to Florence are university graduates, only 9% of those admitted to the hospital were college educated; and in the 26–40 age group, where it would be expected that most would have long since finished their schooling and have established careers, there was a high percentage of students and persons who were unemployed.

Most of the patients, and in particular the women, were traveling on their own rather than with friends or on an organized tour. Most also had only very loosely structured itineraries. It is also noteworthy that more than half of the patients were not new to psychiatric institutions; *i.e.*, they had had at least one prior contact with a psychiatrist or psychologist, although not necessarily one followed up by either therapy or hospitalization. Psychiatric precedents were most common among patients whose symptoms were classified as mental (*i.e.*, altered sense of reality and changes in perception) rather than those with primarily physical, (*i.e.*, psychosomatic) complaints. A picture thus emerges of the "typical" patient as single, relatively young, sensitive, impressionable, traveling alone (or perhaps with one companion), encountering the great works of art and architecture on a one-to-one basis without the mediation of a hired guide.

Some case histories

Before presenting some of the conclusions this author and her colleagues have drawn about the nature of the psychological crisis in Stendhal syndrome, it is useful to consider a few case histories:

Caterina. Caterina, an unmarried 20-year-old nursery school teacher from Switzerland, arrived at the psychiatric ward of the hospital of Santa Maria Nuova accompanied by a *carabiniere* (military policeman). She had been found at sunset in the Boboli Gardens, splendid Renaissance gardens, now a public park, that rise on a hill behind the Pitti Palace. It was not clear how long Caterina had been wandering among the Boboli's fountains, grottoes, and shaded avenues. A park attendant, preparing to close the gates, asked her to leave, but she seemed to be confused and did not comply with his request. She was carrying a diary full of pressed flowers and drawings of an almost childlike naïveté, which she refused to part with.

When she was questioned upon arrival at the hospital, Caterina said of herself that she was "a very special person." The doctors learned that she was an aspiring artist, was traveling alone, and had been in Florence for about a week, during which time she had been, she said, "just about everywhere." She appeared detached from reality, slightly confused, and very much in need of a rest. Her vaguely bohemian manner of dress—she wore a long, flowing skirt—lent her an air of being unconcerned with fashion.

Because she was such an intensely visual rather than verbal person—and because she spoke little Italian—the doctors thought that her drawings, to which she was so obviously attached, might provide insights into

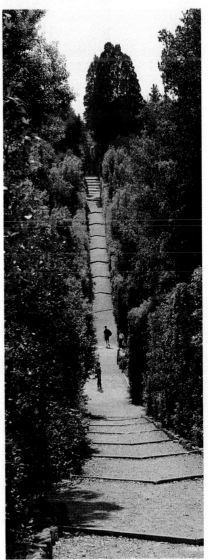

Florence's Boboli Gardens, behind the Pitti Palace, date from 1550 and are among the most admired gardens of the Renaissance world. With their grottoes, fountains, and shaded alleyways, the gardens remain a place full of surprises. One of the patients treated for Stendhal syndrome was discovered there, wandering and confused, after closing time.

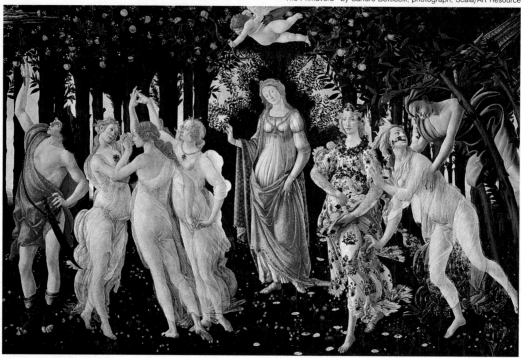

"The Primavera," or "Allegory of Spring" (above), and its companion work, "The Birth of Venus," by Sandro Botticelli (1445–1510) are displayed together in Room 10 of the Uffizi Gallery. According to one contemporary guidebook, the majority of those visiting the museum "come for the Botticelli." Generations of art historians and critics have commented on the confrontation between the intellectual and the sensual—complex imagery intermingling with graceful languor—that imbues this artist's works. Certainly the seductive appeal of his paintings remains undiminished by time.

her personality that were otherwise unobtainable. A striking feature of the drawings was that some bore the names "Spring," "Venus," and "Botticelli." The doctors learned that the highlight of Caterina's stay in Florence, as for so many visitors, had been her visit to the Uffizi Gallery and specifically to the room that contains two of Botticelli's most celebrated works, "The Birth of Venus" and "The Primavera." The press of the museum's crowd, Caterina's eager anticipation of seeing the Botticelli paintings, and her general state of exhaustion due to her ambitious itinerary of sightseeing may have contributed to her extreme emotional reaction to these pictures—although it should be noted that even the most jaded art historians have testified to being deeply affected by these works. It was the beauty of Botticelli's paintings that inspired Caterina's own drawings, in which, the doctors felt, she seemed to be trying to project parts of herself. Although one cannot say for sure, it may have been that Caterina, in her intense preoccupation with Botticelli, was experiencing within herself a conflict between her intellectual and sensual natures not unlike that experienced by Botticelli himself and expressed so clearly in his art.

Despite the language problem, the doctors were able to learn something of Caterina's early life. She had been a delicate child with a small appetite, and her growth lagged behind that of her contemporaries. As she grew up, she was always considered bright and capable, and she was eager to learn. But, Caterina told the doctors, she had suffered from several "breakdowns" that coincided with important changes or transitions in her life, such as going from grammar school to high school.

During her hospital stay, Caterina was encouraged to speak of herself in terms of images, since this seemed to be her primary means of self-

182

expression. She also benefited from a mild tranquilizer. She made a good recovery and was able to leave the hospital after five days.

Kamil. Kamil, a young painter from Prague, was traveling in Italy with a friend. Their itinerary, which Kamil himself had meticulously planned down to the last detail, included Trieste, Verona, Milan, Florence, and Venice. Although he was hitchhiking and carrying his clothes in a rucksack, Kamil made it clear that he did not want to be seen as just another of the many unwashed youths traveling around Europe on a shoestring.

Kamil and his friend had planned to spend only three days in Florence, during which time they intended to make use of "every precious moment." Both of them felt keenly that because of the political situation in Czechoslovakia at the time, they might never again have an opportunity to travel abroad. Thus, Kamil viewed this trip as probably the only opportunity he would ever have to see the art treasures of Italy that he had studied with such great pleasure in his student years at the Academy of Fine Arts in Prague. In expressing the importance of the trip, Kamil conveyed a seriousness and intensity that seemed deeply ingrained in his character.

These traits probably were not surprising in view of what the doctors were able to learn of his life in Prague. Kamil came from a prominent family, known not only in Prague but throughout Czechoslovakia. His father was a well-known and widely read writer; his mother, a scientist. He had grown up in a family of "committed intellectuals."

On their last scheduled day in Florence, Kamil and his friend had gone to the church of Santa Maria del Carmine—particularly to see the frescoes by Masaccio in the Brancacci Chapel in the church's west transept. Probably the most famous of these paintings—although it was not mentioned specifically by Kamil—is "The Expulsion of Adam and Eve from Paradise." For any viewer, the passion with which this event is depicted, the palpable sense of tragedy in Masaccio's rendering, cannot go unnoticed. To the eye of an artist as sensitive as Kamil, however, the aesthetic experience of "The Expulsion" could well be emotionally overwhelming.

In fact, it was just this kind of profound experience Kamil described. He expressed himself fluently in Italian and was able to give the doctors a vivid account of what had happened. Immediately upon leaving the church, he had felt ill. "When we came out onto the steps," he said, "we were exhausted, completely drained of energy as if we had come out of ourselves, coming out of that church." Once outside, he lay down on the ground; he felt that to take even one step would be impossible. He said he felt as if he were "dissolving" physically. He did not know how long he lay there without moving. He was aware that his friend was still with him but did not know if the friend was experiencing these same sensations. Only one image kept recurring in his mind: his own bed at home in Prague. The thought of the bed was comforting; it gave him a sense of security that enabled him to survive this potentially disintegrating experience.

In his treatment at the hospital, Kamil talked much of Masaccio, an artist who seemed to hold a key place in his esteem. He said he could "*only* admire" the works of the other Florentines, whereas Masaccio's paintings had a depth and substance found nowhere else. In addition to talking with

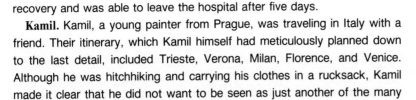

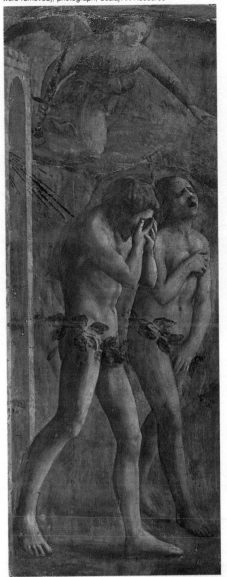

"The Expulsion of Adam and Eve from Paradise" before cleaning and restoration, completed in 1989 (the fig leaves, not by Masaccio, were removed); photograph, Scala/Art Resource

Few who go to Florence consider the trip complete without seeing the celebrated fresco cycle by Masaccio in the Brancacci Chapel of Santa Maria del Carmine. Even the young Michelangelo went to view—and copy—these works. In "The Expulsion of Adam and Eve from Paradise" (c. 1428), the grief of the two intensely human figures is almost palpable. Everyone who sees them is touched by their tragic sense of loss. One of the author's patients, a young Czechoslovak artist, was nonetheless unprepared for their tremendous emotional impact.

the doctors, Kamil's treatment involved rest and the administration of a mild tranquilizer. He returned to Prague on his release from the hospital.

Brigitte. Brigitte was a young woman who appeared at Santa Maria Nuova in the spring of 1986. It was her first time in Florence. She had at first consulted a general practitioner there for symptoms of extreme fatigue, dizziness, and rapid heartbeat. The doctor found nothing physically wrong with her, except that she was a bit depressed and had a vague sense of unreality; a psychiatric consultation was suggested.

When she was questioned by the psychiatrists, Brigitte acknowledged that her discomfort stemmed from more than just being among the enormous crowds of tourists in Florence; there were also "inner events" that were disturbing her. The hospital staff found her to be intelligent and extremely receptive to their questions and their interest in helping her. Of her early life they learned that she had been quite excitable as a child, having a passionate nature, but her emotions had always been kept in check by strict discipline at home, particularly by her father, and at school.

The city of Florence made a remarkably strong impression on her, and much suppressed emotion was now emerging. The encounter with Florentine art in particular stimulated in Brigitte an intense latent sensuality. "We are unprepared, we of the North, for these upsets," she said, referring to the interplay of the spiritual and the sensual so manifest in the art of Italy. Her northern European "Protestant, puritanical upbringing" had not prepared her for this encounter with the southern, Mediterranean sensibility. She expressed surprise that even a religious painter such as Fra Angelico, whose works seem to embody purity and ingenuousness, expresses in his colors "a strong, violent sensuality. He has these reds, these blues . . . almost like Matisse . . . these juxtapositions of very bright colors. . . . In the North everything is more veiled . . . whereas [in Italy] the spiritual life seems to be tied to the sexual life. Spirituality and sensuality coexist in the Latin personality," she said.

Brigitte's therapy consisted primarily of talking with the doctors about her feelings; this opportunity to express herself and interact with a therapist produced a marked improvement. She realized that until her experience in Florence she had never known real emotional freedom. She discovered in her brief psychotherapy the extent to which her feelings had been repressed; as a result of it, she was able to grow as a person.

Franz. Franz was a mature Bavarian bachelor—a civil engineer by trade. One of his hobbies was playing in a string quartet. He was cultured and well-mannered but somewhat affected. He had been to Italy on earlier trips, but this visit was to be a sort of "grand tour," on which he intended to see the art treasures and immerse himself in Italian culture.

Franz's visits to the Uffizi Gallery had a tremendous impact on him. He returned several times. On the first day, he had walked from room to room, feeling dazed, "his head and his heart on fire." He said that he saw colors he had never seen before and felt as if he were being "assailed by their chromatic waves." On subsequent visits to the museum, he had experienced strange mixtures of emotion—exhaustion and excitement, joy and panic. Some pictures seemed to exert special attractions, and these

A crowd gathers in front of the Uffizi to await its opening. A visit to the famed gallery is a highlight on the itinerary of most tourists. The museum's collection is certainly one of the most precious in the world, offering examples of painting from the 13th through the 18th century and including works by most of the significant Italian artists of the Florentine school. Although many may try, it is virtually impossible to see everything in a single visit. For the unwary, the press of crowds, the heat, and the sheer sensory overload can easily overwhelm.

Katharine W. Hannaford

184

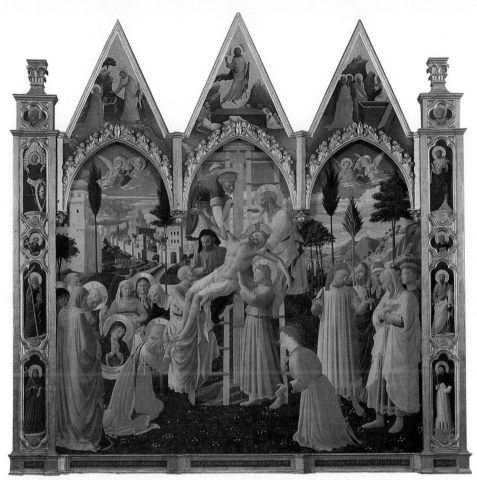

he went to see again and again, each time with a new appreciation, each time noting different details. He experienced a state of exaltation, as if a new "self" were being born out of these turbulent emotions.

One day, stopping before Caravaggio's "The Young Bacchus," he was seized by an attraction not unlike sexual attraction, which, he said, made him feel at once good and bad. He experienced physical symptoms, which he described as a heaviness, or oppression, in his chest, sweating, and faintness. He sought medical help but was advised that the problem was psychological rather than physical. He was thus referred to the psychiatrists at Santa Maria Nuova.

The doctors learned than while in Florence Franz had slept little and badly. At night he was flooded with indescribable emotions, assailed by nameless longings. Upon questioning him about his childhood and family background, they learned that he was the youngest of five children and had been brought up in a well-ordered atmosphere of bourgeois respectability. The crisis that he had experienced in the Uffizi they believed to be basically a crisis of identity, in which unresolved elements of his psychosexual growth had been set free and were struggling to be integrated into his personality. In his lifelong attempt to suppress homosexual inclinations, which were deeply at odds with his respectable upbringing, Franz had at the same time repressed the passionate side of his own nature. The aesthetic experiences he had undergone at the Uffizi had awakened dormant passions within him and forced him to confront this hidden side of himself.

Even in the works of a deeply religious painter such as Fra Angelico, spiritual and sensual elements coexist, as one woman suffering from Stendhal syndrome noted. Visiting the Museum of San Marco, she was struck by this gentle artist's juxtaposition of very bright colors, in which she saw a "strong, violent sensuality" that was foreign and disconcerting to her. During her hospitalization in Florence, she was able to become more accepting of the sexual aspect of her own nature, which her "Protestant, puritanical upbringing" had denied.

"Deposition" by Fra Angelico; photograph, Scala/Art Resource

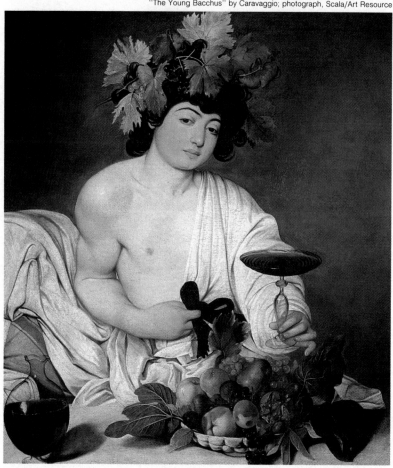

In the course of many visits to the Uffizi, a mature Bavarian traveler found a particular fascination in Caravaggio's "The Young Bacchus" (1593). Contemplating the painting, he began to experience disquieting physical symptoms—tightness of the chest, sweating, and faintness. Worried, he consulted a physician, who advised him that the problem was not physical but psychological. Later, in psychotherapy, he was able to understand that his ambivalence about his own sexual orientation was at the root of the turbulent emotions aroused by "Bacchus."

Franz was well enough to continue his trip after his release from the hospital. Upon his return home, he worked with a therapist who spoke his language and was able to explore his conflicts in more depth. A few months after his departure from Florence, Franz sent a letter of thanks to his doctors there. It was an optimistic message in which he indicated that his newly acquired self-knowledge was enabling him to live life more fully.

Isabelle. Isabelle, a cultivated and refined young French woman, a teacher of art history, was visiting the Uffizi Gallery with a group of her pupils. In one gallery, the Corridoio Vasariano, or Vasari Corridor, which contains portraits of famous people and self-portraits of many artists, she was aware that she felt a particular aversion to certain paintings. She was suddenly overcome with a desire to deface them. So strong was this impulse that she actually feared she might not be able to restrain herself from committing these violent and destructive acts. When she arrived at the hospital, she was agitated and in a state of depression.

In their initial observation of Isabelle, the doctors thought she might be suffering from intense separation anxiety, sharpened by being so far from home and exacerbated by an acute awareness of death, which had been heightened in the portrait gallery by her realization that these people, so very alive in their pictures, were long since dead.

186

In further discussions, more information was elicited about Isabelle's early life. She had been raised in an atmosphere of harmoniousness and gentility. As an infant and young girl, Isabelle had suppressed the cruder human needs and instincts, which in her family would have been unacceptable. In her relationship with her mother, Isabelle's own emotions had been repudiated. Later Isabelle had tried to find a socially acceptable outlet for her crude needs and brute urges, which she had apparently found in her appreciation of art. The doctors felt that in the experience of personally confronting the works of art she had studied and admired for so long, Isabelle's repressed feelings came to the surface and opened the way for an attack of hostility and resentment. She then felt "split" by two opposing feelings toward the works of art: on the one hand, a sincere interest and appreciation of the aesthetic qualities, which very likely represented the idealized qualities of her mother, and, on the other hand, deeply buried hostility emerging in overwhelming feelings of frustration and rage. Upon leaving the hospital, she continued her traveling.

Psychiatric profiles

In studying the 106 cases of tourists admitted to Santa Maria Nuova, from which the above five are drawn, the psychiatrists have discovered three general psychiatric profiles. (The clinical manifestations, however, often overlap.) These are: (1) patients with a predominant disturbance of thought, linked to alterations in their perception of reality; (2) patients with predominant disturbances of affect, or mood; and (3) patients with panic crises and somaticized anxiety, manifest in physical symptoms.

The first group includes all those who were suffering from altered perceptions of sounds or colors; some had frank hallucinations. Patients in this thought-disturbance category experienced delusions of persecution, often combined with anxiety and feelings of guilt.

In the second group, those with disturbances of affect, the doctors observed depressive anguish; a sense of uselessness, emptiness, or inadequacy; or, in contrast, euphoria, exaltation, and feelings of omnipotence, often marked by impaired judgment and a limited capacity for reality testing.

Patients in the third group had all the symptoms of generalized panic disorder, experienced variously as shortness of breath, faintness, trembling, sweating, nausea, chest pain, rapid heartbeat, and visual disturbances, along with fears of dying, choking, or going insane.

As mentioned above, there have been no Italian travelers among the Stendhal syndrome patients. Thus emerges perhaps the most important common factor shared by the patients—the feeling of being "lost" in a foreign country. It is well known that such an experience can induce a psychic crisis—bringing out troubling emotions that have long been repressed. A special part seems to be played by the fact that the individual is removed from his or her cultural context and, even more important, is in a situation where linguistic barriers cause an acute sense of isolation. They are in acute need of the familiar; they need to hear their own language. For this reason, the psychiatric staff encourages patients to call home or contact the consulate in Florence of their home country.

The author has compiled all available data on the cases of Stendhal syndrome seen over a 10-year period at the hospital in Florence, including the type of trip (whether travel was independent or on an organized tour) and the age, sex, marital status, and nationality of patients. The doctors at Santa Maria Nuova have been able to draw some conclusions about the relationship between the type of disturbance experienced by the individual traveler and his or her previous psychiatric history and to correlate these factors with the outcome; i.e., whether the person was able to continue the journey after leaving the hospital or went home to familiar territory instead.

Sex and age of patients

sex	age in years (%)			total* (%)
	26 and under	26–40	over 40	
women	14 (33)	18 (43)	10 (24)	42 (100)
men	21 (35.5)	24 (40.5)	14 (24)	59 (100)
total	35 (34.5)	42 (41.5)	24 (24)	101 (100)

*5 unknown

Outcome and previous psychiatric history

previous history	outcome of hospital stay (%)			total* (%)
	continued trip	returned home	other	
no	13 (33.5)	22 (56.5)	4 (10)	39 (100)
yes	9 (18)	30 (60)	11 (22)	50 (100)

*17 unknown

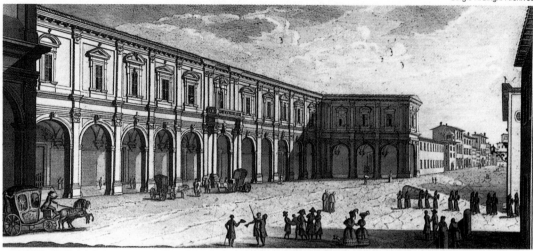

In the heart of Florence, slightly to the east of the Duomo, is Santa Maria Nuova, the city's oldest hospital, dating to the late 13th century. The engraving shows an early 18th-century view of the building. Today the hospital has 353 beds, with 10 in the psychiatric unit. In or near Florence there are five other hospitals— the Careggi Hospital being the largest, with 2,000 beds—but Santa Maria Nuova probably sees the most foreign patients.

Outcome

For tourists who experience strong reactions and are hospitalized, the length of the hospital stay is a variable that seems to be related to several factors, including the sex of the patient, the type of trip, the history of psychiatric episodes, and the type of psychic disturbance. Typically, men's hospitalizations were brief—53% of the men remained for less than four days, whereas only 30% of the women had comparably short stays. Understandably, patients with prevalent disturbances of thought more often had longer hospitalizations than those suffering from acute affective disturbances—the former representing a clinically more severe form of illness. Length of stay was also related to the type of trip—the frequency of hospital stays of eight days or more was greater among those not traveling in organized tours—probably because these travelers were not committed to a fixed itinerary.

Patients differed widely in clinical outcome. In most cases there was either rapid recovery or improvement or an unchanged condition at the time of discharge. Age seems to have been an important factor here. Generally, the younger the patient, the better the chance for a rapid resolution of the problem. The percentage of recoveries after a brief stay in the hospital diminished as the patient's age increased—14% of those under 26 improved rapidly and were discharged, as compared with 10% of those aged 26–40 and 4% of those over 40. Analysis with mathematical models has also highlighted the fact that a close correlation exists between clinical outcome and type of psychic disturbance; patients with predominant disturbances of thought were 7.7 times more likely to be unchanged in their condition upon discharge than patients with predominantly affective disturbances.

A significant moment of reckoning occurred at the time of the discharge from the hospital, since it was at that time that the patient was forced to choose whether to return home (to yield, to seek the familiar conditions of everyday life) or to go on with the trip (risking rekindling of the isolation or rootlessness they experienced so profoundly in Florence). The author and her colleagues observed that those patients with disturbances of thought

188

Photographs, (below) Sergio Ardinghi Archives; (below right) courtesy of Graziella Magherini

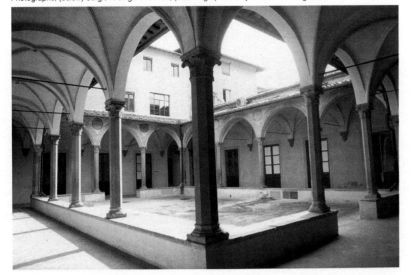

A contemporary view of Santa Maria Nuova shows the cloister of the large hospital complex. Graziella Magherini (below) continues to collect data on tourists treated for Stendhal syndrome. She is in touch with colleagues in other cities, including Venice and Jerusalem, where similar disturbances in visitors viewing great art treasures have been described. She and others hope to learn a great deal more about the emotional breakdowns that can be triggered in susceptible individuals by encounters with deeply moving works of art.

who had had previous psychiatric problems were the most likely to be unable to continue their travels.

Confrontations: art and the self

One constant factor emerges from the study of the various cases seen at Santa Maria Nuova: an identity crisis and, consequently, a crisis in the cohesion of the "self." In each case history there is an underlying link between three factors—personal history, journey, and sudden contact with art. Each factor plays a unique and contributory part. To begin with, there must be a susceptible individual—a person of extreme sensitivity, possibly a deeply conflicted individual or, in some cases, one who has a history of psychiatric problems. Second, there is the trip itself. Travel per se does not necessarily provoke crisis, but a journey can be destabilizing in that it involves a suspension of habitual roles and daily codes of conduct and the removal from one's familiar cultural and linguistic contexts.

Finally, to these is added the confrontation with great art, itself a powerful stimulus of emotions and unconscious experiences. The human mind, when face to face with a work of art, is forced to make an elaboration, a link between emotional experience and thought formation. At this critical juncture everyone encounters an interval, a moment—at an unconscious level—of uncertainty, fatigue, and confusion. It is a moment of transition that, depending on the circumstances and the personality of the person in question, can be the cause of a psychological breakdown or of mental and emotional growth.

Nonetheless, one must point out that there is a great deal more to be learned about the travelers who have such profound reactions to great art. It should be emphasized that 106 patients constitute a small cohort; firm conclusions can be drawn only from study of much larger groups. It is hoped that interest in and ongoing study of the cases that occur in Florence—and in other cities that are major cultural centers attracting vast numbers of tourists each year—will further illuminate this fascinating phenomenon.

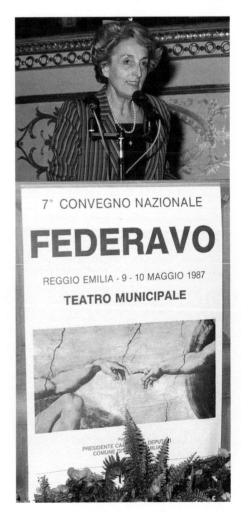

7° CONVEGNO NAZIONALE

FEDERAVO

REGGIO EMILIA - 9 - 10 MAGGIO 1987

TEATRO MUNICIPALE

189

Life-Style, Habits, and Health:
Medicine Learns from the Mormons

by Joseph L. Lyon, M.D., M.P.H.

Joseph L. Lyon, M.D., M.P.H., is Associate Professor, Department of Family and Preventive Medicine, University of Utah School of Medicine, Salt Lake City.

(Opposite page) Mormon family at the evening meal. Photograph, Patsy Lynch

Since ancient times it has been believed that life-styles and personal habits have an effect on human health. It is not surprising, therefore, that practices thought to be associated with good health have been incorporated into religions, both ancient and modern, in the form of various rules, laws, and prohibitions. Perhaps the best known in the Western world is the Law of Moses, set down in the Old Testament book of Leviticus. It included detailed rules on a variety of subjects from dietary practices to childbirth, from treatment of lepers to disposal of human waste. Mosaic law specifically forbade the Jews to eat the flesh of many animals, including pigs, camels, birds of prey, certain insects, and shellfish, all of which were characterized as "unclean" (Leviticus, chapter 11). The proscription against the eating of blood (Leviticus 17:12) was ultimately interpreted to mean that food animals had to be slaughtered in such a way that the blood was properly drained from the carcass.

A conflict over the observance of the Jewish dietary requirements, recorded in the first chapter of the book of Daniel, prompted one of the first recorded tests of the health effects of the Mosaic law. According to this account, when Jerusalem fell in 587 BC, Daniel and several other well-born young Jewish men were taken captive by King Nebuchadnezzar and brought to serve in the king's household. They were well treated and offered the finest food and wine available, that which the king himself ate. Daniel protested that the king's food, although the best in the land, would nevertheless defile him and his companions because it was not approved by the Law of Moses. He persuaded the king's steward to bring the captives only vegetables and to permit them to drink water rather than wine. After 10 days "they were better in appearance and fatter in flesh" (Daniel 1:15) than those men who had eaten the king's delicacies. Thus, the king permitted the Jews to continue eating their special diet.

Studying disease in modern times

In the present century, life expectancy of people in most parts of the world has increased quite dramatically. In the U.S., for example, it rose

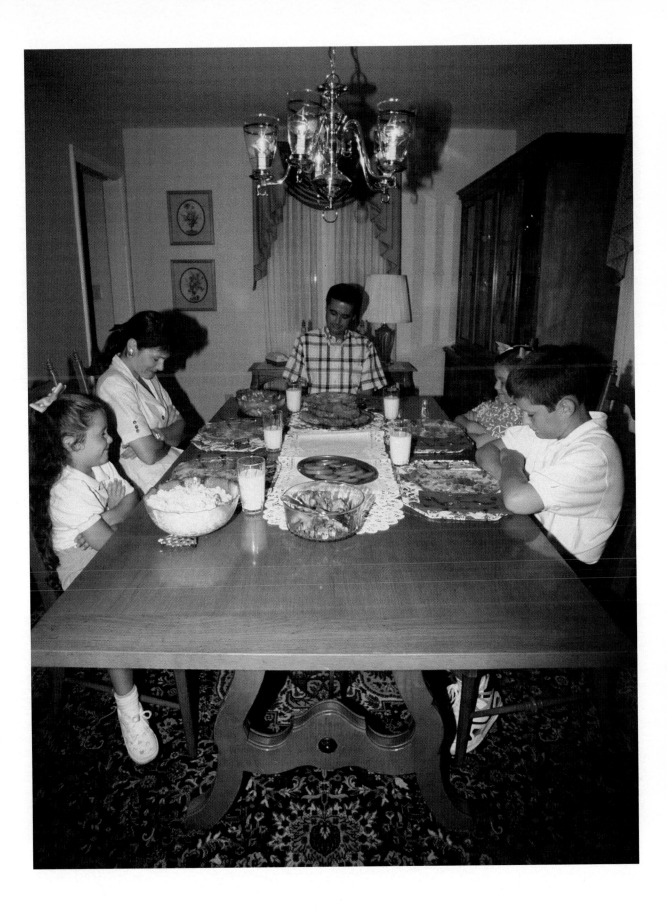

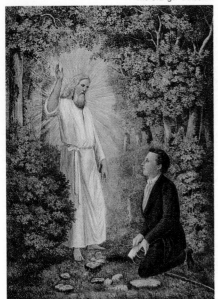

A lithograph depicts the seminal event in Mormon history: the angel Moroni revealing to Joseph Smith the golden "plates" on which the Mormon scriptures were inscribed. Smith founded the first Mormon church in Fayette, New York, in 1830. Religious persecution forced his followers to move steadily westward, to settle eventually in Utah. Their pilgrimage is depicted below by a Mormon artist who himself made the journey in 1857.

from around 50 years in 1900 to about 75 years presently. The increased longevity of Americans—and the peoples of most other developed countries—is almost entirely due to the conquest of infectious diseases. Today heart disease, cancer, and strokes account for about 60% of all U.S. deaths. These are chronic, and to a large extent incurable, conditions. Beginning in the 1940s epidemiologists—scientists who study the incidence of disease in large population groups—began to search for the causes of these chronic disorders. Several large groups of people were enrolled in long-term studies to determine the causes of heart disease. One of the longest running and most comprehensive such investigations is the now famous Framingham Heart Study, in which about 5,000 adult residents of the town of Framingham, Massachusetts, originally took part. The ongoing study has reached important conclusions about how diet, physical activity level, smoking, alcohol consumption, stress, body weight, and hypertension contribute to the risk for heart disease. Other groups have been instrumental in providing important information about the effects of smoking on lung and other types of cancer—in the ongoing study of British physicians, for example, in which a majority of the doctors in the U.K. have been followed medically since 1953. The common thread running through the findings from these various investigations is that life-style and personal habits do influence an individual's risk of acquiring chronic diseases. At the same time, it has also been recognized that some of these diseases "run in the family"—that is, they are more common among the parents and siblings of one family than another—thus, it is presumed that heredity also plays a part in their development.

Studies of diseases in large human populations are difficult and costly and can be quite time consuming because thousands of individuals must be identified and followed medically for 10 or more years. Hereditary studies

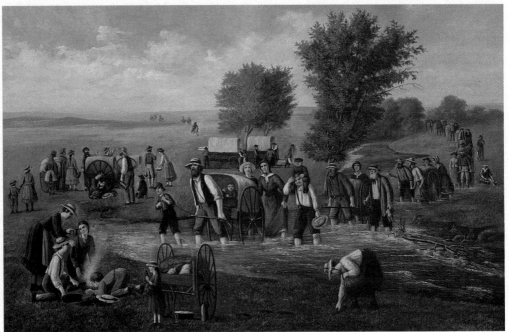

"The Handcart Company" by C.C.A. Christensen, 1900, oil on canvas; collection, Museum of Church History and Art, Salt Lake City

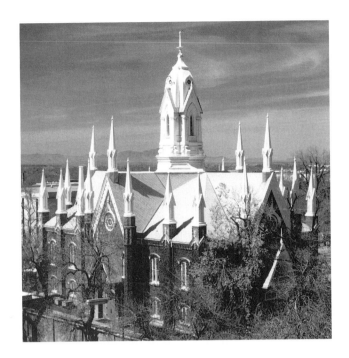

of chronic diseases pose even greater problems because accurate, detailed pedigrees (records of the ancestry of individuals) must be constructed. The process involves identifying thousands of cousins, uncles and aunts, and parents and grandparents of a given individual with a particular disease and then accurately determining their cause of death. This may mean that an investigator will have to determine the cause of a death that may have occurred 100 or more years ago.

The Mormons of Utah: "living laboratory" for epidemiologists

In searching for suitable populations to study, a number of epidemiologists have been especially attracted to the state of Utah, home to a large group of members of the Church of Jesus Christ of Latter-day Saints. This church, whose members are known both as Mormons—after one of their books of scripture—and as Latter-day Saints (often abbreviated to LDS), was founded in 1830 in upstate New York. Religious persecution, however, drove the church west. From the late 1840s until about 1900, the Mormons created new settlements throughout the intermountain West (present-day Utah, Idaho, Nevada, Wyoming, Oregon, and California). While the original settlers of Utah were virtually all LDS church members, the opening of the mining industry, after the coming of the railroad in 1869, brought in substantial numbers of non-Mormon settlers. By 1920 only 55% of the state's population were LDS. Later, with the closing of many mines, the proportion of the population who were LDS once again increased, and by 1950 Mormons constituted 70% of Utah's population. This proportion has remained fairly constant.

As a population group the Mormons of Utah are of particular interest to medical scientists because they are extremely homogenous in their ethnic backgrounds and life-styles. The vast majority are the descendants of

193

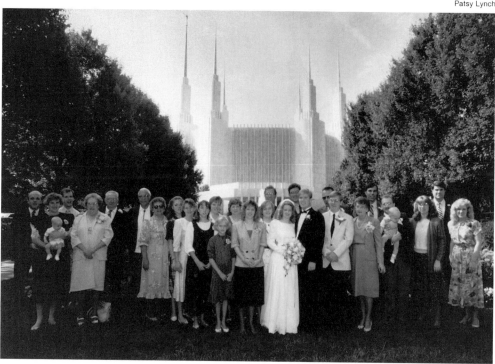

The families of a newly married Mormon couple pose for a formal portrait outside the Washington, D.C., temple. Although plural marriages were once a common Mormon practice, they have long been banned and, in fact, lifelong monogamy is the rule for LDS church members. The bond of marriage—like other family ties—is believed to be eternal, transcending even death. The tracing of one's family tree—which is for many non-Mormons simply an indulgence of curiosity—is for LDS church members virtually a religious mission.

immigrants from England, Germany, and Scandinavia. They can be characterized as middle-class in income and education level—79% of adults are high-school graduates and 27% have college educations. Because of the emphasis in Mormonism on the sanctity of marriage (the controversial practice of plural marriage was officially halted in 1890), the average adult member of the church in Utah is likely to be married and to remain married. Only about 2% of LDS adults are not or have not been married (compared with 10% of the state's non-LDS population), and about 93% marry once (80% among the non-LDS). The average Mormon family, with about 4.1 children, is larger than that of non-Mormon counterparts in Utah and nearly double the size of the average American family.

As a religious group with unique practices, the LDS are of special interest to epidemiologists. Since 1833 the church has promulgated a health code called the Word of Wisdom. This health law, which was handed down in the form of a revelation to LDS church founder Joseph Smith, enjoins church members to abstain from all forms of alcohol and tobacco and "hot drinks" (coffee or tea). According to the text of the revelation, those who obey these commandments shall have "health in their navel and marrow to their bones." It is furthermore promised that they "shall run and not be weary, and shall walk and not faint." The Word of Wisdom specifically encourages the eating of fruits and grains. All forms of meat are also allowed but are to be eaten "sparingly." Since the early part of the 20th century, strict adherence to the Word of Wisdom has been viewed as a requirement for full participation in the church.

The diet of the contemporary Mormon population of Utah is roughly comparable to the average American diet. The LDS diet is slightly lower in

194

calories, however, because of the proscription on alcohol, and both LDS and non-LDS in Utah consume a slightly lower proportion of calories as fat than is the average in the U.S. As a result of the prohibitions against drinking and smoking, which are widely but not universally adhered to by church members, consumption of all forms of alcoholic beverage by the adult population of Utah is about half that of the United States population as a whole, and only about 15% of adults in Utah smoke, compared with 30% of those living elsewhere in the country.

Another distinction that makes the LDS population of Utah of particular interest to epidemiologists grows out of the Mormon belief that family ties, including marriage, are eternal and that religious ordinances such as baptism can be performed by living church members for their deceased ancestors. These rituals are performed on an individual rather than a group basis, with a living church member experiencing the rite by proxy, as it were, for a specific ancestor. A woman church member can perform this function only for female relatives, a man only for his male forebears. This practice has led the LDS church to assemble the world's largest collection of data that identify specific individuals.

The records that have been collected by the church come from virtually every country in the world and date back as far as the 14th century. They include parish registers, tax roles, emigration documents, censuses, and birth, death, and marriage certificates. They are used by church members to construct and verify family trees and are available to the public through the Genealogical Society of Utah, a private, nonprofit corporation affiliated with the LDS church. Copies of most records are on microfilm, and some have been transferred to compact optical discs suitable for use in a personal computer. Microfilm negatives of the vast accumulation of genealogical data collected over the years are stored in an immense underground vault in Little Cottonwood Canyon, east of Salt Lake City. This archive, cut out of solid granite, has an area of more than 0.6 hectare (1.5 acres) and houses (on microfilm) the equivalent of more than two billion pages of records.

Church members are encouraged to use these records to construct and submit to the LDS Church Family History Library detailed pedigree charts that contain the names and birth, marriage, and death dates of all of their ancestors for the preceding three generations. Additional records maintained by the Genealogical Society of Utah include a file of all church members who have died since 1941 and a file containing the records (birth dates, parents' names, spouse's name) of all living members of the LDS church worldwide. (There are large LDS populations in Canada, Mexico, the U.K., New Zealand, and Samoa.)

Investigating disease through church records

Beginning in 1972 epidemiologists, taking advantage of these extensive records, began several large-scale studies of the health of LDS church members living in Utah. Because of the law proscribing cigarette smoking, and the known association between cigarette smoking and lung cancer, there was considerable interest in determining if cancer rates (for lung as well as other cancers) were lower among the LDS. The first study, which

The extensive collection of genealogical records that has been assembled over the years by the LDS church is housed in the Family History Library in Salt Lake City. The records are maintained by the Genealogical Society of Utah, a nonprofit organization established in 1894; they are open to the general public, Mormon and non-Mormon alike. Church members are encouraged to use the library's resources to construct detailed family trees called pedigree charts. These contain the names of all of a given individual's ancestors, going back at least three generations, and include the dates and places of each person's birth and death.

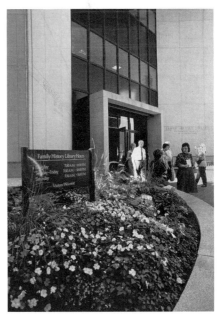

Brad Nelson—Nelson-Bohart & Associates

195

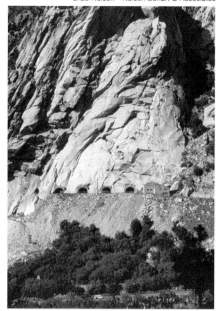

Brad Nelson—Nelson-Bohart & Associates

Microfilm copies of all of the LDS church's genealogical records are stored in an immense rock-cut vault in Little Cottonwood Canyon, east of Salt Lake City. This vast underground archive houses the equivalent of more than two billion pages of records.

was under the direction of this author (and published in the *New England Journal of Medicine* in 1976), serves as an example of the many others that have since been conducted through the use of the records of the Genealogical Society of Utah.

Since 1966 every new case of cancer occurring in Utah has been identified and registered by a state cancer registry. In the author's 1976 study, the records of this Utah Cancer Registry were compared (by church personnel) against the membership records of the LDS church. The process of record matching was done originally by hand but subsequently by a computer algorithm. It involved associating the names of about 80,000 Utahans known to have had cancer with the more than one million individuals in the church's genealogical files. Since neither of these two sets of records shares a unique number that could be matched—for example, a Social Security number—the computer had to examine each name in both files and also the birth dates and other information in order to determine if the two records identified the same individual. Because the church is concerned with protecting the confidentiality of members' records, after the linking was completed, all information that could identify a specific person was removed.

Since its founding Salt Lake City—and subsequently all outlying settlements—has been divided into units called wards. These are geographic and administrative districts similar to parishes. Each church member is also recorded as a member of his or her ward. The data from each ward provide an accurate count of the number of church members living within a specific area. Annually the number of members in each ward is reported to church headquarters, providing a count by geographic area of the LDS population.

Combining the information from the linked cancer registry and genealogical records and the LDS population count provided the rates of cancer for LDS in the state of Utah. Subtracting the LDS cancer cases from the total number of cases reported in Utah, and the LDS population from the total population of the state, produced the rates of disease in the LDS and non-LDS living in Utah. These rates were adjusted so that any differences in age between the two population groups would not influence the survey results.

Strikingly low Mormon cancer rates

Between 1967 and 1975 there were 12,175 new cases of cancer (of all types—with the exception of nonmelanotic skin cancer, which is not reportable) in the LDS population of Utah. On the basis of cancer rates for the rest of the U.S., more than 16,000 cases would have been expected. The rate in the LDS was 74.3%—or nearly three-fourths—of the overall U.S. cancer rate. Much of this difference was accounted for by the lower proportion of cigarette smokers among the LDS. For example, among church members cancer of the lung, the cancer that has the strongest association with cigarette smoking, occurred at a rate that was approximately one-third of that expected in the U.S. population in general.

The number of cases of cancer of the uterine cervix (cervical cancer) was also smaller than expected in the LDS population. The incidence of cervical cancer was about 45% lower among LDS women than among women

196

living elsewhere in the U.S. In 1976, when the original study was done, cervical cancer was not believed to be related to cigarette smoking. Further, because most of the large follow-up studies of smokers had not included women, there were no data on the association between smoking and the development of cervical cancer. Since 1983, however, when the author's original study was published, more detailed studies in Utah and elsewhere have established the fact that this malignancy is indeed associated with cigarette smoking. But merely to note an association between two factors, such as smoking and the development of cervical cancer, is not necessarily to determine a cause-and-effect relationship. A major barrier to a more conclusive demonstration of causality was the fact that the cells of the uterine cervix are never actually exposed to cigarette smoke. This same point had been raised in the 1960s, when follow-up studies of smokers found them to be at increased risk for cancers of the kidneys and pancreas. It was later established that both of these organs concentrate and secrete tobacco products carried by the bloodstream and are thereby indirectly exposed to the carcinogenic properties of tobacco smoke. In 1985 work by Nancy Haley of the American Health Foundation in Valhalla, New York, established the fact that many of the chemicals in cigarette smoke enter the bloodstream through the lungs and are secreted by the cells lining the female genital tract. This observation provided a plausible explanation for the decreased risk of cancer of the uterine cervix seen in LDS women.

The pedigree chart of one member of the author's family, shown below, indicates that the author is the youngest of six children, all of them sons. Like many other Utah Mormons, the Lyons are descended from settlers who moved to the United States from Great Britain and Scandinavia.

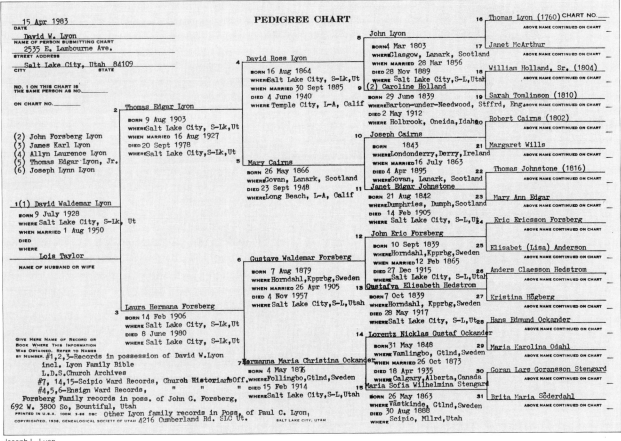

Joseph L. Lyon

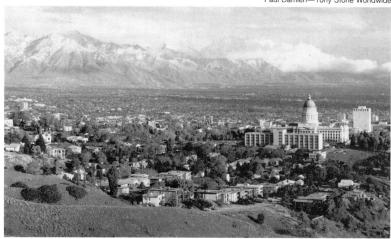

Since 1972 epidemiologists at the University of Utah and elsewhere have taken advantage of the records maintained by the Genealogical Society of Utah to study the incidence of disease in the LDS and non-LDS populations of the state. The Mormons are of particular interest to medical scientists because of religious practices that influence their life-style and habits—e.g., abstention from the use of alcohol and tobacco. As a result of these practices, the LDS tend to have strikingly lower rates of most cancers (graph, opposite page). One exception to this rule is the incidence of cancer of the lip, which is higher in Utah—in which a large proportion of the population ski— than in the rest of the U.S. High rates of lip cancer are seen in both LDS and non-LDS. Since this form of cancer is related to exposure to sunlight, the higher rates are attributed in part to the especially intense ultraviolet light that is reflected off the snow-covered slopes in Utah, to which skiers are exposed.

In the 1976 study other cancers that occurred at rates well below those expected and that were not associated with cigarette smoking were cancers of the stomach, colon (large intestine), rectum, and female breast. The lower rates of breast cancer are partially explained by the earlier age at first pregnancy of women church members as compared with non-LDS women. (Many factors appear to be associated with increased risk of breast cancer, including diet and family history of the disease. Women who have their first child relatively early in their lives have lower rates of breast cancer than women who delay childbearing or are childless.) No explanation has been found for the lower rates of cancers of the digestive tract in the LDS population.

Skin and prostate cancers—exceptions to the rule

Two cancers were found to occur more often in Utah than in the U.S. as a whole. These were cancer of the lip, a cancer related to excess exposure to sunlight, and cancer of the male prostate gland. There was little difference in incidence between church members and nonmembers. The researchers were unable to explain the apparently higher than average rates of prostate cancer in men who live in Utah. And although the incidence of lip cancer is known to rise with increased exposure to sunlight, the risk for people living in Utah is so disproportionately large (more than three times that seen in other areas of the U.S.—or even when compared only with neighboring Colorado) that some other explanation must be considered. It may be that the large proportion of the Utah population who ski receive much greater sunlight exposure—from very intense ultraviolet rays reflected off snow— than skiers in other areas of the United States.

Another study of cancer in the LDS, conducted by epidemiologists at the University of Utah (published in August 1982 in the *American Journal of Epidemiology* by J.W. Gardner and this author), examined fatal cancers occurring in adult LDS church members between 1966 and 1970. There were 1,819 cancer cases among men and 1,561 cancer cases among women during this five-year interval. The study examined cancer risk among those who were active participants in the LDS church compared with those who

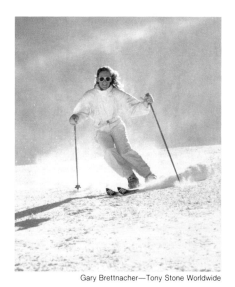

were not. The investigators made the basic assumption that an individual's level of religious participation would correlate with his or her adherence to the Mormon life-style and observance of the tenets of the Word of Wisdom. They used data from the records of deceased church members to classify individuals as to their participation in the church. A similar study of about 12,000 LDS church members living in California (conducted by James E. Enstrom of the University of California at Los Angeles and published in the *Journal of the National Cancer Institute,* December 1989) obtained information directly from church members by questionnaires sent out in the mail. Both of these studies found that LDS who were actively involved in the church—and thus more likely to abstain from smoking—had much lower rates of lung cancer. Other cancers associated with tobacco use (*e.g.,* oral cancers and cancer of the larynx, esophagus, and urinary bladder) were also much lower in the more active group.

Cancer in Utah

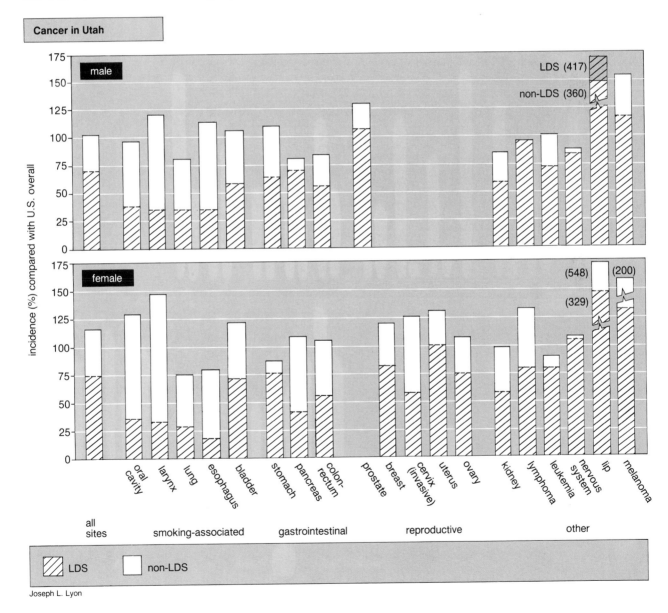

Joseph L. Lyon

One study conducted by the epidemiologists at the University of Utah examined cancer risk among LDS who were active participants in the church compared with those who were not, on the assumption that the level of participation would correlate with adherence to the church's prohibitions against smoking and drinking. The researchers found that those who were actively involved had significantly lower rates of lung cancer and several other cancers known to be associated with tobacco use.

Many benefits of abstinence

The adverse effects of tobacco and alcohol on the human body are not limited solely to their potential as carcinogens. One of the surprising findings from the early studies of cigarette smokers (the long-running study of British physicians and a 1966 study of U.S. veterans) was that smokers were at higher risk than nonsmokers of dying of heart disease. Over the past 15 years it has also been documented that women who smoke during pregnancy have smaller than average babies, who are thus more likely to be unhealthy or die within their first year of life. The adverse effects of alcohol have, of course, been well known for some time. They include increased risk of accidental death and, in those who drink excessively, death from cirrhosis of the liver. Women who drink even moderately during pregnancy increase their risk of giving birth to babies with the specific congenital malformations known as fetal alcohol syndrome.

Cancer rates and adherence to Mormon life-style

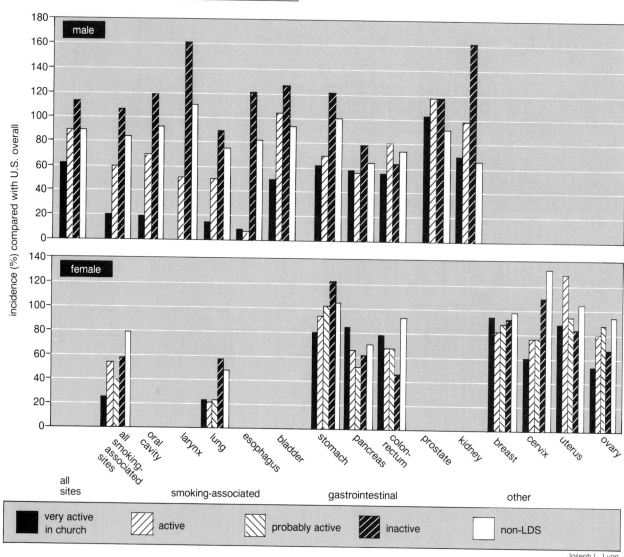

Joseph L. Lyon

By linking death certificates for specific causes to the membership records of deceased LDS church members, researchers have also examined the risk of heart disease, stroke, and cirrhosis of the liver among the LDS. These studies show that LDS in Utah are about 40% less likely than their non-LDS neighbors or others living elsewhere in the U.S. to die of a heart attack. Smoking, however, is only one of several factors involved in the development of heart disease, and the fact that most church members are nonsmokers does not completely account for this difference in deaths from heart attack. Other possible explanations may be that church members exercise more regularly or that fewer of them are obese.

The LDS experience slightly fewer deaths from strokes than the rest of the population. This is one area where the health code of the church confers little protection. Cigarette smoking is probably only a weak factor in the causation of death from strokes, and alcohol consumption—except for binge drinking—also is not closely correlated with stroke mortality.

As expected, the LDS were shown to have lower rates of death from cirrhosis of the liver. This finding undoubtedly reflects the habit of abstention from alcohol among LDS who observe the church's health code.

It has been suggested that because of the contributing effects of air pollution, people who live in cities have higher rates of death from lung disease than people in rural areas. The effects of cigarette smoking in conjunction with air pollutants have not been well evaluated. Members of the LDS church were shown to have the same lung cancer rates whether they lived in urban or rural areas of the state, but the same was not true for nonmembers living in Utah. Among the latter, lung cancer rates were nearly twice as high in urban areas as in rural ones. This finding suggests that the harmful effects of cigarette smoking exacerbate the ill effects of urban air pollution and that the cessation of cigarette smoking is likely to be more beneficial in reducing lung cancer rates than the cleaning up of polluted air.

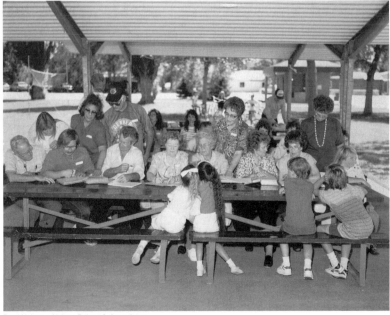

Brad Nelson—Nelson-Bohart & Associates

Attending a reunion in Midvale, Utah, in the summer of 1990, a few members of one large Mormon family take time to look over documents that show how they are related. These traditional gatherings of extended Mormon families have provided epidemiologists with unique opportunities to interview large numbers of related individuals in their pursuit of a better understanding of how familial factors influence the development of disease.

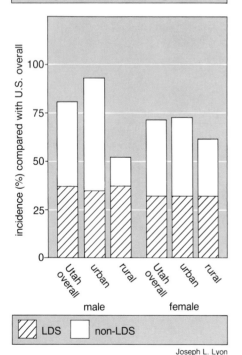

Smoking, air pollution, and lung cancer

Joseph L. Lyon

Do the Mormons perhaps enjoy better health than non-Mormons because church members have a built-in, hereditary resistance to heart disease and some cancers? Several studies have addressed this question and found that it is not so. The health of LDS church members living in California, Hawaii, and New Zealand has also been studied by epidemiologists. In Hawaii and New Zealand large numbers of church members are of Polynesian, rather than European, ancestry, yet they enjoy the same health benefits as are found among the LDS in Utah. This finding seems to confirm the view that the protection from certain diseases among the LDS is conferred by life-style rather than genetics.

Very few epidemiological studies have examined the possible health risks of coffee and tea drinking. One of the difficulties of research on coffee is that a large proportion of people who drink coffee are cigarette smokers, and disentangling the effects of coffee from those of cigarettes has been difficult. Studies of other population groups in the U.S. have found that coffee drinkers are at increased risk of dying from heart attacks and pancreatic cancer. No studies have been done in Utah to determine whether the low incidence of deaths from heart disease among the LDS can be partly explained by their tendency to abstain from coffee drinking. Pancreatic cancer rates are also about 40% lower among the LDS than in the rest of the U.S., and a recent study in Utah did confirm an association between coffee drinking and this disease.

Gardner's discovery: a rare cancer in LDS families

Studies that seek to determine the contribution of heredity to any particular disorder rely on the compilation of accurate information about the occurrence of specific medical conditions in relatives of a person who has the disease in question. Generally one individual is identified as having an unusual illness, or there is evidence that the illness is present in several family members of an individual who has the disease. The genetic epidemiologist must then begin by identifying all the members of that individual's immediate family and determining if any of them has the disease. If more family members are affected than would be expected on the basis of statistical probabilities, the investigator may then look for disease in cousins, uncles, aunts, great-uncles, and great-aunts of the affected individual. This kind of investigation can be extremely time consuming. Most people do not know offhand the names of all of their cousins, especially second or third cousins, or remember accurately the names of great-grandparents and their various siblings. Often many or all of the members of the older generation have already died.

One excellent example of a study of an inheritable disease that proved the value of the church's genealogical records was the identification of a rare genetic syndrome called Gardner's disease. This is a condition characterized by multiple abnormal growths, known as polyps, in the colon, which develop when individuals are in their thirties. People with the disorder also get abnormal bony growths, called exostoses, on the roof of the mouth. The polyps, if not removed surgically, eventually develop into a fatal cancer.

The syndrome was first identified in the 1940s by Eldon J. Gardner, a geneticist then working at the University of Utah. Gardner became interested when a student told him about a family in which many had died of cancer before age 50. He then contacted the family and began constructing the pedigree. This entailed interviewing all living family members and then checking the information against church genealogy records. Using these records, Gardner was also able to expand the pedigree to include distant family members not known to the original family. It was also necessary for him to confirm the cause of death in each case to more precisely determine the actual medical problems that led to the death. It took him about four years to collect and confirm the necessary data.

Once Gardner had constructed the complete pedigree and had determined accurate dates of birth and death and causes of death, it was clear to him that the family was suffering from an unusually high number of deaths from colon cancer. Further investigation identified the more subtle features of the syndrome, including polyps, exostoses, and certain benign growths of the skin. The identification of Gardner's syndrome demonstrated the usefulness of this kind of genetic study and also some of the problems. The main limitation was the availability of information about family members and their causes of death. Clearly, to facilitate studies of diseases that might be inherited, better data were needed.

Uncovering cancer "clusters"

Since 1894 the church had been promoting genealogical research to further the goal of baptizing the ancestors of church members who lived before the founding of the Mormon religion. In the 1960s, with the advent of fairly sophisticated data processing systems, the church requested that each member construct a pedigree chart and a family-group sheet going back four generations. Beginning in 1974 these family-group sheets (which contain the names of each ancestor, his or her spouse, and all of their children) were obtained from the Genealogical Society of Utah and entered into a computer data base. The project was funded by the National Cancer Institute (NCI) and was under the direction of Mark Skolnick, a population geneticist. It involved the inputting of over 1.2 million names of individuals, most of whom had lived in Utah from 1847 onward.

After the names were entered into the data base, substantial work was required for linking the files so that, for example, a great-grandfather in one family could be associated with his siblings and their spouses and the descendants of those marriages traced. These records were then linked to the records of cancer cases identified by the Utah Cancer Registry. Because the state cancer registry had begun registering cases only in 1966, this step of the process covered only members of the present generation. Once this process had been completed, the data were analyzed to determine whether there were certain family groups in which more cancers occurred than would be expected. Researchers were surprised to discover that cancer of the prostate gland, a malignancy that occurs only in men, demonstrated the strongest familial clustering. In one family all five of the brothers had suffered from this disease. Up to this time, prostate cancer had not been believed to run in families. Subsequent studies in Utah and in

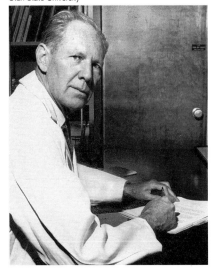

In his now-classic study "Cancer of the Digestive Tract in One Family Group" (1950), geneticist Eldon J. Gardner (above) made use of the LDS genealogical records to trace several generations of a family in which many suffered from a rare genetic syndrome—subsequently named Gardner's disease—that predisposed them to developing colon cancer. (Below) Mark Skolnick (right) and Randall Burt, population geneticists at the University of Utah, examine the pedigree of a large LDS family with a heritable condition similar to that described by Gardner, also leading to an increased risk of colon cancer.

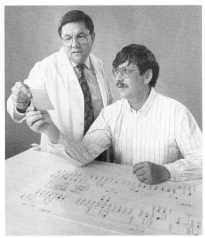

Medical scientists have long known that some diseases "run in the family." They have been aided in studying such conditions not only by Mormons in Utah but also by other culturally cohesive or genetically isolated groups in whom the transmission of a disorder from one generation to another can readily be traced. The smiling youngsters at right are members of one huge extended family in Venezuela that has made an enormous contribution to the search for the gene that causes Huntington's disease, a progressive—and inevitably fatal—neurological disorder. (Below) Amish families in rural Pennsylvania, who have for generations married within their own community, constitute a genetically distinct population that has allowed researchers to gain insight into a number of inherited conditions; e.g., several forms of dwarfism.

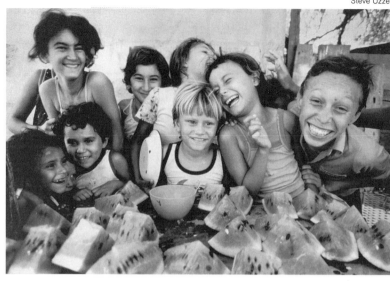

other areas of the country, however, have confirmed the observation that there is a familial predisposition to prostate cancer. This finding suggests that there may be specific genes that, if inherited, increase a man's risk for developing prostate cancer. It could also mean that common environmental factors, such as diet, shared by family members early in life are important determinants of prostate cancer risk.

This NCI-funded project also confirmed the observation made in many earlier studies that breast cancer in women also tends to cluster in families. It has been generally assumed that this phenomenon reflects a genetic predisposition, but common environmental factors shared by sisters and their mother have not yet been studied. It is possible that a strong nongenetic risk factor—for example, older age at first pregnancy—could also run in a family and be mistaken for an inherited gene. This same study yielded evidence that other common cancers, such as cancer of the colon, also might cluster in families.

Additional studies in Utah have followed the approach used by Gardner but have been facilitated by the computerization of family-group sheets and death certificates. Another form of hereditary colon polyps that leads to increased risk of colon cancer was identified by Randall Burt, Lisa Cannon-Albright, and colleagues at the University of Utah in 1988. Initially, the researchers had discovered three individuals, all close relatives, who were suffering from the same type of colon cancer. Family members were contacted, and a pedigree of the extended family was constructed. The records maintained by the Genealogical Society of Utah facilitated this process, helping to identify distant cousins and confirming birth and death dates. This pedigree now contains more than a thousand individuals. Physicians have examined a large number of them and found that they have a higher than expected incidence of colon polyps, which, if not removed, have the potential to become cancerous. The pattern of inheritance is different from that seen in Gardner's syndrome, and fewer family members are affected than in those families with the gene for Gardner's syndrome. Further studies

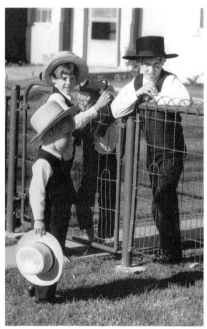

of this very large family are now under way to better characterize the mode of inheritance and, if possible, to identify and locate the gene responsible for this condition.

Heart disease: an experiment in prevention

Deaths from cardiovascular disease in LDS families have also been studied. By reviewing the death certificates for the state of Utah, investigators from the University of Utah identified persons who had died of a heart attack before age 55. Contact was then made with family members of the deceased, and pedigrees were constructed. These pedigrees were then linked to determine if distant cousins shared a common ancestor who might have contributed a gene that predisposed them to early death from a heart attack. Some families were identified as having an inherited tendency to die of heart disease. Thorough investigations of these families followed. Family members were asked to go to a clinic and to submit to a complete physical examination, electrocardiography, and blood testing for cholesterol and other blood lipid levels. Very high levels of serum cholesterol were found in younger members of some of the high-risk families. Given the known association of coronary heart disease with increased levels of serum cholesterol, this finding was considered to be the reason for the preponderance in these families of early deaths from heart attacks.

In a subsequent step of the investigation, family members received dietary counseling to determine if dietary intervention could influence the inherited tendency for high cholesterol levels. The researchers were able to demonstrate that it was possible to lower cholesterol levels by dietary means in people at high risk of dying of a heart attack. This accomplishment suggests that the inherited tendency toward heart attacks operates through well-established nongenetic risk factors (*e.g.,* diet, cigarette smoking) and

While the Mormons of Utah may not be unique in having contributed to medical science, there is at least one respect in which they stand out from other groups that have helped to advance the understanding of human disease—the extraordinary spirit of cooperation they bring to such enterprises. Through their willing participation in epidemiological studies, LDS families have benefited not only themselves but the "human family" as a whole.

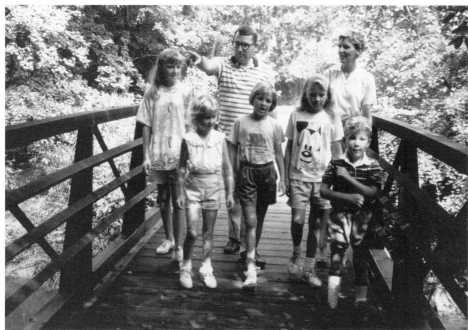

Patsy Lynch

that changes in an environmental factor such as diet can decrease the risk of heart disease in an individual with a genetic predisposition.

Willing cooperation in medical research

The Mormon population of Utah is by no means the only distinctive group to be studied by epidemiologists. Almost any geographically or culturally isolated population that has encouraged intermarriage within the group is fertile ground for the study of both environmental and genetic factors that influence the incidence of disease. Seventh-day Adventists, who, like the Mormons, are urged to abstain from alcohol and tobacco, but who follow a vegetarian diet as well, have proved to be a veritable gold mine of information for epidemiologists. Among the many findings in one study of Adventists living in California was that, on average, they live seven years longer than other Americans and have low rates of each of the 10 disorders that are the leading causes of death in the U.S. One Canadian Mennonite community in which virtually all members trace their descent to a few common ancestors has an unusually high incidence of the neurological condition known as Tourette syndrome; further studies of these families may enable researchers to identify genes responsible for the disorder. Geneticists studying the Amish have found that two unusual forms of dwarfism occur with unexpected frequency in this highly inbred population.

In at least one respect, however, the Mormons of Utah are, if not unique, at least outstanding. This characteristic is their willingness to cooperate with medical researchers. When called upon by doctors to participate in exhaustive physical examinations and blood drawing, large numbers of LDS generally come forward. The response rate when epidemiologists seek participants for studies runs as high as 90%, even for individuals who are only distant cousins of a family being studied. Summer family reunions, a common occurrence among large LDS families in Utah, have afforded investigators unprecedented opportunities to interview many related individuals and to draw hundreds of blood specimens on the spot. The attitude of cooperation even seems to have affected the non-Mormon population of Utah; when asked to participate in medical studies as controls, 80–90% of those contacted willingly show up to answer questions and submit themselves to all kinds of medical tests. In most medical research the participation rate of control subjects selected randomly from the general population runs about 40–60%.

Many observers have made attempts to characterize the Mormon "group personality." One social anthropologist who undertook to do so is John L. Sorenson of Brigham Young University, Provo, Utah. Sorenson noted, among other characteristics, that Mormons tend to be pragmatic, like to do things as a group, and wish generally to be thought well of by each other and by the world at large. It is always risky to make sweeping generalizations about a group of individuals, no matter how cohesive, but some combination of the traits observed by Sorenson may well explain the extraordinary willingness of the LDS of Utah to participate in medical research that, as it continues, will likely benefit not only themselves but all of humankind.

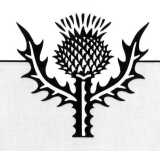

ENCYCLOPÆDIA
BRITANNICA

MEDICAL
UPDATE

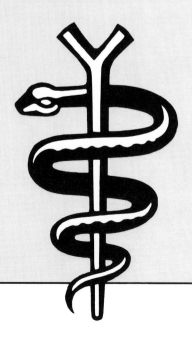

From the 1990 Printing of *Encyclopædia Britannica*

The purpose of this section is to introduce to continuing *Medical and Health Annual* subscribers selected *Macropædia* articles or portions of articles that have been completely revised or rewritten in the most recent edition of the *Encyclopædia Britannica*. It is intended to update the *Macropædia* coverage of topics concerning medicine or health, and it offers a longer and more comprehensive treatment than can be accomplished by the *Annual's* yearly review of re-

cent developments in various medical specialties and allied health fields.

The articles chosen from the 1990 *Britannica* printing are Human EMOTION and PERSONALITY. Both are the work of distinguished scholars and represent the continuing dedication of *Encyclopædia Britannica* to bringing texts that provide authoritative interpretation and examination of timely issues to the general reader.

Human Emotion

An emotion, as it is commonly known, is a distinct feeling or quality of consciousness, such as joy or sadness, that reflects the personal significance of an emotion-arousing event. In modern times the subject of emotion has become part of the subject matter of several scientific disciplines—biology, psychology, psychiatry, anthropology, and sociology. Emotions are central to the issues of human survival and adaptation. They motivate the development of moral behaviour, which lies at the very root of civilization. Emotions influence empathic and altruistic behaviour, and they play a role in the creative processes of the mind. They affect the basic processes of perception and influence the way humans conceive and interpret the world around them. Evidence suggests that emotions shape many other aspects of human life and human affairs. Clinical psychologists and psychiatrists often describe problems of adjustment and types of psy-

chopathology as "emotional problems," mental conditions that an estimated 1 in 3 Americans, for example, suffers from during his or her lifetime.

The subject of emotion is studied from a wide range of views. Behaviorally oriented neuroscientists study the neurophysiology and neuroanatomy of emotions and the relations between neural processes and the expression and experience of emotion. Social psychologists and cultural anthropologists study similarities and differences among cultures by the way emotions are expressed and conceptualized. Philosophers are interested in the role of emotions in rationality, thought, character development, and values. Novelists, playwrights, and poets are interested in emotions as the motivations and defining features of fictional characters and as vehicles for communicating the meaning and significance of events.

The article is divided into the following parts:

Definitions and humanistic background

DEFINITIONS

Emotion has been defined as a particular psychological state of feeling, such as fear, anger, joy, and sorrow. The feeling often includes action tendencies and tends to trigger certain perceptual and cognitive processes. Most experts agree that emotion is a causal factor or influence in thoughts, actions, personalities, and social relationships.

The concept of emotion that will be developed here is a multiaspect, or multilevel, one, considering structure and functions at the levels of neurophysiology, emotion expression, and emotion experience (feeling). It should be noted, however, that not all of the numerous definitions that can be found in emotion literature fit into this multilevel concept. The definitions, which reflect differences in the

The multilevel concept

interests and theoretical orientations of the authors, can be reduced to three categories concerned with structure and three concerned with functions. The three structural categories are the three levels, or aspects, that are included in the multilevel concept. The first of these categories of definition focuses on the neurophysiological processes underlying or accompanying emotions, the second on expression, or emotional behaviour, and the third on the subjective experience, or conscious aspect, of emotion.

Of the three categories of definition related to functions, the first defines emotions in terms of their adaptive or disruptive influences. The second category defines emotion in terms of motivation and considers it as part of the same class of phenomena that contains physiological drives, such as pain, thirst, and the need for elimination. The third category concerned with functions consists of definitions that attempt to distinguish between emotion and other psychological processes.

A multilevel definition of emotion essentially subsumes definitions that focus on one of the three structural categories of neural processes, expressive behaviour, and subjective experience, and elaborations and extensions of such a definition would consider concerns of the three categories related to functions. In summary, the foregoing consideration of the various categories of definitions suggests that a multilevel concept comes closest to a consensus viewpoint among emotion theorists and provides a way of resolving the complex issue of definition. Thus, a specific emotion is a particular set of neural processes that gives rise to a particular configuration of expressive behaviours and a particular feeling state or quality of consciousness that has both motivational and adaptive functions. Under some circumstances extremely intense emotion may become disruptive.

HUMANISTIC BACKGROUND

Orators, literary artists, and philosophers have recognized emotions as part of human nature since recorded history. Homer's *Iliad* contains vivid descriptions of the emotions of the characters; the goddess Athena frequently goes among Agamemnon's troops playing upon their emotions, attempting to allay their fears and bolster their courage for battle. Ancient philosophers discussed the emotions at length, and from these discussions it appears that the basic meanings of emotion concepts are timeless. For example, in the *Rhetoric,* Aristotle described the significance, causes, and consequences of the experiences of anger, fear, and shame in much the same way as contemporary writers. He observed that anger is caused by undeserved slight, fear by the perception of danger, and shame by deeds that bring disgrace or dishonour. His understanding of the relations among emotions also has a modern ring. In contrasting the young and the old, he said of the young,

Aristotle's views

> And they are more courageous, for they are full of passion and hope, and the former of these prevents them fearing, while the latter inspires them with confidence, for no one fears when angry, and hope of some advantage inspires confidence.

Literature. The use of emotion words in literary works can be seen as serving several purposes. They help define the motivations and personalities of the characters in a play or novel, and they help the reader to understand and identify with characters and to experience vicariously their emotions.

Shakespeare, for example, was a master at expressing emotion through his characters and eliciting emotions from the audience. His work also contains quite accurate descriptions of emotional expressions. An example in *Henry V* is the king's effort to ready his soldiers for battle:

> Then imitate the action of the tiger;
> Stiffen the sinews, summon up the blood,
> Disguise fair nature with hard-favour'd rage;
> Then lend the eye a terrible aspect;
> Let it pry through the portage of the head
> Like the brass cannon; let the brow o'erwhelm it
> As fearfully as doth a galled rock
> O'erhang and jutty his confounded base,
> Swill'd with the wild and wasteful ocean.
> Now set the teeth and stretch the nostril wide,
> Hold hard the breath and bend up every spirit
> To his full height.
>
> (Act III, scene 1)

In modern times James Joyce used emotion words and words with emotional connotation to powerful effect. In *A Portrait of the Artist as a Young Man,* much of Stephen Dedalus' mood and character are revealed in a few lines describing a time when he was drinking with his cronies and trying to overcome his sense of alienation from his father:

James Joyce's use of emotion

> His mind seemed older than theirs: it shone coldly on their strifes and happiness and regrets like a moon upon a younger earth. . . . Nothing stirred within his soul but a cold and cruel and loveless lust. His childhood was dead or lost and with it his soul capable of simple joys, and he was drifting amid life like the barren shell of the moon.

According to the literary critic Rosemarie Battaglia, the emotion-arousing words cold, cruel, loveless, dead, lost, and barren resonate with a sense of Stephen's withdrawal from his social world.

Other modern writers have made frank use of psychological concepts of emotion and emotion-related processes, particularly those introduced by Sigmund Freud. Thus, for example, the author's characters may be motivated by unconscious processes, feelings they cannot label and articulate because the fundamental underlying ideation associated with the feelings has been repressed.

Philosophy. Using Aristotle's system of causal explanation, the 16th-century British philosopher John Rainolds defined emotion as follows: the efficient cause of emotions is God, who implanted them; the material cause is good and evil human things; the formal cause is a commotion of the soul, impelled by the sight of things; and the final cause is seeking good and fleeing evil. The American philosopher L.D. Green's commentary on Rainolds' thesis indicates that Rainolds was not faithful to Aristotle's own discussions of emotion.

One thing that Aristotle did advocate was moderation of emotions, allowing them to have an effect only at the right time and in the right manner. Rainolds noted that the Aristotelian thinker Cicero saw emotions as beneficial—fear making humans careful, compassion and sadness leading to mercy, and anger whetting courage. These thoughts about emotion are similar to those of some modern theorists.

For Rainolds, the emotions are the active, energizing aspects of human nature. Although the intellect exercises control over emotions, intellect can have no impact without emotion. Rainolds was specifically concerned with the effects of emotion on rhetoric, but he saw rhetoric as a principal means of influencing human behaviour and affairs. He believed that

> the passions [emotions] must be excited, not for the harm they do but for the good, not so they twist the straight but that they straighten the crooked; so they ward off vice, iniquity, and disgrace; so that they defend virtue, justice, and probity.

Benedict de Spinoza in the 17th century described emotions in much the same way as Rainolds did, but he discussed them in relation to action rather than to language. He saw emotions as bodily changes that result in the amplification or attenuation of action and as processes that can facilitate or impede action. For Spinoza, emotion also included the ideas, or mental representations, of the bodily changes in emotion.

Spinoza's idea of emotion and bodily change

The philosophers Blaise Pascal and David Hume reversed Rainolds' position by assuming the primacy of emotion in human behaviour. Hume said that reason is the slave of the passions (emotions), and Pascal observed in *Pensées* that "the heart has reasons that reason does not know." Although Hume believed that passions (emotions) rule reason or intellect, he thought the dominant passion should be moral sentiment. Some contemporary psychologists trace morality to empathy and empathy to a number of discrete emotions, including sadness, sorrow, compassion, and guilt.

Since Rainolds lectured on emotions at Oxford, philosophers have considered many questions related to emotions: Are they active or passive? Can they be explained by neurophysiological processes and reduced to material phenomena? Are they rational or nonrational? Are they voluntary or involuntary? Characterizing or categorizing emotions according to these dichotomies has resulted in yet other classifications or distinctions.

Ultimately, emotion concepts resist definition by way of dichotomous distinctions. Emotions are generally active and tend to generate action and cognition, but extreme fear may cause behavioral freezing and mental rigidity. Emotion can be explained on one level in terms of neurochemical processes and on another level in terms of phenomenology. Emotions are rational in the sense that they serve adaptive functions and make sense in terms of the individual's perception of the situation. They are nonrational in the sense that they can exist in the brain at the neurochemical level and in consciousness as unlabeled feelings that may be independent of cognitive-rational processes. Emotions are voluntary in that their expression in older children and adults is subject to considerable

Rational and nonrational emotions

modification and control via cognition and action, and willful regulation of expression may result in regulation of emotion experience. Emotions are involuntary in that an effective stimulus elicits them automatically, without deliberation and conscious choice. Nowhere is this more evident than in infants and young children, who have little capacity to modulate or inhibit emotion by means of cognitive processes.

One contemporary American philosopher, Amélie O. Rorty, espouses a three-part causal history for emotions, which includes (1) the formative events in a person's past, including the development of habits of thought, (2) sociocultural factors, and (3) genetically determined sensitivities and patterns of response. These are essentially the same factors that are recognized by psychologists, who frequently reduce the list to two: (1) experience as mediated by culture and learning and (2) genetic determinants that unfold with ontogenetic development. The first of these two causal factors indicates that individual differences in interpretations of an event or situation lead to different emotions in different persons.

Some philosophers are concerned with the question of the rationality of emotion as judged on the basis of causes and consequences. One resolution is in terms of appropriateness: an emotion is appropriate if the reasons for it are adequate, regardless of the reasons against it. There may be a sense, however, in which emotions are intrinsically nonrational because they can come into a person's consciousness without that person having considered all of the relevant reasons for them. In the final analysis, caution should be used in judging the rationality of emotions.

James Hillman's conception

Another contemporary philosopher, James Hillman, has been notably effective in using classical philosophical principles to explain emotions. He has delineated 12 ways that emotion has been conceptualized in philosophy and psychology. These include conceptions of emotion as a distinct entity or trait, an accompaniment of instinct, energy for thought and action, a neurophysiological mechanism and process, mental representation, signal, conflict, disorder, and creative organization. This philosopher found each of these conceptions incomplete or incorrect and returned to Aristotle's system of four causes in an effort to integrate the information from each of the foregoing approaches to defining and studying emotions.

For Hillman, the efficient cause of emotion, described psychologically, consists of conscious or unconscious mental representations (perceptions, images, or thoughts) and conflicts between physiological or psychological systems or between a person and the environment. The efficient cause described physiologically includes genetic endowment and the neurochemical and hormonal processes involved in emotion activation. Hillman stated that the material cause of emotion is energy. He argued that matter, the ultimate source of energy, is relative and that emotion, as the psychological aspect of general energy, is going on all the time and is a two-way bridge uniting subject and object.

In considering the formal cause, one may see emotion as a pattern of neurophysiological and expressive behaviours and subject–object relations. Hillman concluded that, in a formal sense, emotion is a total pattern of the soul:

> Emotion is the soul as a complex whole, involving constitution, gross physiology, facial expression in its social context as well as actions aimed at the environment.

The final cause, or purpose, of emotion, according to Hillman, can be thought of in terms of what it achieves: survival (energy release, homeostatic regulation, and action on the stimulus and environment), signification (qualification of experience, expression, communication, and values), and improvement (emergence of energy into consciousness, facilitation of creative activity, and strengthening of the organization of self and behaviour). Hillman integrated these various descriptions of final cause in the concept of change. Emotion occurs in order to actualize change; "emotion itself is change."

HOW PSYCHOLOGY CONCEIVES EMOTIONS

In 1872, emotion studies received a boost in scientific status when Charles Darwin published his seminal treatise *The Expressions of the Emotions in Man and Animals.*

Twelve years later, the American philosopher and psychologist William James, one of the pioneers of psychology in the United States, published what was to become a famous and controversial theory of emotions. In it James proposed that an arousing stimulus (such as a poignant memory or a physical threat) triggers internal physiological processes as well as external expressive and motor actions and that the feeling of these physiological and behavioral processes constitutes the emotion. Thus, people are happy because they smile, sad because they cry, angry because they frown, and afraid because they run from danger.

A few years later the Danish physician Carl Lange published a more constricted theory, maintaining that emotion is a function of the perception of changes in the visceral organs innervated by the autonomic nervous system. Although there were distinctively individual components in the theories of James and Lange, the theories became linked in the minds of psychologists and the combination became known as the James–Lange theory.

The James–Lange theory

The James–Lange theory was seriously challenged by the American physiologist Walter B. Cannon, who showed that, among other things, animals whose viscera were separated from the central nervous system still displayed emotion expression. Cannon contended that bodily changes were similar for most kinds of emotions, whereas the James–Lange theory implied a different bodily pattern of response for different emotions. The James–Lange theory has remained a more or less permanent fixture in behavioral science nevertheless, and most psychology textbooks summarize the theory and Cannon's criticisms of it. Some theories of emotion are classified as neo-Jamesian, and most theories can be identified or classified on the basis of their similarities and differences with the landmark James–Lange theory.

Psychological theories of emotion can be grouped into two broad categories—biosocial and constructivist. Although this system of categorization is an oversimplification, it provides a way for the student of emotion to get a perspective on a particular theory. A contemporary textbook, for example, describes 20 psychological theories of emotion, and there are many others that it does not consider.

Biosocial and constructivist theories

Many of the differences between the two categories of emotion theory stem from different assumptions regarding the relative importance of genetics and life experiences. Biosocial theories assume that emotions are rooted in biological makeup and that genes are significant determinants of the threshold and characteristic intensity level of each basic emotion. In this view, emotional life is a function of the interaction of genetic tendencies and the evaluative systems, beliefs, and roles acquired through experience. Constructivist theories assume that genetic factors are inconsequential and that emotions are cognitively constructed and derived from experience, especially from social learning. The constructivists' crucible for emotions is formed by the interactions of the person with the environment, especially the social environment. Thus, according to the constructivists, emotions are a function of appraisals, or evaluations, of the world of culture, and of what is learned. (For examples of both types of theory and some of the research generated by each, see below *Contemporary approaches to emotion.*)

The importance of emotions

The use of emotion concepts is common in literature and philosophy, as was discussed above, and there is widespread agreement among scientists that emotions are important in individual development, physical and mental health, and human relations. Experts in different disciplines emphasize different reasons for the importance of emotions.

EVOLUTIONARY-BIOLOGICAL PERSPECTIVES

Darwin and emotion expressions

Darwin included emotions, in particular emotion expressions, in his studies of evolution. He considered continuity or similarity of expression in animals and human beings as further evidence of human evolution from lower forms. His finding that certain emotion expressions are innate and universal was seen as evidence of the "unity of the several races." Thus, the expressions, or the language of the emotions, provide a means of communication among all human beings, regardless of culture or ethnic origin.

In his work *The Expression of the Emotions in Man and Animals,* Darwin made an explicit value judgment regarding the significance of emotion expressions:

> The movements of expression in the face and body, whatever their origin may have been, are in themselves of much importance for our welfare. They serve as the first means of communication between the mother and infant; she smiles approval, and thus encourages her child on the right path, or frowns disapproval. We readily perceive sympathy in others by their expression; our sufferings are thus mitigated and our pleasures increased; and mutual good feeling is thus strengthened. The movements of expression give vividness and energy to our spoken words. They reveal the thoughts and intentions of others more truly than do words, which may be falsified.

From his studies of emotion expressions, Darwin concluded that some emotion expressions were due to the "constitution of the nervous system," or our biological endowment. The implication is that these expressive movements are part of human nature and have played a role in survival and adaptation. Darwin thought other expressions were derived from actions that originally served biologically adaptive functions (*e.g.,* preparation for biting became the bared teeth of the anger expression). Although he noted that expressive movements may no longer serve biological functions, he made it quite clear that they serve critical social and communicative functions.

PSYCHOLOGICAL VIEWS

Significance of emotions

From the very beginning of scientific psychology, there were voices that spoke of the significance of emotions for human life. James believed that "individuality is founded in feeling" and that only through feeling is it possible "directly to perceive how events happen, and how work is actually done." The Swiss psychiatrist Carl Gustav Jung recognized emotion as the primal force in life:

> But on the other hand, emotion is the moment when steel meets flint and a spark is struck forth, for emotion is the chief source of consciousness. There is no change from darkness to light or from inertia to movement without emotion.

Psychologists did not rally to the Darwinian thesis on the evolutionary-adaptive functions of emotions in significant numbers until the 1960s. Several influential volumes following this theme were published in the 1960s and '70s. For example, the American psychologist Robert Plutchik echoed Darwinian principles in several of the postulates of his theory: emotions are present at all levels of animal life, and they serve an adaptive role in relation to survival issues posed by the environment.

The American psychologist Silvin Tomkins believed that the emotions constitute the primary motivational system for human beings. He held that even physiological drives such as hunger and sex obtain their power from emotions and that the energizing effects of emotion are necessary to sustain drive-related actions. In this way, he argued that emotions are essential to survival and adaptation.

Infant emotions

Other theorists and researchers that follow the Darwinian principles of the survival value and adaptive value of emotions have emphasized their role in human development and in the development of social bonds, particularly mother–infant or parent–child attachment. These researchers have shown that even the very young infant has a repertoire of emotion expressions translatable into messages calling for nourishment and affection, both essential ingredients of healthy development. The distress expression is the infant's all-out cry for help, the sadness expression an appeal for empathy, and the smile an invitation to stimulating face-to-face interactions. (For discussion of empirical evidence of the importance of emotions in child development, social relations, cognitive processes, and mental health, see below *The functions of emotion.*)

Contemporary approaches to emotion

Contemporary psychologists are concerned with the activation, or causes, of emotion, its structure, or compo-

nents, and its functions or consequences. Each of these aspects can be considered from both a biosocial and a constructivist view. On the whole, biosocial theories have been relatively more concerned with the neurophysiological aspects of emotions and their roles as motivators and organizers of cognition and action. Constructivists have been relatively more concerned with explaining the causes of emotion at the experiential level and cognition-emotion relations in terms of cognitive–linguistic processes.

STRUCTURES AND PROCESSES OF EMOTION ACTIVATION

The question of precisely how a particular emotion is triggered has been one of the most captivating and controversial topics in the field. To address the question properly, one must necessarily break it down into more precise parts. Emotion activation can be divided into three parts: neural processes, bodily (physiological) changes, and mental (cognitive) activity.

While it is easy for people to think of things that make them happy or sad, it is not yet possible to explain precisely how the feelings of joy and sadness occur. Neuroscience has produced far more information about the processes leading to the physiological responses and expressive behaviour of emotion than about those that generate the conscious experience of emotion.

Neural processes. An emotion can be activated by causes and processes within the individual or by a combination of internal and external causes and processes. For example, within the individual, an infection can cause pain, and pain can activate anger.

The findings of neuroscience indicate that stimuli are evaluated for emotional significance when information from primary receptors (in the visual, tactual, auditory, or other sensory systems) travels along certain neural pathways to the limbic forebrain. Scientific data developed by Joseph E. LeDoux show that auditory fear conditioning involves the transmission of sound signals through the auditory pathway to the thalamus (which relays information) in the lower forebrain and thence to the dorsal amygdala (which evaluates information).

The brain's involvement

Evidence from neuroscience suggests that emotion activated by way of the thalamo-amygdala (subcortical) pathway results from rapid, minimal, automatic, evaluative processing. Emotion activated in this way need not involve the neocortex. Emotion activated by discrimination of stimulus features, thoughts, or memories requires that the information be relayed from the thalamus to the neocortex. Such a circuit is thought to be the neural basis for cognitive appraisal and evaluation of events.

This two-circuit model of the neural pathways in emotion activation has several important theoretical implications. The neurological evidence indicating that emotion can be activated via the thalamo-amygdala pathway is consistent with the behavioral evidence that very young infants respond emotionally to pain and that adults can develop preferences or make affective judgments in responding to objects before they demonstrate recognition memory for them. This suggests that in some instances humans may experience emotion before they reason why.

It might be expected that in early human development most emotion expressions derive from automatic, subcortical processing, with minimal cortical involvement. As cognitive capacities increase with maturation and learning, the neocortex and the cortico-amygdala pathway become more and more involved. By the time children acquire language and the capacity for long-term memory, they may process events in either or both pathways, with the subcortical pathway specializing in events requiring rapid response and the cortico-amygdala pathway providing evaluative information necessary for cognitive judgment and more complex coping strategies.

Physiological processes. Many theorists agree that feedback from physiological activity contributes to emotion activation. There is disagreement over the kind of feedback that is important. Some think that it is a visceral feedback—coming from the activity of the smooth-muscle organs such as the heart and stomach, which are innervated by the autonomic nervous system. Others believe that it is feedback from the voluntary, striated muscles, especially of the face, which are innervated by the somatic nervous system.

Cognitive processes. Constructivist theorists and researchers have been concerned with the causes of emotion at the cognitive-experiential level and with the relations between cognitive processes and emotion. This research has focused on two topics: the relations between appraisals, or evaluations, and emotions and the relations between causal attributions and emotions.

Emotion appraisal

Magda B. Arnold was the first contemporary psychologist to propose that all emotions are a function of one's cognitive appraisal of the stimulus or situation. She maintained that before a stimulus can elicit emotion it has to be appraised as good or bad by the perceiver. She described the appraisal that arouses emotion as concrete, immediate, undeliberate, and not the result of reflection. Her position was adopted and elaborated by others, some of whom assumed that cognitive activity, whether in the form of primitive evaluative perception or symbolic processes, is a necessary precondition of emotion. Biosocial and constructivist theorists agree that cognition is an important determinant of emotion and that emotion–cognition relations merit continued research.

Research by the American psychologists Phoebe C. Ellsworth and Craig A. Smith on the relations between appraisals and specific emotions show that people tend to appraise situations in terms of elements such as pleasantness, anticipated effort, certainty, responsibility, control, legitimacy, and perceived obstacle. Researchers have found that each discrete emotion tends to be associated with a distinctive combination of appraisals. For example, a perceived obstacle (barrier to a goal) that is due to someone else's responsibility is associated with anger, a perceived obstacle that is the person's own responsibility is associated with guilt, and a perceived obstacle characterized by uncertainty is associated with fear. This study was based on subjects' retrospective accounts of emotion-eliciting situations, and therefore the data cannot confirm the view that appraisal causes emotion. However, the assumption that emotion and appraisal are causally related seems reasonable.

Another approach to explaining the causes of emotions is that of attribution theory. The central idea of this theory, according to the American psychologist Bernard Weiner, is that the perceptions of the causes of events can be characterized in three principal ways which affect many emotional experiences. The perceived causes of events (*e.g.,* success and failure) are characterized by their locus (internal or external to the person), stability (a trait of the person or a temporary condition), and controllability (under the person's control or not).

Attribution theory

Research has shown that different patterns of causal attribution are associated with different emotions, including anger, guilt, shame, and the more complex phenomena of pity, pride, gratitude, and hopelessness. Pity is attributed to the perception of uncontrollable and stable causes—people feel pity for a person who has an affliction due to a genetic defect or accident. Anger is attributed to external and controllable events—people feel anger when an affront or injury is caused by someone's lack of concern or thoughtlessness. Guilt is attributed to the perception of internal and controllable causes—people feel guilt for wrongdoing they could have avoided. Children aged five to 12 understand the emotional consequences of revealing the causes of their actions; they know that their teachers might be angry at their failure if they have not tried hard enough and that teachers might feel pity for students who lack the ability to learn efficiently and perform well.

Coping with emotions

Psychologists researching cognitive activation have studied the relations between the ways people cope with stressful encounters and the emotions they experience after their efforts to resolve the problems. In one study emotions were assessed by asking subjects to indicate the extent to which they experienced emotions on four scales: worried/fearful, disgusted/angry, confident, and pleased/happy. Coping was assessed by subjective ratings on eight scales: confrontive coping ("stood my ground and fought"), distancing ("didn't let it get to me"), self-control ("tried to keep my feelings to myself"), seeking social support ("talked to someone"), accepting responsibility ("criticized myself"), escape–avoidance ("wished the situation would go away"), planful problem solving ("changed or grew as a person"), and positive reappraisal. Four of these ways of coping were associated with the quality of emotion that followed the effort to cope. Planful problem solving and positive reappraisal tended to increase happiness and confidence and to decrease disgust and anger. Obversely, the subjects reported that confrontation and distancing techniques increased their disgust and anger and decreased their happiness and confidence. Because these data were retrospective, there can be no firm conclusion that a particular way of coping causes a particular emotion experience. Nevertheless, the observed relations among ways of coping and subsequent emotion experiences are reasonable and in line with theoretical expectations.

The controversy as to whether some cognitive process is a necessary antecedent of emotion may hinge on the definition of terms, particularly the definition of cognition. If cognition is defined so broadly that it includes all levels or types of information processing, then cognition may confidently be said to precede emotion activation. If those mental processes that do not involve mental representation based on learning or experience are excluded from the concept of cognition, then cognition so defined does not necessarily precede the three-week-old infant's smile to the high-pitched human voice, the two-month-old's anger expression to pain, or the formation of the affective preferences (likes or dislikes) in adults.

Multimodal theory. Evidence suggests that a satisfactory model of emotion activation must be multimodal. Emotions can, as indicated above, be activated by such precognitive processes as physiological states, motor mimicry (imitation of another's movements), and sensory processes and by numerous cognitive processes, including comparison, matching, appraisal, categorization, imagery, memory, attribution, and anticipation. Further, all emotion activation processes are influenced by a variety of internal and external factors.

THE STRUCTURE OF EMOTIONS

In the discussion of the structure of emotions it is not always possible to ignore the function of emotions, which is discussed in the following section. The separation, however, is conducive to sorting out the complex field of emotions.

Biosocial and constructivist views

Both biosocial and constructivist theories of emotions acknowledge that an emotion is a complex phenomenon. They generally agree that an emotion includes physiological functions, expressive behaviour, and subjective experience and that each of these components is based on activity in the brain and nervous system. As noted above, some theorists, particularly those of the constructivist persuasion, hold that an emotion also involves cognition, an appraisal or cognitive-evaluative process that triggers the emotion and determines or contributes to the subjective experience of the emotion.

The physiological component. The physiological component of emotion has been a lively topic of research since Cannon challenged the James–Lange theory by showing that feedback from the viscera has little effect on emotional expression in animals. Cannon's studies and criticisms were regarded by many as too narrow, failing to, among other things, consider the possible role of feedback from striated muscle systems of the face and body.

Role of the nervous system. Since the popularization of the James–Lange theory of emotion, the physiological component of emotion has been traditionally identified as activity in the autonomic nervous system and the visceral organs (*e.g.,* the heart and lungs) that it innervates. However, some contemporary theorists hold that the neural basis of emotions resides in the central nervous system and that the autonomic nervous system is recruited by emotion to fulfill certain functions related to sustaining and regulating emotion experience and emotion-related behaviour. Several findings from neuroscience support this idea. Neuroanatomical studies have shown that the central nervous system structures involved in emotion activation can exert direct influences on the autonomic nervous

Findings of neuroscience

system. For example, efferents from the amygdala to the hypothalamus may influence activity in the autonomic nervous system that is involved in defensive reactions. Further, there are connections between pathways innervating facial expression and the autonomic nervous system. Studies have shown that patterns of activity in this system vary with the type of emotion being expressed.

Roles of the brain hemispheres.   There is some evidence that the two hemispheres of the brain are related differently to emotion processes. Early evidence suggested that the right (or dominant) hemisphere may be more adept than the left at discriminating among emotional expressions. Later research using electroencephalography elaborated this initial conclusion, suggesting that the right hemisphere may be more involved in processing negative emotions and the left hemisphere more involved in processing positive emotions.

The expressive component.   The expressive component of emotion includes facial, vocal, postural, and gestural activity. Expressive behaviour is mediated by phylogenetically old structures of the brain, which is consistent with the notion that they served survival functions in the course of evolution.

Involvement of brain structures.   Emotion expressions involve limbic forebrain structures and aspects of the peripheral nervous system. The facial and trigeminal nerves and receptors in facial muscles and skin are required in expressing emotion and in facilitating sensory feedback from expressive movements.

Early studies of the neural basis of emotion expression showed that aggressive behaviour can be elicited from a cat after its neocortex has been removed and suggested that the hypothalamus is a critical subcortical structure mediating aggression. Later research indicated that, rather than the hypothalamus, the central gray region of the midbrain and the substantia nigra may be the key structures mediating aggressive behaviour in animals.

Importance of facial expression *Neural pathways of facial expression.*   Of the various types of expressive behaviour, facial expression has received the most attention. In human beings and in many nonhuman primates, patterns of facial movements constitute the chief means of displaying emotion-specific signals. Whereas research has provided much information on the neural basis of emotional behaviours (*e.g.,* aggression) in animals, little is known about the brain structures that control facial expression.

The peripheral pathways of facial emotion expression consist of the seventh and fifth cranial nerves. The seventh, or facial, nerve is the efferent (outward) pathway; it conveys motor messages from the brain to facial muscles. The fifth, or trigeminal, nerve is the afferent (inward) pathway that provides sensory data from movements of facial muscles and skin. According to some theorists, it is the trigeminal nerve that transmits the facial feedback which contributes to the activation and regulation of emotion experience. The impulses for this sensory feedback originate when movement stimulates the mechanoreceptors in facial skin. The skin is richly supplied with such receptors, and the many branches of the trigeminal nerve detect and convey the sensory impulses to the brain.

The innateness and universality of emotion expressions.   More than a century ago Darwin's observations and correspondence with friends living in different parts of the world led him to conclude that certain emotion expressions are innate and universal, part of the basic structure of emotions. Contemporary cross-cultural and developmental research has given strong support to Darwin's conclusion, showing that people in literate and preliterate cultures have a common understanding of the expressions of joy, surprise, sadness, anger, disgust, contempt, and fear. Other studies have suggested that the expressions of interest and shyness and the feelings of shame and guilt may also be innate and universal.

The experiential component.   There is general agreement that various stimuli and neural processes leading to an emotion result not only in physiological reactions and expressive behaviour but also in subjective experience. Some biosocial theorists restrict the definition of an emotion experience to a feeling state and argue that it can be acti-

vated independently of cognition. Constructivist theorists view the experiential component of emotion as having a cognitive aspect. The issue regarding the relation between emotion feeling states and cognition remains unresolved, but it is widely agreed that emotion feeling states and cognitive processes are typically highly interactive.

Emotion experiences, the actual feelings of joy, sadness, anger, shame, fear, and the like, do not lend themselves to objective measurement. All research on emotion experience ultimately depends on self-reports, which are imprecise. There are few instances where feelings and words are perfectly matched. Yet, most students of emotions, whether philosopher or neuroscientist, ultimately want to explain emotion experience.

The physiological structure of emotion experience.   Little is known about the neural basis of emotion experience. Critical reviews have shown that there is little evidence to support the position that activity in the autonomic nervous system provides the physiological basis for emotion experience. However, there is some evidence to support the hypothesis that sensory feedback from facial expression contributes to emotion experience. Neural basis of emotion experience

Cognitive models of emotion experience have influenced conceptions of the underlying neural processes. Explanations of emotions in terms of appraisal and attributional processes led some researchers to suggest that conscious experiences of emotions derive from the cognitive processes that underlie language. This led to the hypothesis that emotion experiences involve interactions between limbic forebrain areas and the areas of the neocortex that mediate language and language-based cognitive systems. However, this view does not take into account the possibility that emotions occur in preverbal infants and may be mediated in adults by unconscious or nonlinguistic mental processes, such as imagery.

Action tendencies in emotion experiences.   Both constructivist and biosocial theorists have emphasized that emotions include action tendencies. The experience, or feeling, of a given emotion generates a tendency to act in a certain way. For example, in anger the tendency is to attack and in fear to flee. Whether a person actually attacks in anger or flees in fear depends on the individual's methods of emotion regulation and the circumstances.

THE FUNCTIONS OF EMOTIONS

In academic discussions of the functions of emotions the focus is usually on the phenomenological, or experiential, aspect of emotions. For purposes of this discussion, however, the functions of emotions are examined in terms of the three structural components—physiological, expressive, and experiential. Structural components of functions

Physiological functions.   The functions of physiological activity that is mediated by the autonomic nervous system and that accompanies states of emotion can be considered as part of the individual's effort to adapt and cope, but, of course, physiological as well as cognitive reactions in extreme emotion usually require regulation (expressed through cognitive processes and expressive behaviour) in order for coping activities to be effective. For example, adaptation to situations that elicit a less extreme emotion such as interest require a quite different physiological and behavioral activity than do situations that elicit intense anger or fear. The heart-rate deceleration and quieting of internal organs that occur in interest facilitate the intake and processing of information, whereas heart-rate acceleration in intense anger and fear prepares the individual to cope by more active means, whether through shouting, physical actions, or various combinations of the two.

Functions of emotion expressions.   Emotion expressions have three major functions: they contribute to the activation and regulation of emotion experiences; they communicate something about internal states and intentions to others; and they activate emotions in others, a process that can help account for empathy and altruistic behaviour. Feedback of facial expression

Role of expressions in emotion experiences.   In *The Expression of the Emotions in Man and Animals* Darwin clearly revealed his belief that even voluntary emotion expression evoked emotion feeling. He wrote: "Even the simulation [expression] of an emotion tends to arouse it in our minds." Thus, Darwin's idea suggested that facial feedback (sensations created by the movements of expressive behaviour) activate, or contribute to the activation of, emotion feelings. A number of experiments have provided substantial evidence that intentional management of facial expression contributes to the regulation (and perhaps activation) of emotion experiences. Most evidence is related not to specific emotion feelings but to the broad classes of positive and negative states of emotion. There is, therefore, some scientific support for the old advice to "smile when you feel blue" and "whistle a happy tune when you're afraid."

Darwin was even more persuasive when speaking specifically of the regulation of emotion experience by self-initiated expressive behaviour. He wrote:

> The free expression by outward signs of an emotion intensifies it. On the other hand, the repression, as far as this is possible, of all outward signs softens our emotions.

Experiments by more contemporary researchers on motivated, self-initiated expressive behaviours have shown that, if people can control their facial expression during moments of pain, there will be less arousal of the autonomic nervous system and a diminution of the pain experience.

Role of expressions in communicating internal states. The social communication function of emotion expressions is most evident in infancy. Long before infants have command of language or are capable of reasoning, they can send a wide variety of messages through their facial expressions. Virtually all the muscles necessary for facial expression of basic emotions are present before birth. Through the use of an objective, anatomically based system for coding the separate facial muscle movements, it has been found that the ability to smile and to facially express pain, interest, and disgust are present at birth; the social smile can be expressed by three or four weeks; sadness and anger by about two months; and fear by six or seven months. Informal observations suggest that expressions indicative of shyness appear by about four months and expressions of guilt by about two years.

The expressive behaviours are infants' primary means of signaling their internal states and of becoming engaged in the family and larger human community. Emotion expressions help form the foundation for social relationships and social development. They also provide stimulation that appears to be necessary for physical and mental health.

Role of expressions in motivating response. One- and three-day-old infants cry in response to other infants' cries but not to a computer-generated sound that simulates crying. Infants as young as two or three months of age respond differently to different expressions by the mother. The information an infant obtains from the mother's facial expressions mediates or regulates a variety of infant behaviours. For example, most infants cross a modified "visual cliff" (an apparatus that was originally used in depth perception study, consisting of a glass floor that gives the illusion of a drop-off) if their mother stands on the opposite side and smiles, but none cross if she expresses fear.

Facial expressions, particularly of sadness, may facilitate empathy and altruistic behaviour. Darwin thought facial expressions evoked empathy and concluded that expression-induced empathy was inborn. Research has shown that, when mothers display sadness expressions, their infants also demonstrate more sadness expressions and decrease their exploratory play. Infants under two years of age respond to their mother's real or simulated expressions of sadness or distress by making efforts to show sympathy and provide help.

Functions of emotion experiences. Psychologists who adopt a strong behaviourist position deny that emotion experiences are matters for scientific inquiry. In contrast, some biosocial theories hold that emotion feelings must be studied because they are the primary factors in organizing and motivating human behaviour. According to these theories, most of the functions attributed to emotion expressions, such as empathy and altruism, are dependent on the organizing and motivating properties of underlying emotion feelings. Emotion experiences have several other functions.

Research has shown that people in widely different literate and preliterate cultures not only recognize basic emotion expressions but also characterize and label them with semantically equivalent terms. It seems reasonable to assume that the common feeling state of a given emotion generates the cues for the cognitive processes that result in universal emotion concepts. Of course, if researchers include contextual factors, such as societal taboos, in their description of an emotion experience, they then find differences across cultures. In any case, although the feeling of a given emotion, say fear, may be constant, people within and across cultures learn to be afraid of quite different things and to cope with fear in different ways.

Experiential influence on cognitive processes. Several lines of research have shown that induced emotion affects perception, learning, and memory. In one study, conducted by Carroll E. Izard and his students, subjects were made happy or angry and then shown happy and angry faces and friendly and hostile interpersonal scenes in a stereoscope. Happy subjects perceived more happy faces and friendly interpersonal scenes, and angry subjects perceived more angry faces and hostile interpersonal scenes. In this case, emotion apparently altered the basic perceptual process. In another study subjects were made happy or sad and then given happy and sad information about fictional persons and later asked to give their impressions and make judgments about the fictional characters. Overall, happy subjects reported more favourable impressions and positive judgments than did sad subjects. These studies provide evidence for the common wisdom that happy people are more likely to see the world through rose-coloured glasses.

Experiential facilitation of empathy and altruism. An extensive series of studies indicated that positive emotion feelings enhance empathy and altruism. It was shown by the American psychologist Alice M. Isen that relatively small favours or bits of good luck (like finding money in a coin telephone or getting an unexpected gift) induced positive emotion in people and that such emotion regularly increased the subjects' inclination to sympathize or provide help.

Experiential relation to increased creativity. Several studies have demonstrated that positive emotion facilitates creative problem solving. One of these studies showed that positive emotion enabled subjects to name more uses for common objects. Another showed that positive emotion enhanced creative problem solving by enabling subjects to see relations among objects that would otherwise go unnoticed. A number of studies have demonstrated the beneficial effects of positive emotion on thinking, memory, and action in preschool and older children.

Explanation of the functions of emotion experiences. There are two kinds of factors that contribute to the enhancing effects of positive emotion on perception, learning, creative problem solving, and social behaviour. Two factors, emphasized by cognitive-social theorists, are related to cognitive processes. First, positive emotion cues positive material in memory, and, second, positive material in memory is more extensive than neutral and negative material. The second set of factors, emphasized by biosocial theorists, are related to the intrinsic motivational and organizational influences of emotion and to the particular characteristics of the subjective experience of positive emotion. For example, these theorists maintain that the experience of joy is characterized by heightened self-esteem and self-confidence. These qualities of consciousness increase the receptibility to information and the flexibility of mental processes. Biosocial theorists consider that the positive emotion induced by experimental manipulations and experimental tasks includes the emotion of interest, which is characterized by curiosity and the desire to explore and learn. The concepts emphasized by biosocial and cognitive-social theories may be seen as complementary.

EMOTIONS AND ADAPTATION

The results of many of the experiments discussed above indicate that emotions have motivational and adaptive properties. Perhaps the most convincing demonstrations

(Marginal notes:)

Mother–infant relations through emotion expression

Commonality of emotion experience

Effects of positive emotion

of this come from studies showing that emotions influence perception, learning, and memory and empathic, altruistic, and creative actions.

Some theorists have viewed emotions more negatively, seeing them as disorganizing and disrupting influences. Researchers in this tradition have also viewed emotions as transient, episodic states. These ideas were fueled by a research emphasis on "emergency emotions," such as rage and panic. These researchers might agree that, although such emotions may serve an adaptive function under certain circumstances, in many situations they can lead to behaviours that prove to be maladaptive and even fatal. As was indicated above, however, emotion expressions can serve critical functions in mother–infant communication and attachment, and emotion experiences, or feeling states, facilitate learning and empathic, altruistic, and creative behaviour.

Although psychologists generally favour viewing emotions as having motivating, organizing, and adaptive functions, the conditions under which emotions become maladaptive warrant further research. Extreme anger and fear can bring about large changes in the activities of internal organs innervated by the autonomic nervous system. When such arousal repeatedly involves the sympathetic nervous system and the hormones of the medulla of the adrenal gland, the individual may develop resistance to mental and physical disorders. When there is repeated arousal involving the sympathetic nervous system and the hormones of the cortex of the adrenal gland, the individual may experience adverse effects.

Biological adaptations

Problems of adaptation and mental health can also be conceived as attributable not to the emotions but to the way a person thinks and acts. For example, if a person decides to break a moral code and consequently feels guilty, the guilt may be adaptive in that it can provide motivation for making amends. In this framework psychological problems or disorders arise because the individual fails to respond appropriately to the emotion's motivational cues while the emotion is still at low or moderate intensity.

THE REGULATION OF EMOTIONS

Several beliefs and attitudes have contributed to the idea that emotions should be brought under rather tight control. Historically, some religious and philosophical literature has treated human passion, a concept which included emotions, as an evil force that could contaminate or even destroy the mind or soul. In this tradition passions became associated with sin and wrongdoing, and their rigorous control was thus a sign of goodness. Even in this tradition, however, some negative emotions were exempt from tight control—guilt as a result of wrongdoing and righteous indignation toward moral transgressions.

Changing views of emotion regulation. Traditionally, scientists have given far more attention to negative emotions and their control than to positive ones. The focus on negative emotions has continued among clinical psychologists and psychiatrists, who are concerned with relieving depression and anxiety. However, as parents have long recognized, there is also a need to regulate positive emotions when, for example, children are having fun at someone else's expense or while neglecting chores and homework.

Developmental processes in emotion regulation. Of central importance in emotion regulation are developmental processes that enable children, as they mature, to exercise an increasingly greater control over affective responses. For example, before an infant can regulate the innate affective behaviour patterns elicited by acute pain, maturation of neural inhibitory mechanisms is required. Further control is realized through techniques that result from cognitive development and socialization, processes involving both maturation and learning.

Regulation in infants

In a study of responses of two- to 19-month-old infants to the pain of diphtheria-tetanus-pertussis (DTP) inoculation, it was found that the physical distress expression occurred as the initial response in all infants at the ages of two, four, and seven months (the ages at which the first three DTPs were administered). The physical distress expression is an all-out emergency response, a cry for help that dominates the physical and mental capacities of the

infant. Beginning at the age of four months and accelerating rapidly between seven and 19 months, the infants became capable of greatly reducing the duration of the physical distress expression. As the duration of the physical distress expression decreased, that for anger expression increased. By 19 months of age, 25 percent of the infants were able to inhibit the distress expression completely. It was inferred that these developmental changes are adaptive for the relatively more capable toddler: whereas the physical distress expression in the younger subjects is all-consuming, anger mobilizes energy for defense or escape.

Other factors in emotion regulation. Several other factors are observable in emotion or mood regulation. First, there is neurochemical regulation by means of naturally occurring hormones and neurotransmitters. Regulation is also attained through psychoactive drugs, many of which were developed to control the prevalent psychological disorders of anxiety and depression. A substantial body of research has shown that anxiety and depression are associated with chemical imbalances in the brain and nervous system. Psychoactive drugs help to correct these imbalances.

Neurochemical regulation

Socialization processes, especially child-rearing practices, influence emotion regulation. Attempts by parents, teachers, and other adults to control emotions may be aimed either at the level of expression or experience or both. Parents may try to control their child's anger expressions before they culminate in "temper tantrums." A father may try to control his son's expressions of fear of bodily injury because he anticipates the shame of his son being seen as a coward. In considering the net effect of socialization on emotion regulation, it is necessary to weigh the effects that the child's unique genetic makeup may contribute to the process.

Cognitive-social theories point to cognitive processes as means of controlling emotion. According to this approach, if it is possible for people to change the way they make appraisals and attributions about the nature and cause of events, their emotion experiences can be changed. This could be manifested, for instance, in a reduction in self-blame and an alteration in negative concepts and outlooks. That cognitive therapy and cognitive techniques for controlling depressive and aggressive behaviour have achieved some success is testimony to the validity of the idea of cognitive control of emotion. That they sometimes fail indicates that it is no panacea and that other factors may be necessary for emotion regulation. As discussed above, theory and empirical data support the notion that expressive behaviour, which is under voluntary control, can be used to regulate emotions.

EMOTIONS, TEMPERAMENT, AND PERSONALITY

Most theorists agree that emotion thresholds and emotion responsiveness are part of the infrastructure of temperament and personality. There has, however, been little empirical research on the relations among measures of emotions, dimensions of temperament, and personality traits.

Emotions and temperament. Most theories of temperament define at least one dimension of temperament in terms of emotion. Two theories maintain that negative emotions form the core of one of the basic and stable dimensions of temperament. Another suggests that each of the dimensions of temperament is rooted in a particular discrete emotion and that these dimensions form the emotional substrate of personality characteristics. For example, proneness to anger would influence the development of aggressiveness, and the emotion of interest would account for the temperament trait of persistence.

Dimensions of temperament

Emotions and personality. A number of major personality theories, such as theories of temperament, identify dimensions or traits of personality in terms of emotions. For example, the German-born British psychologist Hans J. Eysenck has proposed three fundamental dimensions of personality: extroversion–introversion, neuroticism, and psychoticism. Extroversion–introversion includes the trait of sociability, which can also be related to emotion (*e.g.,* interest, as expressed toward people, versus shyness). Neuroticism includes emotionality defined, as in temperament

Eysenck's fundamental dimensions

theory, as nonspecific negative emotional responsiveness. Psychoticism may represent emotions gone awry or the absence of emotions appropriate to the circumstances.

Several studies have shown that measures of positive emotionality and negative emotionality are independent, are not inversely related, and have stability over time. Further, it has been shown that positive and negative emotionality have different relations with symptoms of psychological disorders. For example, negative emotionality correlates positively with panic attack, panic-associated symptoms and obsessive-compulsive symptoms; that is, the higher the degree of negative emotion, the more likely that the attack or symptoms will occur. Conversely, positive emotionality correlates negatively with these phenomena. Although several of the same negative emotions characterize both the anxiety and depressive disorders, a lack of positive emotion experiences is more characteristic of depression than of anxiety.

Continuity of emotion expressiveness. Some studies have shown that specific emotions, identified in terms of expressive behaviour and physiological functions, have stability. One study showed that a child's expression of positive and negative emotion was consistent during the first two years of life. Other studies have shown stability of wariness or fear responses, indicating that a child who is fearful at one age is likely to be fearful in comparable situations at a later age. In a study of infants' responses to the pain of DTP inoculation, it was found that the child's anger expression indexes at ages two, four, and six months accurately predicted his or her anger expression in the inoculations at 19 months of age. Similar results were obtained for the sadness expression.

A study of mother–infant interaction and separation found that infants' expression at three to six months of age were accurate predictors of infant emotion expressive patterns at nine to 12 months of age. Emotion expression patterns have also shown continuity from 13 to 18 months of age during brief mother–infant separation.

Conclusion

The emotions are central to the issues of modern times, but perhaps they have been critical to the issues of every era. Poets, prophets, and philosophers of all ages have recognized the significance of emotions in individual life and human affairs, and the meaning of a specific emotion, at least in the context of verbal expression, seems to be timeless. Although art, literature, and philosophy have contributed to the understanding of emotion experiences throughout the ages, modern science has provided a substantial increase in the knowledge of the neurophysiological basis of emotions and their structure and functions.

Research in neuroscience and developmental psychology suggests that emotions can be activated automatically and unconsciously in subcortical pathways. This suggests that humans often experience emotions without reasoning why. Pre-cognitive aspects Such precognitive information processing may be continuous, and the resulting emotion states may influence the many perceptual-cognitive and behavioral processes (such as perceiving, thinking, judging, remembering, imagining, and coping) that activate emotions through pathways involving the neocortex.

The two recognized types of emotion activation have important implications for the role of emotions in cognition and action. Subcortical, automatic information processing may provide the primitive data for immediate emotional response, whereas higher-order cognitive information processing involving the neocortex yields the evaluations and attributions necessary for the appropriate emotions and coping strategy in a complex situation.

Biosocial and constructivist theories agree that perception, thought, imagery, and memory are important causes of emotions. They also agree that once emotion is activated, emotion and cognition influence each other. How people feel affects what they perceive, think, and do, and vice versa.

Emotions have physiological, expressive, and experiential components, and each component can be studied in terms of its structure and functions. The physiological compo-

nent influences the intensity and duration of felt emotion, expressions serve communicative and sociomotivational functions, and emotion experiences (feeling states) influence cognition and action.

Research has shown that certain emotion expressions are innate and universal and have significant functions in infant development and in infant–parent relations and that there are stable individual differences in emotion expressiveness. Emotion states influence what people perceive, learn, and remember, and they are involved in the development of empathic, altruistic, and moral behaviour and in basic personality traits.

BIBLIOGRAPHY.   Studies of philosophical and cultural views on emotion include JAMES HILLMAN, *Emotion: A Comprehensive Phenomenology of Theories and Their Meanings for Therapy* (1960), a contemporary philosopher's explanation of emotions in terms of Aristotle's system of causes and a review of other approaches; AMÉLIE OKSENBERG RORTY (ed.), *Explaining Emotions* (1980), a collection of philosophical essays on the causes, meaning, and consequences of emotions; and ROM HARRÉ (ed.), *The Social Construction of Emotions* (1986), a collection of studies on the role of language and culture in the cognitive construction, *i.e.,* learning, of emotions.

The significance of emotions is the subject of many analyses, beginning with CHARLES DARWIN, *The Expression of the Emotions in Man and Animals* (1872, reprinted 1979), a classical work that placed human emotions in evolutionary perspective and presented the first evidence for their innateness and universality in human beings; CARROLL E. IZARD, *Human Emotions* (1977), a discussion of each of the fundamental emotions of human experience in terms of their unique organizing and motivational influence on cognition and action; SUSANNE K. LANGER, *Mind: An Essay on Human Feeling,* 3 vol. (1967–72), a philosopher's view of the significance of feelings in the evolution of human mentality; GEORGE MANDLER, *Mind and Body: Psychology of Emotion and Stress* (1984), a cognitive, or constructivist, view of the role of emotions in mental and bodily processes; ROBERT PLUTCHIK, *Emotion, a Psychoevolutionary Synthesis* (1980), a look at emotions in evolutionary perspective; and SILVAN S. TOMKINS, *Affect, Imagery, Consciousness,* vol. 1, *The Positive Affects* (1962), a brilliant essay on emotions as the primary motivational system of human beings.

The following works reflect some contemporary approaches to the study of emotions: MAGDA B. ARNOLD, *Emotion and Personality,* vol. 1, *Psychological Aspects* (1960), emphasizes the role of cognitive appraisal in emotion and sets the stage for later cognitive-social, or constructivist, theories of emotion; NICO H. FRIJDA, *The Emotions* (1986), is a comprehensive cognitive-social view of emotions; JOSEPH J. CAMPOS *et al.,* "Socioemotional Development," chapter 10 in MARSHALL M. HAITH and JOSEPH J. CAMPOS (eds.), *Infancy and Developmental Psychobiology,* 4th ed. (1983), pp. 783–915, provides a comprehensive review of theory and research on emotional development; ROBERT N. EMDE, THEODORE J. GAENSBAUER, and ROBERT J. HARMON, *Emotional Expression in Infancy: A Biobehavioral Study* (1976), is an influential contribution to the study of expressions; NATHAN A. FOX and RICHARD J. DAVIDSON (eds.), *The Psychobiology of Affective Development* (1984), presents a collection of reviews of theory and research papers on the biological aspects of emotional development; CARROLL E. IZARD, JEROME KAGAN, and ROBERT B. ZAJONC (eds.), *Emotions, Cognition, and Behavior* (1984), is a collection of research papers by leading psychologists on the relations between emotions, cognition, and actions; CARROLL E. IZARD and C.Z. MALATESTA, "Perspectives on Emotional Development I: Differential Emotions Theory of Early Emotional Development," chapter 9A in JOY DONIGER OSOFSKY (ed.), *Handbook of Infant Development,* 2nd ed. (1987), pp. 494–554, provides a detailed theory of emotional development and a review of related research; JOSEPH E. LEDOUX, "Emotion," chapter 10 in FRED PLUM (ed.), *Higher Functions of the Brain* (1987), pp. 419–59, in *Handbook of Physiology,* section 1, vol. 5, discusses brain mechanisms and neural pathways involved in the activation, expression, and experience of emotion; MICHAEL LEWIS and LINDA MICHALSON, *Children's Emotions and Moods: Developmental Theory and Measurement* (1983), explores a cognitive-social view of the development of emotions; PHOEBE C. ELLSWORTH and CRAIG A. SMITH, "From Appraisal to Emotion: Differences Among Unpleasant Feelings," *Motivation and Emotion,* 12(3):271–302 (September 1988), surveys research on the relations between appraisal processes and emotions and presents a new theory of cognition–emotion relations; H. HILL GOLDSMITH *et al.,* "What Is Temperament? Four Approaches," *Child Development,* 58(2):505–29 (April 1987), reviews theories of temperament with attention to temperament–emotion relations; ALICE M. ISEN, KIMBERLY A. DAUBMAN, and GARY P. NO-

WICKI, "Positive Affect Facilitates Creative Problem Solving," *Journal of Personality and Social Psychology,* 52(6):1122–31 (June 1987), exemplifies research showing how positive emotion facilitates creative thinking, empathy, and altruism; CARROLL E. IZARD, ELIZABETH A. HEMBREE, and ROBIN R. HUEBNER, "Infants' Emotion Expressions to Acute Pain: Developmental Change and Stability of Individual Differences," *Developmental Psychology,* 23(1):105–13 (January 1987), studies change and continuity in children's emotion expressions; WILLIAM JAMES, "What Is an Emotion?" *Mind,* 9:188–205 (1884), provides a classic definition of emotion that remains influential today; JEROME KAGAN, J. STEVEN REZNICK, and NANCY SNIDMAN, "Biological Bases of Childhood Shyness," *Science,* 240:167–71 (April 1988), summarizes a series of studies on biological bases and the continuity of shyness; and ROGER SPERRY, "Some Effects of Disconnecting the Cerebral Hemispheres," *Science,* 217:1223–26 (September 1982), discusses the effects of disconnecting cerebral hemispheres on mental and emotional experience.

CARROLL E. IZARD. Unidel Professor of Psychology, University of Delaware, Newark, Del. Author of *Human Emotions.* Coauthor of *Emotions, Cognition, and Behavior.*

Personality

The term personality has been defined in many ways, but as a psychological concept two main meanings have evolved. The first pertains to the consistent differences that exist between people: in this sense, the study of personality focuses on explaining relatively stable human psychological characteristics. The second meaning emphasizes those qualities that make all people alike and that distinguish psychological man from other species; it directs the theorist to search for those regularities among all people that define the nature of man as well as the factors that influence the course of lives. This duality may help explain the two directions that personality studies have taken: on the one hand, the study of ever more specific qualities in people, and, on the other, the search for the totality of psychological functions that emphasizes the interplay between organic and psychological events within people and those social and biological events that surround them. The dual definition of personality is interwoven in most of the topics discussed below. It should be emphasized, however, that no single definition is universally accepted within the field.

The study of personality can be said to have its origins in the fundamental idea that people are distinguished by their characteristic individual patterns of behaviour—the distinctive ways in which they walk, talk, furnish their living quarters, or express their urges. Whatever the behaviour, personologists—as those who engage in the systematic study of personality are called—examine how people differ in the ways they express themselves and attempt to determine the underlying causes of these differences. Although other fields of psychology examine many of the same functions and processes, such as attention, thinking, or motivation, the personologist places primary emphasis on how these different processes fit together and become integrated so as to give each person a distinctive identity, or personality. The systematic psychological study of personality has emerged from a number of different sources and disciplines, including psychiatric case studies that focused on lives in distress, philosophy, which explores the nature of man, and physiology, anthropology, and social psychology.

This article is divided into the following sections:

Personality theories

The systematic study of personality as a recognizable and separate discipline within psychology may be said to have begun in the 1930s with the publication in the United States of two textbooks, *Psychology of Personality* (1937) by Ross Stagner and *Personality: A Psychological Interpretation* (1937) by Gordon W. Allport, followed by Henry A. Murray's *Explorations in Personality* (1938), which contained a set of experimental and clinical studies, and by Gardner Murphy's integrative and comprehensive text, *Personality: A Biosocial Approach to Origins and Structure* (1947). Yet personology can trace its ancestry to the ancient Greeks, who proposed a kind of biochemical theory of personality.

PHYSIOLOGICAL TYPE THEORIES

The idea that people fall into certain personality type categories in relation to bodily characteristics has intrigued numerous modern psychologists as well as their counterparts among the ancients. The idea that people must fall into one or another rigid personality class, however, has been largely dismissed. Two general sets of theories are considered here, the humoral and the morphological.

Humoral theories. Perhaps the oldest personality theory known is contained in the cosmological writings of the Greek philosopher and physiologist Empedocles and in related speculations of the physician Hippocrates. Empedocles' cosmic elements—air (with its associated qualities, warm and moist), earth (cold and dry), fire (warm and dry), and water (cold and moist)—were related to health and corresponded (in the above order) to Hippocrates' physical humours, which were associated with variations in temperament: blood (sanguine temperament), black bile (melancholic), yellow bile (choleric), and phlegm (phlegmatic). This theory, with its view that body chemistry determines temperament, has survived in some form for more than 2,500 years. According to these early theorists, emotional stability as well as general health depend on an appropriate balance among the four bodily humours; an excess of one may produce a particular bodily illness or an exaggerated personality trait. Thus, a person with an excess of blood would be expected to have a sanguine temperament—that is, to be optimistic, enthusiastic, and excitable. Too much black bile (dark blood perhaps mixed with other secretions) was believed to produce a melancholic temperament. An oversupply of yellow bile (secreted by the liver) would result in anger, irritability, and a "jaundiced" view of life. An abundance of phlegm (secreted in the respiratory passages) was alleged to make people stolid, apathetic, and undemonstrative. As biological science has progressed, these primitive ideas about body chemistry have been replaced by more complex ideas and by contemporary studies of hormones, neurotransmitters, and substances produced within the central nervous system, such as endorphins.

Morphological (body type) theories. Related to the biochemical theories are those that distinguish types of personalities on the basis of body shape (somatotype). Such a morphological theory was developed by the German psychiatrist Ernst Kretschmer. In his book *Physique and Character,* first published in 1921, he wrote that among his patients a frail, rather weak (asthenic) body build as well as a muscular (athletic) physique were frequently characteristic of schizophrenic patients, while a short, rotund (pyknic) build was often found among manic-depressive patients. Kretschmer extended his findings and assertions in a theory that related body build and personality in all people and wrote that slim and delicate physiques are associated with introversion, while those with rounded heavier and shorter bodies tend to be cyclothymic—that is, moody but often extroverted and jovial.

Despite early hopes that body types might be useful in classifying personality characteristics or in identifying psychiatric syndromes, the relations observed by Kretschmer were not found to be strongly supported by empirical studies. In the 1930s more elaborate studies by William H. Sheldon in the United States developed a system for assigning a three-digit somatotype number to people, each digit with a range from 1 to 7. Each of the three digits applies to one of Sheldon's three components of body build: the first to the soft, round endomorph, the second to the square, muscular mesomorph; and the third to the linear, fine-boned ectomorph. Thus, an extreme endomorph would be 711, an extreme ectomorph 117, and an average person 444. Sheldon then developed a 20-item list of traits that differentiated three separate categories of behaviours or temperaments. The three-digit temperament scale appeared to be significantly related to the somatotype profile, an association that failed to excite personologists.

Also during the 1930s, personality studies began to consider the broader social context in which a person lived. The American anthropologist Margaret Mead studied the patterns of cooperation and competition in 13 primitive societies and was able to document wide variations in those behaviours in different societies. In her book *Sex and Temperament in Three Primitive Societies* (1935), she showed that masculinity is not necessarily expressed through aggressiveness and that femininity is not necessarily expressed through passivity and acquiescence. These demonstrated variations raised questions about the relative roles of biology, learning, and cultural pressures in personality characteristics.

PSYCHOANALYTIC THEORIES

Freud. Perhaps the most influential integrative theory of personality is that of psychoanalysis, which was largely promulgated during the first four decades of the 20th century by the Austrian neurologist Sigmund Freud. Although its beginnings were based in studies of psychopathology, psychoanalysis became a more general perspective on normal personality development and functioning. The field of investigation began with case studies of so-called neurotic conditions, which included hysteria, obsessive-compulsive disorders, and phobic conditions. Patients with hysterical symptoms complained of acute shortness of breath, paralyses, and contractures of limbs for which no physical cause could be found. In the course of interviews, Freud and his early coworker and mentor, the Austrian physician Josef Breuer, noted that many of their patients were unsure of how or when their symptoms developed and even seemed indifferent to the enormous inconvenience the symptoms caused them. It was as if the ideas associated with the symptoms were quarantined from the consciousness and lay neglected by normal curiosity. To explain this strange pattern Breuer and Freud made two assumptions. The first was based on the general scientific position of determinism, which was quite prevalent in 19th-century science: although no apparent physical causes could be implicated, these neurotic symptoms were nevertheless caused, or determined, perhaps not by one but by multiple factors, some of which were psychologically motivated. The second assumption entailed unconscious psychological processes; that is, ideas continue to be active, to change, and to influence behaviour even when they are outside of awareness. One source for this assumption was the observation of posthypnotic suggestion, which seemed to imply that past experiences, surviving outside of consciousness as latent memories, could be activated by a signal from the environment and could then influence behaviour even though the hypnotized person was unaware of the reasons for his behaviour.

Breuer and Freud believed that the specific motivation for these neurotic symptoms lay in the patient's desire to obliterate from memory profoundly distressing events that were incompatible with the patient's moral standards and thus in conflict with them. These events were considered to have been sexual in nature, and further exploration convinced Freud that his patients had had even earlier troublesome sexual experiences—usually seductions—the memories of which had lain dormant until awakened by a more recent sexual encounter. Freud reasoned that the earlier experience imparted to the later one its pathogenic force. Freud at first accepted many of the experiences reported by his young, impressionable patients as actual seductions. He later came to believe that many of the narrations were fantasies. On the basis of this conviction, Freud formulated a theory indicating that personality is shaped by such experiences as well as by other traumatic or frustrating events. He postulated that the fantasies about sexual traumas were expressions of a sexual drive. Thereafter in his therapeutic method, the search for actual sexual trauma was replaced by an exploration of the ways in which patients' sexual inclinations, already present in childhood, were expressed in behaviour. Neurosis and personality in general came to be viewed as outcomes of conflict between sexual motivations and defenses against them, the conflict being rooted in early child development.

Freud assumed that his patients were motivated to ward off those fantasies that had an exciting as well as a repelling quality about them. Freud described various psychological devices (defense mechanisms) by which people tried to make the fantasies bearable. For example, in the obsessive-compulsive condition, which refers to persistent unwelcome ideas or recurrent irresistible urges to perform certain acts, such as incessant hand washing, the defense maneuvers are called isolation and displacement. They consist in separating (isolating) a fantasy from its corresponding emotion, and then attaching (displacing) the emotion to another, previously trivial idea; for instance, to the hand washer it is the hands that are dirty rather than the desires. Freud also noted that people who rely on isolation and displacement are otherwise characterized by nonpathological personality qualities such as perfectionism, indecisiveness, and formality in interpersonal contacts. To Freud the fantasies were the mental representations of basic drives, among which sex, aggression, and self-preservation were paramount. These drives, moreover, required taming as the child matured into an adult, and the taming process involved blocking out of consciousness some of the ideas associated with the expression of those drives. Other methods of defense include repression, a kind of withholding of conflicting ideas from recall; projection, the attribution to others of one's own rejected tendencies; and reaction formation, turning into its opposite a tendency rejected in oneself—as in excessive generosity as a defense against avarice. The basic conflict between drives and control processes, which Freud believed to be the basis of several neuroses, was also invoked to explain both dream content and the "psychopathology of everyday life"—the ordinary slips of the tongue (sometimes called Freudian slips) and errors such as forgetting intentions or misplacing objects.

These primary human drives, moreover, were seen to undergo transformations as part of psychological and physical growth. This formulation widened the realm of sexuality beyond reproduction, by proposing that genital activity does not encompass all of sexuality, because sexual activity can be observed long before biological maturity and can occur without leading to reproduction. The theory further proposed that sexual maturation develops in a sequence of stages as parts of the body successively yield sensual pleasure to the child, beginning with the mouth, followed by the anus, and then the genitals. Social demands for inhibition and control of the drives centre about the functions of these zones, and it is from this process of socialization that personality is said to emerge. For example, the extent to which the personality expresses power, responsibility, compliance, and defiance seems to coincide with anal expressions of the sexual drive and is related to the process of obtaining control over anal functions.

The conflict between the drives—conceptualized as a wholly unconscious structure called the id—and the drive control processes—conceptualized as a largely unconscious structure called the ego—results in the creation of a characteristic style for mediating conflicts, which is assumed to be formed prior to adolescence. While learning and experience are recognized as conspicuous factors in the shaping of these behaviours, the theory also gives prominence to possibly inborn differences in the strength of drives and of the control processes.

Among the controlling functions of the ego are identifications and defenses. Children are inclined to behave like the significant adult models in their environment, Freud postulated. These identifications give identity and individuality to the maturing child. Moreover, the process of self-criticism is part of the ego controls (Freud called it the superego) and acts as an internal and often unconscious conscience that influences moral values.

Jung. The Swiss psychiatrist Carl Gustav Jung, an early adherent of Freud's theories, questioned the degree of emphasis that Freud gave to sexual motivations in personality development. Jung accepted the significant effect of the unconscious processes, but unlike Freud he preferred to emphasize that behaviour is motivated more by abstract, even spiritual, processes than by sexual drives. Jung also focused more on individual differences; in particular he developed a typology of reaction styles, distinguishing between two basic means of modulating basic drives, introversion and extroversion. Introversion was defined as preoccupation with one's inner world at the expense of social interactions and extroversion as a preference for social interplay for living out inner drives (collectively termed libido). The existence of these two types receives empirical support from most studies of traits (see below).

Adler. The Austrian psychiatrist Alfred Adler, another of Freud's early followers, also disputed the importance of sexual motives. Adler described a coping strategy that he called compensation, which he felt was an important influence on behaviour. In his view people compensated for a behavioral deficiency by exaggerating some other behaviour: a process analogous to organic processes called hypertrophy, in which, for example, if one eye is injured, the other eye may compensate by becoming more acute. In Adler's view, a person with a feeling of inferiority related to a physical or mental inadequacy would also develop compensating behaviours or symptoms. Shortness of stature, for example, could lead to the development

of domineering, controlling behaviours. Adler assigned a prominent place to family dynamics in personality development. Children's position in their family—their birth order—was seen as determining significant character traits.

Erikson. Freud's emphasis on the developmental unfolding of the sexual, aggressive, and self-preservative motives in personality was modified by the American psychoanalyst Erik H. Erikson, who integrated psychological, social, and biological factors. Erikson's scheme proposed eight stages of the development of drives, which continue past Freud's five stages of childhood (oral, anal, phallic, latency, and genital) and through three stages of adulthood. The stages proceed in leaps according to what is called an epigenetic process. The term epigenesis, borrowed from embryology, refers to the predetermined developmental sequence of parts of an organism. Each part has a special time for its emergence and for its progressive integration within the functioning whole. Each phase of emergence depends upon the successful completion of the preceding phase. According to Erikson, environmental forces exercise their greatest effect on development at the earliest stages of growth, because anything that disturbs one stage affects all of the following stages. As if controlled by a biological timetable, each given stage must be superseded by a new one, receding in significance as the new stage assumes dominance. A constant interleaving at critical periods—in which some parts emerge while others are suppressed—must proceed smoothly if personality problems are to be avoided.

The Freudian theory of development with Erikson's modifications provides for a succession of drive-control (inner and environmental) interactions. These can be fit into a schema of polar attitudes that develop in progressive stages of a person's life, creating a conflict at each stage which should be resolved to avoid extremes of personality development. Erikson thus evolved his eight stages of development, which he described as: (1) infancy: trust versus mistrust; (2) early childhood: autonomy versus shame and doubt; (3) preschool: initiative versus guilt; (4) school age: industry versus inferiority; (5) puberty: identity versus identity confusion; (6) young adulthood: intimacy versus isolation; (7) middle adulthood: generativity versus stagnation; and (8) late adulthood: integrity versus despair.

The impact of psychoanalysis. There is little doubt that psychoanalysis had a profound influence on personality theory during the 20th century. It turned attention from mere description of types of people to an interest in how people become what they are. Psychoanalytic theory emphasizes that the human organism is constantly, though slowly, changing through perpetual interactions, and that, therefore, the human personality can be conceived of as a locus of change with fragile and indefinite boundaries. It suggests that research should focus not only on studies of traits, attitudes, and motives but also on studies that reflect the psychoanalytic view that personality never ceases to develop and that even the rate of personality modification changes during the course of a life. Although the theory holds that conflict and such basic drives as sex and aggression figure prominently in personality development and functioning, their presence may be neither recognizable nor comprehensible to persons untrained to look for those motives. However, personality characteristics are relatively stable over time and across situations, so that a person remains recognizable despite change. Another feature of psychoanalytic theory is the insistence that personality is affected by both biological and psychosocial forces that operate principally within the family, with the major foundations being laid early in life.

The data on which psychoanalytic theory rests came from the psychoanalysts' consulting rooms, where patients in conflict told their life stories to their analysts. No provision is made in that setting for experimental manipulation, for independent observation, or for testing the generality of the formulations. As a consequence, although much of the theory has found its way into accepted doctrine, psychoanalysis cannot claim a body of experimentally tested evidence. Nevertheless, psychoanalytic theory provides at least a preliminary framework for much of personality research involving motives and development.

Role model identification

Erikson's eight stages of development

The basis of psychoanalytic theory

TRAIT THEORIES

Contemporary personality studies are generally empirical and based on experiments. While they are more precise, and thus may be more valid than much of psychoanalytic theory, experiments perforce have a narrower scope than the grand sweep of psychoanalysis. In the 1940s many investigators focused on intensive studies of individual traits and of combinations of traits that seemed to define personality types, such as the "authoritarian personality." Others, like the American psychologists David C. McClelland and John W. Atkinson, studied the characteristic presence of certain needs identified by Murray, such as the need for achievement or affiliation. The method used to measure these needs was to examine the fantasy productions of Murray's Thematic Apperception Test (TAT) and to relate the motive score to other behavioral indexes such as personal history, occupational choice, speed of learning, and persistence of behaviour following failure.

Stability of traits.   Traits such as sociability, impulsiveness, meticulousness, truthfulness, and deceit are assumed to be more or less stable over time and across situations. Traits refer not to single instances of a behaviour, such as lying, but to persistent although not unvarying behaviour that, according to some personologists, implies a disposition to respond in a particular, identifiable way. According to Allport's 1937 textbook, traits represent structures or habits within a person and are not the construction of observers; they are the product of both genetic predispositions and experience. It can be generally stated that traits are merely names for observed regularities in behaviour, but do not explain them. Nevertheless, the study of how traits arise and are integrated within a person forms a major area of personality studies.

In the English language there are several thousand words representing traits, many of them close in meaning to others (for example, meticulous, careful, conscientious). Most of the measurement studies employ self-report (personality) inventories that require people to describe themselves by checking relevant adjectives or answering questions about typical behaviours that they are conscious of displaying. In some measurements, observers rate the behaviour of others. Psychologists such as Hans J. Eysenck in the United Kingdom and Raymond B. Cattell in the United States have attempted to reduce the list to what they could consider to be the smallest possible number of trait clusters. The statistical technique of factor analysis has been favoured for this task, since it explores the correlations among all of the trait names and identifies clusters of correlations among traits that appear to be independent of (uncorrelated with) each other. Common to almost all the trait systems are variables related to emotional stability, energy level, dominance, and sociability, although different investigators choose different names for these factors. Eysenck, for example, has reduced the trait names to but three higher-order factors—introversion-extroversion, neuroticism, and psychoticism—and has attempted to explore the biological roots of each factor.

Deviation from trait theory.   The idea that traits represent relatively stable behaviours has received criticism from psychologists who point out that behavioral consistency across situations and across time is not the rule. For example, in a study of children's moral development, the American psychologists Hugh Hartshorne and Mark A. May in 1928 placed 10- to 13-year-old children in situations that gave them the opportunity to lie, steal, or cheat; to spend money on themselves or on other children; and to yield to or resist distractions. The predictive power of personal and educational background was low, and children were not found consistently honest or dishonest, distractible, or altruistic. The most powerful predictor of children's behaviour was what other children around them were doing.

In the 1960s and '70s some psychologists, including Walter Mischel and Albert Bandura in the United States, recalled the Hartshorne and May study and variations of it to support their view that behaviour is controlled not by hypothetical traits but according to the degree of regularity of external stimuli. They believe that personality traits are consistent only if the situation is consistent and that they

vary once the situation changes. In their view, behavioral consistency does not reflect stable personality traits; the environment evokes and shapes the illusion of such traits. This would be in keeping with the view of social learning theorists that personality, like other elements of a person's psychological makeup, is largely a learning phenomenon related to such factors as the imitation of role models. Social learning theory would also contend that personality is more susceptible to change than would trait theory.

Although it has been demonstrated that behaviour is seldom entirely consistent, it also has been shown that it reflects considerable consistency. Even in the Hartshorne and May study some children showed consistently honest or dishonest behaviour, and behavioral consistency was found to increase with age.

Support for personal consistency is bolstered by studies of what has been called the fundamental attribution error. The investigators, most of them social psychologists, report that, in observing the behaviour of others, people exaggerate the role of internal causes and invoke traits as a primary cause (*e.g.*, "John acted the way he did because he is honest"). In assigning cause to their own behaviour, however, people more often cite external causes such as the particular situation. These tendencies are accompanied by another discovered regularity: in seeking sources for their own behaviour, people are likely to favour internal causes (and thus agree with an observer's judgment) when they consider a behaviour to be desirable (*e.g.*, success, as in "I was successful because I am skillful"), and they invoke external, situational causes in judging a behaviour they deem undesirable (*e.g.*, failure, as in "I failed because the test was unfair"). There are, of course, limits to the regularity with which these generalizations hold. Because people tend to know their own characteristics better than observers do, they are generally more aware than observers are of any divergences from their usual behaviour.

Although people may assume the existence of traits in themselves, they do not, in analyzing a specific situation, see themselves as a mere collection of trait names. Consequently, they are not for the most part perplexed by, and often do not recognize, cross-situational inconsistency in their own behaviour. But in observing another person's behaviour, most people attribute high consistency to that person, as if many positive traits could be inferred from the attribution or observation of one positive trait. For example, the American social psychologist Solomon Asch has shown that a physically attractive person will tend to be judged as having many other desirable qualities. Asch also demonstrated that, in forming impressions of the personal characteristics of others, observers are most influenced by their first impression. The reason first impressions seem to be almost indelible is that they carry an excessive amount of new information, which has a high degree of unpredictability. That is, the more new information contained in an event, the more attention it attracts. Since impressions about a person tend to be integrated into a single characterization, an observer may be jarred by recognizing an undesirable fact about an attractive person and may try either to ignore that fact or to mitigate (rationalize) it. These propensities make up a "common sense psychology," in the words of Fritz Heider, an American psychologist. This "naive" psychology, as he called it, consists of a set of rules that guide most people's impressions of other people and of social situations. These rules are used constantly to interpret one's own and other people's behaviour and to predict behaviour under certain conditions. The psychoanalytic view, however, seriously challenges this. Psychoanalysis has no problem explaining that those who put to death countless people in the Nazi death chambers, for example, could also be devoted parents, whereas common sense psychology would have difficulty with this. For the psychoanalyst, a personality may be integrated, but it is rarely seamless and regular. People generally make two types of errors in judging personality: they impute more personality consistency to others than the actors themselves would allow, and they often ignore the operation of unconscious psychological processes that can explain at least some of the inconsistencies.

Much work on trait structure and impression formation

Eysenck's three basic traits

Variations in trait identification

has concerned adjectival words that describe traits, and the fact that these studies have been carried out principally in the United States and western Europe has led some anthropologists, such as the American Robert LeVine, to remark that modern personality trait theory is ethnocentric. For example, the folk-psychological concepts and the trait matrices derived from factor analyses include culture-specific assumptions about personal experiences, such as the distinctions between mind and body, natural and supernatural, and intellect and morality, which do not exist in the folk traditions of many non-Western peoples. Unlike most other cultures, Western thought assumes that a high degree of personal autonomy is desirable and that the most important emotional and personal relations are with a marital partner. For some psychologists these cultural differences point to the need for a less culture-bound approach to personality trait theory.

Ethno-centric trait theory

MODERN TRENDS IN PERSONALITY STUDIES

Sex differences. Despite the physical differences between males and females the finding of behavioral differences between the sexes is controversial. Behaviours associated with sex roles depend heavily on the social and cultural context, and studies of stereotypic male and female roles are therefore understandably ambiguous. Yet some findings indicate small but consistent differences. While there are no differences in measured IQ, itself regarded as a culture-bound assessment, females do better than males on verbal tasks. Girls generally begin to speak earlier than boys and have fewer languageproblems in school and in the course of maturation. Males generally exhibit greater skill in understanding spatial relations and in solving problems that involve mathematical reasoning. Beginning at the toddler stage, the activity level of males is generally higher than that of females. A related finding is that boys are more likely to be irritable and aggressive than girls and more often behave like bullies. Men usually outscore women in antisocial personality disorders, which consist of persistent lying, stealing, vandalism, and fighting, although these differences do not appear until after about the age of three. A study by the American anthropologists Beatrice B. Whiting and Carolyn P. Edwards found that males were consistently more aggressive than females in seven cultures, suggesting that there is a predisposition in males to respond aggressively to provocative situations, although how and whether the attacking response occurs depends on the social and cultural setting.

Aggression. Humans are perhaps the only species of animal that does not have an internal inhibition against slaughtering other members of the species. It has been theorized that man, like other animals, is motivated by an aggressive drive, which has significant survival value, but lacks internal inhibitions against killing his fellow men. Inhibitions, therefore, must be imposed externally by society. Social learning theorists emphasize the decisive effects of situations in triggering and controlling aggression. They account for the poor predictability of aggressive behaviour in man by noting that the environmental context is generally unpredictable. Yet research has shown that an aggressive act is most likely to be produced by a person with a history of aggressive behaviour.

The tendency of man to kill his own kind

Genetic aspects. While social learning theorists emphasize the active shaping of personality by external social influences, experimental evidence has accumulated that genetic factors play a prominent role, if not in the transmission of specific behaviour patterns, then in the readiness of people to respond to environmental pressures in particular ways. In observations of animals, it is commonplace to find in different breeds of dogs wide divergences in behaviour that are attributed to genetic differences: some are friendly, others aggressive; some are timid, others bold (of course there may also be wide variations within a given breed). Among human infants observed in a neonatal nursery, there are also clearly observable differences in activity, passivity, fussiness, cuddliness, and responsiveness. These patterns, which some authorities say may be genetically influenced, shape the ways in which the infant will interact with the environment and can be considered an expression of personality.

In systematic studies of humans, studies of twins and adopted children have been used to try to evaluate environmental and genetic factors as determinants of a number of behaviour patterns. These studies have shown that genetic factors account for about 50 percent of the range of differences found in a given population. Most of the remaining differences are attributable not to the environment that is common to members of a family but to the environment that is unique to each member of the family or that results from interactions of family members with one another. In the United States, behaviour geneticists such as Robert Plomin report that, in behaviours describable as sociability, impulsiveness, altruism, aggression, and emotional sensitivity, the similarities among monozygotic (identical) twins is twice that among dizygotic (fraternal) twins, with the common environment contributing practically nothing to the similarities. Similar findings are reported for twins reared together or separately.

Personality studies of twins

The study of the genetic aspects of personality is a relatively new undertaking. Almost all populations studied have been from industrialized Western nations whose rearing environments are more nearly alike than different. It is known that the more homogeneous the environment, the stronger the genetic contribution will appear. As with the psychology of traits, cross-cultural studies are required to test the validity of the claims of behaviour genetics.

Cognitive controls and styles. Psychologists have long been aware that people differ in the consistent way in which they receive and respond to information. Some make careful distinctions between stimuli, whereas others blur distinctions, and some may typically prefer to make broad categories, whereas others prefer narrow ones for grouping objects. These consistencies in an individual seem to be fairly stable across time and even across situations. They have been referred to as cognitive controls. Combinations of several cognitive controls within a person have been referred to as cognitive style, of which there can be numerous variations.

Cognitive control studies explore constraints within a person that limit the influence of both environment and motivation, and as such they are expressions of personality. In the 1940s and '50s several studies explored the extent to which personal needs or drives determine what one perceives. In one study, children from rich and poor families were asked to adjust a circle of light to the size of several coins of increasing value and to the size of cardboard disks. All of the children overestimated the size of the coins, although not of the neutral disks, but the poor children overestimated the sizes more than did the rich children. The assumption that need influences such judgments has been widely held. Even Shakespeare, in *A Midsummer Night's Dream,* noted, "Or in the night, imagining some fear, / how easy is a bush supposed a bear." But there are limits to the distorting power of drives, and the experimental demonstration of the influence of motives has been difficult to confirm, perhaps because the formal components of cognition—the workings, for example, of attention, judgment, or perception—and individual difference in their expression have been neglected by personologists. Investigators of cognitive controls examine the psychological limits on the distorting effects of needs and of external reality. For example, in estimating the size of a disk, some people are more exact than others, and the extent to which a need can distort size judgments will consequently be limited by the perceiver's preference for strict or relaxed standards of comparison.

Limits of psychological drive distortion

The American psychologists George S. Klein and Herman Witkin in the 1940s and '50s were able to show that several cognitive controls were relatively stable over a class of situations and intentions. For example, the psychologists found a stable tendency in some people to blur distinctions between successively appearing stimuli so that elements tended to lose their individuality (leveling) and an equally stable tendency in other individuals to highlight differences (sharpening). This organizing principle is apparent in judgments of the size of a series of objects, as well as in memory, where it may manifest itself in a blurring of elements in the recall of a story. Another much studied cognitive control is called field dependence-field independence. It pertains to the extent to which people are influenced by inner (field-independent) or environmental (field-dependent) cues in orienting themselves in space and the extent to which they make fine differentiations in the environment. The more field-independent people are, the greater is their ability to articulate a field. There are no general intellectual capacity differences between field-dependent and field-independent people, but there is a tendency for field-dependent people to favour careers that include working with other people, such as teaching or social work. Field-independent people are more often found in careers that involve abstract issues such as mathematics. Cultural differences have also been found. Some Eskimo live and hunt in an environment with little variation, and a high degree of articulation of the field (field independence) would favour survival; some farmers of Sierra Leone, however, who inhabit an area of lush vegetation and many varieties of shape, require less differentiation of the field.

Characteristics of field dependence–field independence

ORIGINS OF PERSONALITY STUDY

In general, information about human personality has come from three different sources of study. The first is biological, conceived to have genetic as well as environmental origins. The second is that of the social realm, including the impact of social forces on the growing child that shape such personal responses as motives, traits, behaviours, and attitudes. The third is the examination of clinical contacts with people who have suffered adaptive and adjustive failures. Some authorities have suggested that a greater degree of integration of all three sources of information and the methods derived from them would accelerate the growth of valid information about personality.

Personality assessment

The measurement of personal characteristics is the subject matter of the field of psychology today called personality assessment. Assessment is an end result of gathering information intended to advance psychological theory and research and to increase the probability that wise decisions will be made in applied settings (*e.g.*, in selecting the most promising people from a group of job applicants). The approach taken by the specialist in personality assessment is based on the assumption that much of the observable variability in behaviour from one person to another results from differences in the extent to which individuals possess particular underlying personal characteristics (traits). The assessment specialist seeks to define these traits, to measure them objectively, and to relate them to socially significant aspects of behaviour.

A distinctive feature of the scientific approach to personality measurement is the effort, wherever possible, to describe human characteristics in quantitative terms. How much of a trait manifests itself in an individual? How many traits are present? Quantitative personality measurement is especially useful in comparing groups of people as well as individuals. Do groups of people from different cultural and economic backgrounds differ when considered in the light of their particular personality attributes or traits? How large are the group differences?

Overt behaviour is a reflection of interactions among a wide range of underlying factors, including the bodily state of the individual and the effects of that person's past personal experiences. Hence, a narrowly focused approach is inadequate to do justice to the complex human behaviour that occurs under the constantly changing set of challenges, pleasures, demands, and stresses of everyday life. The sophisticated measurement of human personality inescapably depends on the use of a variety of concepts to provide trait definitions and entails the application of various methods of observation and evaluation. Personality theorists and researchers seek to define and to understand the diversity of human traits, the many ways people have of thinking and perceiving and learning and emoting. Such nonmaterial human dimensions, types, and attributes are constructs—in this case, inferences drawn from observed behaviour. Widely studied personality constructs include anxiety, hostility, emotionality, motivation, and introversion-extroversion. Anxiety, for example, is a concept, or construct, inferred in people from what they say, their facial expressions, and their body movements.

Personality constructs

Personality is interactional in two senses. As indicated above, personal characteristics can be thought of as products of interactions among underlying psychological factors; for example, an individual may experience tension because he or she is both shy and desirous of social success. These products, in turn, interact with the types of situations people confront in their daily lives. A person who is anxious about being evaluated might show debilitated performance in evaluative situations (for example, taking tests), but function well in other situations in which an evaluative emphasis is not present. Personality makeup can be either an asset or a liability depending on the situation. For example, some people approach evaluative situations with fear and foreboding, while others seem to be motivated in a desirable direction by competitive pressures associated with performance.

MEASURING CONSTRUCTS

Efforts to measure personality constructs stem from a variety of sources. Frequently they grow out of theories of personality; anxiety and repression (the forgetting of unpleasant experiences), for example, are among the central concepts of the theory of psychoanalysis. It is understandable that efforts would be made to quantify one's degree of anxiety, for example, and to use the score thus obtained in the assessment of and in the prediction of future behaviour. Among the major issues in the study of personality measurement is the question of which of the many personality constructs that have been quantified are basic or fundamental and which can be expected to involve wasted effort in their measurement because they represent poorly defined combinations of more elemental constructs; which measurement techniques are most effective and convenient for the purpose of assessment; and whether it is better to interview people in measuring personality, or to ask them to say, for example, what an inkblot or a cloud in the sky reminds them of.

Efforts to measure any given personality construct can fail as a result of inadequacies in formulating or defining the trait to be measured and weaknesses in the assessment methods employed. An investigator might desire to specify quantitatively the degree to which individuals are submissive in social and competitive situations. His effectiveness will depend on the particular theory of submissiveness he brings to bear on the problem; on the actual procedures he selects or devises to measure submissiveness; and on the adequacy of the research he performs to demonstrate the usefulness of the measure. Each of these tasks must be considered carefully in evaluating efforts to measure personality attributes.

Problems in measuring personality constructs

The methods used in personality description and measurement fall into several categories that differ with regard to the type of information gathered and the methods by which it is obtained. While all should rely on data that come from direct observations of human behaviour if they are to have at least the semblance of scientific value, all may vary with regard to underlying assumptions, validity, and reliability (consistency, in this case).

ASSESSMENT METHODS

Personality tests provide measures of such characteristics as feelings and emotional states, preoccupations, motivations, attitudes, and approaches to interpersonal relations. There is a diversity of approaches to personality assessment, and controversy surrounds many aspects of the widely used methods and techniques. These include such assessments as the interview, rating scales, self-reports, personality inventories, projective techniques, and behavioral observation.

The interview. In an interview the individual under assessment must be given considerable latitude in "telling his story." Interviews have both verbal and nonverbal (*e.g.*, gestural) components. The aim of the interview is to gather information, and the adequacy of the data gathered depends in large part on the questions asked by the interviewer. In an employment interview the focus of the interviewer is generally on the job candidate's work experiences, general and specific attitudes, and occupational goals. In a diagnostic medical or psychiatric interview considerable attention would be paid to the patient's physical health and to any symptoms of behavioral disorder that may have occurred over the years.

Two broad types of interview may be delineated. In the interview designed for use in research, face-to-face contact between an interviewer and interviewee is directed toward eliciting information that may be relevant to particular practical applications under general study or to those personality theories (or hypotheses) being investigated. Another type, the clinical interview, is focused on assessing the status of a particular individual (*e.g.*, a psychiatric patient); such an interview is action-oriented (*i.e.*, it may indicate appropriate treatment). Both research and clinical interviews frequently may be conducted to obtain an individual's life history and biographical information (*e.g.*, identifying facts, family relationships), but they differ in the uses to which the information is put.

Although it is not feasible to quantify all of the events occurring in an interview, personality researchers have devised ways of categorizing many aspects of the content of what a person has said. In this approach, called content analysis, the particular categories used depend upon the researchers' interests and ingenuity, but the method of content analysis is quite general and involves the construction of a system of categories that, it is hoped, can be used reliably by an analyst or scorer. The categories may be straightforward (*e.g.*, the number of words uttered by the interviewee during designated time periods), or they may rest on inferences (*e.g.*, the degree of personal unhappiness the interviewee appears to express). The value of content analysis is that it provides the possibility of using frequencies of uttered response to describe verbal behaviour and defines behavioral variables for more-or-less precise study in experimental research. Content analysis has been used, for example, to gauge changes in attitude as they occur within a person with the passage of time. Changes in the frequency of hostile reference a neurotic makes toward his parents during a sequence of psychotherapeutic interviews, for example, may be detected and assessed, as may the changing self-evaluations of psychiatric hospital inmates in relation to the length of their hospitalization.

Sources of erroneous conclusions that may be drawn from face-to-face encounters stem from the complexity of the interview situation, the attitudes, fears, and expectations of the interviewee, and the interviewer's manner and training. Research has been conducted to identify, control, and, if possible, eliminate these sources of interview invalidity and unreliability. By conducting more than one interview with the same interviewee and by using more than one interviewer to evaluate the subject's behaviour, light can be shed on the reliability of the information derived and may reveal differences in influence among individual interviewers. Standardization of interview format tends to increase the reliability of the information gathered; for example, all interviewers may use the same set of questions. Such standardization, however, may restrict the scope of information elicited, and even a perfectly reliable (consistent) interview technique can lead to incorrect inferences.

Rating scales.   The rating scale is one of the oldest and most versatile of assessment techniques. Rating scales present users with an item and ask them to select from a number of choices. The rating scale is similar in some respects to a multiple choice test, but its options represent degrees of a particular characteristic.

Rating scales are used by observers and also by individuals for self-reporting (see below). They permit convenient characterization of other people and their behaviour. Some observations do not lend themselves to quantification as readily as do simple counts of motor behaviour (such as the number of times a worker leaves his lathe to go to the restroom). It is difficult, for example, to quantify how charming an office receptionist is. In such cases, one may fall back on relatively subjective judgments, inferences, and relatively imprecise estimates. The rating scale is one approach to securing such judgments. Rating scales present an observer with scalar dimensions along which

those who are observed are to be placed. A teacher, for example, might be asked to rate students on the degree to which the behaviour of each reflects leadership capacity, shyness, or creativity. Peers might rate each other along dimensions such as friendliness, trustworthiness, and social skills. Several standardized, printed rating scales are available for describing the behaviour of psychiatric hospital patients. Relatively objective rating scales have also been devised for use with other groups. Rating scales often take a graphic form:

To what degree is John shy?

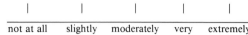

A number of requirements should be met to maximize the usefulness of rating scales. One is that they be reliable: the ratings of the same person by different observers should be consistent. Other requirements are reduction of sources of inaccuracy in personality measurement; the so-called halo effect results in an observer's rating someone favourably on a specific characteristic because the observer has a generally favourable reaction to the person being rated. One's tendency to say only nice things about others or one's proneness to think of all people as average (to use the midrange of scales) represents other methodological problems that arise when rating scales are used.

Self-report tests.   The success that attended the use of convenient intelligence tests in providing reliable, quantitative (numerical) indexes of individual ability has stimulated interest in the possibility of devising similar tests for measuring personality. Procedures now available vary in the degree to which they achieve score reliability and convenience. These desirable attributes can be partly achieved by restricting in designated ways the kinds of responses a subject is free to make. Self-report instruments follow this strategy. For example, a test that restricts the subject to true-false answers is likely to be convenient to give and easy to score. So-called personality inventories (see below) tend to have these characteristics, in that they are relatively restrictive, can be scored objectively, and are convenient to administer. Other techniques (such as inkblot tests) for evaluating personality possess these characteristics to a lesser degree.

Self-report personality tests are used in clinical settings in making diagnoses, in deciding whether treatment is required, and in planning the treatment to be used. A second major use is as an aid in selecting employees, and a third is in psychological research. An example of the latter case would be where scores on a measure of test anxiety—that is, the feeling of tenseness and worry that people experience before an exam—might be used to divide people into groups according to how upset they get while taking exams. Researchers have investigated whether the more test-anxious students behave differently than the less anxious ones in an experimental situation.

Personality inventories.   Among the most common of self-report tests are personality inventories. Their origins lie in the early history of personality measurement, when most tests were constructed on the basis of so-called face validity; that is, they simply appeared to be valid. Items were included simply because, in the fallible judgment of the person who constructed or devised the test, they were indicative of certain personality attributes. In other words, face validity need not be defined by careful, quantitative study; rather, it typically reflects one's more-or-less imprecise, possibly erroneous, impressions. Personal judgment, even that of an expert, is no guarantee that a particular collection of test items will prove to be reliable and meaningful in actual practice.

A widely used early self-report inventory, the so-called Woodworth Personal Data Sheet, was developed during World War I to detect soldiers who were emotionally unfit for combat. Among its ostensibly face-valid items were these: Does the sight of blood make you sick or dizzy? Are you happy most of the time? Do you sometimes wish you had never been born? Recruits who answered these kinds of questions in a way that could be taken to mean that they suffered psychiatric disturbance were detained

The clinical interview

Uses of rating scales

Self-report personality tests

for further questioning and evaluation. Clearly, however, symptoms revealed by such answers are exhibited by many people who are relatively free of emotional disorder.

Rather than testing general knowledge or specific skills, personality inventories ask people questions about themselves. These questions may take a variety of forms. When taking such a test, the subject might have to decide whether each of a series of statements is accurate as a self-description or respond to a series of true-false questions about personal beliefs.

Several inventories require that each of a series of statements be placed on a rating scale in terms of the frequency or adequacy with which the statements are judged by the individual to reflect his tendencies and attitudes. Regardless of the way in which the subject responds, most inventories yield several scores, each intended to identify a distinctive aspect of personality.

The Minnesota Multiphasic Personality Inventory

One of these, the Minnesota Multiphasic Personality Inventory (MMPI), is probably the personality inventory in widest use in the English-speaking world. Also available in other languages, it consists in one version of 550 items (e.g., "I like tall women") to which subjects are to respond "true," "false," or "cannot say." Work on this inventory began in the 1930s, when its construction was motivated by the need for a practical, economical means of describing and predicting the behaviour of psychiatric patients. In its development efforts were made to achieve convenience in administration and scoring and to overcome many of the known defects of earlier personality inventories. Varied types of items were included and emphasis was placed on making these printed statements (presented either on small cards or in a booklet) intelligible even to persons with limited reading ability.

Most earlier inventories lacked subtlety; many people were able to fake or bias their answers since the items presented were easily seen to reflect gross disturbances; indeed, in many of these inventories maladaptive tendencies would be reflected in either all true or all false answers. Perhaps the most significant methodological advance to be found in the MMPI was the attempt on the part of its developers to measure tendencies to respond, rather than actual behaviour, and to rely but little on assumptions of face validity. The true-false item "I hear strange voices all the time" has face validity for most people in that to answer "true" to it seems to provide a strong indication of abnormal hallucinatory experiences. But some psychiatric patients who "hear strange voices" can still appreciate the socially undesirable implications of a "true" answer and may try to conceal their abnormality by answering "false." A major difficulty in placing great reliance on face validity in test construction is that the subject may be as aware of the significance of certain responses as is the test constructor and thus may be able to mislead the tester. Nevertheless, the person who hears strange voices and yet answers the item "false" clearly is responding to something—the answer still is a reflection of personality, even if it is not the aspect of personality to which the item seems to refer; thus, careful study of responses beyond their mere face validity often proves to be profitable.

Reactions to the testing environment

Much study has been given to the ways in which response sets and test-taking attitudes influence behaviour on the MMPI and other personality measures. The response set called acquiescence, for example, refers to one's tendency to respond with "true" or "yes" answers to questionnaire items regardless of what the item content is. It is conceivable that two people might be quite similar in all respects except for their tendency toward acquiescence. This difference in response set can lead to misleadingly different scores on personality tests. One person might be a "yea-sayer" (someone who tends to answer true to test items); another might be a "nay-sayer"; a third individual might not have a pronounced acquiescence tendency in either direction.

Acquiescence is not the only response set; there are other test-taking attitudes that are capable of influencing personality profiles. One of these, already suggested by the example of the person who hears strange voices, is social desirability. A person who has convulsions might say "false" to the item "I have convulsions" because he

believes that others will think less of him if they know he has convulsions. The intrusive potentially deceiving effects of the subjects' response sets and test-taking attitudes on scores derived from personality measures can sometimes be circumvented by varying the content and wording of test items. Nevertheless, users of questionnaires have not yet completely solved problems of bias such as those arising from response sets. Indeed, many of these problems first received widespread attention in research on the MMPI, and research on this and similar inventories has significantly advanced understanding of the whole discipline of personality testing.

The MMPI as originally published consists of nine clinical scales (or sets of items), each scale having been found in practice to discriminate a particular clinical group, such as people suffering from schizophrenia, depression, or paranoia. Each of these scales (or others produced later) was developed by determining patterns of response to the inventory that were observed to be distinctive of groups of individuals who had been psychiatrically classified by other means (e.g., by long-term observation). The responses of apparently normal subjects were compared with those of hospital patients with a particular psychiatric diagnosis—for example, with symptoms of schizophrenia. Items to which the greatest percentage of "normals" gave answers that differed from those more typically given by patients came to constitute each clinical scale.

In addition to the nine clinical scales and many specially developed scales, there are four so-called control scales on the inventory. One of these is simply the number of items placed by the subject in the "cannot say" category. The L (or lie) scale was devised to measure the tendency of the test taker to attribute socially desirable attributes to himself. In response to "I get angry sometimes" he should tend to mark false; extreme L scorers in the other direction appear to be too good, too virtuous. Another so-called F scale was included to provide a reflection of the subjects' carelessness and confusion in taking the inventory (e.g., "Everything tastes the same" tends to be answered true by careless or confused people). More subtle than either the L or F scales is what is called the K scale. Its construction was based on the observation that some persons tend to exaggerate their symptoms because of excessive openness and frankness and may obtain high scores on the clinical scales; others may exhibit unusually low scores because of defensiveness. On the K-scale item "I think nearly anyone would tell a lie to keep out of trouble," the defensive person is apt to answer false, giving the same response to "I certainly feel useless at times." The K scale was designed to reduce these biasing factors; by weighting clinical-scale scores with K scores, the distorting effect of test-taking defensiveness may be reduced. Types of control scales

In general, it has been found that the greater the number and magnitude of one's unusually high scores on the MMPI, the more likely it is that one is in need of psychiatric attention. Most professionals who use the device refuse to make assumptions about the factualness of the subject's answers and about his personal interpretations of the meanings of the items. Their approach does not depend heavily on theoretical predilections and hypotheses. For this reason the inventory has proved particularly popular with those who have strong doubts about the eventual validity that many theoretical formulations will show in connection with personality measurement after they have been tested through painstaking research. The MMPI also appeals to those who demand firm experimental evidence that any personality assessment method can make valid discriminations among individuals.

In recent years there has been growing interest in actuarial personality description—that is, in personality description based on traits shared in common by groups of people. Actuarial description studies yield rules by which persons may be classified according to their personal attributes as revealed by their behaviour (on tests, for example). Computer programs are now available for diagnosing such disorders as hysteria, schizophrenia, and paranoia on the basis of typical group profiles of MMPI responses. Computerized methods for integrating large amounts of personal data are not limited to this inventory and are applicable to other inventories, personality tests (*e.g.,* inkblots), and life-history information. Computerized classification of MMPI profiles, however, has been explored most intensively.

The MMPI has been considered in some detail here because of its wide usage and because it illustrates a number of important problems confronting those who attempt to assess personality characteristics. Many other omnibus personality inventories are also used in applied settings and in research. The California Psychological Inventory (CPI), for example, is keyed for several personality variables that include sociability, self-control, flexibility, and tolerance. Unlike the MMPI, it was developed specifically for use with "normal" groups of people. Whereas the judgments of experts (usually psychiatric workers) were used in categorizing subjects given the MMPI during the early item-writing phase of its development, nominations by peers (such as respondents or friends) of the subjects were relied upon in work with the CPI. Its technical development has been evaluated by test authorities to be of high order, in part because its developers profited from lessons learned in the construction and use of the MMPI. It also provides measures of response sets and has been subjected to considerable research study.

The California Psychological Inventory (margin note)

From time to time, most personality inventories are revised for a variety of reasons, including the need to take account of cultural and social changes and to improve them. For example, a revision of the CPI was published in 1987; the inventory itself was modified to improve clarity, update content, and delete items that might be objectionable to some respondents. Because the item pool remained largely unchanged, data from the original samples were used in computing norms and in evaluating reliability and validity for new scales and new composite scores. The descriptions of high and low scorers on each scale have been refined and sharpened, and correlations of scale scores with other personality tests have been reported.

Other self-report techniques. Beyond personality inventories, there are other self-report approaches to personality measurement available for research and applied purposes. Mention was made earlier of the use of rating scales. The rating-scale technique permits quantification of an individual's reactions to himself, to others, and, in fact, to any object or concept in terms of a standard set of semantic (word) polarities such as "hot-cold" or "good-bad." It is a general method for assessing the meanings of these semantic concepts to individuals.

Another method of self-report called the Q-sort is devised for problems similar to those for which rating scales are used. In a Q-sort a person is given a set of sentences, phrases, or words (usually presented individually on cards) and is asked to use them to describe himself (as he thinks he is or as he would like to be) or someone else. This description is carried out by having the subject sort the items on the cards in terms of their degree of relevance so that they can be distributed along what amounts to a rating scale. Descriptive items that might be included are "worries a lot," "works hard," and "is cheerful."

Typical paper-and-pencil instruments such as personality inventories involve verbal stimuli (words) intended to call forth designated types of responses from the individual. There are clearly stated ground rules under which he makes his responses. Paper-and-pencil devices are relatively easy and economical to administer and can be scored accurately and reliably by relatively inexperienced clerical workers. They are generally regarded by professional personality evaluators as especially valuable assessment tools in screening large numbers of people, as in military or industrial personnel selection. Assessment specialists do not assume that self-reports are accurate indicators of personality traits. They are accepted, rather, as samples of behaviour for which validity in predicting one's everyday activities or traits must be established empirically (*i.e.,* by direct observation or experiment). Paper-and-pencil techniques have moved from their early stage of assumed (face) validity to more advanced notions in which improvements in conceptualization and methodology are clearly recognized as basic to the determination of empirical validity.

Evaluation of self-reports (margin note)

Projective techniques. One group of assessment specialists believes that the more freedom people have in picking their responses, the more meaningful the description and classification that can be obtained. Because personality inventories do not permit much freedom of choice, some researchers and clinicians prefer to use projective techniques, in which a person is shown ambiguous stimuli (such as shapes or pictures) and asked to interpret them in some way. (Such stimuli allow relative freedom in projecting one's own interests and feelings into them, reacting in any way that seems appropriate.) Projective techniques are believed to be sensitive to unconscious dimensions of personality. Defense mechanisms, latent impulses, and anxieties have all been inferred from data gathered in projective situations.

Personality inventories and projective techniques do have some elements in common; inkblots, for example, are ambiguous, but so also are many of the statements on inventories such as the MMPI. These techniques differ in that the subject is given substantially free rein in responding to projective stimuli rather than merely answering true or false, for example. Another similarity between projective and questionnaire or inventory approaches is that all involve the use of relatively standardized testing situations.

While projective techniques are often lumped together as one general methodology, in actual practice there are several approaches to assessment from a projective point of view. Although projective techniques share the common characteristic that they permit the subject wide latitude in responding, they still may be distinguished broadly as follows: (1) associative techniques, in which the subject is asked to react to words, to inkblots, or to other stimuli with the first associated thoughts that come to mind; (2) construction techniques, in which the subject is asked to create something—for example, make up a story or draw a self-portrait; (3) completion techniques, in which the subject is asked to finish a partially developed stimulus, such as adding the last words to an incomplete sentence; (4) choice or ordering techniques, in which the subject is asked to choose from among or to give some orderly sequence to stimuli—for example, to choose from or arrange a set of pictures or inkblots; (5) expressive techniques, in which the subject is asked to use free expression in some manner, such as in finger painting.

Hidden personality defense mechanisms, latent emotional impulses, and inner anxieties all have been attributed to test takers by making theoretical inferences from data gathered as they responded in projective situations. While projective stimuli are ambiguous, they are usually administered under fairly standardized conditions. Quantitative (numerical) measures can be derived from subjects' responses to them. These include the number of responses one makes to a series of inkblots and the number of responses to the blots in which the subject perceives what seem to him to be moving animals.

Inkblot techniques (margin note)

The Rorschach Inkblot Test. The Rorschach inkblots were developed by a Swiss psychiatrist, Hermann Rorschach, in an effort to reduce the time required in psychiatric diagnosis. His test consists of 10 cards, half of which are in colour and half in black and white. The test is administered by showing the subject the 10 blots one at a time; the subject's task is to describe what he sees in the blots or what they remind him of. The subject is usually told that the inkblots are not a test of the kind he took in school and that there are no right or wrong answers.

Rorschach's work was stimulated by his interest in the relationship between perception and personality. He held that a person's perceptual responses to inkblots could serve as clues to basic personality tendencies. Despite Rorschach's original claims for the validity of his test, subsequent negative research findings have led many users of projective techniques to become dubious about the role assigned the inkblots in delineating relationships between perception and personality. In recent years, emphasis has tended to shift to the analysis of nuances of the subject's social behaviour during the test and to the content of his verbal responses to the examiner—whether, for example, he seeks to obtain the assistance of the examiner in "solving" the inkblots presented to him, sees "angry lions" or "meek lambs" in the inkblots, or is apologetic or combative about his responses.

Over the years, considerable research has been carried out on Rorschach's inkblots; important statistical problems in analyzing data gathered with projective techniques have been identified, and researchers have continued in their largely unsuccessful efforts to overcome them. There is a vast experimental literature to suggest that the Rorschach technique lacks empirical validity. Recently, researchers have sought to put the Rorschach on a sounder psychometric (mental testing) basis. New comprehensive scoring systems have been developed, and there have been improvements in standardization and norms. These developments have injected new life into the Rorschach as a psychometric instrument.

The Holtzman Inkblot Test

A similar method, the Holtzman Inkblot Test, has been developed in an effort to eliminate some of the statistical problems that beset the Rorschach test. It involves the administration of a series of 45 inkblots, the subject being permitted to make only one response per card. The Holtzman has the desirable feature that it provides an alternate series of 45 additional cards for use in retesting.

Research with the Rorschach and Holtzman has proceeded in a number of directions; many studies have compared psychiatric patients and other groups of special interest (delinquents, underachieving students) with ostensibly normal people. Some investigators have sought to derive indexes or predictions of future behaviour from responses to inkblots and have checked, for example, to see if anxiety and hostility (as inferred from content analyses of verbal responses) are related to favourable or unfavourable response to psychotherapy. A sizable area of exploration concerns the effects of special conditions (e.g., experimentally induced anxiety or hostility) on the inkblot perceptions reported by the subject and the content of his speech.

Thematic Apperception Test (TAT). There are other personality assessment devices, which, like the Rorschach, are based on the idea that an individual will project something of himself into his description of an ambiguous stimulus. The TAT, for example, presents the subject with pictures of persons engaged in a variety of activities (e.g., someone with a violin). While the pictures leave much to one's imagination, they are more highly specific, organized visual stimuli than are inkblots. The test consists of 30 black and white pictures and one blank card (to test imagination under very limited stimulation). The cards are presented to the subject one at a time, and he is asked to make up a story that describes each picture and that indicates the events that led to the scene and the events that will grow out of it. He is also asked to describe the thoughts and feelings of the persons in his story.

Although some content-analysis scoring systems have been developed for the TAT, attempts to score it in a standardized quantitative fashion tend to be limited to research and have been fewer than has been the case for the Rorschach. This is especially the state of affairs in applied settings in which the test is often used as a basis for conducting a kind of clinical interview; the pictures are used to elicit a sample of verbal behaviour on the basis of which inferences are drawn by the clinician.

In one popular approach, interpretation of a TAT story usually begins with an effort to determine who is the hero (i.e., to identify the character with whom the subject seems to have identified himself). The content of the stories is often analyzed in terms of a so-called need-press system. Needs are defined as the internal motivations of the hero. Press refers to environmental forces that may facilitate or interfere with the satisfaction of needs (e.g., in the story the hero may be physically attacked, frustrated by poverty, or suffer the effects of rumours being spread about him). In assessing the importance or strength of a particular inferred need or press for the individual who takes the test, special attention is given to signs of its pervasiveness and consistency in different stories. Analysis of the test may depend considerably on the subjective, personal characteristics of the evaluator, who usually make to interpret the subjects' behaviour in the testing situation; the characteristics of his utterances; the emotional tone of

the stories; the kinds of fantasies he offers; the outcomes of the stories; and the conscious and unconscious needs speculatively inferred from the stories.

Word stimulus responses

Word-association techniques. The list of projective approaches to personality assessment is long, one of the most venerable being the so-called word-association test. Jung used associations to groups of related words as a basis for inferring personality traits (e.g., the inferiority "complex"). Administering a word-association test is relatively uncomplicated; a list of words is presented one at a time to the subject who is asked to respond with the first word or idea that comes to mind. Many of the stimulus words may appear to be emotionally neutral (e.g., building, first, tree); of special interest are words that tend to elicit personalized reactions (e.g., mother, hit, love). The amount of time the subject takes before beginning each response and the response itself are used in efforts to analyze a word association test. The idiosyncratic, or unusual, nature of one's word-association responses may be gauged by comparing them to standard published tables of the specific associations given by large groups of other people.

Sentence-completion techniques. The sentence-completion technique may be considered a logical extension of word-association methods. In administering a sentence-completion test, the evaluator presents the subject with a series of partial sentences that he is asked to finish in his own words (e.g., "I feel upset when . . . "; "What burns me up is . . . "). Users of sentence-completion methods in assessing personality typically analyze them in terms of what they judge to be recurring attitudes, conflicts, and motives reflected in them. Such analyses, like those of TAT, contain a subjective element.

Behavioral assessment. Objective observation of a subject's behaviour is a technique that falls in the category of behavioral assessment. A variety of assessments could be considered, for example, in the case of a seven-year-old boy who, according to his teacher, is doing poorly in his schoolwork and, according to his parents, is difficult to manage at home and does not get along with other children. The following types of assessment might be considered: (1) a measure of the boy's general intelligence, which might help explain his poor schoolwork; (2) an interview with him to provide insights into his view of his problem; (3) personality tests, which might reveal trends that are related to his inadequate social relationships; (4) observations of his activities and response patterns in school; (5) observations of his behaviour in a specially created situation, such as a playroom with many interesting toys and games; (6) an interview with his parents, since the boy's poor behaviour in school may by symptomatic of problems at home; and (7) direct observation of his behaviour at home.

Types of assessment

Making all of these assessments would be a major undertaking. Because of the variety of data that are potentially available, the assessor must decide which types of information are most feasible and desirable under a given set of circumstances. In most cases, the clinician is interested in both subjective and objective information. Subjective information includes what clients think about, the emotions they experience, and their worries and preoccupations. Interviews, personality inventories, and projective techniques provide indications of subjective experience, although considerable clinical judgment is needed to infer what is going on within the client from test responses. Objective information includes the person's observable behaviour and usually does not require the assessor to draw complex inferences about such topics as attitudes toward parents, unconscious wishes, and deep-seated conflicts. Such information is measured by behavioral assessment. It is often used to identify behavioral problems, which are then treated in some appropriate way. Behavioral observations are used to get information that cannot be obtained by other means. Examples include the frequency of a particular type of response, such as physical attacks on others or observations by ward attendants of certain behaviours of psychiatric patients. In either case, observational data must meet the same standards of reliability as data obtained by more formal measures.

The value of behavioral assessment depends on the behaviours selected for observation. For example, if the goal of assessment is to detect a tendency toward depression, the responses recorded should be those that are relevant to that tendency, such as degrees of smiling, motor activity, and talking.

Baseline observations

A type of behavioral assessment called baseline observations is becoming increasingly popular. These are recordings of response frequencies in particular situations before any treatment or intervention has been made. They can be used in several ways. Observations might be made simply to describe a person's response repertoire at a given time. For example, the number of aggressive responses made by children of different ages might be recorded. Such observations also provide a baseline for judging the effectiveness of behaviour modification techniques. A similar set of observations, made after behaviour modification procedures have been used, could be compared with the baseline measurement as a way of determining how well the therapy worked.

Behavioral observations can be treated in different ways. One of these is to keep track of the frequency with which people make designated responses during a given period of time (*e.g.,* the number of times a psychiatric patient makes his own bed or the number of times a child asks for help in a novel situation). Another approach involves asking raters to support their judgments of others by citing specific behaviour (critical incidents); a shop foreman, for example, may rate a worker as depressed by citing incidents when the worker burst into tears. Critical incidents not only add validity to ordinary ratings, but they also suggest behavioral details that might be promising predictors of success on the job, response to psychiatric treatment, or level of academic achievement.

Behavioral observations are widely made in interviews and in a variety of workaday settings. Employers, supervisors, and teachers—either formally or informally—make use of behavioral observations in making decisions about people for whom they have responsibility. Unfortunately the subject may know he is being studied or evaluated and, therefore, may behave atypically (*e.g.,* by working harder than usual or by growing tense). The observer may be a source of error by being biased in favour of or against the subject. Disinterested observers clearly are to be preferred (other things being equal) for research and clinical purposes. The greater the care taken to control such contributions to error, the greater the likelihood that observations will prove to be reliable.

Cognitive assessment. The types of thoughts experienced by individuals are reflective of their personalities. Just as it is important to know what people do and how their behaviour affects others, it is also necessary to assess the thoughts that may lie behind the behaviour. Cognitive assessment provides information about thoughts that precede, accompany, and follow maladaptive behaviour. It also provides information about the effects of procedures that are intended to modify both how subjects think about a problem and how they behave.

Cognitive assessment can be carried out in a variety of ways. For example, questionnaires have been developed to sample people's thoughts after an upsetting event. Beepers (electronic pagers) have been used to signal subjects to record their thoughts at certain times of the day. There are also questionnaires to assess the directions people give themselves while working on a task and their theories about why things happen as they do.

Methods of recording people's thoughts

The assessment of thoughts and ideas is a relatively new development. It has received impetus from the growing evidence that thought processes and the content of thoughts are related to emotions and behaviour. Cognitive assessment provides information about adaptive and maladaptive aspects of people's thoughts and the role their thoughts play in the processes of planning, making decisions, and interpreting reality.

Bodily assessment. Bodily responses may reveal a person's feelings and motivations, and clinicians pay particular attention to these nonverbal messages. Bodily functions may also reflect motivations and concerns, and some clinicians also pay attention to these. Sophisticated devices have been developed to measure such physiological changes as pupil dilation, blood pressure, and electrical skin responses under specific conditions. These changes are related to periodic ratings of mood and to other physiological states that provide measures of stability and change within the individual. Technological advances are making it possible to monitor an individual's physiological state on a continuous basis. Sweat, heartbeat, blood volume, substances in the bloodstream, and blood pressure can all be recorded and correlated with the presence or absence of certain psychological conditions such as stress.

Personal facts. One type of information that is sometimes overlooked because of its very simplicity consists of the subject's life history and present status. Much of this information may be gathered through direct interviews with a subject or with an informant through questionnaires and through searches of records and archives. The information might also be gathered by examining the subject's personal documents (*e.g.,* letters, autobiographies) and medical, educational, or psychiatric case histories. The information might concern the individual's social and occupational history, his cultural background, his present economic status, and his past and present physical characteristics. Life-history data can provide clues to the precursors and correlates of present behaviour. This information may help the investigator avoid needlessly speculative or complex hypotheses about the causation of personality traits when simple explanations might be superior. Failure on the part of a personality evaluator to be aware of the fact that someone had spent two years during World War II in a concentration camp could result in misleading inferences and conjectures about the subject's present behaviour.

Techniques for gathering personal information

RELIABILITY AND VALIDITY OF ASSESSMENT METHODS

Assessment, whether it is carried out with interviews, behavioral observations, physiological measures, or tests, is intended to permit the evaluator to make meaningful, valid, and reliable statements about individuals. What makes John Doe tick? What makes Mary Doe the unique individual that she is? Whether these questions can be answered depends upon the reliability and validity of the assessment methods used. The fact that a test is intended to measure a particular attribute is in no way a guarantee that it really accomplishes this goal. Assessment techniques must themselves be assessed.

Evaluation techniques. Personality instruments measure samples of behaviour. Their evaluation involves primarily the determination of reliability and validity. Reliability often refers to consistency of scores obtained by the same persons when retested. Validity provides a check on how well the test fulfills its function. The determination of validity usually requires independent, external criteria of whatever the test is designed to measure. An objective of research in personality measurement is to delineate the conditions under which the methods do or do not make trustworthy descriptive and predictive contributions. One approach to this problem is to compare groups of people known through careful observation to differ in a particular way. It is helpful to consider, for example, whether the MMPI or TAT discriminates significantly between those who show progress in psychotherapy and those who do not, whether they distinguish between law violators of record and apparent nonviolators. Experimental investigations that systematically vary the conditions under which subjects perform also make contributions.

Although much progress has been made in efforts to measure personality, all available instruments and methods have defects and limitations that must be borne in mind when using them; responses to tests or interview questions, for example, often are easily controlled or manipulated by the subject and thus are readily "fakeable." Some tests, while useful as group screening devices, exhibit only limited predictive value in individual cases, yielding frequent (sometimes tragic) errors. These caveats are especially poignant when significant decisions about people are made on the basis of their personality measures. Institutionalization or discharge, and hiring or firing, are weighty personal matters and can wreak great injustice when based on faulty assessment. In addition, many personality assessment techniques require the probing of private areas

Limitations in personality measurement methods

of the individual's thought and action. Those who seek to measure personality for descriptive and predictive reasons must concern themselves with the ethical and legal implications of their work.

A major methodological stumbling block in the way of establishing the validity of any method of personality measurement is that there always is an element of subjective judgment in selecting or formulating criteria against which measures may be validated. This is not so serious a problem when popular, socially valued, fairly obvious criteria are available that permit ready comparisons between such groups as convicted criminals and ostensible noncriminals, or psychiatric hospital patients and noninstitutionalized individuals. Many personality characteristics, however, cannot be validated in such directly observable ways (*e.g.,* inner, private experiences such as anxiety or depression). When such straightforward empirical validation of an untested measure hopefully designed to measure any personality attribute is not possible, efforts at establishing a less impressive kind of validity (so-called construct validity) may be pursued. A construct is a theoretical statement concerning some underlying, unobservable aspect of an individual's characteristics or of his internal state. ("Intelligence," for example, is a construct; one cannot hold "it" in one's hand, or weigh "it," or put "it" in a bag, or even look at "it.") Constructs thus refer to private events inferred or imagined to contribute to the shaping of specific public events (observed behaviour). The explanatory value of any construct has been considered by some theorists to represent its validity. Construct validity, therefore, refers to evidence that endorses the usefulness of a theoretical conception of personality. A test designed to measure an unobservable construct (such as "intelligence" or "need to achieve") is said to accrue construct validity if it usefully predicts the kinds of empirical criteria one would expect it to—*e.g.,* achievement in academic subjects.

Predictiveness of personality measures

The degree to which a measure of personality is empirically related to or predictive of any aspect of behaviour observed independently of that measure contributes to its validity in general. A most desirable step in establishing the usefulness of a measure is called cross-validation. The mere fact that one research study yields positive evidence of validity is no guarantee that the measure will work as well the next time; indeed, often it does not. It is thus important to conduct additional, cross-validation studies to establish the stability of the results obtained in the first investigation. Failure to cross-validate is viewed by most testing authorities as a serious omission in the validation process. Evidence for the validity of a full test should not be sought from the same sample of people that was used for the initial selection of individual test items. Clearly this will tend to exaggerate the effect of traits that are unique to that particular sample of people and can lead to spuriously high (unrealistic) estimates of validity that will not be borne out when other people are studied. Cross-validation studies permit assessment of the amount of "shrinkage" in empirical effectiveness when a new sample of subjects is employed. When evidence of validity holds up under cross-validation, confidence in the general usefulness of test norms and research findings is enhanced. Establishment of reliability, validity, and cross-validation are major steps in determining the usefulness of any psychological test (including personality measures).

Clinical versus statistical prediction. Another measure of assessment research has to do with the role of the assessor himself as an evaluator and predictor of the behaviour of others. In most applied settings he subjectively (even intuitively) weighs, evaluates, and interprets the various assessment data that are available. How successful he is in carrying out his interpretive task is critical, as is knowledge of the kinds of conditions under which he is effective in processing such diverse data as impressions gathered in an interview, test scores, and life-history data. The typical clinician usually does not use a statistical formula that weighs and combines test scores and other data at his disposal. Rather, he integrates the data using impressions and hunches based on his past clinical experience and on his understanding of psychological theory and research. The result of this interpretive process usually includes some

form of personality description of the person under study and specific predictions or advice for that person.

The degree of success an assessor has when he responds to the diverse information that may be available about a particular person is the subject of research that has been carried out on the issue of clinical versus statistical prediction. It is reasonable to ask whether a clinician will do as good a job in predicting behaviour as does a statistical formula or "cookbook"—*i.e.,* a manual that provides the empirical, statistically predictive aspects of test responses or scores based on the study of large numbers of people.

Evaluating the evaluator

An example would be a book or table of typical intelligence test norms (typical scores) used to predict how well children perform in school. Another book might offer specific personality diagnoses (*e.g.,* neurotic or psychotic) based on scores such as those yielded by the different scales of the MMPI. Many issues must be settled before the deceptively simple question of clinical versus statistical prediction can be answered definitively.

When statistical prediction formulas (well-supported by research) are available for combining clinical information, however, experimental evidence clearly indicates that they will be more valid and less time-consuming than will a clinician (who may be subject to human error in trying to simultaneously consider and weigh all of the factors in a case). The clinician's chief contributions to diagnosis and prediction are in situations for which satisfactory formulas and quantified information are not available. A clinician's work is especially important when evaluations are required for rare and idiosyncratic personality characteristics that have escaped rigorous, systematic empirical study. The greatest confidence results when both statistical and subjective clinical methods simultaneously converge (agree) in the solution of specific clinical problems.

BIBLIOGRAPHY. Definitions of personality as a psychological concept, with treatment of related issues, are found in the following reference works: ROM HARRÉ and ROGER LAMB (eds.), *The Dictionary of Personality and Social Psychology* (1986); RICHARD L. GREGORY (ed.), *The Oxford Companion to the Mind* (1987); RAYMOND J. CORSINI *et al.* (eds.), *Concise Encyclopedia of Psychology* (1987); and JONATHAN L. FREEDMAN, *Introductory Psychology,* 2nd ed. (1982).

Major theories of personality are surveyed in CALVIN S. HALL and GARDNER LINDZEY, *Theories of Personality,* 3rd ed. (1978); and in NATHAN BRODY, *Personality: In Search of Individuality* (1988). ROGER BROWN, *Social Psychology, the Second Edition* (1986); and IRWIN G. SARASON, *Personality: An Objective Approach,* 2nd ed. (1972), review and evaluate contemporary personality studies and research methods. The best presentation of psychoanalytic ideas remains Freud's own, available in many translated selections.

Discussions of the variety of currently held views on personality include JAMES F. MASTERSON, *The Search for the Real Self: Unmasking the Personality Disorders of Our Age* (1988); and ARTHUR PEACOCKE and GRANT GILLETT (eds.), *Persons and Personality: Contemporary Inquiry* (1987). Adaptation of personality in social interaction is explored in JOEL ARONOFF and JOHN P. WILSON, *Personality in the Social Process* (1985); ALAN S. WATERMAN, *The Psychology of Individualism* (1984); ROBERT A. LEVINE, *Culture, Behavior, and Personality: An Introduction to the Comparative Study of Psychosocial Adaptation,* 2nd ed. (1982); NANCY CANTOR and JOHN F. KIHLSTROM, *Personality, Cognition, and Social Interaction* (1981); and NANCY CANTOR and JOHN F. KIHLSTROM (eds.), *Personality and Social Intelligence* (1987). Issues of personality development from childhood through adulthood are interpreted in ROBERT L. LEAHY (ed.), *The Development of the Self* (1985); LAURENCE R. SIMON, *Cognition and Affect: A Developmental Psychology of the Individual* (1986); LAWRENCE S. WRIGHTSMAN, *Personality Development in Adulthood* (1988); and ERIK H. ERIKSON, *Childhood and Society,* new anniversary ed. (1985).

Some general approaches to personality assessment are surveyed in ANNE ANASTASI, *Psychological Testing,* 6th ed. (1988); and LEE J. CRONBACH, *Essentials of Psychological Testing,* 4th ed. (1984). JAMES V. MITCHELL, JR. (ed.), *The Ninth Mental Measurement Yearbook,* 2 vol. (1985), describes numerous psychometric tests, including personality assessment instruments.

PHILIP S. HOLTZMAN. Esther and Sidney R. Rabb Professor of Psychology, Harvard University, Cambridge, Mass. Coauthor of *Assessing Schizophrenic Thinking* and others.
IRWIN G. SARASON. Professor of Psychology, University of Washington, Seattle. Author of *Personality: An Objective Approach.* Coauthor of *Abnormal Psychology.*

WORLD
OF
MEDICINE

Alphabetical review of
recent developments
in health and medicine

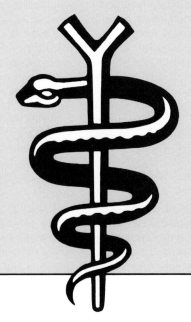

Accidents and Safety

Accidents continue to be the fourth-leading cause of death among Americans and the leading cause of death among those younger than 38 years old. They claimed 94,000 American lives in 1989 and resulted in untold millions of injuries. Nearly 47,000 of those deaths resulted from traffic accidents, and young males continued to be overrepresented in traffic deaths.

Falls, also a major cause of accidental death, accounted for over 12,000 deaths in 1989. More than half of the fatal falls occurred at home, and most of those involved persons 75 years old or older.

Poisonings by solids and liquids claimed more than 5,000 lives in 1989. A majority of the poisoning deaths occurred among adults between the ages of 25 and 44, many as a result of suicide or illicit drug use.

Despite gains made in fire safety since the introduction of laws requiring smoke detectors, home fires claimed more than 3,000 lives in the U.S. in 1989, about 600 of them among children younger than 5 years old and about 1,000 among persons over 65. Fire-safety experts suggest that the old and very young are overrepresented among fire victims because they have a more difficult time escaping when fire breaks out.

An issue currently being debated is that of safety seats for infants and small children on airplanes. Babies under the age of two now fly free if they are held on an adult's lap. In a plane accident—as in a car accident—the child is almost certain to be ripped from the adult's arms. The controversy centers around the question of whether the immense cost involved would be justified by the small number of lives likely to be saved. A U.S. Federal Aviation Administration (FAA) study estimated that requiring these seats would add an average of $185 to a family's cost of flying with an infant, making such travel unaffordable for 20% of families with young children. In addition, over the previous 14 years only two lives would have been saved by mandatory safety seats. Nevertheless, the National Transportation Safety Board (NTSB) has recommended that the FAA require the seats. This is seen as especially controversial because the NTSB has recommended against requiring seat belts on school buses. It may be a year before the FAA reaches a decision.

Other issues currently receiving special attention—restraint systems in automobiles, a new treatment for spinal cord injuries, accidental poisoning of children, and prevention of skateboarding injuries—are discussed below.

Safety belts and air bags—gaining in usage

There is new hope that the number of traffic deaths in the U.S. will be reduced. With model year 1990 began the equipping of every new automobile sold in the U.S. with either a driver's-side air bag or "passive" restraints—belts that automatically wrap themselves

Civil Aeromedical Institute, FAA

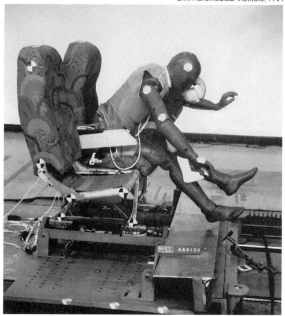

Dummies in an airplane crash test demonstrate the potential for injury to a small child held on an adult's lap. A proposed rule would require infant safety seats, but the costs—and cost effectiveness—of such a measure are still under debate.

around the driver and front-seat passenger. This came about largely because of a decision handed down in 1984 by the U.S. Department of Transportation (DOT) to settle a decades-long debate on how to protect drivers and passengers from traffic accidents.

The safety belt first appeared in U.S.-made automobiles more than 30 years ago. One problem with the belts became apparent almost as soon as they were introduced—most drivers and passengers refused to wear them. Consumers commonly complained that the belts wrinkled their clothes, were uncomfortable, or were simply too difficult and time-consuming to snap on and adjust.

Over the years automakers worked to make safety restraints easier to use and more comfortable. Buckles were moved to the side to avoid digging into a driver's body, and belts were made to adjust automatically to each person's size. Many were designed so they would lock into position only on impact, eliminating the need for the belt to be tight at all times.

Studies of traffic accidents, meanwhile, confirmed that safety belts were indeed effective. The belts helped prevent the "secondary collision"—which occurs when the car stops moving but passengers are carried forward by their own momentum and slam into the car's interior—that is responsible for a large share of traffic-accident injuries. Researchers in traffic safety have concluded that three-point (lap-and-shoulder) belts could prevent nearly half of all traffic fatalities and almost two-thirds of the serious injuries.

Given the combination of those figures, the fact that only about 15% of drivers and passengers wore the belts, and the high cost to society of traffic accidents (estimated at more than $72 billion annually in medical bills, lost wages, property damage, and insurance expenses), government officials finally proposed that drivers and passengers be protected, like it or not. Exactly how to provide that protection became the focus of a 20-year debate that pitted the powerful auto and insurance industries against each other.

The federal government first proposed in 1969 that beginning with the 1974 model year, air bags or passive belts be required on all cars. Through petitions to DOT and court challenges, automobile manufacturers succeeded in delaying this deadline several times; DOT eventually dropped the requirements completely. In 1983, however, the U.S. Supreme Court ordered a review of the issue, and the battle lines were drawn again.

Automakers were afraid the high cost of air bags would depress sales of new cars. The air bags would add at least $500 to the price of each car, they insisted, and would cost as much as $1,500 to reinstall after being deployed. The automakers were justified in believing that consumers did not want to pay the price. General Motors had offered air bags on some cars during model years 1974 through 1976. Even at a below-cost price of $300, consumers bought only 10,000 of a planned production of 300,000.

Automakers also pointed out, correctly, that air bags are not as effective as the three-point belts they were already installing in all cars. Air bags are deployed only in frontal and near-frontal crashes of more than 40 km/h (25 mph) into another car or 19 km/h (12 mph) into a fixed object. They would not be deployed (or useful) in side, rollover, or rear-end collisions and

would therefore prevent only about a third of traffic fatalities, as opposed to nearly half that could be prevented by belts. Worse yet, the automakers pointed out, air bags could discourage belt use by providing drivers with a false sense of security.

While passive belts would be cheaper (at a cost of about $50 per car to manufacturers), automakers pointed out that consumers—thinking that the belts would not be detachable in case of fire or water-immersion emergencies—might not use them. They offered as evidence their experience with interlocks, which prevented a car from starting unless passengers were buckled up. Many drivers simply buckled the belts behind their backs or paid to have the system overridden. Even if consumers used passive restraints, the benefits would be slow in coming; it would take more than 10 years for new cars equipped with passive restraints to replace cars then in use.

Auto companies argued that if DOT wanted drivers and passengers to be restrained, it should use the approach already taken in most other industrial countries: simply pass laws requiring drivers and passengers to use the restraints already provided. This, the automakers insisted, would provide protection immediately. New York state passed such a law in 1984, and 26 states currently require front-seat drivers and passengers to buckle up. All states require that young children ride in child safety seats.

Insurance companies and some safety advocates argued that belt laws alone would not be effective because compliance rates varied widely and were as low as 20% in some areas; only passive restraints would protect the majority of drivers and passengers. Insurance companies further argued that air bags would save more lives than three-point restraints, which, though more effective in theory, often in practice are

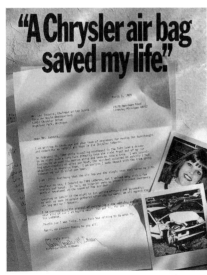

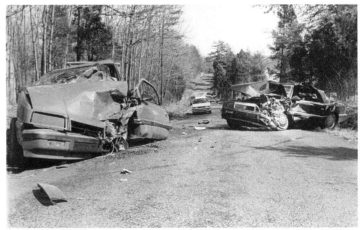

Drivers of the air-bag-equipped automobiles below walked away virtually uninjured from what could have been a fatal head-on collision. Recognizing that safety is now a prime concern of consumers, several U.S. automakers are promoting safety features as part of their marketing strategies.

(Left) Chrysler Corporation; (right) Mike Hensdill/Culpeper Star-Exponent

not worn. Nevertheless, according to one study, despite polls in which nearly half of the respondents said they would unbuckle their passive restraints, close to 90% of drivers actually wear them.

After weighing all these arguments, U.S. Secretary of Transportation Elizabeth Dole ruled in 1984 that passive restraints had to be phased in: 10% of all cars built in model year 1987 would have to be equipped with passive restraints or air bags. The figure would rise to 25% for model year 1988, 40% for model year 1989, and 100% for model year 1990. However, the requirements would be rescinded if states representing two-thirds of the nation's population passed belt-use laws by Sept. 1, 1989.

The requirements stayed in place, and automakers have since produced four types of passive protection. In one, a motorized shoulder belt rides a track along the driver's or passenger's door, wrapping across the person's body from the door-side shoulder to the opposite hip once the door has been closed. The lap belt is separate and must be buckled manually. These belts are standard on many new Toyotas, Fords, and Chryslers. A second system also uses a two-point shoulder belt, which is attached to the door and swings into place when the door is closed. This system is standard on many new Chryslers, Peugeots, and Volkswagens. A third system uses a three-point belt connected at two points on the door and at another point near the passenger's hip. The belts swing into place when the door is closed. These systems are standard on many new Hondas and General Motors cars.

The fourth system is the air bag. In a higher-speed crash an electronic sensor detects the impact in less than $3/100$ of a second. By $6/100$ of a second an explosive reaction has filled the air bag. The bag is fully inflated for about $1/10$ of a second—just when the passenger would have moved forward into it—and prevents him or her from striking the car's interior. In some cars the same sensor also causes the safety belts to tighten and lock. The air bag then deflates in about another $1/10$ of a second, so that the driver can see.

Though air bags are still expensive, their price could drop to about $300 in the next few years with mass production. Turning necessity into a virtue, some manufacturers have begun using them as a selling point. Chrysler announced that from model year 1990 driver's-side air bags would be standard equipment on all cars. Ford followed suit; about 40% of its 1990 cars had driver's-side air bags, and its goal was to have driver's- and passenger-side air bags as standard equipment by the mid-'90s. General Motors equipped about 15% of its 1990 cars with air bags for drivers but intends to install them in all its models by 1995 and increasingly to add air bags for passengers. Threatening these plans was the possibility of a shortage of critical components. A series of flash fires

at equipment factories occurred during the past year when the chemical used as the air bag inflater ignited during the manufacturing process, and some factories had to halt production. Since reengineering a car designed for air bags so that it could use passive safety belts would take months and cost millions of dollars, suppliers were investigating alternative propellants.

It is not only the automakers who are responding to the DOT requirements. Surveys indicate that Americans have become generally more health- and safety-conscious; many consumers have become particularly concerned about automobile safety and are, in fact, looking for safety features instead of avoiding them. A 1987 poll showed that 92% of Americans believe safety belts save lives, and 70% favor belt-use laws. The same poll showed that 75% of those surveyed claim they always or nearly always buckle up; the observed rate of belt use has in fact risen to nearly half of all drivers.

Sensing the trend, automakers are actively promoting the safety features of their cars. Volvo spends fully half of its advertising budget on safety-oriented ads. If these ads are successful, and if consumers continue to rate safety as an important factor when buying cars, the long and often bitter debate about how to force drivers to use seat belts could fade into insignificance. The vast majority of drivers may well decide on their own initiative to buckle up.

New treatment for spinal cord injuries

Perhaps the most tragic of nonfatal accidents are spinal cord injuries that leave victims paralyzed. Each year nearly 10,000 Americans suffer acute spinal cord injuries that lead to some degree of paralysis. A recent breakthrough in drug therapy offers doctors and victims new hope for treating these injuries effectively.

In March 1990 scientists at the National Institutes of Health (NIH) announced that high doses of the steroid drug methylprednisolone can, if administered quickly, reduce neurological damage caused in a spinal cord injury. Researchers emphasized that the drug does not cure spinal cord damage but can limit the subsequent paralysis; even minor improvements can make a great deal of difference to the victim. Persons whose injuries might have left them in a wheelchair could, with the drug therapy, be able to walk with crutches. Those who might have otherwise been completely paralyzed might maintain the use of their hands.

To be most effective, the drug must be administered in high doses within eight hours of the injury. Doctors estimate that about 95% of spinal-injury victims are treated in a hospital within that time limit; the drug would therefore be beneficial in a majority of cases.

The drug appears to work by reducing swelling in injured spinal tissue, thereby preventing cell degeneration. Tissue degeneration occurs over several hours after an injury; thus, the earlier the drug is admin-

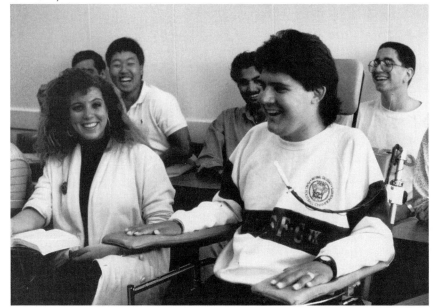

Rendered quadriplegic as a result of a 1985 football injury, Marc Buoniconti is now a student at the University of Miami, Florida. He is also one of 200 patients participating in the Miami Project, a pioneering research effort seeking a "cure" for paralysis. A recent development in critical care treatment of spinal cord injury may offer more immediate hope for those newly injured; researchers reported in 1990 that steroid treatment, if given within eight hours of an injury, can reduce that injury's severity and may lessen the individual's disability.

istered, the more likely it will be beneficial. For this reason doctors are considering training paramedics to administer the drug at the scene of an accident.

Because the results of the research were so dramatic, the NIH broke with its usual policy and issued a special alert to make physicians aware of the drug's potential before the study was published in a medical journal.

Accidental poisoning—easily prevented

Deaths from accidental poisoning increased in 1989, and many of the deaths were among the young age groups. Nevertheless, during the past three decades, most of the news on accidental poisonings involving children has been good. The number of children who die by accidental poisoning has dropped from 450 in 1961 to several dozen per year at present. Many factors have figured in the reduction. Federal labeling requirements have made more parents aware of the products that are poisonous; child-resistant caps have made it much more difficult for children to open containers of dangerous products; and poison-control centers have given parents a way to get correct first-aid information quickly in a poisoning emergency. In recent years manufacturers and government officials have been exploring the use of bittering agents, which are colorless and odorless but make liquids taste so bitter that children are more likely to spit them out than swallow them.

Still, tens of thousands of children each year are involved in nonfatal poisonings, which can be harmful and frightening, as well as injurious. The best efforts of manufacturers and safety advocates cannot overcome parental failure to observe poison-prevention suggestions.

Children are natural explorers, and much of what they find they immediately put in their mouths. By the time they are crawling, some children are capable of opening unprotected cabinets. Parents should either lock up cabinets (a variety of inexpensive, easily installed locking systems are available) or remove toxic products completely from lower shelves and cabinets. One of the most popular storage areas for cleaners—under the sink—is also one of the first places children like to explore, if only to imitate their parents.

When children begin walking, parents need to remove all toxic products, such as medicines, perfumes, nail polish, and alcohol, from drawers and nightstands. Even child-resistant caps are not foolproof; some precocious children can open these containers, and parents should not leave them where children can get at them.

Many older people who suffer from arthritis or diminished hand strength specifically request medications without child-resistant caps. When parents take their children to visit elderly relatives or friends, they should be aware of what medications are in the house and where they are stored. Any within reach should be moved to a safe location.

When children need to take a medication, parents should avoid the temptation to refer to it as candy or a goodie to induce them to swallow it. This may only tempt them to go looking for more "candy" later.

Many poisonings result from simple confusion about the contents of a makeshift container. For this reason parents should keep all household products in their original containers, complete with warnings and directions for proper use. Too often, parents put toxic cleaners into a glass or soda bottle for a small cleaning job, turn their backs for a moment, and return to find

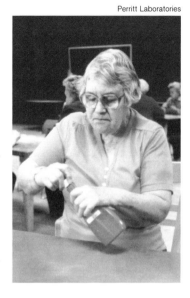

So-called child-resistant caps meant to prevent youngsters from consuming dangerous substances may be virtually impossible for many adults to open, especially if they have arthritis. When an adult fails to replace the cap properly—or cannot replace it at all— young children in the household are still at risk of poisoning.

that a child has taken a drink. Similarly, paints, paint thinners, or other toxins should not be placed, even temporarily, in a glass or coffee cup.

When a parent suspects that a child may have been poisoned, the first step is to call the local poison-control center. (Parents should have the number next to or on the phone at all times.) In areas where there is no poison-control center, parents should call the local hospital or dial 911.

Tips for skateboarding safety

After enjoying brief popularity in the 1960s, skateboards reappeared in the late 1980s to stay. As the number of skateboards sold rose dramatically, so did the number of injuries suffered by those riding them. In 1983 the Consumer Product Safety Commission reported 16,000 injuries associated with skateboards; by 1986 that figure had risen to over 80,000. About 75% of these injuries are to the arms and legs. Many are wrist sprains and fractures suffered when riders stick out their hands to break a fall. Of particular concern to safety advocates are head and neck injuries, which account for 17% of the injuries.

Not surprisingly, the majority of those suffering these injuries are young males, the group among which skateboarding is most popular. For many, skateboarding is a serious endeavor, involving hours of practice on increasingly difficult daredevil stunts. Falls are part of the process of learning.

While safety experts concede that falls from skateboards and the resulting injuries cannot be eliminated, they do suggest ways to reduce the risks. The first is to buy a good-quality skateboard—sturdy, well balanced, and designed for the weight of the intended rider. Riders should also immediately purchase protective equipment, such as a well-fitting bicycle helmet, knee pads, elbow pads, wrist guards, and ankle

guards. The cost of this gear can exceed $200 easily, but injuries can cost considerably more.

Skateboarding enthusiasts suggest that those just taking up the sport learn with an experienced partner. A partner can hold onto a novice as he or she first rides the skateboard and gets a sense of how to balance on it. An experienced rider can also show a novice how to turn the board safely by shifting body weight and how to jump off without falling or twisting an ankle.

Those who participate in the sport also need to be choosy about where they ride; about half of all falls are caused by rough and irregular surfaces that jolt the skateboard. Riders should look for smooth riding surfaces away from traffic and pedestrians.

—Tom D. Naughton

Aging

The health care of older persons continues to reflect research and clinical advances in a variety of areas. For example, the impact of vision and hearing disturbances on health and function of older persons is becoming more clearly identified. The substantial psychological effects of care giving for persons with Alzheimer's disease upon the care giver are becoming recognized. Ethical issues, such as whether to resuscitate terminally ill persons, particularly those living in nursing homes, and whether the withdrawal of feeding is ever appropriate, have been examined by both health researchers and public officials.

In this update, four common syndromes (Parkinsonism, urinary incontinence, falls, and dementia) are focused upon because recent research has resulted in changes in the clinical care of older persons who are afflicted with them. In addition, a major economic issue currently causing considerable turmoil in the United States—the financing of long-term care— is addressed.

Parkinson's disease: advances in drug treatment

Parkinson's disease is the most common of several progressively disabling illnesses causing neurological decline; it is characterized by decreases in normal movements, rigidity, and tremor. The incidence is estimated to be about one person in 1,000 in the over-50 population; in 75% of cases onset occurs between ages 50 and 65.

Parkinson's disease often begins as general slowing of all voluntary motions and may progress to loss of facial expressions (masklike facies), loss of normal motions such as arm swinging while walking, and a short, shuffling gait. At the late stages of the disease, some victims may appear "frozen" in their own bodies. In addition to significant neurological dysfunction, personality changes are common in Parkinson's disease, especially depression and dementia. Although the usual cause of Parkinson's disease is unknown,

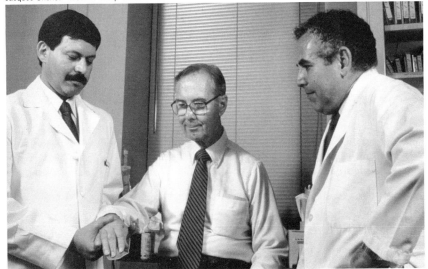

Physicians examine a patient with Parkinson's disease who appears to have benefited from the drug L-deprenyl, an agent from a new class of drugs known as monoamine oxidase B inhibitors. Early trials have shown that the drug delays clinical manifestations of the disease, such as stiffness and palsy, and is well tolerated by the majority of patients taking it.

autopsy studies have shown there is a characteristic loss of neurons (nerve cells) in the part of the brain called the substantia nigra.

It is important to distinguish Parkinson's disease from forms of parkinsonism with other causes. For example, the same symptoms may occur in persons who have had strokes in the substantia nigra (the same area of the brain that is involved in Parkinson's disease). Parkinsonism may also occur after a specific type of encephalitis ("sleeping sickness"), an infectious inflammation of the brain. Although this was an important cause earlier in this century, postencephalic parkinsonism is rare now. Drug-induced parkinsonism may occur with some psychiatric medications that are often used to control behavior in agitated or demented older persons; symptoms are usually reversible when the drug is stopped. Other rare causes of parkinsonism are carbon monoxide poisoning and manganese toxicity.

At some point drug therapy is necessary for most persons with the disease. One survey found that about 75% of patients require drug treatment within two years. Such therapy is based on correcting the neurochemical imbalance that is believed to be the cause of the disorder. The crucial deficit is a lack of dopamine, a neurotransmitter that is produced in the substantia nigra; there is also a relative overabundance of another neurotransmitter, acetylcholine. Therefore, one therapeutic approach attempts to decrease acetylcholine through the use of anticholinergic medications, such as trihexyphenidyl (*e.g.*, Artane, Tremin) and benztropine mesylate (Cogentin). Another approach is to increase dopamine. The latter can be accomplished by a variety of classes of drugs. The antiviral drug amantadine hydrochloride (Symmetrel) enhances the release of dopamine from nerve cells but is usually only temporarily effective.

The most common medication used today is a drug that combines levodopa (L-dopa) and carbidopa; the former is a chemical precursor of dopamine and the latter a chemical that allows efficient entry of L-dopa into the brain by preventing its metabolism before it reaches the part of the brain where it is needed. Although this combination drug (Sinemet) is usually successful in managing many parkinsonism symptoms, some patients may experience serious side effects, especially dizziness, involuntary movements, delusions, and cardiac effects such as abnormal heartbeats. Moreover, after several years of use, the drug appears to be less effective, probably because the disease has progressed.

Bromocriptine (Parlodel) and other similar drugs, which act by directly stimulating the nerve cell receptor for dopamine and thereby substituting for the neurotransmitter, may be effective when patients are no longer responsive to the levodopa-carbidopa combination, and they may also cause fewer movement side effects. Such drugs are very expensive, however, and eventually patients become refractory to their benefits as well.

Recent studies have demonstrated the benefit of a new class of drugs, monoamine oxidase B inhibitors, in the treatment of Parkinson's patients. The first drug to be studied in this class was L-deprenyl (selegiline), which is remarkably well tolerated. Although deprenyl's mechanism of action is unknown, one theory suggests that it prevents death of cells in the substantia nigra and thereby delays clinical manifestations of the disease. Consistent with this theory, one study demonstrated that only 24% of Parkinson's patients treated with deprenyl progressed to the point of needing levodopa within a year, compared with 44% of patients who did not receive the drug. Several small studies have also suggested that there may be some benefit

235

in patients with more advanced disease, but these effects appear to be long lasting in only a minority of patients.

Another treatment for Parkinson's disease that has been widely reported upon but is in only the experimental stage is the transplantation of fetal nerve tissue to the brain. In this procedure fetal cells that produce dopamine are implanted directly in the area of the brain where they are needed. At present only a few patients have had the procedure, and not all have benefited. Recently, testing of this new approach in Sweden has resulted in at least one patient's experiencing apparently sustained clinical improvement, and Swedish researchers are continuing their investigations. In the U.S., however, the government has banned the expenditure of federal funds for the research involving the transplantation of fetal tissue into human patients.

Incontinence: focus on a neglected problem

Urinary incontinence is defined as the involuntary loss of urine that is severe enough or frequent enough to cause social or health problems. Women, especially those who have had several children, are twice as likely as men to have incontinence, but the prevalence increases with age in both sexes. A persistent and unfortunate misconception has been that incontinence is normal with aging. Although age-related changes may predispose older people to the problem, normal aging is not a cause per se.

Recently the U.S. National Institutes of Health (NIH) held a consensus development conference to address this common, costly, and too often unacknowledged problem. The panel members—urologists, gerontologists, internists, gynecologists, nurses, psychotherapists, and other health care professionals from across the country—arrived at many conclusions. Among them were that urinary incontinence leads to social isolation and stigmatization; that fewer than half of the 10 million Americans afflicted have received evaluation or treatment; that most cases can be cured or improved; and that health care professionals have paid little attention to the problem, as have medical and nursing education programs. The panel also provided recommendations for appropriate evaluation and treatment.

The extent of the incontinence problem depends in large part upon the population that is being surveyed. For example, in older persons living in the community, 15 to 30% are incontinent, but only 20 to 25% of those persons would be considered to have a severe problem. In nursing homes, however, approximately 50% of the residents are affected.

Incontinence is a symptom of many different diseases, and the seriousness and appropriate management of this symptom depend upon the specific cause. Therefore, before the problem can be addressed properly, the nature and likely cause must be established. The first step is to determine whether the problem

is of new onset and might be easily reversible. This type of transient incontinence often occurs in older persons who are hospitalized and may be related to an acute illness or a new medication. If, on the other hand, incontinence is persistent, it may be one of three basic types.

Stress incontinence, a disorder that occurs almost exclusively in women, is characterized by the leakage of small amounts of urine when abdominal pressure is increased, such as with coughing or sneezing. Previous pregnancies that may relax the muscles supporting the bladder and urinary system, hormone deficiency after menopause, and pelvic surgery can all predispose to the development of stress incontinence.

Several approaches have been successful in managing this type of incontinence. These include performing pelvic exercises in which the woman repeatedly contracts the muscles of the vagina that surround the bladder outlet; these exercises should be repeated several times a day. Biofeedback is another method that helps control stress incontinence. The use of specialized visual or auditory equipment shows incontinent persons how well they are controlling the muscles that inhibit voiding and enables them to relearn the exertion of voluntary control over the contraction of these bladder and pelvic muscles. When such conservative measures fail, surgical therapy may be necessary to restore normal anatomy and continence. The most common surgical procedure, a bladder neck suspension, seeks to restore the normal anatomical positioning of the bladder and urethra. Several techniques for achieving this restoration with minimal risk and success rates exceeding 90% have been reported.

The second type of incontinence—urge incontinence—occurs commonly in persons with neurological disease (e.g., strokes, Parkinson's disease, spinal cord injuries) but can also be due to local conditions such as cystitis or bladder tumors. In other cases of this type, no specific cause is found. Whatever the cause, the common factor is an overactive bladder muscle that contracts involuntarily when the bladder is not completely full. Hence, the actual amount of urine that is lost tends to be small. If a treatable cause is not found, biofeedback or bladder relaxant medications such as oxybutynin hydrochloride (Cystrin, Ditropan), may be very valuable in controlling urge incontinence.

Overflow incontinence, the third type, is due to obstruction of the urinary system or poor contraction of the muscles of the bladder. Prostate enlargement, diabetes, and certain medications (including some antidepressants, sedatives, and antihistamines) are common causes of overflow incontinence. If an obstruction is present and can be relieved, the incontinence will often resolve. For example, prostate surgery may cure overflow incontinence in some older men. Occasionally a catheter, which is a long rubber or plastic tube that is inserted into the opening of the urethra and threaded into the bladder, is necessary to control urinary overflow.

A fourth type of incontinence is caused not by a pathological condition but rather by the individual's inability to get to the toilet. This condition has been termed functional incontinence. Diseases that cause immobility such as arthritis or strokes are frequently the cause, but dementia, psychological unwillingness, and environmental barriers also have been implicated in functional incontinence. A regular schedule of voiding, which may require assistance, is usually the approach to treatment. In rare cases management of the problem requires a catheter.

Many cases of urinary incontinence are due to more than one of the various subtypes, especially in frail older persons. In these situations a behavioral approach to management may be most useful. A recent study has demonstrated that a behavioral therapy program based on hourly checking and prompting of nursing home patients to void regularly, then providing praise to reinforce the accomplishment, decreased the number of "wet episodes" per day in the residents by 26%; the behavioral approach also increased patient-initiated requests for assistance in toileting.

Because the problem of incontinence had long been neglected, the NIH consensus committee acknowledged that there remain gaps in knowledge. Directions for future investigation cited by the panel members included basic research on mechanisms underlying each type, elucidation of risk factors through epidemiological studies, determination of effective preventive measures, determination of relative efficacy of cures—i.e., behavioral versus pharmacological versus surgical treatments—through randomized clinical trials, and development of new and innovative therapeutic methods.

Falls: preventing their huge toll

Approximately one-third of older Americans living in the community sustain a fall each year; half of these persons fall more than once. Most falls occur at home, primarily in the living room and bedroom during daytime activities. Environmental factors contribute to approximately half of all falls, indoors as well as outside the home. Throw rugs, low-lying tables, stairways, poorly lighted areas, and pets are a few of the potential hazards in the older person's home environment that can contribute to falling. Slippery surfaces, curbs, uneven pavement, and moving vehicles are common outdoor hazards. Among older persons living in nursing homes, the likelihood of falling is even higher, exceeding 50% annually.

Although the vast majority of these falls have no serious repercussions, 5–10% of falls result in serious injuries to muscles, tendons, skin, and joints. Another 5% of falls result in fractures, the most serious of which are hip fractures; an estimated 170,000 Americans over the age of 65 sustain this potentially devastating injury. Hip fractures are often the precipitating factor in the move from the community to a nursing home and are associated with mortality rates approaching 25% during the first year after the fracture. Falling may precipitate other adverse consequences, most notably the fear of falling and accompanying social withdrawal.

Some falls may result from acute medical events such as strokes or seizures, but these causes are uncommon and account for fewer than 10% of falls. More important causes of falls are chronic medical disorders, especially arthritis (which limits normal range of motion), diabetes (because of a decrease in sensation in the legs and feet), and neurological diseases. Additional conditions that contribute to falls are disturbances of the vestibular system in the ear (which is responsible for balance), disturbances of the visual system that affect the older person's ability to see obstacles and changes in the terrain, and disturbances of the proprioceptive system (a part of the nervous system that orients the person in space, especially during position changes and on unstable ground). Often older people who sustain falls are afflicted with multiple conditions.

Drugs that disturb gait and balance are another important cause of falls. Medications can contribute to falls and fractures in several ways. Medicines that affect the central nervous system (e.g., tranquilizers) can cause drowsiness and incoordination. Other drugs, including some blood pressure medicines, cause blood pressure to drop upon standing (postural, or orthostatic, hypotension).

The medical approach to the older person who has fallen or is at risk has changed dramatically in the past few years. Previously, the evaluation relied

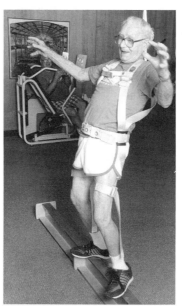

Because falls take such a major toll on the elderly, physicians are now examining their causes and the best ways to prevent them. The medical approach to the older person at risk should include functional assessment of gait, balance, and posture. The man at left is taking a test to determine the effects of an exercise program on his balance.

Medical Media, Durham Veterans Administration Medical Center on thorough medical and neurological examinations, with laboratory testing as indicated. Although these evaluations are still conducted, much greater emphasis has been placed on functional evaluation of gait. Such evaluations may be conducted in a physician's office and consist of a series of maneuvers in which the older person's gait, balance, and posture in daily life are reproduced and scored. On the basis of the results, rehabilitative and environmental changes can be recommended. For example, muscle-strengthening exercises and physical therapy coupled with assistive devices (such as grab bars) might be recommended for an older person who has difficulty getting into and out of a bathtub. The new approach also relies to a much greater extent on practical evaluation of the home environment, which can be done with self-administered questionnaires, *e.g.,* the National Safety Council's "Home Safety Checklist" or the U.S. Consumer Product Safety Commission's "Home Safety Checklist for Older Consumers," or through a formal home evaluation, usually done by a visiting nurse.

In addition, several recent studies have attempted to delineate in a precise manner the actual risk of falling that an individual older person may have. By providing an estimate of risk, the older person and his or her family will have better information for judging whether the current living situation is safe. If it is not, it is then important to determine what appropriate measures can be taken to improve safety to the extent that will enable the older person to remain as independent as possible.

Surprising prevalence of Alzheimer's disease

Dementia, probably the most feared complication associated with aging, is characterized by progressive intellectual impairment that is disabling or hampers an individual's ability to function. Although memory dysfunction (*i.e.,* forgetfulness) typically is the foremost complaint (often coming from a family member rather than the patient), other deficits are also identifiable, including loss of higher intellectual capabilities (*e.g.,* ability to do calculations), loss of language (*e.g.,* speech with very little content), loss of visual-spatial capabilities (*e.g.,* getting lost), lack of spontaneity and initiative, and deterioration of personality. Before dementia can be diagnosed, deficits in several of these areas must be established.

Dementia is a syndrome and has a variety of causes. A form of dementia known as multi-infarct dementia is the result of numerous strokes, usually in the deep parts of the brain. This type of dementia can be distinguished by the presence of risk factors for stroke, physical findings of previous strokes, and a stepwise pattern of deterioration. Dementia also may be associated with other diseases, including Parkinson's disease, chronic alcoholism, vitamin B_{12} deficiency, and certain metabolic diseases. Sometimes psychiatric

illnesses, particularly depression, may give the appearance of dementia, only to respond to antidepressant therapy with resolution of the dementia symptoms. The major cause of dementia, however, is Alzheimer's disease, a degenerative disease of unknown cause.

The results of a major recent study have caused the medical community to reconsider the prevalence rates of Alzheimer's disease. The research, which was conducted by a team from Harvard Medical School, surveyed more than 3,600 people living in East Boston; it was one of the few U.S. studies to date that had sampled subjects from the community. The method of determining the frequency of the disease was also unique. First, the investigators administered a brief memory test to 81% of those in the community over 65 years of age. On the basis of this test, older persons were divided into three groups—those with good, intermediate, and poor memory function. Samples of subjects from each of these three groups (a total of 467) were then selected for a thorough clinical neuropsychological evaluation. Laboratory tests were also performed. The overall results revealed that the probability of dementia was considerably more common than previously believed. Moreover, a striking relationship between age and dementia was demonstrated. Among the 65–74-year-old group, 3% had dementia; this figure rose to 47% in the group aged 85 and older. In this unique study Alzheimer's disease was believed to be the sole cause of dementia in 84% of demented persons who were evaluated.

Several problems in the design of the Harvard re-

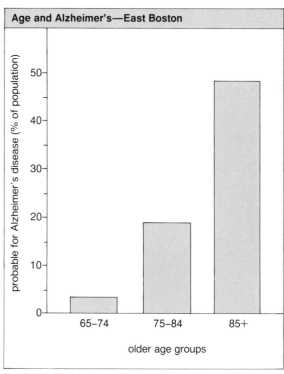

Age and Alzheimer's—East Boston

probable for Alzheimer's disease (% of population)

older age groups

From Denis A. Evans *et al.,* "Prevalence of Alzheimer's Disease. . .," *JAMA,* Vol. 262, no. 18 (Nov. 10, 1989), pp. 2551–56. Copyright 1989, American Medical Association

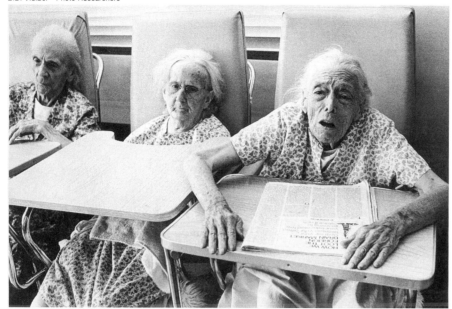

Older persons afflicted by dementia, immobility, and incontinence constitute the majority of long-term residents of nursing homes. Such incapacitating conditions are responsible for a substantial burden of suffering. Research could elucidate the causes of many of the disorders that are so common in the elderly, which would enable physicians to discover methods of prevention and to provide appropriate treatment; the staggering costs of long-term care could also be reduced substantially.

searchers' study have been acknowledged; the new findings therefore require further confirmation. As the investigators noted, they were unable to adequately determine whether the loss of cognitive function was associated with loss of social or occupational functioning. Furthermore, the research has been criticized because the study did not include brain-imaging tests of the subjects, such as computed tomography (CT) scanning or magnetic resonance imaging (MRI), to establish a specific cause of dementia.

The role of extensive diagnostic laboratory tests, which are used mainly to determine reversible dementias—those caused by disorders other than Alzheimer's disease—is questionable. This is especially true in light of the East Boston results and other recent research suggesting that the potentially reversible causes of dementia are much less common than previously thought. A recent review of all published studies of dementia estimated that only 11% of dementias were reversible, either partially (8%) or fully (3%). Because many of these studies were done in teaching hospitals that have special referral centers, which tend to see unusual cases, the true prevalence of reversible dementias may be even lower.

On the basis of published reports, the most common causes of reversible dementia are drugs, depression, and disturbances in metabolism, such as thyroid disease. These three categories account for 70% of all reversible dementias and usually can be detected by a careful history and physical examination and a few simple blood tests. At present, therefore, the most important diagnostic steps in evaluating memory problems and dementia are a thorough history and physical examination with particular attention to the mental status assessment.

The role of brain-imaging tests in evaluating dementia, however, continues to be controversial. The tests that are presently available in some clinical settings have the potential for creating remarkably detailed images of the brain; some tests used in research settings appear to provide a picture of physiological disturbances that may accompany Alzheimer's or other disease states. The reliability of these tests for differentiating between the causes of dementia is still being clarified, however. For example, images generated by CT scans cannot provide a diagnosis of dementia, although CT images can exclude other diagnoses. MRI can aid in a diagnosis of multi-infarct dementia, but its overall clinical value is uncertain. Some of the abnormalities that are believed to be associated with strokes may also occur in normal persons.

Newer brain-imaging tests—including the single photon emission computerized tomography (SPECT) and positron emission tomography (PET) scanning—may be more accurate in specifically diagnosing Alzheimer's disease. However, further investigation is necessary before these diagnostic methods can become routine in clinical practice.

A particular concern is that the elaborate information these methods provide is of little ultimate value in determining therapy. For now, there is no effective treatment for Alzheimer's disease. (The treatment of multi-infarct dementia is to attempt prevention of further strokes, usually by the use of aspirin.) Knowing that a patient has Alzheimer's disease and having an awareness of its characteristic, progressive loss of intellectual capabilities may be useful to some patients and their families in planning care-giving and living arrangements.

Although research into potential drug treatments

239

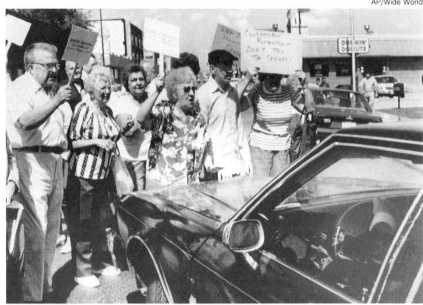

In August 1989 angry senior citizens confronted U.S. Rep. Dan Rostenkowski in Chicago. The Illinois legislator had been a chief proponent of an act passed by Congress in 1988 (subsequently repealed) that was aimed at expanding health care benefits for older Americans. The proposed funding of the federal program provoked a bitter outcry—particularly from the higher-income elderly who were slated to bear the major share of the costs through an annual surcharge on their income taxes. How to provide for the long-term care of the elderly will remain a foremost national concern until adequate solutions are found.

for Alzheimer's disease has accelerated, currently no medication has been demonstrated to be consistently effective to the extent that it could be recommended for general clinical use. Nevertheless, at least 16 drugs in the U.S. are currently being investigated in clinical trials nationwide. Even if one or more of these drugs prove to be effective, none is likely to reverse the memory loss of severely demented patients. More likely, these drugs will slow or halt the progression of memory loss or perhaps provide modest improvement in some cognitive function.

Financing long-term care: critical U.S. problem

Long-term care refers to the medical and social support services needed to optimize the physical, social, and psychological function of frail older persons who usually have multiple chronic illnesses. In the U.S. this care may be provided at home by community services such as home health care agencies that provide intermittent skilled nursing and rehabilitative services, in hospices that are designed to provide care for the last six months of life or less, and in nursing homes.

Contrary to popular belief, only a small percentage of older persons (5% of all persons 65 years of age or older) live in nursing homes. However, with advancing age this rate rises from 1% of those in the 65–74-year-old group to 22% of those 85 and older. Furthermore, the latter group is the fastest growing segment of the population. It is estimated that one in five people living in the U.S. who survives to old age will at some point reside in a nursing home.

The nursing home population comprises those who are recovering from an acute illness and usually have short stays (less than three months) and those who are long-term residents. To date, Medicare coverage

has focused benefits primarily on the first group. As of late 1990, Medicare covered 100% of the first 20 days, all but $67.50 per day for days 21 through 100, and nothing beyond 100 days of care. Although long-term nursing home residents are entitled to the same benefits, Medicare coverage quickly expires, and the burden of nursing home costs falls upon the older person's savings and retirement pensions or on other family members' finances. Long-term-care residents are not eligible for public assistance until they "spend down" personal resources and qualify for welfare programs such as Medicaid. As a result, Medicare provides only 2% of all nursing home revenues, the remainder being split between private revenues of older persons and their families and state-administered welfare programs.

A small minority of older persons have private health insurance policies that provide coverage for long-term care (the latest available figures showed fewer than 2% had private insurance in 1986). This option has been limited because of the low income of most older persons; the high premium costs of such insurance, which range from $2,500 per year for a 65-year-old person to $8,500 per year for an 80-year-old for a good policy; the incorrect assumption by many older persons that Medicare or current private insurance policies (so-called Medigap insurance) will cover these costs; and the belief that "it won't happen to me."

In 1988 the U.S. Congress enacted a law that increased coverage for nursing home stays to 80% for the first eight days and 100% for the 9th through the 150th day of each calendar year. However, the increased premiums to be paid by senior citizens to provide the expanded benefits stimulated a public outcry, which resulted in the law's repeal.

A variety of alternative solutions for the problem of financing long-term care have been proposed, most of which rely on some combination of public and private funding. An executive panel of the Ford Foundation's Project on Social Welfare and the American Future has recommended a plan that provides federal government coverage of long-term care, but only after a waiting period of two or three years. During that waiting period older persons would have to bear the cost of this care either personally or through the purchase of private insurance. A federal subsidy would help lower-income persons to purchase insurance to cover expenses incurred during the waiting period. Another proposal suggests increasing governmental funding of home care services—so that older persons could be kept in the community rather than in nursing homes—and providing federal support for a limited segment of the institutionalized population. For example, a one-year nursing home benefit would be provided for those who are likely to return to the community or who have dependents (e.g., a spouse) who are living in the community and who require financial support.

A number of obstacles must be surmounted for any plan for elderly long-term care to be successful. In the case of government-sponsored funding, steps will have to be taken to limit the enormous potential costs of providing comprehensive coverage. Private policies (and to a lesser extent government funding) must take into consideration the effect of inflation on long-term-care costs. Most policies are indemnity plans that offer a fixed payment per day of institutionalization. When the plan is purchased, the amount offered may adequately cover the costs of the nursing home, but two decades later, when the plan is to be used, the costs may have risen considerably.

Nevertheless, nationally there has been a surge of activity in the development and marketing of private long-term-care insurance. In some communities hospitals and civic and religious organizations have taken leadership roles in selecting good policies for their constituents and members; a few of these organizations have taken on the administrative responsibilities of organizing the marketing of policies.

Finally, the medical community can help lower the costs of long-term care by conducting research on ways to improve the care of persons who will require it. Persons with disorders such as Alzheimer's disease and other dementias, immobility, and incontinence are responsible for the bulk of long-term-care costs. If the devastating effects of these disorders upon function and independent living can be reduced, considerable cost savings can be achieved. Thus, some have suggested that any federal plan to finance long-term care should include a component that funds research on improving the health and function of the ever growing elderly population.

—David B. Reuben, M.D.

AIDS

Seven years after researchers first isolated and identified the organism that causes AIDS (acquired immune deficiency syndrome)—the virus now known as HIV, or human immunodeficiency virus—the disease has been reported in more than 150 countries. In some parts of the world—particularly central Africa, where the virus spreads primarily via heterosexual intercourse and contaminated blood products—infection rates approach 20–30% of the population, threatening an entire generation. In the U.S. and Europe, where the epidemiological pattern differs significantly from that in Africa, infection rates remain relatively low. Reports from Asian countries present a mixed picture. In Thailand, for example, the number of people reported to have tested positive for HIV went from slightly over 100 in 1988 to more than 14,000 in early 1990, according to one estimate. Public health officials in that country fear that the disease is spreading rapidly from drug abusers into the heterosexual community at large. In China, where officials had previously insisted that all AIDS cases involved foreigners, an outbreak of the disease was reported in 1990 among drug abusers in Yunnan province. And in one of the past year's most shocking and tragic reports, several hundred infants in Romania were discovered to have been infected with HIV as a result of the outdated and widely discredited medical practice of giving blood transfusions to thin or anemic babies. Reuse of unsterilized medical equipment was also cited as a factor in the spread of the disease.

Some scientists believe the AIDS epidemic is already on the decline in the U.S., while others predict increasing numbers of cases well into the 21st century. Such widely divergent forecasts of the direction of the epidemic—along with disagreement about its scope and extent—have made it difficult for public health officials to anticipate the need for health care and social services. It is clear that, in the U.S. at least, the disease has shifted from one mostly affecting homosexual males to one increasingly affecting drug abusers and their sexual partners, children of HIV-infected mothers, and inner-city minority and poor populations. Still unclear, however, is whether this shift poses an added risk to the heterosexual population at large—another subject of considerable debate. Congress has so far refused to fund a controversial National Institutes of Health (NIH) proposal for a survey of U.S. sexual practices, designed to aid in making such projections.

Also still unknown is how the nation—and indeed the world—will cope with the enormous costs of treating people with AIDS. Estimates from the U.S. Public Health Service indicate that the average lifetime cost of treating a single individual with AIDS is now in excess of $75,000. On the basis of Centers for Disease Control (CDC) estimates of the number of new AIDS

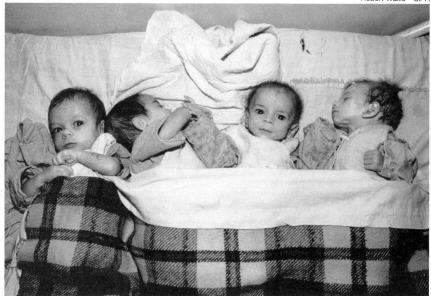

Unlike American babies with AIDS, most of whom are born to HIV-infected mothers, these tiny Romanian AIDS victims—presumably healthy at birth—acquired the infection as a result of outdated and unsanitary medical practices.

Robert Wallis—SIPA

cases expected in coming years, the cumulative costs of treating all persons with AIDS in the U.S., from the time of diagnosis until the time of death, will be $4.3 billion in 1990 and could reach $7.8 billion by 1993. Significantly, these costs will not be borne equally in all areas of the country. One study indicated that fewer than 5% of all U.S. hospitals currently treat more than 50% of all AIDS cases.

Despite the many uncertainties about the outlook for the future, several developments over the past year provided grounds for optimism. The creation of new drugs that may be helpful alone or in combination with zidovudine, more commonly known as AZT (azidothymidine; Retrovir); the increasing usefulness of genetically engineered test animals that incorporate features of the human immune system; a remarkable string of advances in the understanding of the molecular biology of HIV; and promising results of experimental vaccine trials in animals—all contributed to a feeling among AIDS researchers that they were at last making headway in their attempt to outwit this subtle, persistent, and deadly disease. This report covers events from mid-1989 through the closing of the Sixth International Conference on AIDS, held in San Francisco in June 1990.

Basic research: mice and mycoplasmas

During the past year some of the most exciting developments in basic research centered around genetically engineered strains of mice that incorporate elements of the human immune system. The mice, first developed in 1988, began almost immediately to live up to their predicted potential as surrogates for human subjects in the testing of drugs to treat AIDS and vaccines that may someday prevent infection.

At Stanford University, researchers Joseph M. Mc-Cune, Irving Weissman, and colleagues created one variety of these mice by transplanting human lymph node and other tissues into mice bred to have the disorder known as severe combined immunodeficiency disease (SCID)—*i.e.,* mice that lack functioning immune systems. McCune demonstrated that the mice were indeed accurate models for testing the effectiveness of anti-AIDS drugs. Another team, led by Donald Mosier of the Medical Biology Institute in La Jolla, Calif., created similar animal models by transplanting human white blood cells into the so-called SCID mice. The mice bred by Mosier showed promise as a means of demonstrating vaccine efficacy.

In other developments, molecular biologists delineated new details of the genetic and biochemical mechanisms critical to the survival and replication of HIV in human cells. This work has led to the design of a new generation of anti-AIDS drugs capable of blocking HIV replication in laboratory-cultured cells, either by providing defective versions of critical viral ingredients, which then become incorporated into viral progeny, or by blocking enzymatic pathways critical to viral reproduction. Application of these and other experimental approaches in living organisms remains a few years away. Nonetheless, their success in cell cultures hints at novel therapeutic approaches that may soon become critical, as HIV has already begun to display resistance to AZT and other first-generation AIDS drugs.

Meanwhile, researchers continued to debate the question of whether other agents—in addition to HIV—play a role in causing or exacerbating AIDS. Research by Robert C. Gallo of the U.S. National Cancer Institute (NCI) suggested that a recently discovered herpesvirus

242

called HHV-6, which can be passed in saliva, may play some part in triggering symptoms in HIV-infected individuals. Perhaps most intriguing, Shyh-Ching Lo and colleagues at the Armed Forces Institute of Pathology in Washington, D.C., identified a new microbe, given the name *Mycoplasma incognitus,* which they believe may be a cofactor in the development of AIDS in many individuals. In terms of taxonomic classification, mycoplasmas fall somewhere between viruses and bacteria. Some mycoplasmas are known to cause disease in humans. At the international conference in San Francisco, Luc Montagnier of the Pasteur Institute in Paris surprised many scientists with a report suggesting that coinfection with *M. incognitus* may be responsible for HIV's lethal effect on T-helper cells (the infection-fighting immune system cells that are the primary target of the AIDS virus). Despite Montagnier's support of this controversial coinfection theory, most scientists remained unconvinced of a direct link between AIDS and the microbe.

AZT: benefits of early treatment

In March 1990 the U.S. Food and Drug Administration (FDA) approved AZT therapy for generally healthy, *i.e.,* asymptomatic, HIV-infected people who have fewer than 500 T-helper cells per cubic millimeter of blood, an early sign that immune function is failing. Doctors had been using the drug to treat full-blown AIDS in adults since its approval in March 1987; under the new treatment protocol, clinicians can prescribe an early course of AZT in an attempt to stave off disease progression and perhaps prolong survival. The FDA's action was prompted by two landmark clinical trials that suggested that early treatment could benefit HIV-infected people who had not yet acquired the panoply of opportunistic infections that signal full-blown AIDS.

Scientists estimate that about one million people in the U.S. may meet the criteria for early AZT therapy. Of course, many have not been tested for HIV and therefore do not realize they are infected. The two studies also indicated that AZT doses of 500 mg per

Reuters/Bettmann Newsphotos

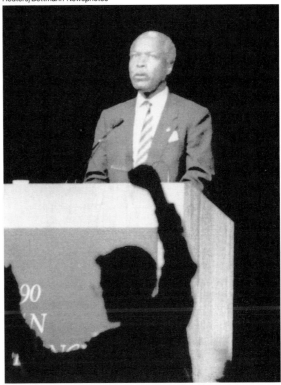

U.S. Secretary of Health and Human Services Louis Sullivan, scheduled to address the Sixth International Conference on AIDS in San Francisco in June 1990, was shouted down by protesters angry about federal policies.

day effectively ward off progression of the disease and cause less severe side effects than the originally approved dose of 1,200 mg. This finding prompted the FDA to approve a dose of 500 mg per day for asymptomatic HIV-infected persons and 600 mg per day for those with symptoms. In many people the higher (1,200-mg) dosage of the drug had caused severe anemia and bone marrow suppression.

The decision to start outwardly healthy people on AZT therapy did not meet with universal approval. Early treatment may delay the onset of disease, but it is still unclear whether the drug will improve a person's chances of living longer. Moreover, long-term AZT therapy is not without risks, including the possible development of resistance to the drug early in the course of the disease, thus precluding its use later on when the illness has become more severe. In May 1990, in an important step toward better treatment of pediatric AIDS, the FDA approved AZT for treatment of children aged three months and older. The drug had not previously been approved for children because information about its safety and efficacy in infants and children was inadequate. Several prominent AIDS researchers had publicly criticized Burroughs Wellcome Co. of Research Triangle Park, N.C., maker of the

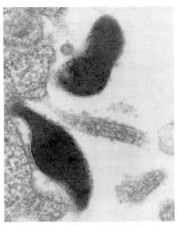

An electron micrograph shows two mycoplasmas (dark-stained bodies) of the variety known as Mycoplasma incognitus, *believed by some researchers to be a cofactor, along with the human immunodeficiency virus, in the development of AIDS.*

Joseph G. Tully and Roger M. Cole, National Institute of Allergy and Infectious Diseases, National Institutes of Health

drug, for its delay in seeking approval for AZT use in HIV-infected children.

Other anti-HIV drugs

Scientists around the world continue their attempts to develop other anti-HIV agents that might be used instead of or in combination with AZT. One such drug still under investigation is dideoxyinosine (ddl). Like AZT, ddl works by blocking replication of the virus. In July 1989 a research team at the NCI, led by Samuel Broder and Robert Yarchoan, reported a small pilot study that demonstrated ddl's promise in shoring up HIV-damaged immune systems. This study showed that the drug boosted the number of T-helper cells and seemed relatively safe. These encouraging findings prompted the FDA and the NIH to open up distribution of the as yet unapproved drug to people with AIDS who could no longer take AZT and who failed to qualify for the official clinical trials of ddl. Under this expanded-access program, private physicians can obtain ddl and other experimental AIDS drugs that show promise in pilot studies for patients who cannot take AZT because of its severe side effects or who have not been helped by it. The maker of ddl, Bristol-Myers Squibb Co., New York City, estimated that about 9,000 people in the U.S. were receiving the drug under the expanded-access program.

The results of some phase I clinical trials of ddl, reported in May 1990, showed that the drug boosted the number of T-helper cells and seemed to reduce the amount of HIV present in the blood. Many of the 71 people who took the drug reported feeling better, and some gained weight. Still, the researchers noted some toxic side effects in certain people, including pancreatitis (a potentially deadly inflammation of the pancreas), and physicians providing ddl under the expanded-access program were urged to monitor patients carefully for signs of adverse effects. Of the several thousand people who took the drug in late 1989 and early 1990, 290 died. Six deaths were believed to have occurred as a direct result of ddl toxicity.

In June 1990 another drug was made available to AIDS patients who were unable to benefit from AZT or ddl. Dideoxycytidine, or ddC, also acts by interfering with viral replication. Its effectiveness and toxicity—as compared with those of AZT and ddl—were still under investigation. Trials of another promising agent, the genetically engineered substance known as soluble CD4, indicated that it slowed viral replication, but more research was needed to prove its effectiveness. Soluble CD4 works by binding with circulating HIV, thus preventing it from attaching to, and infecting, T cells.

AIDS activists have long held out hope for another experimental drug, called compound Q, which is derived from the root of a Chinese cucumber plant. At the international meeting in June, Martin Delaney of Project Inform, a San Francisco-based organization,

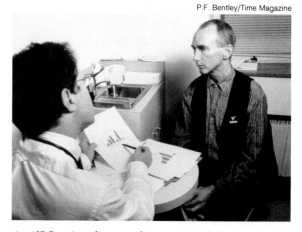

P.F. Bentley/Time Magazine

An AIDS patient discusses the experimental drug compound Q with his physician. He is a participant in a trial of the drug being conducted by the AIDS activist group Project Inform.

presented preliminary data from a trial of the drug conducted by the group. In that study of 46 HIV-infected people, treatment with compound Q appeared to boost T-cell levels. However, FDA-approved clinical trials of compound Q have yet to demonstrate its efficacy, and many scientists were skeptical of the Project Inform study results.

Attacking opportunistic infections

In early 1990 the FDA approved the drug fluconazole (Diflucan) to treat two opportunistic fungal diseases that commonly strike people with AIDS: cryptococcal meningitis, a life-threatening infection of the central nervous system, and candidiasis, a yeast infection that may cause sores in the mouth and throat. Fluconazole showed fewer side effects when compared with amphotericin B (Fungizone), a standard drug used previously to treat such fungal diseases in AIDS patients.

Recombinant erythropoietin (Epogen), a genetically engineered blood factor, was approved by the FDA in June 1989 for treatment of anemia in people with chronic kidney failure. The FDA was allowing distribution of erythropoietin as a treatment of anemia in AIDS patients who are taking AZT, although its efficacy for this use was still undergoing evaluation. Researchers in England and the U.S. were testing a drug known as 566C, an oral antimalarial, as a treatment for pneumocystis pneumonia, a form of bacterial pneumonia that is the leading cause of death in AIDS patients. Several already available drugs are known to be effective in suppressing pneumocystis pneumonia, but the new agent has been shown, in animal tests at least, to kill the organism that causes the deadly lung infection.

Ongoing search for a vaccine

The prospects for developing a vaccine that can protect against HIV infection or prevent the onset of

AIDS symptoms continued to improve in 1989 and 1990. Fundamental problems remain, however, including an incomplete understanding of the biological mechanisms that confer immunity against HIV and the failure of scientists to identify a single "signature" sequence of antibody-inducing amino acids common to all strains of HIV.

Vaccine studies are difficult to evaluate for a disease such as AIDS because of its long latency period (the time between infection and onset of disease) and unpredictable progression. Ideally, in testing a potential vaccine, protection should be measured by following vaccination with a "challenge" dose of HIV—a practice that would be highly unethical with human test subjects. Instead, several research teams have concentrated on testing vaccines in animals, although that research has been hampered because only humans are known to become ill from HIV. Chimpanzees, however, while they do not develop symptoms of AIDS, are susceptible to infection with HIV, and they have been used in successful vaccine experiments in the United States and France. In both cases, animals that were given vaccines made from subunits of the virus did not become infected when they were subsequently injected with HIV.

A virus that is related to HIV, the simian immunodeficiency virus, or SIV, which produces an AIDS-like disease in monkeys, has also been the focus of several vaccine trials. Ronald C. Desrosiers and colleagues at the New England Regional Primate Research Center in Southborough, Mass., created a vaccine from chemically deactivated SIV. In August 1989 they reported that the vaccine had prevented symptoms in all of six monkeys challenged and had completely prevented SIV infection in two of them. Similar results were re-

Scientists are now able to transplant elements of the human immune system into specially bred immunodeficient mice. The mice are then used to test AIDS drugs and vaccines that are not yet ready for human trials.

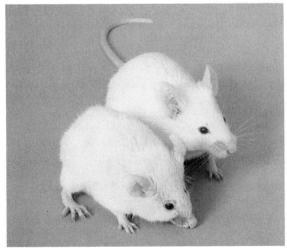

The Jackson Laboratory

ported by Michael Murphy-Corb and co-workers at the Delta Regional Primate Research Center in Covington, La., using a vaccine made from detergent-inactivated SIV. At the international meeting in June, more recent results from these laboratories and new data from the California Primate Research Center in Davis appeared to verify that vaccines made from killed, whole SIV can protect macaque monkeys against low-dose SIV infection.

In another important development researchers at the New England facility, using a cloned form of SIV, were able to produce the infection in monkeys. Previous experiments with SIV had relied on virus isolated from infected animals. With the ability to produce it in the laboratory, researchers expected that they would be able to make changes in the virus and then observe how such changes would affect the nature or severity of the resulting disease. Although the results of these experiments have been encouraging, significant hurdles remain before the work can be applied to trials of a human vaccine. Researchers have also employed strains of the genetically engineered mice mentioned above as surrogate subjects in trials of vaccines designed for humans. It is still unknown whether protection against HIV in mice is predictive of protection in humans.

In the meantime, the first AIDS vaccine to be cleared by the FDA for testing in humans, made by Micro-GeneSys, Inc., of West Haven, Conn., moved into its fourth year of testing in government-sponsored clinical trials. Thus far, more than 200 HIV-negative individuals have received the vaccine, which is made from a genetically engineered replica of a protein, gp160, found on the surface of HIV. The trials have been expanded to include a number of people already infected with HIV to see if the vaccine can prolong the latency period. Although no data regarding either protection or extended latency have been released, the vaccine appears safe and has triggered enhanced immune responses in more than half of the patients tested, according to Robert Redfield, principal investigator for the study at the Walter Reed Army Medical Center and Walter Reed Army Institute of Research, both in Washington, D.C. Other limited trials in humans in the United States and England also show evidence of immune enhancement, but it may be years before scientists can determine whether these cellular responses translate into actual protection against HIV infection.

In June researchers at San Francisco-based Genentech, Inc., said their experimental vaccine—made from a fragment of the AIDS virus called gp120—had protected two chimpanzees from HIV infection for more than six months. Also in June, investigators from Johns Hopkins University, Baltimore, Md., and MicroGeneSys reported that another viral fragment—gp41—may improve the efficacy of some AIDS vaccines. Hopkins researchers also reported that promising immune re-

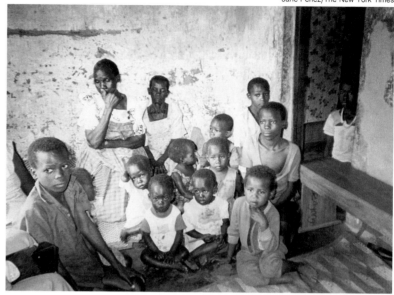

A 69-year-old Ugandan widow whose three sons and their wives have died of AIDS is now left to care for her 12 orphaned grandchildren. An estimated 800,000 of Uganda's population of 17 million are believed to be infected with the virus that causes the disease. There, as in other parts of central Africa, AIDS threatens an entire generation.

sponses had been stimulated by a vaccine made by inserting an HIV gene into the vaccinia virus, which is commonly used to trigger protection against smallpox.

A vaccine made from killed whole viruses, created in 1987 by polio-vaccine developer Jonas Salk and first described by him at the 1989 international AIDS meeting in Montreal, successfully induced immune responses in most of the approximately 70 HIV-positive individuals who took part in a California study under a state law that allows clinical trials within the state. In 1990 the FDA approved plans for expanded testing of the vaccine, including controlled trials expected to begin by the end of the year.

The epidemic: static or growing?

In 1990 the World Health Organization (WHO) estimated that from 8 million to 10 million people throughout the world were infected with HIV. Slightly more than 260,000 AIDS cases had been reported in 156 countries as of June 1990. The pattern of transmission in Europe continued to mirror that seen in the U.S., with homosexuals and intravenous (IV) drug abusers making up the bulk of the reported cases. By contrast, in Africa and some Caribbean countries the major routes of transmission are heterosexual sexual activity and exposure to infected blood products. WHO also predicted a potential AIDS crisis in Asia, where the number of HIV-infected people had risen dramatically—from almost nil two years ago to an estimated total of about 500,000. Experts on the situation in Asia noted that there had been a rapid rise in HIV infection among IV drug abusers and female prostitutes, especially in Thailand and India.

The CDC estimates that there will be a total of 390,000 to 480,000 AIDS cases reported in the United States by the end of 1993, but not everyone accepts these figures. Dennis Bregman and Alexander Langmuir, researchers at the University of Southern California, believe that the incidence of new AIDS cases has peaked and is declining rapidly; they predict that about 200,000 cases will have occurred in the U.S. by the mid-1990s. CDC scientists, citing the spread of HIV infection among groups other than homosexual men, feel that the 200,000 figure seriously underestimates the scope of the problem. The CDC view was echoed in a report by a National Research Council (NRC) panel, presented at the international AIDS conference in San Francisco. The NRC does not see the epidemic as peaking or leveling off in the 1990s but rather as spreading to new, previously unaffected population groups—in particular, women, adolescents, and non-IV drug abusers.

Indeed, a recent study of U.S. teenagers applying for the military showed that the rate of HIV infection among this group is higher than previously suspected. Donald S. Burke and colleagues of the Walter Reed Army Medical Center found that about one out of every 3,000 male and female teenage applicants tested positive for HIV, with the prevalence of HIV higher in black adolescents than in whites. Public health authorities see drug abuse, and in particular cocaine abuse, as a potential avenue for the spread of HIV among heterosexuals. Researchers at the University of California at San Francisco found that addicts who injected cocaine were more likely than other IV drug addicts to frequent so-called shooting galleries and share needles—a finding that could translate into increasing HIV infection among this group of drug abusers. Experts cite the epidemic spread of crack cocaine as another factor in the transmission of HIV in the heterosexual population, especially where addicts exchange sexual favors for drugs.

246

Discrimination: increasingly evident

Despite a growing public awareness about the nature of AIDS—including the broadening recognition that HIV cannot be transmitted by casual contact and that AIDS can strike individuals of every social class and sexual preference—discrimination against people with AIDS has become an ever more visible and troubling aspect of the epidemic. In the U.S. AIDS activists—and many scientists as well—were particularly disturbed by the federal immigration policy that prevented many HIV-infected foreign citizens from attending the international conference in San Francisco.

Nearly all persons with AIDS have, as a result of their illness, experienced discrimination either in the workplace, at school, or in their access to medical or dental care. One large study published in the *Journal of the American Medical Association* predicted that discrimination in the area of health care delivery would grow as the epidemic moved from the homosexual community to intravenous drug abusers. The problem of medical discrimination strikes at the very heart of the private-insurance-based health care system in the United States. Social scientists examining the dynamics of AIDS discrimination in the past year noted with increasing alarm the inherent conflict between the principles of insurance underwriting—which is based on identifying individuals at high risk for disease or death—and the basic social principle of nondiscrimination.

Confidentiality: still an issue

At the core of all questions of health care discrimination lies the issue of confidentiality. Many U.S. hospitals ignore HIV testing policies promulgated by the CDC that were designed to ensure confidential HIV testing for persons being admitted to hospitals. Similar concerns have been raised with regard to the confidentiality of HIV test results at outpatient clinics. Yet while there may be lapses of confidentiality, the medical establishment and AIDS activists are now in agreement in their endorsement of expanded testing for HIV. With incontrovertible evidence that AZT and other drugs can improve the quality of life for many HIV-infected individuals, testing is now regarded as crucial to identifying those who may benefit from early treatment. Toward this end, the FDA in April 1990 reversed its long-standing opposition to the concept of diagnostic AIDS tests that can be performed at home and mailed to a laboratory for analysis. The agency had begun accepting applications from companies interested in licensing such tests. Final FDA approval of these tests, which some authorities say will radically increase the number of individuals willing to be tested, will depend in part on satisfying the FDA's requirement that confidentiality can be maintained and that adequate counseling will be provided over the phone to those who test positive for HIV infection.

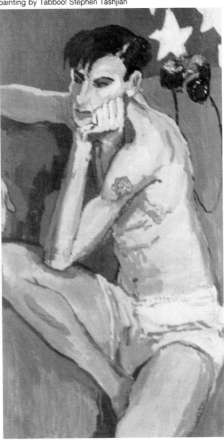

This portrait was part of an exhibit called "Witnesses: Against Our Vanishing," a collective expression of anger and grief by New York City artists, whose community has been particularly hard hit by the AIDS epidemic.

Nowhere does the issue of confidentiality remain more an issue than in the arena of contact tracing—the controversial efforts by public health officials to identify the sexual partners of HIV-positive people. While contact tracing has long been a mainstay of the CDC's effort to control the spread of sexually transmitted diseases (STD) such as syphilis and gonorrhea, the practice takes on new significance with AIDS, a disease that has spawned unprecedented examples of STD-based discrimination. This apparent conflict between individual rights and the public good has prompted many public health officials and civil libertarians to push for improved guarantees of protection against AIDS-related discrimination. In one positive step toward this objective, the Americans with Disabilities Act was signed into law in July 1990. The new law extends antidiscrimination protection for people with disabilities, including HIV infection, to the private sector in employment, public accommodations, transportation, and public services.

—Kathy A. Fackelmann
and Rick Weiss

247

Biomedical Patents: Profits and Pitfalls

by Edmund L. Andrews, M.S.J.

For a medical researcher who daily presses at the frontiers of knowledge, the idea of applying for a patent—at least, until fairly recently—would probably have seemed remote and irrelevant, not to mention tedious. Nowhere, however, has the importance of patents become more evident in the past decade than in the biomedical sciences. The variety of devices that has emerged from discoveries in this field covers an enormous range—from implantable timed-release drug dispensers to machines that generate three-dimensional images of organs inside the living body to a syringe with a retractable sleeve that prevents accidental needle sticks. Patents are also granted to innovative processes, from novel techniques for detecting tumors to computer programs that tell cardiac pacemakers when to stimulate the heart.

The financial implications of such biomedical innovations are awesome. Patent holders—corporations, universities, and individual researchers—regard their patents as "intellectual property," which is every bit as precious as real property. Indeed, a single biomedical patent can be more valuable than a major manufacturing plant or a parcel of prime real estate.

A tale of two drugs

A graphic demonstration of the importance of patent protection can be seen in the sharply contrasting experiences of two pharmaceutical companies that developed enormously profitable new drugs. In 1976 researchers for what is now called SmithKline Beecham Corp. developed a revolutionary antiulcer drug called Tagamet (cimetidine). Traditional ulcer medications had typically depended on a coating action, lining the stomach to prevent its acid secretions from burning through the stomach wall. Although temporarily soothing, these drugs did little to promote healing. Tagamet did something quite different, blocking the release of the gastric acids that cause ulcers in the first place. Because SmithKline obtained a strong patent, the company enjoys monopoly control of Tagamet through 1996. The result is that its revenues from this drug alone total more than $1 billion a year.

By contrast, Amgen Inc., a biotechnology firm in Thousand Oaks, Calif., had quite a different—and sobering—experience with a drug patent. Amgen was the first company to use gene-splicing technology successfully to produce a form of erythropoietin (EPO), a hormone that stimulates red-blood-cell formation. The drug, Epogen, which is used to combat anemia, won limited approval from the U.S. Food and Drug Administration in 1989 for use in kidney dialysis patients. It is eventually expected to be used to fight anemia in persons with cancer and AIDS. The sales of the drug already total about $300 million a year, and the market is expected to reach $2 billion. Amgen, however, has become embroiled in an acrimonious patent dispute that is confounding its pioneering work. A rival biotechnology firm, Genetics Institute Inc. of Cambridge, Mass., has challenged Amgen with a related patent. Although a federal court concluded that Amgen was in fact first with the crucial scientific breakthrough, the court also ruled that the rival company has a competing patent that Amgen must respect. In mid-1990 the dispute was still in litigation, but it seemed almost certain that Amgen would be forced to offer its competitor a license on the gene-splicing technology, sharing both the rights to the process and the huge profits.

The lesson is clear: patents can be enormously important; they can also become the focus of bitter battles that have surprising outcomes. Despite the federal ruling against Amgen, however, the general trend in the past decade has been toward dramatically strengthened patent rights. Indeed, individual inventors have recently won millions of dollars in infringement suits against major corporations. Corporate battles involving a number of multibillion-dollar claims will probably be decided within the next year.

The newfound strength of patent holders has very specific origins. Throughout most of U.S. history, patent disputes were decided by the same federal courts that decide other national issues. In general, the nonspecialist judges in these courts tended to be skeptical about the breadth of many patent claims out of concern for the monopoly power such claims confer. In 1982, however, Congress formed a new, centralized appeals court in Washington, D.C., known as the U.S. Court of Appeals for the Federal Circuit. This court was given exclusive responsibility for hearing all appeals on patent cases. Because the judges who serve on this court have specialized knowledge of patent and trademark law, the court's decisions have tended to clarify many murky areas and have significantly strengthened patent claims in general.

The patent process

To understand both the potential and the pitfalls of patents, especially as they affect biomedical research, it helps to know something about what they are and how they work. The basic U.S. patent law was first established by Congress in 1790. Thomas Jefferson, then secretary of state, was given responsibility for administering the new system. Under the law, a person who invented a product or a process that was new, useful, and nonobvious could obtain a patent giving him or her the right to stop anybody else from making, using, or selling that invention in the United States for 14 years. (The period of exclusive rights was changed to 17 years in 1816.)

In essence, patents were conceived of as a covenant between society and individual inventors, and they are designed to achieve two goals simultaneously and benefit both parties to the covenant. First, by granting a person a temporary monopoly, patents provide financial incentive for innovation and creativity. At the same time, however, the inventor must agree to publicly disclose exactly how his or her invention works. Thus is achieved the second goal—facilitating the spread of knowledge so that people can build on each other's advances. Indeed, the U.S. patent files constitute one of the greatest technological libraries of all time, a library that is accessible to anyone.

In the United States patents are issued by the Patent and Trademark Office, a part of the Department of Commerce, based in Crystal City, Va. It employs roughly 1,400 examiners, who review every patent application that is submitted. Each examiner is a specialist in the particular technology he or she reviews. In 1989 it handled 160,000 applications and awarded 102,712 patents—a 24% increase over the preceding year. Because biomedical products and devices fall into dozens of technical classifications, it is virtually impossible to say how many such patents are issued in a given year.

In some respects the Patent and Trademark Office has not changed since it was first created. Patents are still stored in boxes on miles of shelves for both the public and government examiners to peruse. However, the agency is well on the way to computerizing its

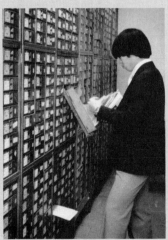

Although they are now in the process of being computerized, the more than 4,750,000 patents on file at the U.S. Patent and Trademark Office are still stored in wooden boxes, as they have been since 1790.

U.S. Patent and Trademark Office

files, a massive task that is expected to be completed in the mid-1990s at a cost of more than $600 million.

Most countries have patent systems of their own, which have goals similar (but not identical) to those of the U.S. system but different procedures. Because U.S. patents are enforceable only in the United States, inventors who want protection abroad must apply for separate patents in the countries where they wish to market their products. Likewise, inventors from other countries who want access to the U.S. market must apply for a U.S. patent.

The American patent system is different from that of almost every other country in one key respect. Elsewhere, inventors obtain patents by being the first to file an application for a particular invention. In the U.S. being "first to file" is irrelevant; inventors must show that they were actually first to invent their device or process. As a result, the approval process is also quite different. The inventor must prove not only that his or her invention is different from anything else submitted to the patent office but that he or she was the first person to come up with the idea. Because disputes frequently arise about who was "first to invent," many inventors immediately document their date of invention by have having their work papers notarized. If a dispute erupts between rival inventors, the patent office launches a legal proceeding, known as an interference, to weigh conflicting evidence.

To help ensure that examiners get all relevant information, inventors are under strict legal obligation to provide such information about previous work in the field and about the way the invention works. If at some later date a court determines that an inventor concealed important information—a violation known as patent fraud—the patent will be permanently invalidated.

Typically, examiners reject every patent application at least once. The inventor must then try to modify the application to overcome the objection or try to persuade the examiner to his or her view. If the patent office issues a final rejection, the inventor may appeal to the agency's board of appeals. If that effort fails, inventors can take disputes to a federal court. The Supreme Court is the ultimate authority, but it very rarely agrees to hear patent cases—an important exception being its 1980 decision to permit patents on genetically engineered bacteria.

The basic requirements an invention must meet in order to be patentable seem simple in theory, but in practice they are anything but straightforward. As noted above, the three main criteria are that an invention be new, be useful, and be nonobvious. But what exactly is "new"? A patent covers more than just the specific details of an invention; it also covers the basic underlying principles. Thus, a patent is a strong form of protection—an imitator cannot evade a patent on a device simply by changing the shape of a part. This very specificity of the law also raises knotty questions; how, for example, does one tell the difference between a cosmetic change to an existing invention and a patentable improvement? To what extent should an old patent cover new variations on the basic principle? Determining whether an idea is obvious in light of earlier inventions is even more difficult. The answer depends on what people who are skilled in the particular technology might think. Interestingly, there is rarely a dispute over usefulness. The philosophy seems to be that the usefulness of an item will be determined by its success in the marketplace.

Because winning patent approval can take years, most inventors thoroughly research the novelty of their ideas before applying. They do this by searching both the patent office files, which contain records of all previously issued patents, and published technical literature. In applying for the patent, the inventor must disclose to the examiner all the relevant technology that has previously addressed the problem at hand—this is known in patent-law terminology as the "prior art." If the inventor knowingly fails to disclose important information, the patent can be invalidated. In the U.S. the patent office keeps all information in an application secret until the patent itself is issued. To protect their rights while the application is under consideration, inventors are allowed to mark their products with the designation "patent pending."

Most inventors hire patent attorneys to shepherd them through the process of winning patent approval. In their applications inventors first explain the problems they are trying to solve and any previous attempts at solutions. They then describe their own invention, providing diagrams and illustrations and explaining how it improves on previous technologies. In the interest of fostering the spread of knowledge, inventors are required to disclose what they believe to be the best mode of making or using the invention and to provide enough information so that anyone skilled in the art of that technology can duplicate it.

The most crucial, and contentious, part of the application comes last: the claims. Having described the new invention, the inventor sets down the basic features he or she feels are entitled to proprietary rights. Typically, an inventor tries to write these claims broadly, so that the patent can cover as many variations as possible. After all, even if a patent can be enforced for 17 years, it has little value if a competitor can engineer around the details presented in the claims.

Typically, an examiner will reject an initial application on the grounds that certain claims seem to have been anticipated by earlier technology. The inventor is given time to respond and either tries to defend a controversial claim or to reword it or simply drops it altogether. It is a slow and sometimes frustrating process, often entailing several rounds of rejection and rebuttal, and the sluggish pace has been criticized by both Congress

and industry as a hindrance to the advancement of innovative technologies. Still, the U.S. patent process is faster than that of Japan, for example, where applications can easily languish for a decade.

Magnetic resonance imaging: a claim —and fortune—lost

Difficult as it is, getting approval from the government examiner can often be easier than enforcing a claim in court. Because fortunes may depend literally on the scope of a single sentence or phrase, precise choice of wording can have enormous consequences in litigation. To illustrate just how tricky claims can be, there is the unfortunate experience of Raymond V. Damadian, the inventor of magnetic resonance imaging (MRI), one of the most spectacular advances in the history of medical imaging. MRI scanners provide doctors with intricately detailed pictures of the soft tissues of the human body; the process is now widely used as a painless and noninvasive method of detecting tumors and other abnormalities. In 1989 the importance of his discovery was attested to when the Patent and Trademark Office inducted Damadian to its National Inventors Hall of Fame, placing him alongside the likes of Thomas Edison and Alexander Graham Bell.

Ironically, Damadian has found himself powerless to enforce his own patent. Indeed, such manufacturers as General Electric Co. and Hitachi Ltd. sell more MRI machinery than Damadian's own company, Fonar Corp., yet they pay him no royalties at all. Why? The answer lies in the language of the claims in the Damadian patent, which outlined the basic principle of magnetic resonance systems but envisioned a somewhat different mode of implementation than what in the course of MRI's wide usage has actually evolved.

MRI technology is based on the fact that atomic nuclei act like tiny bar magnets, aligning themselves in a specific direction in the presence of an electromagnetic field. (For medical purposes, the nuclei most commonly probed are those of ordinary hydrogen contained predominantly in water and fats in the body.) An MRI scanner consists of a large cylindrical magnet that surrounds a patient with an electromagnetic field oriented in one direction. The device then delivers a crosswise burst of radio waves, causing the hydrogen nuclei to line up perpendicular to the first magnetic field. When the radio-frequency energy is removed, the nuclei gradually "relax," or reorient themselves, to the original position and, in the process, give off a distinctive radio signal.

In 1971 Damadian was the first person to demonstrate that magnetic resonance signals given off by cancerous tissue were different from those of healthy tissue. He quickly conceived of building a scanning system that could survey the human body in order to detect cancer, and he obtained a patent for such a system in 1974. In 1977, amid widespread skepticism from many in the scientific community, Damadian built and tested a prototype machine. Today MRI equipment and services constitute a billion-dollar industry.

The problem with the Damadian patent, however, was that it proposed a scanner that would compare the signals from normal body tissues to a "standard" signal emitted by cancerous tissue. Ultimately, however, instead of comparing normal-tissue signals against cancer-tissue signals, the scanners employed a computer to plot the signals given off by different tissues and create from them a detailed visual image. To detect cancer, therefore, doctors study the images plotted from the signals rather than the signals themselves. This proved to be a pivotal distinction when Damadian tried to enforce his patent against a subsidiary company of Johnson & Johnson that manufactured a computerized image-producing machine. Although a federal jury in Boston decided in favor of the inventor, its verdict was overturned by the judge, who concluded that detecting cancer by MRI depended upon inferences "from the shapes and locations of images." Because Damadian had not spelled this out in his patent, the judge ruled, he was out of luck.

Biotechnology: patent "nightmare"

By far the thorniest problems, however, arise in the "brave new world" of biotechnology. The field is still so new that the patent office is having trouble finding and training examiners capable of understanding the technical issues. Beyond that, the technology has posed a profusion of questions that never arose in other technologies and that have become the subject of enormous debate.

Many biotechnology companies are applying genetic engineering technology to create new sources of vital proteins, such as human growth hormone, insulin, and enzymes that dissolve blood clots. To do this,

researchers must first identify the gene that codes for a particular protein and then "splice" that gene into the DNA of a "host" cell, usually a bacterium or an animal cell. These cells then reproduce in laboratory culture mediums and form billions of tiny, living factories capable of producing commercially valuable substances.

The patent problems have become a nightmare, however. On a practical level biotechnology patents have created a major backlog at the patent office. Although the agency typically approves the average patent in about 18 months (a major improvement from several years ago), biotechnology applications often languish for three to four years. The main reason is that the patent office has enormous difficulty retaining skilled examiners, who, because of their technical expertise, can make considerably more money in private industry. Under pressure from Congress and from industry, the agency added hundreds of new examiners to its total corps in the late 1980s, and it specifically targeted the biotechnology area for improvement. Complaints about claim approvals, however, are still common.

Aside from the slow pace of approvals, another source of concern to biotechnology companies is that too much work is being handled by relatively inexperienced examiners, creating uncertainty for companies worried about enforcing their rights in court. In response, the patent office recently launched an educational program for its employees conducted by the Industrial Biotechnology Association, an industry trade group.

The more fundamental problem, however, is that the biotechnology business raises questions that no one has ever had to address before. None of these issues is beyond solution, but they are all contentious and probably will be decided only as they work their way through the judicial system.

"It'll never work out. She's patented, he isn't."

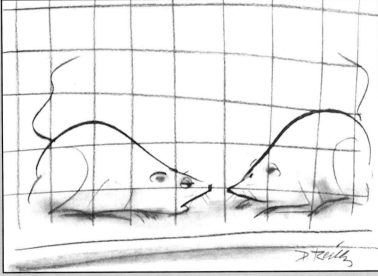

Altered cells and modified mice

To date, the most important biotechnology decision is the Supreme Court's 1980 decision in the case of *Diamond* v. *Chakrabarty*. There the justices ruled that it was possible to patent a living creature—in this case a genetically altered bacterium that, because of its ability to break down crude oil, was potentially useful in cleaning up oil spills. The case was of critical importance because biotechnology products are produced by novel organisms, created not by nature but by laboratory scientists through genetic engineering. If the Supreme Court had ruled differently, the burgeoning industry would have formed much more slowly— or perhaps not at all.

The Chakrabarty decision also paved the way for inventors to patent new strains of animals. The patent office concluded that a principle applied to single-celled organisms also applied to larger, more complex organisms. Thus, in April 1987 it issued a patent on a mouse created at Harvard University that carried a cancer gene. Although popular interest has been drawn principally to the prospect of patented farm animals—such as cows genetically altered to produce more milk—the most immediate applications are expected to be in medical research. Several companies are trying to develop mice that will contract AIDS and can thus serve as models of the human disease. Others are hoping to breed animals that would become sources of valuable drugs.

Nevertheless, a number of difficult issues remain unresolved. For example, if a scientist isolates a gene that produces a vital human hormone, should the patent cover small variations on that gene? On the one hand, a host of slightly different genes will also produce the hormone, and a patent that covers only one specific DNA sequence could be easily circumvented by technicians who could design insignificant modifications of the sequence. On the other hand, some modified versions might produce the hormone more efficiently or with slight improvements in quality. To what extent, then, should the basic patent control other patents?

Process versus product: a paradox

Another vexing issue concerns the process for making drugs based on recombinant DNA technology. Roughly speaking, the process for creating all such drugs is very similar—the gene for a protein is copied, inserted into a "vector" (a segment of DNA that serves as a carrier), and spliced into the DNA of a host cell. Patent-office examiners have been understandably reluctant to view the process itself as particularly new or patentable. They have preferred to issue patents on the specific DNA sequences and host cells. Although such patents provide protection in the U.S., they leave a loophole that benefits foreign companies. To circumvent a firm's U.S. patent on a gene, all a competitor has to do is create a product using that gene in another country. The firm can then import the resulting drug into the U.S. and market it without fear of legal action. Interestingly, U.S. law does allow a company to block imports of a product made abroad by a patented process—but a patented gene and host cell do not constitute a "process." A proposed new law, the Biotechnology Patent Protection Act of 1990, would exclude from the U.S. market biotechnology products made from U.S.-patented components (*i.e.*, genes and host cells) by companies that have not obtained permission to use those components.

Perhaps the most troubling issue that has developed regarding competing biotechnology patent claims centers on the question: Is it more important to be first in identifying a particular protein or to be first in producing that protein through genetic engineering? From a commercial viewpoint, the key breakthrough is isolating the gene, which then allows a manufacturer to produce large quantities of a useful protein. Companies that are first on this score are entitled to a patent on both the isolated gene and the host cell that actually produces the protein.

This is quite different from getting a patent on the protein substance itself, however. As events have unfolded, some companies have been able to get patents on specific proteins by purifying them from natural sources and identifying their structure and characteristics. In some cases the two different patents—one on the gene and host cell, one on the particular protein— have been granted to rival companies.

This is the question in the previously mentioned dispute between Amgen and Genetics Institute. It was an Amgen scientist who was the first to isolate the gene to make erythropoietin. Genetics Institute did not succeed in isolating the gene until nine months later, but it was the first to purify a tiny amount of the natural protein, and it obtained a patent on the protein.

As a practical matter there was little real use for the purified natural protein, but both companies needed to use the patented gene and host cell to make a marketable amount of protein. Logically, therefore, Amgen should have been in the dominant position. It was not, however, because of a long-standing legal principle that holds that a patent on a compound covers that compound regardless of how it is made. As a result, therefore, a federal court ruled in late 1989 that Amgen was infringing on its rival's patent—even though Amgen researchers had never used the purified natural material that earned Genetics Institute its patent.

To some extent equivocal situations like this one are the natural result of revolutionary technologies that raise novel issues. Eventually court decisions on disputed claims will make the ground rules in biotechnology clearer. In the meantime, however, companies navigating these uncharted waters can expect some rough sailing.

Asthma

Although a precise definition of asthma is difficult to formulate, there is general agreement that it is a chronic disease of the air passages, causing them to constrict too readily and too much in response to a variety of stimuli. When tested in clinical studies, the airways of asthmatic persons respond much more to such pharmacological agents as histamine and methacholine than do the airways of normal subjects. This phenomenon, known as airway hyperreactivity or hyperresponsiveness, is considered a cardinal feature of asthma. Despite the common reference to *bronchial* asthma, the condition affects all parts of the airway, both larger and smaller than bronchi.

Magnitude of the problem

Asthma is more prevalent in certain countries, *e.g.,* New Zealand, Australia, and the U.K., than in others, *e.g.,* the U.S. and Sweden. The disease is thought to be rare in rural Africa and among the Eskimos, and its prevalence is lower in village communities than in large industrial cities.

In the U.S., despite the lower international ranking, asthma must now be considered a major national health problem. It affects between 7 million and 20 million people, 2 million to 5 million of whom are children. Recent national statistics show that (1) between 1970 and 1987 the prevalence of asthma increased 33%, from 30.2 to 40.1 per 1,000; (2) hospitalization for asthma also rose, indicating an increase in severity; and (3) the death rate for asthma almost doubled from 1979 to 1987, with mortality rates rising fastest among blacks and those older than 65. Health care costs for asthma sufferers recently were estimated at more than $4 billion per year. The increasing illness and death rates for asthma are particularly alarming in view of the greater availability of effective medications and falling death rates for other diseases.

Major features of asthma

The symptoms of asthma are typically intermittent and include wheezing, a feeling of tightness in the chest, difficulty in breathing, and cough. Either spontaneously or with appropriate treatment, these symptoms are completely reversible—hence, the description reversible airway disease is applied to the condition. The majority (90%) of persons with asthma are atopic; *i.e.,* they produce antibodies (known as immunoglobulin E, or IgE) in response to particular protein substances (allergens) derived from inhaled airborne particles, such as dander, house dust, and pollen, or from certain foods. This form of asthma is known as extrinsic (or allergic) asthma, as opposed to intrinsic (or nonallergic) asthma, which afflicts people who show no such allergic response. Extrinsic asthma usually appears in childhood, while the intrinsic variety often begins in adult life. Asthma can be provoked by a wide variety of factors that can be either allergic or nonallergic, or chemical or nonchemical, as described below.

Airway abnormalities in an asthma attack include (1) bronchospasm, or muscular constriction of the bronchi, perhaps the most widely recognized and most easily reversible of all changes; (2) excessive secretion of mucus by glands and cells within the airways; (3) swelling of the mucosal (mucus-producing) cells of the airway lining and the thin layer beneath them, due to leakage of blood plasma into the airway tissues; (4) increased presence of cells involved in the inflammatory response, especially the white blood cells known as eosinophils and neutrophils; and (5) damage to the cellular lining, or epithelium, of airway passages.

All of these abnormalities contribute to the principal functional alteration: an increase in airway resistance to the flow of air. Airways progressively narrow and some close, but the lungs as a whole are overinflated. These changes, in turn, lead to increases in the work of breathing and in the oxygen cost of breathing (*i.e.,* the portion of the body's total oxygen consumption needed to supply the muscles of breathing). Uneven distribution of air and blood in the smallest openings of the airways, the alveoli, results in reduced oxygenation of blood. In a more severe, prolonged attack, a condition termed status asthmaticus, the muscles of breathing (the diaphragm and the muscles between the ribs) become fatigued, allowing accumulation of lactic acid (a metabolic waste product) in the blood and tissues and resulting in respiratory failure, the failure of the lungs to rid the body of carbon dioxide.

Protein substances from plant pollen (shown highly magnified) are common provoking factors in extrinsic, or allergic, asthma, the form experienced by the great majority of asthma sufferers.

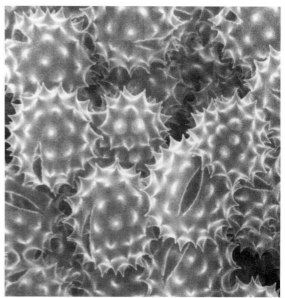

David Scharf—Peter Arnold, Inc.

Kinds of asthma and contributory factors

The age of the victim, the place or situation in which an asthma attack is likely to occur, and the type of provoking stimulus all contribute to the ways that asthma can be classified and to its evaluation and treatment. Some of the more important of these aspects are discussed below.

Childhood asthma. Asthma is the most common chronic disease of childhood. In developed countries it is more common in children than in adults and more common in boys than in girls. Generally the prognosis for asthma starting in childhood is better than that for the disease beginning in adulthood. More specifically, people with mild episodic or seasonal wheezing that starts in mid childhood tend to lose their disease as they grow older, while those with more frequent, early-onset symptoms or with severe, chronic, perennial asthma are less likely to improve with the years. Recurring cough and wheezing may follow bronchiolitis (inflammation of the bronchioles, smaller branches of the bronchi) due to respiratory syncytial virus infection, a prevalent childhood affliction in winter months, but these asthmalike symptoms do not necessarily progress to full-blown atopic asthma.

Occupational asthma. Asthma may be triggered by exposure to sensitizing concentrations of any of a wide spectrum of substances found in the work environment. These include enzymes (*e.g.,* subtilisin, a bacterial protein used in detergent manufacturing), animal danders, plant proteins (*e.g.,* in oils and particles from Western red cedar, oak, and other woods; pollen), metals (*e.g.,* platinum salts), and other chemicals (*e.g.,* isocyanates, used in plastics and adhesives manufacture). In most instances such sensitization results in nonspecific airway hyperreactivity, or heightened sensitivity to a variety of stimuli. A positive reaction to experimental exposure to the suspected agent is the most reliable demonstration of the particular sensitization and, hence, of the provoking agent of asthma in a given individual. Once the cause has been identified, avoiding exposure to it provides the best chance for symptomatic improvement.

Drug-induced asthmas. A number of drugs may bring on or worsen asthma in susceptible individuals. Examples are aspirin and related drugs; beta-adrenergic blocking agents, or beta blockers (*e.g.,* propranolol); and certain food and beverage additives, including tartrazine yellow dye and bisulfite compounds, which are widely used as preservatives. Aspirin-induced asthma, the best known form of drug-induced asthma, typically develops within minutes to a few hours after taking aspirin or another analgesic with a similar mode of action (*e.g.,* ibuprofen). Such drugs are sometimes classified as nonsteroidal anti-inflammatory agents. People with aspirin-induced asthma usually also have preexisting chronic watery nasal secretion, nasal polyps, and sinusitis.

Exercise-induced asthma. Most asthmatics suffer a transient worsening of symptoms after vigorous exercise. The asthmatic difficulty usually begins during the exercise and peaks after the activity ceases. Even in the absence of exercise, asthma may be brought on by hyperventilation (increased rate and depth of breathing), especially of dry air. Asthma induced by exercise or hyperventilation is believed to result from loss of water from the lining of the airway, leading to increased concentration of dissolved substances in the liquid that coats the respiratory tract and the release of asthma mediators from certain cells in the vicinity called mast cells. (Very dilute watery solutions, such as tap water, may also trigger airway constriction by changing the concentration of dissolved substances in the airway.) The higher the ventilation level associated with the exercise and the colder (hence, drier) the air breathed in, the greater the risk of exertional asthma. Thus, ice hockey, cross-country skiing, and snow shoveling are more provocative than walking and swimming in an indoor heated pool.

Exercise-induced asthma can almost always be avoided by the regular use of antiasthma medications to prevent attacks. In fact, many athletes continue to participate in vigorous sports—some at the Olympic level—despite being diagnosed as asthmatic.

Other provoking factors. Sulfur dioxide, an air pollutant, is an intense respiratory irritant; in contact with

Occupational asthma can be a hazard in the silk-screening industry, where workers face chronic exposure to sensitizing chemicals. Usually the sensitization results in heightened reactivity to a variety of asthma-provoking stimuli.

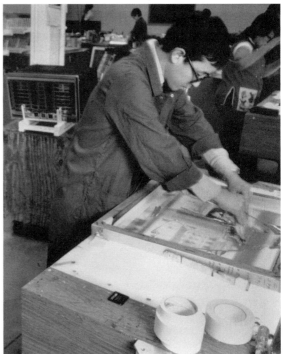

Cathy Melloan

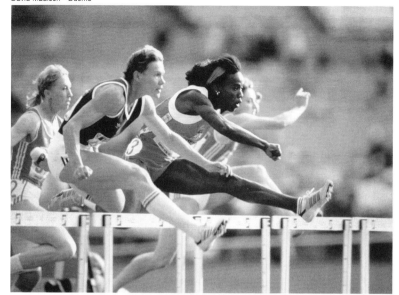

Winner of two gold medals in the 1988 summer Olympic Games, Jackie Joyner-Kersee (third from left) was little hampered by her chronic asthma, kept under control with daily and pre-exercise medications and a modified training approach. In addition to asthma, Joyner-Kersee has allergies to several foods and inhaled substances.

the moist lining of the airway, it is chemically transformed to sulfuric acid. Curiously, in another context sulfur dioxide is sometimes added to beverages and foods as a preservative. Either inhaled or ingested, the compound can provoke severe attacks in asthmatic people. Increased airway responsiveness may also result from other industrial- and automotive-associated pollutants such as ozone and nitrogen dioxide or from various components in cigarette smoke. Respiratory infections, including viral and *Haemophilus influenzae* bacterial infections, can worsen asthma in children and adults. Gastroesophageal reflux (backup of stomach contents into the esophagus), with aspiration of stomach acid into the lungs, can provoke airway constriction. Emotional stress may also be a factor in asthmatic attacks. While virtually no case of asthma is "all in the mind," psychological factors may play a role in modifying the disease, and the importance of interactions between the immune and nervous systems is being increasingly recognized.

Cardiac asthma: a special case

For more than 150 years, physicians have recognized that victims of severe heart failure may complain of a sudden suffocating breathlessness, often associated with wheezing and cough and usually striking at night. This complex of symptoms, termed cardiac asthma, has long been considered to have a cause different from that of bronchial asthma. The asthmalike attack in heart failure has been thought to result from a sudden increase in blood pressure in the small vessels of the lungs, causing plasma to leak out of the blood vessels into the air spaces and thus reducing access of oxygen to the lung capillaries.

Although this traditional view of the causation of cardiac asthma still appears valid today, recent studies

suggest that some element of airway hyperreactivity—the dominant feature of bronchial asthma—may be present. If such a suspicion is confirmed, future therapy for cardiac asthma may include bronchodilators, although the essential treatment will remain that of heart failure.

New understanding of the asthmatic response

New pieces of the asthma puzzle have recently been discovered. Although the full mechanisms of the asthmatic response are still incompletely understood, several important insights into the nature of bronchial asthma emerge:

● It has been found that exposure of atopic asthmatics to allergens provokes two distinct reactions: an immediate airway-obstructive response peaking within minutes and spontaneously resolving within one or two hours, and a late asthmatic response (late-phase reaction) developing four to eight hours after exposure and lasting from one day to several days. In laboratory animals the immediate response is characterized by airway constriction, tissue swelling, and engorgement of blood vessels. Mast cells, a type of inflammatory cell involved in allergic reactions and found in large numbers in the respiratory tract, are associated with this reaction. The late response, which mirrors more closely the findings in severe chronic asthma in humans, has as its main feature an acute influx of inflammatory cells, with neutrophils and eosinophils predominating. The latter laboratory findings, confirmed by similar results in humans dying of status asthmaticus, underscore the importance of inflammation in the development of asthma.

● Another insight derives from the fact, mentioned above, that hyperreactivity of the airways to provoking stimuli is a key abnormality in asthma. This hyper-

255

reactivity now is believed to be correlated with, and possibly due to, the inflammatory changes seen in the late response.

• A variety of cellular and noncellular mediators participate in producing inflammation in the asthmatic airways. They include the already mentioned eosinophils, neutrophils, and mast cells, and others such as the epithelial cells lining the airways, the macrophages (which engulf foreign particles and bacteria), and the T lymphocytes, or T cells (the mainstay of the immune response). The noncellular mediators comprise a large variety of locally produced compounds that are capable of reproducing, partially or completely, the picture of asthma in airway tissue. Among them are substances known as amines, *e.g.*, histamine and serotonin; powerfully active compounds such as prostaglandins and related products that are derived from essential fatty acids; another, recently identified substance called platelet-activating factor; peptides (small proteins), especially a group called tachykinins; enzymes (proteins that catalyze chemical reactions); and reactive oxygen species, which are highly toxic molecules that derive their reactivity from their oxygen atoms. The identification of these mediators has made it possible to work toward counteracting their effects or production in individuals who are afflicted with asthma.

• It has long been known that lung tissue is influenced by both major components of the unconsciously controlled, autonomic nervous system: the adrenergic system, whose signals are transmitted by release of the neurotransmitters epinephrine and norepinephrine, and the cholinergic system, whose signals are transmitted by acetylcholine. It has recently become apparent that the dominant neurological component of airway relaxation in humans is neither adrenergic nor cholinergic but a different system whose likely transmitter is a neuropeptide (a peptide produced, stored, and released by nerve cells) known as vasoactive intestinal polypeptide (VIP). So named because it was first isolated from intestine and because of its ability to dilate blood vessels, VIP is also a potent relaxant of airway smooth muscle; is present in nerve fibers and nerve terminals supplying airway smooth muscle, glands, and blood vessels; and binds to specific receptors on these structures. In a recent study of five subjects with asthma, sections of their airways showed no VIP-containing nerves. By contrast, the vast majority of sections from nine control subjects without asthma revealed a rich innervation with VIP. The investigators concluded that deficiency of VIP in asthmatic airways may be an important factor in their hyperreactivity to irritants and bronchoconstrictors. This report must be confirmed by direct evidence of impaired VIP production and a corresponding genetic defect in asthmatic lungs to prove that the lack of VIP is a primary cause.

• An increasing number of biologically active neuro-peptides have been found in the lungs. A few, like VIP, relax airway smooth muscle and may modulate asthmatic responses. Others, notably the tachykinin peptides—*e.g.*, substance P—constrict airway smooth muscle, stimulate bronchial secretion, and increase vessel wall permeability (leakage of plasma from the blood vessels). These peptides occur predominantly in sensory nerves supplying the airway epithelium and other structures. It is speculated that through a local reflex mechanism, these sensory neuropeptides may contribute to the occurrence of asthma whenever airway epithelium is damaged.

• Airway neuropeptides have been found to be inactivated locally by an enzyme, neutral endopeptidase (enkephalinase), that is present in various other tissues. This enzyme has been shown to degrade bronchial relaxant peptides (*e.g.*, VIP) and bronchial constrictor peptides (*e.g.*, substance P). Thus, by selectively limiting the biological activity of airway neuropeptides, neutral endopeptidase (and other peptidases) may play a key role in regulating airway function in both normal subjects and subjects with asthma.

• Airway epithelium once had been regarded simply as a passive covering of the airways. Much like vascular endothelium (the corresponding lining of blood

For most antiasthma drugs, the preferred method of delivery is inhalation. Below, the correct delivery position of the inhaler is demonstrated. The spray is inhaled slowly over 5 seconds and the breath held for 5 to 10 seconds more.

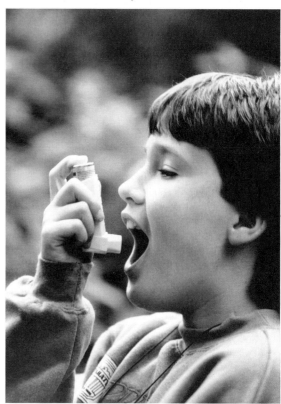

vessels), which has been discovered to have several major metabolic activities, airway epithelium is now believed capable of modulating airway function in important ways. Upon irritation or another form of activation, airway epithelial cells can release potent substances that contract airway smooth muscle. Airway epithelium normally produces a substance, epithelium-derived inhibitory (or relaxant) factor, that reduces the tone of airway smooth muscle. This factor corresponds to, but is apparently distinct from, the endothelium-derived relaxant factor made by blood vessel lining. The existence of this epithelial substance explains why removal or extensive injury of airway epithelium results in accentuated responses to inducers of airway spasms and diminished responses to several relaxants.

Today's treatment: drugs of choice

A variety of effective drugs are available for reversing, or at least ameliorating, the airway constriction of an asthma attack. Fewer drugs, however, are successful against airway hyperreactivity and inflammation, and none alters the chronic nature of the disease. Antiasthma drugs in common use are beta$_2$-adrenergic agonists, theophylline, anticholinergics, corticosteroids, and cromolyn and related drugs. For all except theophylline, the preferred method of administration is in the form of an inhaled aerosol delivered directly to the site of the reaction—a method that increases efficacy and reduces systemic side effects.

Selective beta$_2$-adrenergic agonists (e.g., albuterol, fenoterol) are the drugs of choice for the immediate relief of bronchoconstriction. They act by stimulating certain receptors of the adrenergic nervous system in a way similar to that of the body's natural chemical mediators. When taken preventively by inhalation, they can also protect against many forms of provocation, including allergens, exercise, histamine and methacholine, and sulfur dioxide.

Theophylline, taken by mouth, is now formulated for sustained release over a period of 12 to 24 hours. Intravenous infusion of the soluble form, theophylline ethylenediamine, may be necessary in more severe and persistent attacks. Concentrations of theophylline in the blood should be monitored so that the drug dosage can be adjusted for best possible effectiveness and safety. Side effects, less common with the newer slow-release preparations than with earlier, short-acting ones, begin with nausea, vomiting, restlessness, and tremor and may include heartbeat irregularities and seizures. Slow-release theophylline is effective in controlling nighttime or early-morning asthma but is less effective than beta$_2$ agonists in preventing exercise-induced asthma. Theophylline's mechanism of action remains uncertain.

Anticholinergic drugs, exemplified by the synthetic atropine-like compound ipratropium bromide, are taken as aerosol inhalants and have few side effects, as they are poorly absorbed into the circulation. As bronchodilators they are less effective in younger patients than in older people with chronic airflow obstruction.

Corticosteroids may be given orally, intravenously, or by inhalation. Although not rapidly acting bronchodilators, they are highly effective against asthma over a period of time, acting at least in part by reducing the inflammatory reaction and the bronchial hyperreactivity of the late response. On a short-term basis, systemic corticosteroids (for example, prednisone, methylprednisolone) are used in severe acute asthma attacks when bronchodilators (beta$_2$ agonists and theophylline) have been unsuccessful. Their long-term use, however, has the potential for serious side effects, and aerosol corticosteroids (triamcinolone acetonide, budesonide), which greatly lower this risk, are much preferred for management therapy. The development of corticosteroid inhalants is one of the most significant advances in asthma therapy in recent years. In view of the mounting evidence that inflammation plays a critical role in asthma, these drugs should be given increased priority in the treatment of chronic asthma.

Cromolyn (sodium cromoglycate) is another drug that may suppress the inflammatory response. Given as an aerosol liquid or powder, cromolyn is thought to "stabilize" mast cells at or near the inner surface of the airway, thereby inhibiting the release of mast-cell mediators. Cromolyn is effective against both the immediate and the late-phase responses to allergens. When used on a regular basis before asthma attacks occur, it reduces or prevents the response to exercise, hyperventilation with cold air, and sulfur dioxide. Nedocromil sodium, closely related to cromolyn in its effects and possibly more potent in some respects, has recently been introduced as a management drug, but clinical experience with it is still too limited to characterize its effectiveness.

Future goals for asthma treatment and control

Current research in asthma has two major goals—better understanding of the disease mechanisms and improved methods of therapy. Active areas of investigation include clarification of the way that airway inflammation is initiated and maintained, of the role of inflammatory mediators, of the interactions between different cellular and noncellular mediators, of the full scope of lung neuropeptides and their participation in regulating airway function and in the origin and modulation of asthma, and of the protective role of airway epithelium and importance of epithelium-derived inhibitory factor.

Advances in therapy and prevention may come from improvements in currently available products such as longer-acting, more selective, and more potent beta$_2$ agonists, corticosteroid preparations, and cromolyn-like drugs. Advances may also derive from lines of drugs based on new knowledge of regulatory neu-

Common cold

ropeptides—for example, the aerosol administration of VIP and VIP-like peptides such as helodermin. VIP and helodermin have anti-inflammatory as well as bronchodilator actions, and their use would provide rational "replacement" therapy because they occur naturally in normal lung tissue and because VIP is deficient in asthmatic airways. Another approach would involve the development of agents that selectively block the release or actions of likely mediators of inflammation in the asthmatic process.

Needed: new focus for therapy and better education

The treatment of asthma all too often is restricted to the immediate relief of acute attacks. This approach is a mistaken one. Physician and patient alike must realize that asthma is a chronic, continually present disease in which undetected airway obstruction and inflammation may exist even during symptom-free periods. Treatment therefore should be aimed at preventing acute attacks or decreasing their frequency and severity and at suppressing the ongoing inflammatory reaction. Many of the drugs used for treating acute asthmatic episodes also have preventive value and should be used regularly for that purpose. Anti-inflammatory drugs such as aerosol corticosteroids and cromolyn should be prescribed early in the course of treatment. It is hoped that other anti-inflammatory agents, derived from current research on mediators and airway neuropeptides, such as those described above, will soon be available for immediate therapy and long-term control of asthma.

Finally, the general public needs to be made aware of the importance of prompt treatment of early signs of asthma attacks, the chronic nature of the disease, its increasing incidence and severity, and the need for a systematic and rational approach to its management.
—Sami I. Said, M.D.

Common Cold

Humankind's most frequent illness is probably the common cold, a runny, stuffy nose due to infection of the cells of the nasal lining by one of a large number of viruses, particularly rhinoviruses and coronaviruses. In recent years investigators at a number of research centers have advanced their understanding of cold-causing agents and have made progress in treating the disease.

Although an individual may experience a succession of colds having similar symptoms, each bout is very likely due to infection with a different virus. Some colds are caused by viruses belonging to quite unrelated viral families; e.g., mild attacks of influenza A or B viruses, reinfections with parainfluenza virus (types 1 to 4) that may have caused more serious illnesses such as croup or pneumonia in early life, or infections with respiratory

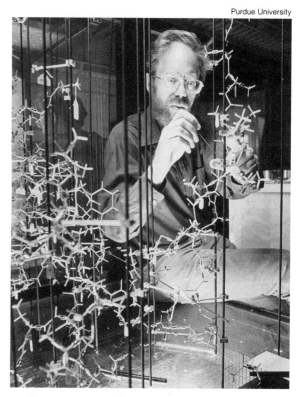

Purdue University researcher Michael Rossmann poses with part of a model of a cold-causing virus. Rossmann's team determined the structure of the viral shell, gaining clues as to how the rhinovirus attacks the nasal lining.

syncytial virus, which can cause bronchiolitis (inflammation of the small airways in the lungs) in infants. The two main causes of colds, however, are rhinoviruses, a group of at least 100 small viruses (picornaviruses) that are biologically related to polioviruses and other enteroviruses, and coronaviruses, a separate family having fewer distinct types but, instead, the ability to reinfect individuals throughout their lives. Rhinoviruses cause at least one-third of colds and coronaviruses about one-sixth.

The structure of a rhinovirus

It has been known since the 1960s that rhinoviruses are extremely small (about 27 nanometers, or billionths of a meter, in diameter) and that their genes are in the form of a long single strand of ribonucleic acid (RNA). The virus particle consists of an outer "shell" of protein made of four types of smaller protein subunits. Each subunit in turn comprises a chain of molecules called amino acids. The subunits assemble into an orderly structure that surrounds the strand of RNA, protects it from damage when outside its host cell, and introduces it into a cell in the process of infection. The viral RNA then takes over the cell's protein-making machinery and makes it produce more viral RNA, protein, and eventually entire virus particles.

258

Studies during the past decade, particularly work focusing on rhinovirus type 14, have greatly refined scientific knowledge of rhinoviruses. Using molecular biological techniques, independent research teams in the United States and the United Kingdom obtained the sequence of nucleotide building blocks that make up the viral genes. This sequence then was used to deduce the corresponding sequence of amino acids encoded by the genes and hence the four subunits of the viral shell. In addition, virus was grown in relatively large amounts and purified, and the conditions were found in which the particles assembled in regular arrays to form crystals. Subsequently, researchers led by Michael Rossmann of Purdue University, West Lafayette, Ind., used X-ray protein crystallography to study the crystalline structure. In essence, they passed a strong beam of X-rays through a crystal. Those X-rays that came near atoms or groups of atoms were deflected from their original paths. Because the atoms in a crystal are regularly arranged, the deflections fell into regular patterns in such a way that the X-rays emerged from the crystals as a series of deflected, or diffracted, beams, which were recorded on photographic film.

From a large number of such diffraction patterns, plus the information already known about other related viruses and about the precise amino acid sequence of the proteins of the crystallized rhinovirus, Rossmann's team was able to make extremely laborious calculations to determine the positions in space of all of the atoms of the protein shell. This effort showed that the shell was constructed symmetrically on an icosahedral plan—as a roughly spherical geometric solid having 12 corners, or vertices, and 20 triangular faces, with the faces formed by protein subunits arranged and linked

together in a regular pattern. The necessary rigidity of the shell arose from the folding up of certain regions of amino acid chains into firm barrel-like structures, but there were also loops of chains rising above the surface of the shell. Although the sequences of rhinoviruses and other picornaviruses vary greatly, they are all constructed in this basic way.

Clues to how rhinoviruses attack

Medical researchers have yet to learn the full reason why rhinoviruses preferentially attack the nasal lining while, for example, polioviruses invade the intestine and the nervous system. Part of the explanation lies in the fact that rhinoviruses enter cells by combining with specific molecules, or receptors, that protrude from the surface of the target cell. Around each of the 12 icosahedral vertices of the rhinovirus particle runs a deep groove, or "canyon," which Rossmann and his colleagues theorized to be involved in the entry of the virus into cells. They suggested that a molecular structure at the bottom of the canyon interacts with protruding cellular receptors, an event that in some way triggers the virus particle to open up and release its genes into the cell. It is clear that antibody molecules that can prevent virus infection attach to amino acid chains on the rim of the canyon and in this way may interfere with the interaction between the virus and the cellular receptor. Adults are often resistant to many rhinoviruses because they have developed such antibodies as a result of previous infections.

Three groups of U.S. scientists recently identified what appeared to be the major rhinovirus receptor molecule. Two of them purified the protein from susceptible cells and then determined its amino acid sequence. The third group had been searching for a

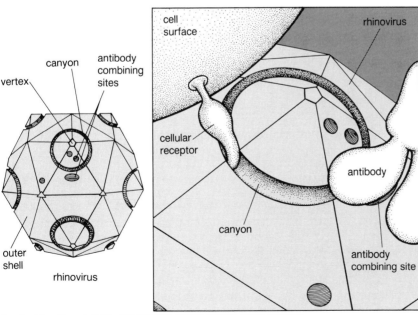

Recent research has shown that the protein shells of rhinovirus particles are constructed on the plan of a regular geometric solid called an icosahedron. Around each of the 12 vertices of the particle runs a groove, or canyon, at the bottom of which lies a structure thought to interact with protruding receptors on susceptible cells of the nasal lining, thereby causing the shell to open and insert its cargo of infectious genes into the cell. Antibody molecules that can interfere with this action may do so by attaching to combining sites near the rim of the canyon, although they are too large to reach the protected structure on the canyon floor.

Based on information provided by M.G. Rossmann and R.R. Rueckert, Purdue University

molecule that made certain cells stick to other cells as part of the immunologic and inflammatory responses the body mounts against infection and tissue damage. When they first found it, they called it intercellular adhesion molecule-1 (ICAM-1). Unexpectedly, it turned out that the amino acid sequences of this molecule and of the virus receptor are the same. Furthermore, it was found that antibody directed against the receptor prevented cells from being infected. Presumably the antibody bound to and covered up the molecule in such a way that the virus could not interact with it.

All three groups agreed that their observations might form a basis for future treatment of rhinovirus infections. For example, antibodies or some other molecule might be used to bind to the cell receptor and so prevent the virus from attacking. On the other hand, receptor molecules prepared in solution as a nasal spray might unite with free virus particles so that they could no longer attach to cells. In either case, the process of infection would be interrupted, an effect that indeed already has been demonstrated in the test tube. Whether it can be turned into a useful therapy remains to be seen.

The search for drugs to fight colds

Two lines of research on antirhinovirus drugs have been pursued in the past 10–15 years. One has been a study of chemical relatives of a compound, arildone, that inactivates viruses and prevents them from opening. Among such compounds synthesized to date, some have proved especially effective against rhinoviruses and others against enteroviruses such as polioviruses. One of these, disoxaril, was shown by means of crystallography to have inserted itself into a region at the base of the canyon in rhinovirus type 14. In that position it prevents the virus particle's opening and releasing RNA and thus initiating infection.

In the second line of research, various pharmaceutical companies pursuing independent screening programs have identified molecules that inactivate rhinoviruses in the laboratory at low concentrations. Four of these compounds were first tested in animals to show that they were not toxic and then were tested in human volunteers at the Medical Research Council's Common Cold Unit, Salisbury, England, to determine whether they would prevent colds induced by rhinoviruses. After several unsuccessful trials it was found that the last of the new molecules to be studied, code numbered R61837 and produced by the Janssen Research Institute in Belgium, did indeed prevent colds, although it was not effective if given after symptoms had appeared.

Both lines of investigation into antirhinovirus substances have since converged in that it is now clear that the compounds tested in volunteers at the Common Cold Unit interact with the same site in the canyon as does disoxaril. Such work represents important advances, for molecules are now known that specifically inactivate at least some common cold viruses, and at least one has effects in the human body. Nevertheless, further work is needed before they can be applied to the prevention or treatment of colds in the general population.

Preventing cold symptoms

Many people find a runny or blocked nose the most unpleasant part of a cold, and most cold remedies are formulated to alleviate these symptoms. If the immediate cause of the symptoms were better understood, it might be possible to devise better remedies.

Recent research has shown that during infection with cold-causing viruses, some of the cells lining the nasal passage are damaged and the hairlike processes (cilia) in the lining that clear the mucus are destroyed. Obviously, that portion of the symptoms brought on by such damage will disappear only when the nasal lining heals and replacement cells are formed. On the other hand, it appears that histamine and related substances, which produce the symptoms experienced in nasal allergies, are found only in low concentrations during colds and that drugs that block the effects of histamine provide little benefit to cold sufferers. In other words, the symptoms of colds are produced in a way different from the similar symptoms of such diseases as hay fever. More recently it was found that bradykinins, natural peptide substances (small proteins) involved in inflammation and released from injured tissue, are present in nasal secretions during colds. When given to healthy volunteers, these substances induced coldlike symptoms. The next step will be to determine whether antibradykinins, which have now been synthesized, will prevent or alleviate cold symptoms.

Both chemical and physical treatments can influence the body's response to invasion by cold viruses, and in regard to the latter approach, it recently was found that local hyperthermia (temperature elevation) of the nasal lining may be beneficial. In an experimental trial, cold sufferers received hyperthermia treatment by inhaling carefully controlled hot, moist air fully saturated with water vapor at 43° C (109° F). (Warm air that is dry is less effective in heating the nasal lining.) A single treatment—administered for at least 20 minutes once a cold had started—improved nasal symptoms. The improvement started immediately, but surprisingly some benefit persisted for several days afterward. Hyperthermia seemed to have no effect on the virus and presumably works by altering the response of the body in some as yet undiscovered way. Although the idea of using the inhalation technique to deliver complementary symptom-relieving or antiviral drugs is attractive, whether it can be done remains to be demonstrated.

—D.A.J. Tyrrell, M.D., D.Sc.

Dentistry

Space-age technology has reshaped the focus of many health-related sciences in recent years, and indeed dentistry is one of these. In North America extensive public education campaigns promoting the importance of good oral hygiene, along with the development of effective measures to combat tooth decay, have so effectively improved the dental health of the population that dental practice has evolved into one that now permits practitioners to focus on novel and elective approaches. These new approaches are ones that are responsive to the needs and desires of patients.

The generalized reduction of tooth decay has allowed dentists to focus on other facets of dentistry, among them cosmetic procedures, the treatment of sport-induced dental injuries, and the oral care of the cancer patient. Further, the promise of painless dentistry—made possible by recent developments in laser technology—may help to extend regular care to those who are so fearful of dental procedures that they hesitate even to enter the dentist's office.

Whiter, brighter teeth

References to the desirability of white teeth go back as far as biblical times ("Your teeth are like a flock of shorn ewes that have come up from the washing . . ."; Song of Solomon 4:2), and a search for magical dental whiteners proceeded through the Middle Ages. A serious scientific approach to tooth whitening was not undertaken until the end of the 19th century, however. At that time a number of different chemicals were proposed for dental bleaching. The objective was to develop a material strong enough to penetrate the crystalline structure of the enamel without damaging the sensitive tissues of the mouth and lips.

Initially, bleaching therapy was intended primarily for "nonvital" teeth, those on which root canal treatment had been performed (sometimes erroneously referred to as "dead" teeth). These devitalized teeth generally become darker with time and may be particularly unattractive when they are located in the highly visible front of the mouth. Since the nerves are no longer present in these teeth, there is no danger of nerve damage from corrosive materials that may be used in various treatments. Because of the many advances in oral hygiene and decay prevention, people are now able to keep their teeth free of caries to an extent that was never previously possible. These teeth, although healthy, are often discolored, particularly as a result of food, beverage, and tobacco stains. Today's focus is therefore on whitening vital rather than nonvital teeth. To achieve this, the active agent must be strong enough to bleach the enamel yet gentle enough not to disturb the underlying dentin and the tooth pulp.

The first modern process for tooth bleaching, which came into general use in the early 1980s, only partially

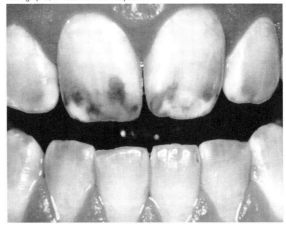

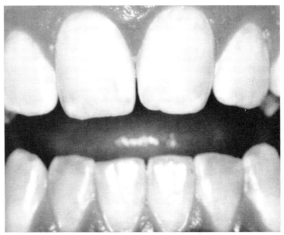

Badly discolored teeth show dramatic improvement as a result of a recently developed bleaching procedure that uses carbamide peroxide—a safe, nonirritating, and extremely effective whitener.

fulfills these conditions. In this procedure a 35% solution of hydrogen peroxide is placed on the teeth, and its rate of chemical activity is increased through the application of heat (71° C [160° F]) and light. Because the solution is quite caustic, care must be taken to keep it from coming into contact with any of the soft tissues of the mouth. The treatment process involves multiple appointments of long duration, and there are the ever present dangers of chemical burn and dessication of the teeth, which could make them fragile and prone to chipping or cracking. The potential hazards of this procedure have prevented its enthusiastic acceptance by both dental practitioners and patients, and it has never been widely used.

The most recent development in tooth whitening involves the use of carbamide peroxide, a slower acting and less reactive derivative of hydrogen peroxide. Carbamide peroxide has been used extensively for more than three decades as an intraoral antimicrobial agent. It has been shown to be nontoxic, nonaller-

261

genic, and a promoter of tissue healing. While the exact mechanism of enamel whitening has not been demonstrated, it is thought that as the peroxide breaks down into water and oxygen, it may dissolve some of the discoloring organic debris that has become lodged in between the crystals of hydroxyapatite (a calcium-containing compound) that form the enamel. The carbamide peroxide is supplied in a stabilized glycerine base that helps it to adhere to oral surfaces. Additional substances in the gel adjust the pH (acid-alkaline balance) of the whitening liquid approximately to neutral, which prevents inadvertent etching (surface roughening), and associated weakening, of the enamel.

After a thorough examination and cleaning, the dentist takes an impression of the teeth and uses it to fabricate thin, flexible, transparent plastic "trays" for the upper and lower dental arches. The trays fit over the teeth and, when filled with carbamide peroxide, keep the bleaching agent in close proximity to the tooth surfaces. The gel-like consistency of the substance prevents saliva from mixing readily with the whitening agent, thus keeping it from becoming diluted and, eventually, swallowed. It takes only an hour or so for the patient to become accustomed to wearing the trays, which are hardly visible and may be worn in public without attracting undue attention. The trays need be removed only at mealtimes. The patient is asked to avoid eating acidic foods for the duration of the treatment because they may slow the whitening process or make the mouth more sensitive to the bleaching agent. At regular intervals, the patient removes the trays briefly to add a few additional drops of the whitening solution. The overall duration of the treatment varies from three to six weeks, depending on the nature of the stains and the patient's compliance in wearing the tray. The patient is monitored weekly by the dentist to evaluate the whitening process. Very rarely, a transient irritation of the gums may be noted. This is generally caused by an ill-fitting or broken tray rather than by the bleaching agent itself.

It has been found that yellow stains respond more quickly and more completely to whitening procedures than do grayish discolorations. While the results of carbamide peroxide treatment are variable, depending on the source of the stain and the depth to which it penetrates the enamel, generally all teeth exposed to carbamide peroxide—including those stained by tetracyclines—will exhibit some whitening. The longevity of the whitening effect has not yet been established, as the procedure is fairly new and recurrences of staining have not yet been observed. Even if it should be found that stains do return after several years, it is a simple matter to rewhiten the teeth with a touch-up procedure. Tooth whitening by means of bleaching is desirable from the point of view of both patients and dentists, as it represents an effective and relatively safe method for improving the appearance of the teeth

without the need for extensive dental procedures. The approximate cost for whitening both upper and lower teeth is about the same as the cost of a single crown.

Laser dentistry: painless, accurate, fast

The whine of the dental drill may soon be a sound of the past, replaced instead by the soft hiss of a laser. Dental lasers promise to revolutionize the removal of decay and the treatment of gum disease; root canal procedures and oral surgery will also undoubtedly be transformed by laser use. Lasers are named for the type of crystal that is electrically charged to emit the characteristic beam. In the case of the dental laser, the medium is a crystal of neodymium: yttrium-aluminum-garnet, called Nd:YAG or, simply, YAG. Carbon dioxide lasers, widely used in dental treatment, are suitable only for soft-tissue surgery. They cannot be used on hard tissues (teeth and bone), as the heat buildup from the laser beam tends to destroy the dental structures.

The YAG laser has the potential for use on both the soft tissues of the mouth and the teeth. The feature that makes the YAG acceptable for use on the teeth is a pulsing mechanism. The pulse lasts about 100 microseconds and is repeated 10–30 times each second. The thermal energy that is delivered to the target structures vaporizes them while concurrently preventing heat from accumulating. This latter feature eliminates the potential for heat damage to the nerves. The ultrashort duration of the laser pulse provides an added bonus—the burst of energy is so short that it does not stimulate the pain-receptor nerves. Therefore, most procedures that utilize laser dentistry can be accomplished without anesthesia, a great boon for those who dread intraoral injections of local anesthetics.

The laser unit is a self-contained apparatus that can be plugged into any electrical outlet. The machine generates two coaxial laser beams that are delivered through a fiber-optic cable to an instrument that is designed in the familiar shape of a dental drill. The YAG beam is in the infrared spectrum and is thus invisible to the human eye. A HeNe (helium-neon) aiming beam provides a red dot that guides the operator precisely to the surgical site. The dentist can adjust the pulse rate and the intensity of the laser emission. Because the normal, healthy tooth surface reflects and scatters the beam, the laser has no effect on healthy enamel. The darker areas of decay and organic debris absorb the beam and are vaporized. As a result of this selectivity of operation, the YAG laser represents the most conservative of all methods for removing decay. The heat of the beam also destroys any residual decay- or infection-causing bacteria that may be present in the teeth or the other oral tissues that are being lased. The patient may experience a slight warming sensation in a tooth that is being treated by YAG laser, but it never reaches the point of pain or even serious discomfort. It should be noted, again, that the use of the

The current rage for skateboarding is international, and so too is the epidemic of resulting injuries. Even though the sport was outlawed in Norway prior to 1989, many, like this Oslo youth, found it hard to resist the thrill. Unfortunately, most skateboarders are blissfully unaware of the potential for trauma, particularly to the skull, jaw, and teeth. While younger children are the most vulnerable to accidents involving the head—and teeth—teenagers are usually the most reckless, and while they have fewer head injuries, these are often more serious.

YAG laser for removing decayed areas of teeth is still experimental in the U.S. The procedure itself is quite new and is available only in some dental practices.

Sensitivity of the dentin (the substance immediately under the enamel on the root surfaces) is reduced or eliminated by the laser as it rearranges the surface crystalline structures, leaving them smoother and more regular and thus more impervious to external stimuli. In fact, this is the first specific treatment that has been made available to patients who suffer from chronic tooth sensitivity—the pain that is elicited by anything cold or sweet touching certain parts of the undecayed tooth surface. When used in soft-tissue surgery, the YAG laser makes a very fine, precise incision. The tissue necrosis that this "laser scalpel" leaves is so minimal that healing occurs at a much faster rate than with conventional surgery. The laser beam also ensures a dry field of operation; as the laser cuts, it cauterizes small blood vessels. Simultaneously, it sterilizes the wound, thus reducing postoperative infections and the resultant need for antibiotics. Furthermore, the dentist has a greatly improved view of the surgical area and can complete the work more quickly and precisely.

It is this latter capacity, elimination of the need to "freeze" the nerves in the affected area, that is potentially the greatest advantage of laser technology in dentistry. It is estimated that almost half of all adults in North America do not seek regular dental care. Many of these people avoid necessary treatment out of fear of pain. In fact, current oral anesthesia techniques are sufficient to eliminate virtually all dental pain. Nonetheless, the memory of unpleasant experiences is sometimes strong enough to overcome logic, and some people are unable to face dental procedures even with the knowledge that reliable anesthetics are available. With the advent of painless laser dental procedures, they may now change their minds.

The speed, accuracy, and broad applicability of laser dentistry indicates that this mode of treatment will be involved in an increasing number of dental procedures in the near future. It is possible that within the next decade or so, the laser will become an integral part of every dentist's equipment.

Skateboarding and dental injuries

Not surprisingly, "epidemics" of injuries have coincided with trends in the popularity of skateboards. A peak occurred in 1977, when over 150,000 accidents involving skateboards were recorded in the United States alone. By 1983, as the sport fell in popularity, this number had decreased to about 16,000. Since then, however, such incidents have been increasing at an alarming rate. In 1985, 36 children died from injuries directly attributable to skateboarding accidents. Very young children, who are comparatively less capable of using their hands and arms to break a fall from a skateboard, tend to suffer the highest percentage of head and neck injuries. Among children under four years of age, 75% of the trauma caused by such a fall is to the head region, where often the teeth are involved. The dental injuries sustained by children in this age group are most likely to deciduous teeth. Thus, if prompt dental attention is provided, ensuring that there has been no damage to the underlying permanent teeth, it is likely that no long-term dental problems will result.

In youngsters aged five to nine, however, recently erupted permanent front teeth are greatly at risk. These teeth tend to be larger than the surrounding ones and more prominent and therefore are likely to be among the first structures of the head that come into contact with an object during an unexpected impact. In skateboard accidents in this age group, fully 50% involve the head region, and the potential for permanent dental damage is very high. Teeth may be chipped, broken, or completely knocked out. Beyond the initial pain and expense that are involved, such ac-

263

cidents may have long-term effects on the individual's appearance and, ultimately, self-confidence.

The pattern of injuries in teens is quite different. Teenagers are using their skateboards on streets and highways, often recklessly and at quite high speeds. Teens are more adept at breaking a fall and therefore sustain more injuries to their legs, arms, and hands; only 15% of their accidents involve the head, but these tend to be much more serious than in younger skateboarders.

Considering the extent and scope of skateboard injuries occurring today, with the risk of serious damage to the skull, jaw, and teeth, the use of a padded helmet and face guard should be mandatory. In American football, both professional and amateur, the mandatory use of helmets (instituted in 1959) has reduced dental and facial injuries by 98%. Furthermore, the injuries that do occur are less severe and thus less costly to treat. Because skateboards can be so dangerous, younger children, whose coordination is not well developed, should not be permitted to use them. And all skateboarders should stay away from traffic.

Dental care of patients with cancer

Cancer treatments create conditions that require special consideration by both the patient and the dentist. The major areas of concern are dental procedures that

Because cancer patients undergoing radiotherapy are vulnerable to infection and have reduced healing capacity, it is important for them to attend to existing dental problems before they begin such treatments.

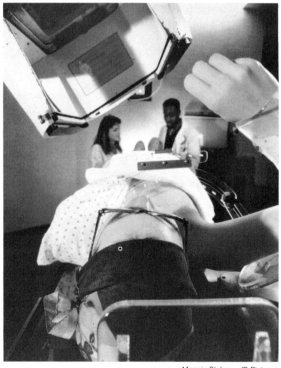

Maggie Steber—JB Pictures

should be done prior to treatment and oral hygiene needs after radiation or chemotherapy. Proper dental care is an area now being addressed more routinely in cancer treatment than it was in the past.

Patients who are about to receive head and neck radiation or chemotherapy or both require a thorough dental evaluation. Severely decayed teeth and those compromised by gum disease need to be extracted as soon as possible; because the individual's ability to withstand infection will be reduced following therapy, the dentist's goal is to eliminate all potential sources of oral infection. The healing capacity of the tissues is also diminished by radiation and drug therapy. For this reason radiotherapy generally is not initiated for at least 14 days after tooth extractions. At that time the dentist assesses the oral tissues, and if any bone remains exposed, therapy needs to be delayed for several more days. The remaining teeth are then cleaned and smoothed, and the patient is instructed in a thorough oral-hygiene regimen. Dentures, both partial and complete, need to be evaluated and corrected so that they will not traumatize the oral tissues. Patients are instructed to remove any dental prosthesis that causes discomfort during cancer therapy.

Following radiation or chemotherapy, both home and office dental care are fairly routine; particular attention needs to be paid to effective oral hygiene and preventive measures. Routine cleanings, X-rays, fillings, and root canal treatments can be safely performed at this time. Crowns, bridges, and dentures pose no medical or dental problems to the patient undergoing cancer treatment. The only dental procedures that are contraindicated are tooth extractions, periodontal (gum) surgery, and surgical endodontics (root canal treatment) within the irradiated area. Occasionally, oral irritations develop during or after cancer drug or radiation treatment. Mouthwashes that contain alcohol or phenol tend to further aggravate the situation. A chlorhexidine rinse will minimize oral infection and reduce inflammation.

One of the major causes of oral discomfort after head or neck radiotherapy is xerostomia, or dry mouth, caused by the deterioration of the salivary glands that occurs as a frequent side effect of the treatment. Lacking their natural lubrication, the oral tissues become irritated and fragile. Anesthetic gels and alcohol-based mouthwashes will exacerbate the problem. A simple and effective mouth rinse is a diluted sodium bicarbonate solution (one teaspoon per liter or quart of water) that can be made at home. Where oral irritation is already present, an ultrasoft toothbrush or a sponge-type cleaner may be substituted for a stiff toothbrush. A program of meticulous oral hygiene is the first and most important step in the oral rehabilitation of patients who have undergone head and neck radiotherapy.

—*George A. Freedman, D.D.S.*

The New Oxford English Dictionary: Keeping Up with Medicine

by Alan M. Hughes, M.A.

People tend to talk of "the dictionary" as they do of the Bible—as though it were unique—yet there are many different dictionaries of varying degrees of authority. The *Oxford English Dictionary* is the largest dictionary of the English language, now occupying 20 volumes of 21,728 pages and holding a unique position in the English-speaking world. It was first published between 1884 and 1928 (in fascicles) and filled 15,488 pages. In 1933 it was reissued in 12 volumes with a new one-volume supplement; the supplement included words that arrived on the scene too late to be included in the main work, such as *appendicitis* (coined in 1886) and *psycho-analyse* (1923).

In 1957 work began on another supplement, again to add words and meanings not included in the parent work. It was soon recognized that the growth of the language was such that one volume would be insufficient; thus, the *Supplement to the Oxford English Dictionary* (incorporating that of 1933) came out in four volumes between 1972 and 1986. It included terms such as (*intravenous*) *drip* (first recorded in 1933), *pathway* (within the nervous system; 1924), and the antibiotic *tetracycline* (1952). It was during the preparation of the first of these four volumes that Oxford University Press, the dictionary's publisher, took on scientifically trained staff for the first time, since scientific vocabulary made up a large proportion of the new words and meanings to be included in the supplement.

What makes the *OED* (as it is commonly known) unique is its historical treatment of each word, phrase, and meaning. Every item included is traced back to its first recorded appearance in the language, and its history is presented by a number of quotations of various dates, beginning with the first known use. This is in addition to the usual information given in a dictionary, such as definitions and etymologies. When other dictionaries give dates from before the mid-20th century, they are usually derived from the *OED*.

A dictionary cannot be kept up-to-date properly by the addition of successive supplements, so in 1983 Oxford University Press established the New Oxford English Dictionary Project. The investment was £10 million. One objective was to produce a second edition that integrated the two works, the *OED* and the *Supplement,* as well as incorporating new material, and this edition was duly published in March 1989 to worldwide acclaim.

Establishing an electronic data base

A major achievement of the second-edition project is not apparent from the printed volumes, however. A second objective was to turn the two works into an electronic data base, so that the whole work would exist in electronic form. The earlier versions of the dictionary had been typeset the old way—in hot metal. By the 1980s, however, computer technology had reached a state of sophistication that made it a highly appropriate tool for the task being undertaken by the New Oxford English Dictionary Project. The establishment of a computer data base would facilitate the integration of the *OED* and *Supplement* and readily enable the editors to annotate and update the text on a regular basis. Creating a data base would also make future electronic versions of the resource possible. (Currently the first edition—that published in 1928—is available commercially on compact disc [CD-ROM]. An electronic form of the second edition is expected to be on the market sometime in the 1990s.)

For the purpose of preparing the new edition, the electronic text was tagged so that, for instance, every etymology is preceded by an etymology tag, <etym>, and followed by an end tag, </etym>. Such tagging enables the electronic text to be readily searched for an etymology. Other tags include parts of speech, subject labels (*Med., Math.,* and so forth), and cross-references. As a result of this kind of breakdown of the text (known as parsing), information is available not only via the alphabetical position of each individual dictionary entry but also by the nature of the information itself. One can, for example, look at all the definitions with a medical subject label (*e.g., Med., Path., Anat., Biochem.*), all the quotations taken from the *Journal of the American Medical Association,* or all the occurrences of the word *neuron* or *neurone.* In the data base these assorted tags are distinguished from each entry's text proper by angle brackets, < >, and do not appear in printed versions of the dictionary.

The project was very much a cooperative one. The management and lexicography took place in Oxford; the keyboarding and tagging of the text were done by International Computaprint Corp. in Tampa, Fla., and Fort Washington, Pa.; IBM donated equipment and loaned both software and personnel; and the University of Waterloo, Ont., assisted in the design of the data-base system and the writing of the parsing

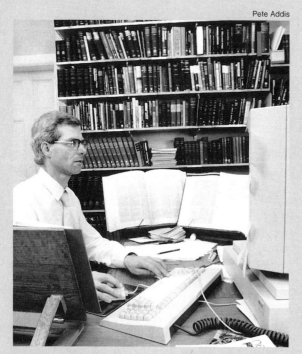

Scientific lexicographer Alan Hughes searches for new medical words by using the electronic data base established to facilitate the preparation of the monumental second edition of the Oxford English Dictionary, *published in 1989.*

software that would enhance the tagging of the text. The software used to edit the text and automatically integrate the *OED* and *Supplement* was written in Oxford by Oxford University Press staff (the integration program received the name OEDIPUS—OED Integration, Proofing, and Updating System). The typesetting was done in Yorkshire, England, and the printing in Massachusetts.

Collecting new words

Although the primary purposes of the project were the integration of the two texts and their conversion into an electronic data base rather than a full-scale revision of the *OED* text, opportunity was taken to add about 5,000 new words and meanings to the *OED2*, as the second edition is now familiarly known. This edition contains about 290,000 main entries and includes 140,000 pronunciations, 220,000 etymologies, and 2,430,000 illustrative quotations. The number of entries added reflects the time devoted to the task and staff available to research and write the entries more than it does the growth per se of the English language.

The actual acquisition of new words and meanings resulted from an ongoing reading program. Paid readers regularly go through selected books, magazines, newspapers, and journals and copy onto 10 × 15-cm (4 × 6-in) slips quotations for any new or unusual lexical item that they come across. The slips are entered into a cumulative quotation file that serves as

a resource for all of the many dictionaries that are published by Oxford University Press.

During the 1980s the reading program was supplemented by commercial data bases of periodicals and books, such as NEXIS and DIALOG. (NEXIS provides on-line access to newspapers, magazines, wire services, and other full-text information from a wide array of fields; DIALOG operates an on-line information retrieval service from professional associations, publishers, government agencies, and many other sources.) These can be useful in seeking early examples of very recent terms, in assessing currency (in some cases), and in supplying additional quotations in order to provide a more complete record, but they are of little help in finding new words. Given the word *enkephalin,* for example, one can use DIALOG to search medical journals to discover when or whether the spelling *encephalin* has been used (*enceph-* rather than *enkeph-* being the usual English representative of the Greek *egkephalos,* "brain"), but one cannot ask DIALOG, "What new terms are there for neurochemical compounds?" Another drawback for lexicographers of such data bases is that they do not by themselves differentiate between different meanings of a word. A drug name such as *tolbutamide* usually has only one meaning, and any occurrence found by means of a data-base search is likely to be relevant. The situation is different, however, with a word like *tolerance.* Even in a medical context there are at least three different meanings the word may have: "diminished response to a drug after continued use," "the ability of an organism to survive despite infection with a pathogen," and "the ability to accept without an immune reaction an antigen that normally causes one." Given a printout of 50 instances of *tolerance* from medical sources, each one has to be read in context by an editor knowledgeable enough to differentiate these three meanings before such a list can be of any use.

The ability to differentiate senses of a medical or scientific term is also required for collecting new words, which makes the job of reading for scientific items something of a specialist activity. A naive reader may well not recognize the noun *flutter* as having a more specific meaning than "quivering" when used in connection with the heart.

The ever enlarging vocabulary of medicine

The first edition of the *Oxford English Dictionary* and its *Supplement* contained about 9,500 medical words. All these were retained in *OED2* and a further 300 were added, most of them in the first half of the alphabet. This reflects the fact that the later part of the alphabet was more up-to-date in the *Supplement;* volume IV (Se–Z) was published in 1986, volume I (A–G) in 1972. One might expect the additions to be recently coined words, but this is so only in a minority of cases. The additions do include recent terms, such as *legionnaires' disease* (the earliest known use being in 1976); *legionella,* its causative bacterium (1979), and *legionellosis,* infection with the bacterium (also 1979); *AIDS* (first recorded in the *Morbidity and Mortality Weekly Report* of the U.S. Centers for Disease Control for Sept. 24, 1982); *endorphin* (1976), a morphinelike compound in the brain; and *enkephalin* (1975), a particular kind of endorphin. But the additions also include many terms that have existed for some time, such as *amniocentesis* (1958), *Delhi belly* (1944), *Kaposi's sarcoma* (1897), and *anorectic* (1894).

The reason for the inclusion of older terms only in a 1989 publication is partly due to the size of the *OED,* paradoxical as that may sound. The last part of the original *OED* was published in 1928, and there have been only three occasions since then when a word could have been added—1933, in the first supplement; 1972–86, in the second *Supplement;* and 1989, in *OED2.* Thus, a word that came to the dictionary editors' attention too late had to wait a considerable time before it could be included. This is in contrast to the situation with the smaller Oxford dictionaries such as the *Little Oxford Dictionary of Current English* (688 pages), the *Concise Oxford Dictionary of Current English* (1,454 pages), and the *Oxford Reference Dictionary* (992 pages). They can be revised more frequently, every five or six years, and can be more up-to-date with the more common words that they include (*amniocentesis,* for example, was in the sixth edition of the *Concise Oxford Dictionary* in 1976, 13 years before it made it into the *OED*).

Another factor is the nature and extent of the literature drawn on for new words and meanings. So much medical literature is published in so many specialties that no dictionary maker can do more than sample it. If a word is widely used, it is soon represented in the *OED*'s quotation files. Such was the case with *enkephalin* and *endorphin;* coined in 1975 and 1976,

Endorphin was one of 300 new medical terms included in OED2. What makes this dictionary unique, aside from its being the largest dictionary of the English language, is that every word is traced back to its first recorded appearance.

endorphin (ɛnˈdɔːfɪn). *Biochem.* [ad. F. *endorphine* (E. Simon: see *Compt. Rend.* (1976) Ser. D. CCLXXXII. 785), f. *endogène* ENDOGENOUS *a.* + *morphine* MORPHINE.] Any of a group of peptides that occur naturally in the brain and bind to the same receptors as does morphine.
  1976 *Proc. Nat. Acad. Sci.* LXXIII. 3942 1 We have reported isolating from a crude extract of (porcine) hypothalamus-neurohypophysis three peptides named endorphins. **1978** *Nature* 22 June 675/1 Recent research has led to the hypothesis that acupuncture produces analgesia through the release of endorphins. **1983** *Oxf. Textbk. Med.* II. xxi. 21/1 Electrical stimulation of nerve trunks or of cutaneous nerves can result in endorphins appearing in the cerebrospinal fluid, presumably indicating activation of pain inhibitory mechanisms.

respectively, they were first represented in the quotation files in 1975 and 1977. *Kaposi's sarcoma,* on the other hand, had been around for many years but was rather obscure until it attracted attention as one of the symptoms of AIDS; it first arrived in the quotation files in 1978, but not until 1983 was the evidence sufficient to make the scientific staff lexicographers decide that an *OED* entry should be written for it.

To include or not to include?

This raises another point: given that a word is represented in the quotation files, what are the criteria for including it in a dictionary? Currency in the language is the short answer, to which quotation files are but a guide. For most dictionaries this means present-day currency; for a historical dictionary like the *OED,* past currency also counts, a point to be addressed below.

Ideally one would like to include in a large dictionary every term current in the language, but this is a practical impossibility. Finite resources and a competitive market mean that some degree of selectivity is necessary even in the largest dictionary. The number of quotations in the quotation file is one criterion for inclusion; it is crude but has the advantage that its application is a clerical rather than a lexicographical task. It is supplemented by the lexicographer's own knowledge, information from textbooks, and the expertise provided by specialist consultants. Sometimes the research for one entry brings to a lexicographer's attention another word that should be included. For example, investigations of the terms *anorectic* and *anorexic* prompted the editors to include the word *anorexigenic* as well. The latter had been represented in Oxford's files by one quotation only and had been passed over in the initial sorting procedure, but research on the other two words showed that *anorexigenic* too had sufficient currency to be included. (It was first used in 1948 in the *Annals of Internal Medicine:* "We chose to decrease the desire for food by administering anorexigenic compounds of a type similar to 'Benzedrine.' ")

A similar case occurs when a derivative of a word already in the *OED* comes to the staff's notice. The 1972 *Supplement* included the noun *agammaglobulinæmia* ("lack of gamma globulin in the blood," first used in 1952), and sooner or later one would expect the adjective *agammaglobulinæmic* to be used, but the editors had no record of that form during the 1960s when the "A" entries for the *Supplement* were being prepared. By the time work on *OED2* was begun, there was such a record, and the term was duly included (with a first quotation dated 1957).

What is meant by a record is an independent record of a word used in context—not an entry in some other dictionary. Other dictionaries are occasionally quoted, usually when they contain the earliest instance of a word that it has been possible to find. (*Anoretic* provides two dictionary references: one to *Gould's Med-*

ical Dictionary of 1926, which contains *anoretic* as a misprint for *anorectic*, and another to *Webster's Third New International Dictionary* of 1961, which includes the word and predates any use of it otherwise discoverable.) But the fact that a medical term occurs in as many as three medical dictionaries does not by itself carry the same weight as three examples of its actual use. The *OED* is a dictionary of record and aims to draw on primary source material. In this respect present policy is stricter than that prevailing during the writing of the original *OED*. The original contained many medical words for which the only source cited was the *Lexicon of Medicine and Allied Sciences,* published by the New Sydenham Society, 1879–89, or less often *An Expository Lexicon of the Terms, Ancient and Modern, in Medical and General Science* by Robert G. Mayne (1860). Examples are *dolichopodous* ("having long feet") and *pareccrisis* ("disordered secretion"). These are not in current medical dictionaries, and they may be considered for omission from a future edition of the *OED* on grounds of insufficient usage.

Not including words previously included is different from omitting words because they have become obsolete, a practice *not* followed by the *OED*. Future editions are likely to retain obsolete words such as *incide* ("to make an incision") and *suffumigation* ("fumigating from below" as a therapeutic technique or a practice of witchcraft).

A factor that does not affect a term's inclusion in the *OED* is its technical nature. Many definitions of scientific words have to contain technical terms if they are to have the precision and information expected of a large dictionary. Many bacterial names, for example, have the terms *Gram-negative* or *Gram-positive* in their definition, and that of AIDS mentions a retrovirus. It is recognized that a full definition of a technical term will sometimes not be fully understandable to a person who has no acquaintance with the field. Medical terms, especially those of pathology and surgery, are among the less problematic in this respect; the hardest definitions to write for a layperson to understand are those in mathematics and petrography.

What the *OED*'s scientific lexicographers do aim for—like any good lexicographers—is not to define a word by using a term that is not itself defined in the dictionary. (This is another factor contributing to a decision to include a word.) In the writing of entries for the *Supplement* and *OED2,* a similar principle was adopted in relation to quotations, though held to less rigorously: if a word occurred in a quotation printed in the dictionary, an endeavor was made to include that word as a dictionary entry.

OED2 versus medical dictionaries

In its coverage of medical terms, how does the 20-volume *OED2* compare with medical dictionaries? As mentioned above, the former contains about 9,800 medical terms; most standard large medical dictionaries contain between 15,000 and 20,000. The widely used *Dorland's Illustrated Medical Dictionary* has 278 entries for words beginning *neuro-; OED2* has 199. Of course, *OED2* is not primarily a medical dictionary but a historical one (indeed the only historical one of the English language as a whole). Medical dictionaries do not tell one, for example, that all the words related to the term *anorexia* date from 1894 or later except for *anorexia* itself, which (as *anorexie*) has been around for almost 400 years and in 1873 acquired the epithet *nervosa*. Similarly one learns from *OED2* that although *Cæsar,* as slang for a cesarean section, is first recorded in 1952, the word was used to mean "a baby delivered by cesarean section" as long ago as 1540; and *HIV,* the virus to which AIDS is attributed, had appeared in print before its formal coinage in a scientific journal.

This last point illustrates Oxford's concern to track each word to its earliest use. During the preparation of *OED2* there was no question about including *HTLV* and its successor *HIV,* and there was no difficulty tracing *HIV* to the issue of *Nature* (May 1, 1986) where the name human immunodeficiency virus and its abbreviation were first proposed. Subsequently, however, it was discovered that the name occurred in print a few weeks earlier as a rumor. *Capital Gay,* a London periodical for homosexuals, reported in its issue of April 11, 1986: "An international committee on viral names has been looking into the problem, and was rumoured to have agreed on 'human immune deficiency virus' (HIDV or HIV)." And this quotation duly appears in *OED2*.

New directions in medical vocabulary

On the basis of the extensive work of selecting words for inclusion in *OED2,* is there a trend discernible in medical terminology? Acronyms are a 20th-century development. An early one, now included in *OED2,* was *bipp* ("bismuth iodoform paraffin paste"), a dressing for wounds used during World War I. Two modern terms suggest a new degree of informality in word formation. *Lumpectomy,* also in *OED2,* is a partial mastectomy and dates from 1972; it is unusual for words ending in *-ectomy* to be formed from an ordinary English word (*lump*) rather than a Greek or Latin stem; a traditionally formed word would have been *thraumectomy,* from Greek *thrauma* ("fragment"). And in 1977 a physical sign was named not after its discoverer but after an entertainer who did not have the condition. The Terry-Thomas sign is a gap between two bones of the wrist, diagnostic of a rotational dislocation of the navicular bone of the hand. It is named after Terry-Thomas, a British comedian whose smile was made more engaging by a prominent gap in his upper front teeth. It joins the ever growing waiting list for inclusion in *OED3,* planned to appear early in the next millennium.

Disasters

It is primarily through television and newspapers that most people in the United States learn about the massive environmental destruction and personal devastation wrought by natural disasters such as hurricanes, earthquakes, volcanic eruptions, tidal waves, and avalanches. The natural tendency is to conclude that disasters are something that happens to other people, in some other, distant part of the world. During a 30-day period in the fall of 1989, however, two dramatic though very different natural disasters hit much closer to home—Hurricane Hugo on the East Coast and the Loma Prieta earthquake in the San Francisco Bay area. Since then many other parts of the world have been struck by other equally catastrophic events—Peru, Iran, and the Philippines sustained heavy losses in earthquakes in 1990 (in Iran alone, about 40,000 people were believed to have been killed)—but it will be some time before the full import of these more recent disasters is known and the extent of the destruction assessed. But in the year or so that has passed since Hurricane Hugo and the California earthquake, the impacts have become evident; both situations have been studied and now provide some meaningful lessons about how to improve public health preparedness for, and response to, natural disasters.

Hurricane Hugo: landfall and after

Hurricane Hugo was the sixth Atlantic hurricane of 1989. On Sunday, September 17, with sustained winds up to 225 km/h (140 mph), Hugo struck the eastern Caribbean islands of Guadeloupe, Antigua, Dominica, Montserrat, and Tortola, among others. On September 18 the storm moved to Puerto Rico and the U.S. Virgin Islands (St. Croix, St. Thomas, and St. John). Hugo hit the continental U.S. at Charleston, S.C., on September

21. Thereafter, downgraded to a tropical storm, Hugo headed northwest through Charlotte, N.C., Charleston, W.Va., and Zanesville, Ohio. The greatest environmental impact was in the Caribbean, where Hugo caused massive damage to airports, public buildings, hospitals, schools, hotels, and residences. Telephone and radio communications and electric service and water supplies were disrupted; food crops were damaged; and additional rainfall, with associated flooding and landslides, compounded the impact of the storm.

The island of St. Croix was particularly hard hit. Eighty percent of the infrastructure was initially reported destroyed. Electric, water, and telephone services were completely disrupted. Initial urgent problems included inadequate security to prevent looting in heavily damaged neighborhoods, inadequate measures to ensure public safety, and lack of vehicles and manpower to distribute food and drinkable water. In addition, the St. Croix Hospital had to be closed and 120 patients evacuated.

The part of the continental United States that sustained the greatest environmental impact was Charleston and the surrounding coastal areas of the state of South Carolina. There were utility disruptions and extensive property destruction, and many roads were blocked by fallen trees and debris; several evacuation centers and bridges were seriously damaged. It was apparent from the amount of structural wreckage that in many cases building codes were inadequate or enforcement of them had been lax. Sand dunes were destroyed and needed to be rebuilt to prevent future flooding. Other noncoastal areas of South and North Carolina sustained relatively smaller amounts of damage, and no major environmental devastation was reported north of Charlotte.

Hurricane Hugo resulted in at least 62 injury-related deaths, the largest number of them in South Carolina

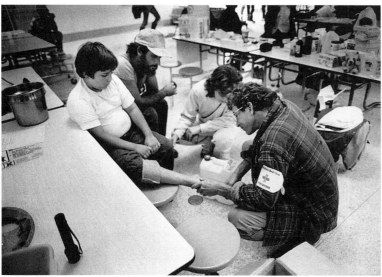

American Red Cross

A Red Cross volunteer helps a youngster injured when Hurricane Hugo struck Charleston, South Carolina, in September 1989. The city was heavily damaged by high winds and flooding; the state sustained 29 storm-related deaths—drownings, people crushed by falling trees and buildings, electrocutions, and people killed in home fires. Still, advance warning of the storm and well-executed evacuation plans were credited with having saved countless lives in low-lying coastal areas along Hugo's path.

(29) and Puerto Rico (9). In South Carolina people were killed both during Hugo's passing (six persons drowned, five were crushed by or in their homes, and two were hit by falling trees) and soon after (nine in house fires, four by electrocution, two from falling trees, and one in an accident with a chain saw). In Puerto Rico associated deaths occurred immediately before (one electrocution), during (two drownings), and soon after (six electrocutions) the hurricane. There were numerous cases of minor injuries (lacerations and puncture wounds from debris) and stress-related physical ailments reported soon afterward. The human toll—in terms of death, injury, and illness—associated with the hazards of recovery after the storm far exceeded those from the winds and high seas during the storm. There were reports of individual cases of disease (gastrointestinal disorders resulting from contaminated food or water; respiratory infections transmitted in the close quarters of temporary shelters), but there were no epidemics. Hundreds of thousands of people were at least temporarily left homeless.

Relief for Hugo's victims

The Federal Emergency Management Agency has the primary responsibility for coordinating the response to domestic disasters. Initially, assessment of the extent of the damage from Hurricane Hugo and coordination of relief efforts were hampered by the loss of ordinary telecommunications; high-frequency radio links had to be established, which involved a delay and meant that access to communications equipment was limited. On September 20 Pres. George Bush declared the U.S. Virgin Islands a disaster area; similar declarations were made for Puerto Rico on September 21, South Carolina on September 22, and North Carolina on September 25. On September 29 Bush signed a $1.1 billion relief package that had been approved by Congress for victims of Hugo in all four areas.

Response to emergency public health needs was a joint effort of state and local governments, federal health agencies, and public and private relief organizations. The United States Public Health Service sent disaster medical assistance teams to St. Croix and assisted in restocking the island's medical supplies. Federal epidemiological surveillance and health care assessment teams were sent to assist the local and state government and health department officials. Surveillance systems for the reporting of illness and injury were established by local and state health departments, which also assumed the chief responsibility for assessing sanitation facilities, controlling disease-causing organisms, assuring food and water safety, evaluating the structural soundness of hospitals and other centers providing medical services, assessing the need for medical equipment and supplies, and providing guidance on health matters to disaster relief workers.

Medical supplies and equipment were provided by AmeriCares, a private, voluntary relief organization made up of U.S. manufacturers and distributors of medical supplies and equipment and pharmaceuticals. Other volunteer agencies also provided food, clothing, and medical and shelter supplies. The American Red Cross provided medical assistance, helped with care of the homeless (including the setting up of temporary shelters), and aided with inquiries about victims.

The Loma Prieta earthquake

The Loma Prieta earthquake, the first major earthquake on the San Andreas Fault since the 1906 San Francisco earthquake, occurred at 5:04 PM on Oct. 17, 1989. Measuring 7.1 on the Richter scale, the quake was felt as far away as Los Angeles and Reno, Nev. It ranked among the strongest earthquakes in the U.S. in the 20th century and resulted in property losses and recovery costs estimated at $10 billion.

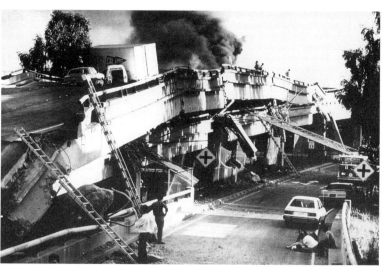

A 1.6-kilometer (one-mile) section of Interstate 880 (Nimitz Freeway) collapsed during the evening rush hour when an earthquake measuring 7.1 on the Richter scale hit the San Francisco Bay area on Oct. 17, 1989. Aided by residents of the nearby community, emergency crews converged on the scene to rescue motorists trapped in crushed vehicles on the freeway's lower deck. The largest number—two-thirds—of a total of 63 confirmed fatalities in the quake occurred at this site.

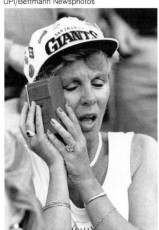

A woman at San Francisco's Candlestick Park waiting for the start of the third game of the 1989 World Series registers shock as she hears of the extensive earthquake that has just struck the city. The ballpark itself was not damaged, and the crowd was evacuated without incident.

The Goodyear Blimp, covering the third game of the World Series at Candlestick Park, quickly provided the world with pictures of the most memorable damage—the I-880 (Nimitz Freeway) collapse in Oakland, the Marina District fire in San Francisco, and the collapse of a section of the Bay Bridge. In terms of total destruction, the Marina District sustained the worst damage. Two factors minimized the effect of the earthquake on the environment: the quality of building construction and the relatively short time of shaking—6–10 seconds. Had the quake lasted as long as the similarly extensive one that occurred in 1988 in Armenia—30 seconds—there would have been far greater soil liquefaction, and many more buildings would have collapsed. An unanticipated environmental impact of the quake was a significant reduction in air pollution in the Bay Area for several weeks afterward, the result of decreased motor vehicle traffic.

There were 63 confirmed fatalities and 3,757 injuries; more than 12,000 persons were left homeless, many of whom were chronically ill or had been staying in shelters for the homeless that sustained quake damage. Nevertheless, Loma Prieta did not result in a disaster in terms of health care. The health care system was probably most strained in Santa Cruz county, where one of the three local hospitals was heavily damaged. No major medical facility was taken out of commission, however, and many successfully implemented their emergency disaster plans.

Quake aftershocks—physical and emotional

Mental health and stress-related problems presented the most significant medical challenge in the aftermath of the quake. Aftershocks upset already frayed nerves, especially among the homeless, the poor, and Armenian children receiving medical care in the Bay Area, who had to relive the terror of the devastating earthquake that had ravaged their homeland the preceding year. It was estimated that the psychological impact alone reduced employee productivity 20–30%

in the Bay Area during the first few weeks after the earthquake. Interestingly, there were large increases in attendance at northern California golf courses, perhaps reflecting a desire to be out-of-doors and away from buildings. The psychological impact was also felt outside the state; even though tourist-oriented attractions were not damaged, Bay Area tourism was affected, and would-be newcomers became reluctant to move to the state. Some businesses, fearful of sustaining worse damage in a future quake, decided to relocate outside the area. Psychological effects were even experienced by residents of other areas of the United States, such as those who live along the New Madrid Fault, which runs along the Mississippi River valley from Tennessee to Illinois; that fault, in 1811–12, generated a series of the most powerful tremors ever known in North America, and another devastating quake has been predicted for the area, possibly in the not-too-distant future.

An initial public health concern in San Francisco was the limited communication available to those responding to the disaster, which may have resulted in a lack of information on the extent of casualties and damage. Another concern was the possibility that aftershocks would cause further damage and more injuries.

Caring for the homeless was a major problem for public health workers. Not only did shelters have to be established for more victims than would usually have been expected, they also had to be maintained for a longer time than anticipated. Besides setting up and managing 45 shelters, the American Red Cross organized damage-assessment teams and two staging areas. Many of the most experienced Red Cross staff were still assisting victims of Hurricane Hugo, however, so local Bay Area chapters had to take charge of the initial response and provide on-the-spot training to many volunteers. The federal response to public health needs was negligible. These needs were met primarily by local sources, with limited assistance from state agencies.

Responding to disaster: lessons learned

There were three major differences between Hurricane Hugo and the Loma Prieta earthquake—differences in the type of disaster, the amount and extent of destruction, and the degree of preparedness at the local, state, and federal levels. For these reasons the public health response to these disasters was in many ways dissimilar. In the case of Hurricane Hugo, ample warning of the storm's approach allowed local and state authorities to conduct effective evacuations and establish temporary shelters. For the Loma Prieta earthquake, however—as is true for nearly all earthquakes—there was no prior warning. In terms of environmental destruction, the level of damage and the total area affected by Hurricane Hugo were far greater than anticipated, whereas the destruction resulting from the Loma Prieta earthquake was more centralized than might have been expected (confined to four or five distinct areas).

Furthermore, in the U.S. there has probably been much more public health preparedness planning for a major earthquake than for a hurricane, at least partly because of the far greater anticipated public health impact of such a catastrophe. Perhaps this, in addition to the relatively smaller amounts of actual destruction, is why the public health response appeared more coordinated for the Loma Prieta earthquake than for Hurricane Hugo. Because of "what was" for Hugo and "what could have been" in the Bay Area, many individuals, organizations, companies, and government agencies are seeking ways to improve public health preparedness for natural disasters.

In terms of future preparedness, more may perhaps be gained from analysis of the overall similarities of the situations created by these two disasters than from a detailed evaluation of the events in each. A parable helps make an important point: According to Mayan legend, after a flood destroyed all of the villages in low-lying areas, the villagers decided to build their homes in the trees. Then a fire destroyed these dwellings. The people rebuilt, this time using mud and brick, but their new homes collapsed during an earthquake. The point is that certain general precautions may be equally crucial to the success of preparedness and response in all natural disasters.

In several respects, what went wrong in the response and relief efforts was similar in Hurricane Hugo and the Loma Prieta earthquake. One problem was in communications. Functioning communication links are all-important to the success of any emergency plan, enabling rapid estimates of disaster-related injuries and fatalities and needs for medical care. Such communications were either nonexistent or insufficient

for the first few days after the Atlantic hurricane and the California quake and continued to be a problem for some time in many areas affected by Hugo. Responders to both disasters also had to spend valuable time sorting through donations, many of which proved inappropriate, such as used winter clothing and perishable foods. The need was much greater for money and canned goods. This problem was not unique to these two disasters but, in fact, because of poor public understanding of what is truly needed, usually occurs in response to disasters.

The actual or potential vulnerability of the local medical care system was another weakness demonstrated during both disasters. Future preparedness planning should provide for backup from other local sources, as well as from state and federal sources, because of the potential for even greater failures of existing local systems than occurred in these two instances.

Both disasters also demonstrated that there is an important impact on public health after, in addition to during, a disaster. Two factors probably account for this: current preparedness planning is adequate to prevent many risks directly caused by a natural disaster (for example, because of advanced warnings and evacuations, people are less likely to drown from storm surges during a hurricane), while, at the same time, both the general public and the disaster responders may not be sufficiently aware of postimpact health risks. In the case of Hugo, for example, thousands of residents of low-lying, flood-prone areas of Puerto Rico were saved by storm warnings and effective evacuation plans. In the 10 days following the storm, however, six men, five of them electric company employees, were electrocuted in accidents involving downed power lines. It was obvious to public health officials who analyzed the reports of these deaths that better precautions need to be taken by utility company

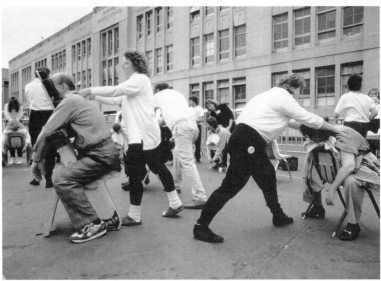

In the aftermath of the quake, overstressed San Franciscans gratefully accept the tension-relieving ministrations of practitioners of holistic massage. In terms of future preparedness, one of the most important lessons learned from the Loma Prieta earthquake was the need for better planning to deal with disaster-related mental and emotional stress.

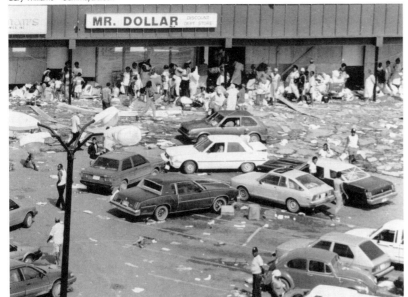

Media coverage of a disaster can significantly influence public response to the need for emergency relief. The focus on looting and disorder on St. Croix in the wake of Hurricane Hugo undoubtedly diminished sympathies for the storm's victims. Considering the extent of the damage and the hurricane's cost to the American Red Cross, overall contributions to support the Hugo relief effort were small, totaling less than $12 million.

employees responding to emergency situations. They suggested educational plans designed to familiarize people with the hazards of downed power lines, for both utility workers and the community at large, and the installation of various kinds of safety devices that would reduce risks to electrical workers.

Perhaps the two greatest public health issues that faced responders in both disasters were caring for the homeless and dealing with disaster-related mental stress. Future planning should include the establishment of more shelters and mental health field services more quickly and for longer periods of time. This effort would involve not only the availability of supplies (tents, trailers, designated public buildings, drinking water, food, clothing, and so forth) and people but also the capability to mobilize these resources within short periods of time.

Such planning should also encompass educating the media about the public health needs and issues when natural disasters strike. Media coverage tremendously influences the general public concern about, and contributions to, disaster relief. Media coverage of Hurricane Hugo may have worked against public health efforts by focusing more on the looting and violence on St. Croix than on the devastation and suffering of the people there. Furthermore, public health needs continue to exist long after the headlines cease. The almost instantaneous television coverage of the Loma Prieta earthquake may have convinced many people that the public health impact was far greater than what had occurred with Hurricane Hugo, whereas the opposite was true. As a result, Hurricane Hugo cost the American Red Cross $72 million and drew only $11.9 million in designated contributions, whereas the Loma Prieta earthquake cost the Red Cross $12

million initially but drew $52.5 million in designated contributions. A related problem is the donation of inappropriate relief supplies, which, as noted above, is not uncommon. Despite Red Cross public service announcements about what is and is not needed to aid disaster victims, people have a tendency to immediately search their attics and basements for unwanted or unused items that they imagine will be helpful. What is needed is a more aggressive public education campaign that would impress people with the true needs, usually for cash contributions and nonperishable foods and, when appropriate, willing volunteers.

Last, these two disasters emphasize that one should never put all one's eggs in the same basket. Occurring as they did within weeks of each other, the hurricane and earthquake put the country's disaster-response system to an enormous test. The system was strained, but it did not collapse. Future preparedness planning may need to pay more attention to striking a balance between responding to one catastrophe and maintaining sufficient reserves against the possibility of other, nearly concurrent disasters.

—Lee M. Sanderson, Ph.D.

Drugs

The pharmaceutical industry is in a state of flux, as it has been for the past several years. In the United States important changes are being made in the way medicines are being discovered, developed, manufactured, marketed, regulated, and paid for.

New drugs: 1989 and '90

The changes are occurring at a time of rapid development and approval of new drugs. The U.S. Food

273

Drugs

and Drug Administration (FDA)—the federal regulatory agency authorized to review and approve applications for the marketing of new drug products—cleared approximately 20 new compounds (drugs that are distinctly different from those already on the market) each year throughout most of the 1980s. In 1989 the agency approved a total of 87 new drugs, 113 biological products, and 265 generic drugs; of the 87 new drugs, 23 were new compounds, 12 of which were approved within the last five weeks of the year.

Only four new compounds in 1989 were considered by the FDA to be major therapeutic advances: clomipramine (Anafranil), an antidepressant manufactured by Ciba-Geigy Corp. for the treatment of obsessive-compulsive disorder; mefloquine (Lariam), an antimalarial agent manufactured by Hoffmann-La Roche; ganciclovir (Cytovene), a Syntex Corp. product used to treat cytomegalovirus retinitis (an eye infection caused by herpesviruses); and Sandoz Pharmaceuticals Corp.'s clozapine (Clozaril), a drug for treatment of schizophrenia that has not responded to other medications on the market.

Two other new compounds approved late in 1989 were among five new cardiovascular agents—Knoll Pharmaceuticals' propafenone (Rythmol) and Eli Lilly & Co.'s indecainide (Decabid). Both are intended for use specifically in treating severe, life-threatening arrhythmias (irregular heart beats). During the year the FDA also recommended that *all* antiarrhythmic drugs be limited to use in serious arrhythmia; in July 1989 results from a highly publicized federally funded study indicated that the use of two other antiarrhythmic agents, encainide (Enkaid) and flecainide (Tambocor), in patients with mild conditions more frequently worsens the condition and can cause death.

Pfizer's fluconazole (Diflucan) was one of a number of key approvals the FDA granted in early 1990. An antifungal product, fluconazole was approved for treatment of cryptococcal meningitis and candidiasis,

fungal infections that afflict many patients with AIDS.

Other important new approvals often involve a newly approved use or dosage form for already marketed drug products. For more than three years Burroughs Wellcome Co.'s zidovudine, more commonly known as AZT (azidothymidine; Retrovir) has been marketed as a toxic but effective therapy for AIDS patients to help prevent the deterioration of their condition. On March 2, 1990, the drug was approved to help prevent AIDS in people who test positive for the presence of the human immunodeficiency virus but who do not show symptoms of AIDS. AZT in a syrup form as well as a new long-term dosage was also approved. The new dosage is half of that previously prescribed and should allow patients to benefit from the drug for longer periods without developing major side effects such as anemia. And on May 3, 1990, AZT was approved as treatment for AIDS virus infections in children aged 3 months to 12 years. It is estimated that as many as 20,000 children in the U.S. under 13 may be infected with the virus.

Drug design by computer

Historically, the basic process for the development of prescription drug products began with the discovery of a chemical, which was followed by its analysis for similarities to existing chemicals, its screening for particular properties and for its physiological effects, and finally its testing—first in test tubes (*in vitro*), then in animals, and then in humans. Now, however, an evolving development strategy called "rational drug design," which has been made possible by the combination of advances in the medical sciences and in computer technology, involves the essential creation of new compounds to address a particular underlying cause of a disease or condition. The pharmaceutical industry has developed computer programs that can examine a series of compounds with similar organic structures and break the structures down into their component

The process of fashioning new compounds that interfere with the activity of an enzyme involved in inflammation illustrates the use of computers in rational drug design. Early on, a computer model of the enzyme (1; detail shown) is constructed from crystallographic data. The enzyme's active site—the region that binds other molecules in the inflammatory process—is further modeled (2). The model is then tested with structures that are likely to fit into and thus block the active site (3). Finally, the more promising structures are studied for their interaction with the entire enzyme (4) and then synthesized and tested as drugs.

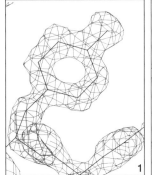 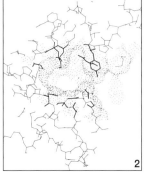 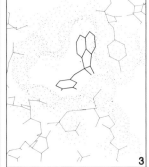 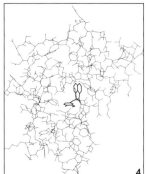

"functional groups." Such programs can predict how various changes in the functional groups will result in different pharmacokinetic effects; *i.e.*, beneficial or adverse actions of the compound in the human body.

One example of a prescription drug produced through rational drug design is the highly publicized cholesterol-lowering drug lovastatin (Mevacor), introduced to the market by Merck & Co. in 1987. Development of the drug has been compared to a "key" created in response to discovery of a disease "lock." That is, after the discovery that people with high cholesterol levels (hypercholesterolemia) have a deficiency of an enzyme that controls the liver's production of cholesterol, lovastatin's development constituted a search for a way to correct the deficiency. The agent works, in part, by reducing liver-generated cholesterol by triggering low-density lipoprotein receptors in the liver.

Drug-testing policy and the critically ill

Fundamental changes in the testing and government preclearance of prescription drugs intended for "critically ill" patients—those with life-threatening illnesses or diseases that are debilitating and for which no other adequate therapy exists—have come about as a result of the AIDS epidemic. Not only AIDS but also certain forms of cancer and Alzheimer's disease are affected by the changes.

The FDA normally requires drug manufacturers that apply for licenses to market new drugs to submit data from two well-controlled, statistically valid studies, documenting the safety and effectiveness of a proposed new drug product. Before a marketing request is granted by the FDA, the drug companies often test their products in 1,000 or more human subjects. However, at the prodding of advocates of AIDS patients— an especially active and politically aware group—the FDA in an October 1989 report announced its relaxation of its drug-approval requirements for products intended for critically ill patients.

For example, the agency generally requires that well-controlled studies include a placebo control group so that results in patients taking the experimental drug can be compared with results from a control group of patients who receive an inactive preparation made to look, smell, and taste like the test product. In testing products for critically ill patients, however, the FDA has acknowledged that once an experimental therapy has demonstrated a modicum of efficacy, administering a placebo is unethical. Consequently, placebo controls are now being limited to the very first group of critically ill patients in whom experimental products are tested. After initial results demonstrate effectiveness, and as testing continues to measure safety and to determine the optimum dosage range, studies may be designed with different controls, such as historical and active controls. Studies with historical controls compare results of the test drug with records of similar patients

in whom the same disease was allowed to progress untreated. Studies with active controls compare test drug results with results in similar patients to whom the standard therapy is administered.

The recent approval by the FDA of AZT for use in children was granted without separate testing for effectiveness in children. Rather, effectiveness was inferred on the basis of demonstrated effects in adults. However, before the approval, data on what doses were likely to be both safe and effective in children were obtained.

In addition, the FDA and drug manufacturers have agreed to initiate discussions on how best to design protocols for studying critical therapies in human patients earlier in the drug-testing process, generally during preclinical safety testing in animals. Other steps have also been taken by the FDA. The agency has formalized a procedure whereby experimental drugs that demonstrate some effectiveness during early testing may be distributed to patients who need them before final approval. A number of drugs distributed under this so-called treatment IND (investigational new drug) procedure have subsequently been approved; clomipramine and fluconazole are two examples.

A similar but even more liberal procedure for distributing unapproved drugs to patients is the "parallel track" testing system. The FDA has cleared one experimental drug, Bristol-Myers Squibb Co.'s dideoxyinosine (ddI), for such testing, under which AIDS patients who cannot tolerate or are not helped by AZT but are not enrolled in formal clinical studies can receive ddI as part of an informal parallel data-collection procedure.

Robots on the assembly line

The manufacturing of pharmaceutical products has changed dramatically over the past decade, particularly within the last five years. The use of automation has proliferated within both testing laboratories and production facilities. Robots, for example, are now used for running various laboratory tests, such as analyses of content uniformity, assays of purity, and dissolution tests. Robots also perform a diversity of functions during the manufacturing process—*e.g.*, monitoring tasks such as checking weights and analyzing contents. In sterile processing functions that must protect against human contamination, such as aseptic capping of bottles, robots have proved particularly useful.

Automated manufacturing advances have brought about a new emphasis on process validation in plant inspections by the FDA's field investigators. Whereas the agency formerly relied upon end-product testing to assure itself that a manufacturing facility was operating properly, the FDA now relies on hardware and software computer validation and other forms of process validation to assure consistent quality. Inspectors want to see documented results from tests by manufacturers to show that manufacturing processes,

275

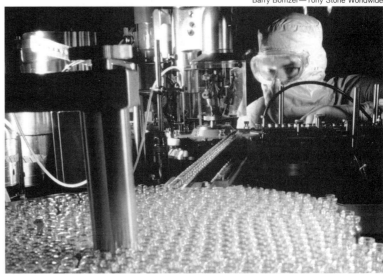

Barry Bomzer—Tony Stone Worldwide

Pharmaceutical bottles are filled under sterile conditions in a manufacturing plant. Contamination-free processing of drugs is just one of the refinements brought about by automation advances in the drug industry—advances that have revolutionized the modi operandi of both processing facilities and testing laboratories.

testing functions, and computer programs are all performing the tasks they are intended to perform.

The move away from a reliance on end-product testing has been crucial for the development and approval of biotechnology products. These substances, many of which are complex proteins, are manufactured within living cells by means of genetic engineering. Such products are made by the insertion of the genetic material of a biological substance—one that naturally occurs in the human body—into a "manufacturing" cell line, such as the bacterium *Escherichia coli*. The FDA wants assurance that such cell lines reproduce what are otherwise scarce products consistently over time and that formulation, toxicology, and stability standards are met throughout the manufacturing process. (Human growth hormone was among the first of the biotechnology products manufactured in this way.)

New approaches to marketing and advertising

The advertising of prescription drugs directly to consumers is a slowly developing trend in the marketing of pharmaceuticals. It has grown out of the confluence of the increasing demand by consumers for greater health care information and the desire of brand name drug makers to create brand loyalty. Until recently, brand name pharmaceutical manufacturers were satisfied to address their ads to prescribers. However, since Congress enacted legislation in 1984 to facilitate FDA approval of generic copies for marketing immediately after expiration of patents on the original "pioneer" products, brand name drug manufacturers have looked for ways to protect their products' market shares from generic competition.

The FDA's advertising regulations have made so-called direct-to-consumer advertising of prescription drugs difficult. A regulatory mandate for "fair balance" in drug advertising requires that promotions mention a product's risks as well as its benefits. Consequently, ads that appear in professional medical journals are usually two or more pages in length because if they list a drug product's uses or benefits, they must also reproduce its professional labeling, which includes copious information on precautions, potential adverse effects, and contraindications; *i.e.,* situations in which the drug should be avoided. Because of the regulatory restrictions, drug advertising generally has been considered too detailed to be effective for the general public.

However, the FDA permits advertisers to omit cautionary information if an ad makes no reference to the product's medical use. Thus, Boots Pharmaceuticals has advertised its Rufen brand of ibuprofen as less expensive than Upjohn Co.'s popular Motrin brand without mentioning the products' most common use: relief from arthritis pain.

Similarly, ads may avoid including voluminous cautionary information if they simply describe a disease for which patients can get treatment from their doctors. Such promotions completely avoid reference to the drug product. This approach is evident in Upjohn's television advertising for its hair regrowth stimulant Rogaine (minoxidil). The ad features a young, balding man who states his intention to see his physician to obtain "help" in reversing his hair loss; the ad does not mention that the "help" he is seeking will come in the form of a drug product. Such ads are designed not to persuade viewers to ask for a product but to prompt them to see their doctors, who have been lobbied by Upjohn salespeople to prescribe Rogaine.

Marion Merrell Dow promotes two products directly to consumers through broadcast ads that do not mention the products by name. An ad for Nicorette (nicotine polacrilex), a nicotine-containing chewing gum, states simply that cigarette smokers who hope to quit can get help from their physicians. An ad for the non-sedating antihistamine product Seldane (terfenadine) advises people suffering from nasal discharge due to cold and allergy to consult their doctors for treatment that avoids the side effect of drowsiness normally attendant to other antihistamines available with and without a prescription. Late in 1989 the company began broadcasting a television ad that named and pictured Nicorette chewing gum and identified it simply as "nicotine gum . . . available only from your doctor."

Not only had the FDA disallowed promotion of a product's benefits without the cautionary information, it also had prohibited ads that included even a hint of the intended use when the product name was given. One manufacturer received a "regulatory letter" in which the FDA reprimanded the firm for running a print ad for a cardiovascular drug that pictured a heart next to the product name without including the complete cautionary information. Before Rogaine was approved, the agency asked Upjohn to change the brand name from Regaine on the grounds that the intended name suggested exaggerated effectiveness. The name change was a request, not a requirement; however, Upjohn felt compelled to comply because its ability to market the product depended upon FDA approval.

A coalition of advertising agencies and a few manufacturers are seeking to have the FDA relax its advertising restrictions. In response to advertisers' arguments that by facilitating drug advertising a relaxation of FDA regulations would increase the flow of health care information to consumers, U.S. Rep. Henry A. Waxman (Dem., Calif.) has repeatedly pointed out that the object of advertising is to sell, not to inform. Waxman chairs the Health and Environment Subcom-

mittee, which is responsible for FDA-related legislation in the House of Representatives.

Physicians and pharmacists also have opposed consumer-directed pharmaceutical ads. They have expressed concern that patients, swayed by a particularly effective ad, might pressure their doctors to prescribe a drug product that is not appropriate. Just as important, most prescription drug manufacturers agree that more liberal advertising of potentially harmful products could place sponsors at a liability risk. On the other hand, many manufacturers agree that they could be forced to increase consumer-directed promotions if they found that their competitors were effectively doing so.

Since the latter half of 1989, the manufacturers of Rogaine, Nicorette, and Seldane have run professional-style print ads in lay publications. The ads are two to three pages long and include cautionary information as well as claims about the products' intended uses. Although the FDA has not formally objected to such ads, regulators have expressed concern that they may not fulfill the regulatory requirement for fair balance to the extent that consumers are unable to comprehend the large volume of cautionary information printed in fine print.

Prescription drug prices

Faced with continually skyrocketing costs of U.S. health care, government and private health care insurers are now coping with upwardly spiraling charges by developing several kinds of cost-containment strategies. One of these has been to restrict reimbursements on prescription drugs. Since Congress established the Medicare program in 1965, the average cost for a prescription drug has risen by a factor of more than

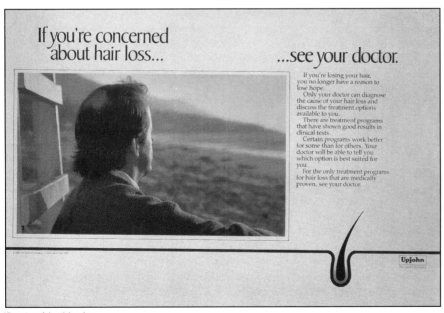

Klemptner Advertising, Inc.

Before granting approval to Upjohn Co.'s antibalding remedy, the FDA requested that the intended brand name, Regaine, be changed because it suggested exaggerated effectiveness. Upjohn complied, calling its product Rogaine. This magazine ad that pitches the hair regrowth stimulant directly to consumers gets around the requirement for mentioning a product's potential side effects as well as its benefits by not including the name at all.

4.6—from $3.59 in the mid-1960s to $16.60 in 1989; throughout the 1980s prescription prices rose at approximately twice the rate of general inflation.

Under many private health care insurance plans that provide prescription drug benefits, beneficiaries having a prescription filled either pay nothing to the pharmacy or pay a fixed "copayment" of a few dollars or a "coinsurance" charge, a small percentage of the price. The pharmacy must then be reimbursed by the insurer for the remainder of the price. Similarly, when prescriptions are filled by pharmacies for beneficiaries of Medicaid, the government health care program for the poor, pharmacists must submit paperwork to their state Medicaid agencies to obtain reimbursement. According to the most recent edition of the *Lilly Digest,* an annual survey of community drugstores published by the pharmaceutical manufacturer Eli Lilly & Co., such third-party payments accounted for 40% of all prescriptions filled in 1989.

Third-party payers generally try to restrict expenditures by limiting reimbursements to pharmacies. For example, many states' Medicaid agencies rely on the average wholesale price (AWP), which is listed in trade publications, to determine a pharmacy's acquisition cost for a given product. However, because the AWP is often inflated and pharmacies can obtain discounts from the manufacturers, Medicaid and private plans often deduct 5 to 10% or more from the acquisition cost in their reimbursements. Obviously, pharmacists have opposed such deductions. Third-party payers have argued that reimbursement deductions are necessary to slow prescription drug price inflation; pharmacists, on the other hand, have countered that increased prices on the drugs they dispense stem principally from the manufacturers.

Several states are now taking a supply-side approach to drug cost containment under Medicaid. For example, the Kansas Medicaid agency has established a bidding program in which pharmaceutical manufacturers that offer the highest price rebates on individual drug products gain placement on a state formulary, which assures that all Medicaid prescriptions for a particular drug will be filled with products made by the bid-winning companies. Manufacturers, however, have been generally resistant to offering Medicaid discounts, and when Kansas first tried to implement its program in 1988, it received bid prices for only six products from three manufacturers. In April 1990 the pharmaceutical firm Merck & Co. broke with the traditional resistance in announcing that it would discount its prices for all products sold under state Medicaid programs; up to eight manufacturers were subsequently expected to propose such programs.

California is taking a different tack. The state's Medi-Cal program in mid-1990 was establishing a volume purchasing program. The plan included buying and warehousing large amounts of prescription drugs from all manufacturers to be dispensed under the program in hopes of obtaining substantial volume discounts in the process.

One cost-containment measure universally used by third-party payers is the provision of incentives for generic substitution. Unless a physician prescribes a particular brand of drug, Medicaid and other programs generally will reimburse pharmacies only for the price of a low-cost generic version of the product. Even if a physician identifies a drug on a prescription form by a brand name, the pharmacist can substitute a generic product unless the physician specifically orders otherwise.

Generic drugs are generally priced one-third to one-half less than the price of their brand name counterparts. Consequently, generic drugs are crucial to prescription drug cost-containment efforts. For this reason the scandal over generic products in the U.S. pharmaceutical industry that occurred in 1989 has had major repercussions.

Generic drugs scandal

The U.S. pharmaceutical industry was rocked when a series of investigations by the FDA uncovered cheating in the procedures for premarket review of generic products. Essentially, two types of misbehavior were found: the offering of illegal gratuities to agency employees to speed generic drug approvals and submissions of false information in support of such approvals.

The earliest sign of a problem came in 1985 when the FDA received an anonymous tip that a male chemist in the agency's generic drug review division was socializing with a female executive from a company called American Therapeutics. Subsequently, Mylan Laboratories—a Pittsburgh, Pa., generic drug producer—complained to the FDA that it felt that the division was prejudiced against its marketing applications. The company alleged that in certain cases it was receiving approvals later than other firms that had submitted marketing applications after Mylan. Acting as a whistle-blower, Mylan then hired a private detective to follow the FDA division chemist. The investigator found papers from a marketing application—which should have been secured within the agency—in a trash can outside the chemist's home. Mylan took this evidence to law-enforcement authorities and to the House Oversight and Investigations Subcommittee, chaired by Rep. John D. Dingell (Dem., Mich.). Beginning in May 1989, Dingell held a series of widely reported hearings on the criminal and congressional investigations into the generic drug industry.

Three agency chemists pleaded guilty and were sentenced for accepting illegal gratuities in connection with the review of generic drug applications. Three former FDA generic division employees pleaded guilty to accepting illegal gratuities for providing information to drug companies about their competitors' applications.

A fourth was charged with perjury. In addition, three generic drug companies and six company officials or agents have pleaded guilty to charges involving the offering of illegal gratuities to government employees. The companies are Par Pharmaceutical, its subsidiary, Quad Pharmaceuticals, and American Therapeutics. The companies' willingness to break the law to speed approval of their marketing applications was apparently due to the fact that newer and more lucrative drugs were coming off patent. It is a huge competitive advantage to market the first or one of the first generic copies of a brand name product, as the first generic versions often retain the largest portion of a particular drug's sales.

The U.S. district attorney for Baltimore, Md., Breckenridge Willcox, announced on March 30, 1990, that the bribery phase of the investigation was complete and the prosecution would then focus on the allegations of fraud and falsification of manufacturing records. "Product substitution" is among the most egregious of the fraudulent acts disclosed to date. Several companies have acknowledged to the FDA that they substituted samples of a brand name product for generic samples in so-called bioequivalence studies, which are carried out to determine whether the generic copies act as safely and effectively in the human body. The resulting deception makes it seem that a generic is bioequivalent to a brand name drug, when actually the brand name product has been tested against itself.

A worker inspects pills at Mylan Laboratories, a small generic drug company that touched off an industry-wide scandal when it charged that the FDA had been stalling in processing its new drug applications.

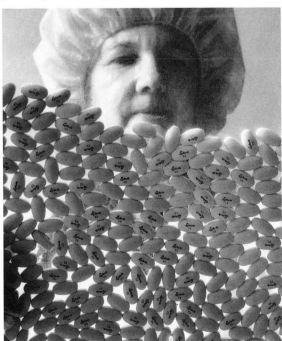

Mylan Laboratories; photograph, Lynn Johnson

The generic company Vitarine Pharmaceuticals admitted perpetrating product substitution in obtaining approval for its version of the SmithKline Beecham Corp.'s antihypertensive diuretic Dyazide. Vitarine's product has since been withdrawn from the market. The generic firm Bolar Pharmaceutical Co. admitted to a product switch in bioequivalence testing of its version of Sandoz Pharmaceuticals Corp.'s antipsychotic drug Mellaril. The generics manufacturer Par admitted to performing a product switch during an FDA inspection to cover up a discrepancy in company records.

As findings of the congressional and criminal investigations became public, the FDA launched a series of inspections. The agency first inspected 13 firms it suspected of fraudulent behavior. Only one, Able Laboratories, was found relatively free of regulatory problems. The FDA then tested the 30 most frequently prescribed generic drugs and their brand name forms. The FDA has reported that its tests of 2,500 individual generic products detected only 27, or 1.1%, that failed to meet required standards.

In further investigations of the 20 leading generic drug manufacturers, record-keeping abnormalities sufficient to cause suspicion of a deliberate attempt to mislead the agency and defraud the premarket review process were found in more than half. Further investigations are proceeding to determine the extent of the fraud. FDA inspections have also uncovered regulatory violations in several major brand name manufacturers' facilities, including those of Eli Lilly & Co. and Abbott Laboratories.

The findings will lead to important changes in the way the FDA regulates both the brand name and the generic drug industries. The agency does not test experimental new drugs or proposed new generic products. It only reviews data from the required tests, which are conducted by manufacturers that apply for marketing approval. Until now, the FDA relied largely on an applicant's word that submitted data accurately reflected studies that were properly conducted. The agency has announced that in the future it will rely less on companies' assurances and more on inspections and spot checks.

The FDA is already revamping its system for reviewing generic drug marketing applications to standardize the process and make it more difficult for individual reviewers to influence the process in arbitrary ways. Furthermore, Congress made it a short-term goal to increase the FDA's resources and enforcement authority over the generic drug industry, and it is expected to consider legislation to enhance FDA regulatory powers over all industries that seek agency approvals, including those of brand name drugs, biological products, medical devices, animal drugs, and cosmetic ingredients.

Although there are instances in which certain generic products have been found unsafe or not equivalent

Engraving from *Transactions of the Clinical Society of London* 7 (1874), pp. 22–28

to brand name drugs, the FDA continues to defend the general safety and effectiveness of most available generic drugs and insists that the publicized malfeasance is limited to a small minority of the industry. The FDA advises patients who are currently taking generic drugs not to stop taking their medicine or switch their medication to a brand name product unless they notice a problem and consult their physicians.

—Louis A. LaMarca

Eating Disorders

In 1694 Richard Morton, an English physician, described an 18-year-old girl who died three months after he first saw her "like a skeleton only clad with skin." He referred to this disorder as a form of nervous consumption ("phthisis nervosa") that came about through "sadness and anxious cares." In 1873 Sir William Gull, Queen Victoria's physician, named and identified the illness anorexia nervosa, which literally means "a nervous loss of appetite." Anorexia nervosa, primarily affecting young women, is now characterized by emaciating weight loss, body image disturbance, and the intense fear of becoming obese. Bulimia nervosa, which literally means "hunger of an ox," is more widespread than anorexia nervosa; it is characterized by episodes of secretive binge eating, usually followed by purging via self-induced vomiting, fasting, excessive use of laxatives or diuretics, or sometimes excessive exercising or fasting.

Although anorexia and bulimia nervosa are defined as separate disorders, some patients have symptoms associated with both syndromes. Approximately one-half of anorexics have engaged in bulimic behavior. Many bulimics previously have experienced symptoms of anorexia nervosa or become anorexic themselves.

Who is affected?

Both anorexia and bulimia nervosa disproportionately affect women; approximately 90–95% of reported cases are female. Traditionally researchers thought that these disorders were largely confined to women of middle and upper socioeconomic classes, but recent studies have documented that anorexia and bulimia nervosa increasingly cross the boundaries of race and class.

Anorexia nervosa typically has its onset between the ages of 12 and the early twenties. Bulimia nervosa is associated with a broad age spectrum; at the Eating Disorders Unit (EDU) of the Massachusetts General Hospital in Boston, for example, the mean age of onset for bulimic patients is between 16 and 18. Bulimic patients, however, are often symptomatic for years before seeking help and, on average, have had their eating disorder for six years before entering the EDU or similar programs for treatment.

A number of studies in the U.S. and Europe have

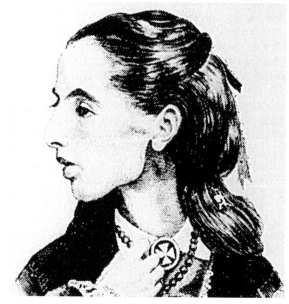

This engraving depicting an emaciated young female patient, identified as "Miss C," appeared in Sir William Gull's first clinical case report of the eating disorder anorexia nervosa. It was Gull who identified and named the disease in 1873.

estimated that the incidence of anorexia nervosa has doubled over the past 20 years. While these studies present compelling evidence that this rise reflects a true increase—not simply improved recognition, earlier hospitalization, or hospitalization for less severe cases—another recent retrospective study in the U.S. found that the incidence of anorexia nervosa has remained unchanged for four decades. Nonetheless, primary care clinicians commonly report that they are seeing more patients with anorexia nervosa now than before the late 1970s. While the true incidence of anorexia nervosa is difficult to determine (probably between 0.1 and 0.5% of young women are affected), any increase is worrisome because anorexia nervosa is linked to a high mortality rate.

While the mortality rate for bulimia nervosa is lower than that for anorexia nervosa (most of those who suffer from bulimia maintain a normal or near-normal weight), the true incidence of this more widespread eating disorder is difficult to determine. Many researchers in the early 1980s estimated that among college-age women the rate varied between 4.5 and 18%. Some of these early studies, however, may have overestimated the true incidence of the syndrome; the investigators used less restrictive criteria than those that are used today—as set forth in the American Psychiatric Association's *Diagnostic and Statistical Manual of Mental Disorders,* third edition, revised (*DSM-III-R,* published in 1987), and they did not readily distinguish between women with bulimic symptoms and those having the full-blown disorder. David E. Schotte and

Albert J. Stunkard at the University of Pennsylvania improved on this methodology in a 1987 study; distinguishing between women with bulimia nervosa and women with bulimic symptoms only, these investigators reported that 1–4% of the population in their survey met the full diagnostic criteria for the disorder, while 15% were found to have bulimic symptoms. Although some researchers have suggested that the prevalence of bulimia nervosa is lower in nonuniversity settings, Harrison G. Pope, Jr., and his colleagues at McLean Hospital, Belmont, Mass., found that 10% of females surveyed at a suburban shopping mall had a lifetime history of bulimia nervosa.

As already noted, eating disorders have gone through several diagnostic renditions in American psychiatry. The currently most widely used criteria for the diagnosis of anorexia nervosa and bulimia nervosa are listed in Table 1, below.

Relentless pursuit of thinness

Anorexia nervosa typically begins during the teenage years when a young woman either is overweight or perceives herself as such. It may start after experiencing a painful event or suffering a disappointment or loss in a relationship. Once present, the course tends to be either brief and self-limiting or protracted with eventual recovery. In the worst case, the disorder may be chronic and unremitting.

A typical pattern of anorexia nervosa has been recognized for some time: the anorexic begins to restrict her food intake, often first eliminating whole food groups or foods high in fat. Usually the diet begins as a simple attempt to shed a few unwanted pounds and then escalates into a relentless pursuit of thinness. Despite her reluctance to eat, the anorexic often becomes preoccupied with dietary restrictions and will spend hours in the kitchen developing elaborate food (or mealtime) rituals. The anorexic may use laxatives, self-induced vomiting, and excessive exercise to hasten weight reduction. Often losing up to 25% of her

---

Table 1: **Diagnostic criteria for eating disorders**

anorexia nervosa
1. weight loss of at least 15% of ideal body weight
2. intense fear of becoming fat
3. disturbance of body image
4. loss of menstruation (amenorrhea) for three consecutive cycles

bulimia nervosa
1. overconcern with body weight and shape
2. eating binges where a large amount of food is consumed in a short period of time
3. a feeling of being out of control during the binge
4. use of a purging method to counteract the effects of the binge; *e.g.,* self-induced vomiting, laxatives, diuretics, exercise, or restrictive eating
5. minimum number of two binge-purge episodes per week for three months

Adapted with permission from the *Diagnostic and Statistical Manual of Mental Disorders,* third edition, revised. Copyright 1987 American Psychiatric Association

---

ideal body weight, the anorexic may achieve a severe weight loss quite rapidly. Even with this tremendous drop in body weight, she continues to perceive herself as fat. In fact, anorexics even find pleasure in exercising this strict control over their weight; they do not see themselves as having a problem with either their eating or their weight. Many anorexics fit the stereotype of the high-achieving perfectionist who is driven to meet unreasonable expectations. While strictly disciplining their food intake and body weight, anorexics attempt to shut down other impulses in the vain hope of gaining control over every aspect of their lives.

Binge eating and shame

In contrast to the anorexic, the bulimic has frequently attempted a variety of diets with little or no success. This frequent dieting may lead to binge eating, the hallmark of bulimia nervosa. Typically, the bulimic consumes junk foods high in calories and carbohydrates at time periods each day set aside specifically for binge eating. Consuming 4,000–5,000 cal in a single binge is not unusual. There have been reports of patients consuming as many as 20,000 cal in a single day. They learn, either accidently or through a friend, about using self-induced vomiting or laxatives to help control their weight. While anorexics take pride in their ability to control their eating, bulimics are often embarrassed by their binge eating, feeling guilt, shame, remorse, and low self-esteem. These feelings contribute to their inability to tell even family members about their disordered eating patterns. Because bulimics are most often of normal body weight, they are more easily able to hide their disorder. In contrast to anorexics, however, they are bothered by their symptoms and tend to seek treatment much more readily. Impulsive behaviors often extend beyond the realm of food for bulimics. Alcohol and drug abuse, stealing and shoplifting, and suicidal behavior may accompany bulimic symptoms. Bulimia nervosa is often a chronic, relapsing disorder. Of patients seeking treatment at the EDU, the probability of recovery within three to four years has been 69%, while the probability of relapse for those who have recovered is 63%.

Contemporary theories

Current American cultural values place tremendous pressure on women to be thin. One study found, for example, that both *Playboy* centerfold models and Miss America winners had progressively smaller hip and bust measurements over a 25-year span from the mid-1950s through the 1970s. This study found progressively lower weights among these women—even though the American population had grown steadily heavier—making it even more difficult for the average woman to achieve this idealized definition of beauty.

Such a pervasive demand to be thin is believed to contribute to the high prevalence of eating disorders.

Eating disorders

In fact, the incidence of eating disorders is even higher in women who participate in activities that traditionally have required a thin figure, such as ballet dancing and long-distance running. Some researchers, however, have argued that the emphasis on being thin is not limited by occupational boundaries. Psychologists Marlene Boskind-White and William C. White (formerly at Cornell University, Ithaca, N.Y.) have suggested that the American male-dominated society teaches women to define themselves by the way in which men perceive them. Articles in women's magazines focus to a major extent on diets and getting trim and also on food and cooking. Although many women strive covetously for a model's figure, only in the late 1980s did a few signs begin to emerge that successful models may differ from the strictly thin standard that has long dominated the fashion industry. These differences may reflect a positive change in the societal emphasis on body weight and shape that will be manifested in the 1990s.

Some feminist theorists hypothesize that many "normal" women are obsessed with "diets, exercise, and poundage" because the growth of their female identity is arrested and in crisis. According to Kim Chernin in the book *The Hungry Self: Women, Eating, and Identity,* women's pursuit of thinness is regarded as a form of male-imposture in which these women try to look like boys or men—lean, muscular, and competitive. She describes how contemporary society teaches young women to be assertive, self-reliant, and able to compete in a man's world. However, she explains, this conflicts with the traditional developmental demands on a young woman. According to Janet L. Surrey of McLean Hospital, traditionally normal male development requires cutting early maternal ties, but the fostering of close relationships continues to play an integral role in healthy female development. The emotional openness, sharing, and cooperation girls need as they grow into adolescence and adulthood clash with the independence that today's society tries to impose.

In the 1970s the late psychoanalyst Hilde Bruch, a primary contributor to the present understanding of eating disorders, documented how anorexics are developmentally stunted. She described the anorexic's sense of ineffectiveness, inappropriate responses to internal body messages, and body-image disturbance and linked these deficits to childhood experiences. When these children reached adolescence, they gained feelings of competence, effectiveness, and control by rejecting their own appetites and remaining thin.

Family characteristics may contribute to the onset or maintenance of an eating disorder. According to Salvador Minuchin, a family therapy pioneer at the Philadelphia Child Guidance Center, the following characteristics are common in many families of anorexics: "enmeshment," in which the complex psychological needs of the anorexic, the parents, and siblings block the normal process of individuation of family members; overprotection; rigidity; lack of conflict resolution; and use of the anorexic daughter to diffuse parental conflict. The parents may be directly or indirectly threatening to separate or divorce, in which case their conflicts very frequently are detoured through the daughter with anorexia nervosa and her symptoms and behavior. Her maturation then may serve to threaten the basic balance of such a family system.

Self-psychology theorists more recently have hypothesized that women with bulimia nervosa undergo a profound disruption of the early parent-child relationship, causing in the child an inability to regulate tension. Thus, unregulated tension builds to intolerable levels and disrupts the bulimic's sense of psychological balance and sense of self. The bulimic attempts to alleviate internal tension by repetitive binge eating and purging. Ego psychologists have suggested that bulimics lack so-called object constancy and suffer a great loss when cut off from the symbiotic relationship with their mother. They resort to binge eating in an attempt to fulfill the need for soothing and nurturing that they once had from their mother.

Biological components: new insights

Researchers have documented a variety of neurochemical abnormalities in anorexic and bulimic patients. In the case of anorexia nervosa, however, starvation itself can cause profound changes in the neuroendocrine

The first published photograph of a patient with anorexia nervosa in an American medical journal (1932) showed a young woman whose treatment included a change of environment, forced feeding, and psychotherapy.

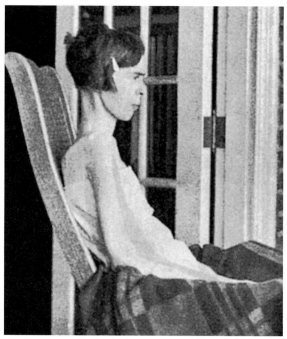

From the *New England Journal of Medicine*, vol. 207, no. 14 (Oct. 6, 1932), pp. 613–617; photograph, The John Crerar Library

system, making it unclear whether alterations in brain chemistry are the result of radical eating changes or help cause the disorder in the first place. This has complicated the search for specific metabolic changes due to anorexia nervosa.

Some hormonal changes in anorexics cannot be attributed to starvation alone since approximately 20 to 25% cease menstruating even before they lose weight. Moreover, serum or urine levels of cortisol, a hormone that is secreted by the adrenal glands and affects a variety of organ systems, are usually diminished in starvation but are noted to be elevated in anorexia nervosa. The elevated level of cortisol may be related to the decreased bone density levels often noted in chronic anorexics.

A neurochemical change commonly found in women with anorexia nervosa involves abnormal levels of the neurotransmitter norepinephrine. Recent evidence suggests that anorexics' chronic self-starvation serves to lower their levels of central nervous system norepinephrine. Since heightened levels of norepinephrine are associated with increased anxiety, researchers hypothesize that anorexics may be lessening their own anxiety by lowering their levels of norepinephrine. This decrease in anxiety may serve as reinforcement to anorexics to continue their self-starvation whenever they begin to feel anxious.

The chronic self-starvation of anorexia nervosa may be perpetuated by yet another change in the anorexic's brain chemistry. Researchers have documented that chronic and extreme dieting elevates brain levels of opioids, neurochemicals synthesized within the body, producing a starvation "high." Theorists suggest that the opioid-induced euphoria may therefore reinforce and perpetuate the anorexic's behavior.

Research on bulimia nervosa has uncovered neurochemical abnormalities in the serotonergic and noradrenergic systems. In animals, elevated serotonin levels have been linked to the feeling of satiety. However, one study with bulimic patients found that bulimics have a low level of serotonin. This low serotonin level may reflect a disturbed satiety mechanism, which reduces the sensation of having just eaten and predisposes bulimics to binge eating. An altered satiety mechanism theory gains further support from the finding that bulimics have abnormally low levels of cholecystokinin, a hormone released from the small intestine, also implicated in the sensation of satiety. Pharmacological evidence, too, has been implicated indirectly in the noradrenergic system. Imiprimine, a powerful drug that blocks the reuptake of norepinephrine (a hormone in the noradrenergic system), has reduced the desire to binge in some bulimics.

Medical complications: widespread and serious
The medical complications of anorexia nervosa are mainly those of starvation. Clinicians can find changes in almost every organ system, including abnormalities in the cardiovascular, hematological, gastrointestinal, renal, endocrine, and skeletal systems. Patients may experience amenorrhea (cessation of menstruation), bone demineralization, elevated growth hormone levels, abnormal temperature regulation, decreased heart rates, decreased blood pressure, arrhythmias, edema (swelling), decreased gastric emptying, constipation, elevated liver enzymes, anemia, low white blood cell counts, and low blood platelet counts. Many of these symptoms may be due to both metabolic changes and inadequate nutrition. Osteoporosis, for example, may develop because of inadequate mineral intake and decreased estrogen, which is a response of the endocrine system to starvation.

The medical problems that accompany bulimia nervosa are mainly due to binge eating and purging. These include ipecac poisoning (from using the emetic syrup of ipecac), decreased potassium in the blood (diuretic induced), abraded knuckles from induced vomiting (Russell's sign), acute stomach dilation or rupture, parotid gland enlargement, dental-enamel erosion, esophagitis, esophageal rupture, decreased potassium in the blood (laxative induced), and aspiration pneumonia. Menstrual irregularities affect over 40% of bulimics.

No easy cures
Eating disorders continue to present formidable barriers to treatment. Anorexics typically deny their illness, viewing their weight loss as the perfect solution to often deep-seated sadness and feelings of inadequacy. Because anorexics feel better by not eating, treatment is seldom initiated without overt coercion, and even the normal course of treatment can be difficult. The anorexic often agrees to receive help not to address her disorder but to appease her family.

However, some families join the anorexic in denying her illness and resist seeking treatment or refuse to accept the clinician's recommendations. A very recent study found that the family's strong misgivings

Table 2: **Medical manifestations of bulimia nervosa**

system affected	complication
endocrine/metabolic	menstrual irregularities
cardiovascular	ipecac poisoning
renal	decreased blood potassium (diuretic induced), edema
gastrointestinal	acute dilation or rupture of the stomach, parotid gland enlargement, dental-enamel erosion, inflammation or rupture of the esophagus, decreased blood potassium (laxative induced)
pulmonary	aspiration pneumonia

about psychiatry may stem from their style of problem solving, previous frustrating experiences with the mental health field, or a fear that family secrets will be revealed.

Although bulimics may resist seeking treatment because of the shame and embarrassment they feel about their eating disorder (and frequently other pathological behaviors), they tend to accept treatment more readily than anorexics. Once they have admitted to their eating disorder and initiated treatment, they may experience difficulty remaining in a program that does not immediately alleviate their symptoms.

Unfortunately, no easy or rapid cure yet exists for either eating disorder. Rather, clinicians today rely on a variety of treatment techniques, often using several simultaneously. A typical treatment regimen for the anorexic employs a combination of individual psychotherapy, nutritional counseling, and family therapy for adolescent patients. Drug treatment may be recommended for those who have concomitant depressive disorder, obsessive-compulsive symptoms, severe anxiety symptoms, or psychosis. Drug treatment is also used when anorexics have not responded to other treatments, but the true effectiveness of antidepressants or other medications has yet to be demonstrated. All anorexics need ongoing medical management, requiring regular visits to an internist, family practitioner, or pediatrician.

An integrated treatment program is also recommended for bulimia nervosa. The syndrome's biological components, cognitive aberrations, and developmental underpinnings respond best to a multidimensional therapeutic approach that typically includes individual psychotherapy, group therapy, family therapy, nutritional counseling, medications, and self-help groups.

One goal is to keep the patient who has an eating disorder free from medical risk despite her often intense resistance to change. In order to accomplish this goal effectively, clinicians must establish early in treatment clear and acceptable guidelines concerning weight and vital medical signs with the patient and her family. Hospitalization may be necessary.

Promising treatments

Three particular treatment modalities are presently considered among the most promising. Recent short-term trials have found the following approaches to be effective.

Psychodynamic approach. In the treatment of anorexia nervosa, Bruch described the individual psychodynamic treatment setting as a stage for the reenactment of traumatic misunderstanding in the patient's past. She described the anorexic as often looking back on her early development as an endless series of concessions to meet other people's expectations and plans. During individual psychotherapy both patient and therapist work to recognize, define, question,

and challenge erroneous attitudes and assumptions so that they can eventually be modified and replaced. This approach to treating patients with eating disorders is employed both in individual psychotherapy and in group therapy.

For bulimia nervosa psychodynamic therapy tries to uncover the meaning of the bulimic symptoms and to determine what functions the symptoms serve for the patient. The therapist helps the patient with bulimia identify anxious and negative emotions and recollect early home or family experiences that were associated with tension release and soothing. The therapist also explores the patient's and family's use of food in achieving psychological balance and family stability.

Group therapy has emerged as a successful and popular treatment intervention for patients with bulimia nervosa. The psychodynamically oriented support group, for example, initially provides a safe forum that allows patients to share their insights about their disorder and to realize that they are not alone. As therapy progresses and as the focus turns toward inner experiences, families, and interpersonal relationships, group members learn more about the role that their own bulimic symptoms play in their lives. Psychodynamically oriented group therapy can foster growth

As awareness of the prevalence of eating disorders has increased, many treatment programs have become available. Meanwhile, ongoing research is providing better understanding of these complex conditions; promising new therapies are likely to emerge.

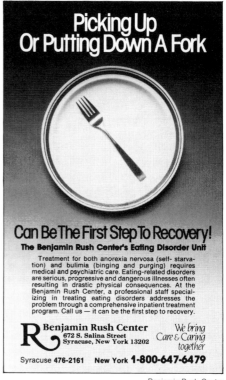

and understanding by untangling the internal conflicts that give rise to bulimic symptoms.

Cognitive-behavioral approach. Cognitive-behavioral psychotherapy for bulimia nervosa was first investigated in the early 1980s; since then it has become among the most widely employed and important treatments. The goals of cognitive-behavioral therapy in bulimia—in both individual and group therapy—are twofold: first, to help the patient control her unwanted binge-and-purge behaviors; second, to change distorted thoughts about food, body shape, and weight. Treatment often includes cognitive restructuring (using techniques developed for treatment of depression), discussion of the association between mood states and binge eating, self-monitoring of relevant thoughts and behavior (often through the use of a mood diary), the establishment of a pattern of regular eating through self-control measures, and the introduction of avoided foods into the patient's diet.

Psychologists Barbara Bauer and Wayne Anderson of the University of Missouri have recently delineated a series of typical irrational beliefs held by many bulimic patients. Therapy involves modifying beliefs such as the following: (1) becoming overweight is the worst thing that can happen to me; (2) there are good foods, such as vegetables and fish, and bad foods, such as sweets and carbohydrates; (3) I must have control over all of my actions to feel safe; (4) I must do everything perfectly, or what I do is worthless; (5) everyone is aware of, and interested in, what I am doing; (6) everyone must love me and approve of what I do; (7) external validation is crucial to me; (8) as soon as a particular event such as graduation or marriage occurs, my bulimic behavior will disappear; and (9) I must be dependent and subservient yet competitive and aggressive.

Drug therapies. Pharmacological studies to date have produced much more encouraging results for treating bulimia nervosa than for treating anorexia nervosa. There have been relatively few controlled drug studies of anorexia nervosa, in large part because anorexics typically deny their illness, are unwilling to gain weight, and are ambivalent about taking anything by mouth. Cyproheptadine, a serotonergic antagonist and appetite stimulant, is the only drug that in a controlled study of anorexic patients has been shown to be effective. However, although patients taking the drug gained a statistically significant amount of weight in comparison with patients taking a placebo, the actual gain was modest and of minimal clinical significance. Several trials using antidepressants have not yielded promising results.

Drug treatment for bulimia nervosa has received increasing attention after several published studies in the late 1980s reported the effectiveness of antidepressant medications. Interest in the use of antidepressants was spurred by the high frequency of concurrent depressive disorder in bulimic patients, by reports of an increased incidence of depression in first-degree relatives, and by positive responses to antidepressants in open clinical trials. With few exceptions, short-term studies of antidepressants have found a significant reduction in symptoms for the majority of bulimic patients. Three classes of antidepressant drugs—tricyclic antidepressants, monoamine oxidase (MAO) inhibitors, and selective serotonergic agents such as fluoxetine—are most commonly used. In recently conducted 6–10 week trials, these drugs, tended to reduce bulimic symptoms by more than 50% in 60–70% of patients, although a much smaller percentage of patients ceased binge eating entirely. In general, antidepressants prescribed in conjunction with psychotherapy are more effective than either treatment administered alone.

Present and future outlook

Follow-up studies of anorexia nervosa show that five years after hospitalization, 30% of anorexics are well, 40% are improved, and 30% remain chronically ill. Several recent outcome studies have documented the mortality rate associated with anorexia nervosa. Researchers have noted a mortality rate of 5% for patients having the disorder for 5 years, a 10-year mortality rate of 6.5%, a 20-year mortality rate of 16%, and a 33-year mortality rate of 18%. To date, there are no published long-term outcome studies of bulimia nervosa.

While anorexia and bulimia nervosa present a major challenge to the health care providers who treat them, research has helped clinicians better understand their complexity. At present, family studies of patients with eating disorders are under way to help increase understanding of the role of genetics in the etiology of these diseases.

Further research investigating the neurochemistry and exploring the central nervous system changes that precede the onset of anorexia and bulimia nervosa is necessary for increased understanding of their mechanisms. For example, research delineating the pattern of sensory responsiveness to certain types of food (*e.g.,* sweet and fatty foods) during childhood or early adolescence may determine early psychobiological markers for an eating disorder in later life.

Investigations of osteoporosis, a relatively recently recognized and severe complication of anorexia nervosa, will reveal mediating mechanisms and appropriate treatment. It is anticipated that these and other research efforts will allow health care professionals to develop new interventions—both pharmacological and nonpharmacological—that will be effective for these all-too-common disorders.

—*David B. Herzog, M.D.,*
Janine K. Stasior, M.S.,
and David S. Stasior, M.D., M.P.P.

Children Exposed to Lead—Clear and Present Danger

by David Bellinger, Ph.D., M.Sc.

To many people the term *lead poisoning* evokes the image of a child in a run-down inner-city building peeling flakes of paint from the walls and eating them. To be sure, such children are at greatest risk of lead poisoning, and the ingestion of leaded paint is responsible for their most concentrated exposure. Like most stereotypes, however, this one has proved to be simplistic. In the past decade dramatic advances in understanding of the epidemiology of childhood lead exposure have led to increasing recognition of a syndrome of "subclinical," or "silent," lead toxicity. Children who have no overt symptoms may nevertheless suffer serious harm from exposure to lead.

Lead in the environment: ubiquitous, persistent

The widespread perception that lead poisoning is no longer a major problem in the U.S. can be traced in part to the implementation of restrictions on the use of lead. In 1977 the Consumer Product Safety Commission limited the amount of lead in paint to 0.06% net weight. Thus, newer buildings are free of the hazard of highly leaded paint. Still, millions of older structures constitute an enormous reservoir of lead.

Another source of hazardous lead exposure in the past was exhaust from internal combustion engines. In 1986 the U.S. Environmental Protection Agency (EPA) reduced to 0.1 g per gal the amount of lead that can be added to gasoline to reduce engine knock. Over the preceding half century, however, as much as three or four grams of lead were added to each gallon, resulting in the dispersion of enormous amounts of lead into the environment via automobile exhaust. From 1975 to 1984 more than one million metric tons of lead were added to the gasoline sold in the U.S.; most of it now resides in the soil and dust of urban areas.

Thus, although laws have been passed curtailing lead use, childhood lead poisoning remains one of the most important pediatric environmental health problems. Indeed, in a recent comparative risk assessment conducted by the EPA's New England region, lead poisoning was included in the category of problems posing the greatest public health risk, sharing this dubious distinction with the hazards of radon exposure indoors and ozone in the outdoor environment.

The ubiquity of exposure distinguishes lead from many other environmental pollutants. Children do not have to live near a lead smelter or a hazardous-waste dump to accumulate unhealthy amounts of lead in their systems. Further, there appears to be a remarkably small margin of safety between "average" lead exposures and those considered hazardous. Analyses of the concentration of lead in the bones of people living millennia ago reveal that today's "average" exposures may be hundreds of times higher than those experienced by humans before lead mining and smelting were begun. Not all ancient societies managed to avoid heavy exposure to lead, however. The Romans used it extensively in their cooking materials and municipal water systems. The English word *plumbing* derives from *plumbum*, the Latin word for "lead." Some historians have even proposed that lead contamination of food and drinking water contributed to the well-documented mental impairment and reproductive disorders that developed among the Roman aristocracy and, ultimately, to the collapse of the empire.

Leaded paint in older, deteriorating buildings continues to be the major source of toxic exposure for young children in the U.S. Since 1977 there have been strict limits on the amount of lead allowed in paint.

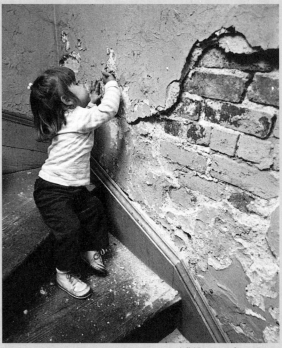

Jeff Albertson—Stock, Boston

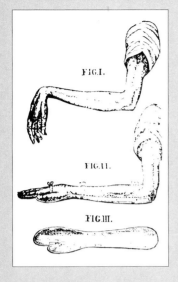

Lead poisoning was known as long as 2,000 years ago to be a cause of wrist-drop, a muscular paralysis in which the affected hand dangles loosely from the wrist. A 19th-century illustration shows a splint developed to correct the condition.

From Richard P. Wedeen, *Poison in the Pot: The Legacy of Lead*

Why children are at greater risk

Young children constitute the group at greatest risk of lead poisoning. Because of their behavior and physiology, they generally experience greater exposure than do adults living in the same environment. For instance, children's blood lead levels rise more than those of adults in response to an increase in dietary or air lead levels because, for each kilogram of body weight, children eat more and breathe a greater volume of air. Most children also engage in some "hand-to-mouth" activity—this is how infants and toddlers typically explore the immediate environment. This common pathway by which children ingest lead-bearing materials, such as household dust or garden soil, poses little hazard to adults. A smaller number of children engage in the behavior known as pica, the pathological ingestion of nonfood items. These children are at especially high risk because they may actually swallow leaded paint chips. A thumbnail-size chip that is 50% lead and weighs one gram will deliver a dose of 50,000 micrograms of lead, far above the presumably safe daily intake of 5 micrograms per kilogram of body weight (The word *safe*, however, should not be interpreted to mean "necessary," "required," or "recommended." Lead has no known biological function, and all exposure is anthropogenic—*i.e.*, due to human activity.)

The metabolism of lead also differs in children and adults. A young person's absorption of lead from the stomach and intestines is more efficient, especially in the presence of certain nutritional deficiencies (*e.g.*, of iron, calcium, and zinc), which are fairly common among children. Furthermore, a greater proportion of the total lead amount in a child's body is metabolically active rather than sequestered (stored) in bone. Whereas lead toxicity in an adult shows up primarily as peripheral nervous system dysfunction (*e.g.*, muscle weakness), its effects in children usually involve the central nervous system. The infant's developing nervous system is especially vulnerable. Because of the incomplete development of the so-called blood-brain barrier, a cellular partition that protects the brain from contact with toxic substances in the blood, lead in circulating blood has greater access to the young brain. Furthermore, the faster rate of cellular metabolism of the immature brain makes it more vulnerable than the adult brain to the adverse effects of lead on cell respiration and oxygen transport. Excessive exposure in critical stages of development may alter the number or organization of connections between nerve cells or the communication between them, possibly resulting in irreversible changes in brain structure and function.

"Acceptable" blood lead levels: changing standards

The toxic effects of various levels of lead exposure range from mild inhibition of certain enzymes to an acute encephalopathy (a disease of the brain). Lead exposure is generally assessed through measurement of the level of lead, in micrograms, per deciliter of blood, a measurement expressed as µg/dL. Acute encephalopathy, which occurs at blood lead levels above 80–100 µg/dL, is characterized by incoordination, confusion, swelling of the brain, and seizures; it may lead to coma or even death. Fortunately, the frequency of symptomatic illness has decreased dramatically over the past 20 years as screening of blood lead levels has become more widely available, facilitating early identification of youngsters at high risk. Another important factor has been the development of more effective means of treatment.

At the same time, however, opinions about how much lead is safe for a child have also changed. In the early decades of the 20th century, conventional wisdom held that a child who did not show signs of encephalopathy was not likely to suffer lasting neurological damage from lead exposure. As recently as the 1960s, a blood lead level of 60 µg/dL was considered the boundary between "normal" and "abnormal." Since then, this boundary level has been revised downward several times, most recently in 1985, when the U.S. Centers for Disease Control (CDC) defined a blood lead level greater than 25 µg/dL as "elevated." Still another revision is considered likely on the basis of accumulating evidence that blood lead levels near or even below 25 µg/dL impair the function of children's blood-forming organs, endocrine system (including vitamin D and calcium metabolism), overall growth, and intellectual development. In early 1990 an EPA advisory board concluded that 10 µg/dL is the maximum permissible blood lead level in children and other sensitive populations.

Those most at risk: urban poor and black

The magnitude of the hazard posed by low-level lead exposure has generally been underappreciated. In a report submitted to the U.S. Congress in July 1988, the Agency for Toxic Substances and Disease Registry (ATSDR) estimated that in 1984 approximately 2.4 million, or 17%, of children aged six months to five years living in urban regions called "standard metropolitan statistical areas" (SMSAs) had blood lead levels above 15 μg/dL. Over the country as a whole, the number was three million to four million children. An estimated 1.5% (200,700) had levels exceeding 25 μg/dL. These are national estimates, and they therefore obscure substantial regional and socioeconomic differences. For instance, in 1986, 11% of the children screened in St. Louis, Mo., met the criteria for "lead toxicity." In the last nationally representative survey of blood lead levels in the U.S. population (the National Health and Nutrition Examination Survey II, or NHANES II, 1976–80), the prevalence of elevated blood lead levels among black children was six times that of white children. Levels were also higher among urban children and those living in poverty. These risk factors appear to work in concert. The mean blood lead level of black children aged six months to five years living in large urban areas was 23 μg/dL—closely approaching the level now regarded as "elevated."

Although worrisome, these figures are a tremendous improvement over those from the 1960s and early 1970s, when one-quarter to one-half the children screened in large, older U.S. cities had blood lead levels above 40 μg/dL. The average level at the completion of the NHANES II survey (1980) was 37% lower than the average when the survey began (1976). This decline appeared to parallel rather closely a concurrent decline in the amount of lead added to gasoline. Presently the average blood lead level of U.S. preschool children is below 10 μg/dL.

Sources of exposure

Five sources, or pathways, account for most childhood exposure to lead: paint, air, soil and dust, food, and water. Some contribute to background exposure, the amount that would be received by anyone living in a given environment. The contributions of other sources to overall exposure depend to some extent on the individual's behavior. The exposures received via the different routes are additive. Thus, while the exposure from any individual source may be low, the cumulative exposure from all may be sufficient to produce an elevated blood lead level.

The ingestion of leaded paint is responsible for most cases of clinical lead poisoning. If a home is in poor repair, even a child who does not practice pica may become ill. Children may be exposed to toxic levels during home renovations in which lead-painted surfaces are disturbed; sanding and scraping liberate large amounts of very small lead particles that are difficult to contain and are readily inhaled or ingested. Efforts to "de-lead," unless conducted with scrupulous care, may actually dramatically increase the short-term hazard. Pregnant women and young children should stay out of the home until these activities, including a thorough cleanup, are completed.

Before the virtual elimination of lead from gasoline, airborne lead derived from the combustion of leaded gasoline provided at least 25% of an individual's exposure. The percentage has declined considerably in recent years and will continue to do so as the number of vehicles using leaded gasoline becomes smaller and smaller. Airborne lead will, however, continue to be an important source of exposure for children living near lead smelters or other industrial sources.

Lead in the soil derives from the deposition, or "fallout," of airborne lead and, even more importantly, from the deterioration of leaded exterior paint. The level of contamination may be particularly high in children's play areas near older houses. Although soil lead levels exceeding 500–1,000 parts per million are currently regarded by the EPA as hazardous to children, the average soil lead concentration in many large cities falls within this range. The EPA is currently funding demonstration projects in Baltimore, Md., Boston, and Cincinnati, Ohio, to determine whether the removal of lead-contaminated soil from around the homes of inner-city children reduces their blood lead levels.

House dust is particularly important because it is the final common pathway to the child from several sources of lead exposure: lead from outdoor soil is tracked inside on shoes; airborne lead enters through windows and doors; lead may be carried home on the clothing of a parent exposed to it at work; and leaded interior paint becomes powdery and chalky with time. Correlations have been established between the amounts of lead in house dust, on children's hands, and in their blood.

The contribution of dietary lead has decreased over the past decade as a result of changes in food canning and processing methods. However, eating vegetables grown in lead-contaminated soil or food prepared or served on improperly fired ceramic ware will add to background dietary lead exposure.

Lead enters drinking water at various points in the distribution system. It may leach out of lead pipes still in place in older homes and out of lead solder used to join copper pipes in newer homes. The process by which lead leaches into water is more efficient when the water is low in mineral content (soft) or acidic. Within a given building, the lead concentration is generally highest in water that stands in the plumbing system overnight. The hazard can be reduced if the tap is left open for a few minutes each morning until this water is flushed from the pipes.

Evidence of intellectual impairment

Because the central nervous system is an important target of lead in children, the impact of subclinical ex-

Amit Bhattacharya, University of Cincinnati Medical Center

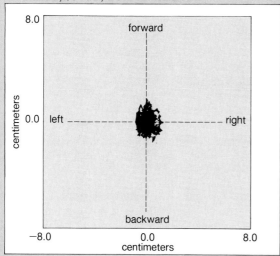

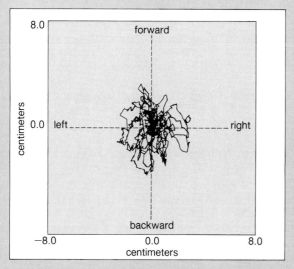

To test their suspicion that poor balance in young children may be an indication of lead exposure, researchers evaluated the ability of six-year-olds to stand still, with their eyes closed, on a postural sway platform. These two "sway plots" compare the area of sway—or deviation from a stationary upright posture—of a youngster with a relatively low blood lead level (top) with that of a child whose blood lead level is quite high (above).

posures on children's intellectual function has been a major focus of investigation. This research effort has been worldwide and includes studies carried out in the U.S., the U.K., Australia, West Germany, Greece, Denmark, Mexico, Yugoslavia, Italy, and Belgium. In 1986 the EPA concluded that a five-point drop in IQ was associated with blood lead levels above 50 µg/dL, a four-point drop with levels of 30 to 50 µg/dL, and a one–two-point drop with levels of 15 to 30 µg/dL. The EPA also concluded that signs of peripheral nervous system dysfunction (slower reaction time, slower nerve-conduction velocity, abnormalities in brain waves

as reflected in electroencephalograms) were evident at levels below 30 µg/dL. Other deficits linked to levels comparable to or below those presently considered toxic were lower reading achievement, hearing impairment, below-normal stature, and poor classroom behavior (*e.g.,* inattentiveness, inability to follow directions, impulsivity, physical aggression). An 11-year follow-up study conducted by Herbert L. Needleman and his colleagues, published in 1990 in the *New England Journal of Medicine,* found that the link between low levels of childhood lead exposure and academic performance may persist into young adulthood. The risks of serious problems such as reading disability and failure to graduate from high school were much greater among those individuals who had had relatively higher levels of lead in the baby teeth they shed at six or seven years of age. Although most public health experts support the hypothesis that subclinical lead exposure produces cognitive impairment in children, not all studies have detected this link; this discrepancy in findings has fueled an ongoing debate over the magnitude of lead's impact on intellectual functioning and the conditions under which that impact is apparent.

Another problem in interpreting such studies is that it is difficult to demonstrate that the intellectual deficits observed in these children are actually due to lead rather than to some other factor or combination of factors, such as poor medical care, inadequate nutrition, or lack of educational opportunities. Studies using laboratory animals can help to resolve this problem of interpretation. Although great care must be taken in extrapolating from animals to humans, it has already been demonstrated that nonhuman primates exposed to lead under experimental conditions display the same types of cognitive and behavioral deficits as those seen in humans exposed to lead under naturalistic conditions.

A further complication is that children who are mentally impaired may behave in ways that increase their exposure to lead (*e.g.,* pica). Lead might therefore be unjustly blamed as the source of the impairment. In order to establish with greater certainty which comes first, lead exposure or intellectual impairment, recent studies have begun testing children at or prior to birth. The tests measure blood lead levels and various indexes of mental functioning over a period of time. In addition to clarifying the issue of causation, these studies are generating a wealth of new information about the impact of fetal lead exposure on a child's early development.

Fetal exposure

The placenta, the highly vascular sac that surrounds the developing fetus, does not afford the fetus much protection from lead. The disastrous impact of mothers' high-dose lead exposure on pregnancy outcome has been known for over a century, evidenced by higher rates of infertility, spontaneous abortion, and stillbirth among women working in lead-related industries. According to some historical reports, lead was voluntarily ingested by some women as a way to terminate unwanted pregnancies.

The ATSDR concluded that lead concentrations of 10 to 15 µg/dL in maternal blood or in umbilical-cord blood are hazardous to the fetus. Exposures of this magnitude, experienced annually by approximately 400,000 fetuses in U.S. SMSAs, have been linked to shorter gestation, reduced birth weight, minor birth defects, and slower growth in the months after birth. Once again, however, not all studies substantiate these associations.

Several studies have found an association between babies' prenatal lead exposure and their achievement of developmental milestones in the first few years of life (*e.g.*, perception, coordination, language acquisition, memory, problem-solving ability). Medical and psychological follow-up of these children has not been carried out over a long-enough period of time to determine whether these deficits are permanent. It may be that over time and with appropriate interventions and support, children are able to compensate for early developmental impairment.

IQ controversy

Many people question the practical significance of a reduction in IQ that is limited to only a few points. And most investigators agree that factors such as parental intelligence and socioeconomic status are more important determinants of children's intellectual functioning than is exposure to lead. On the other hand, a factor that has even a modest impact at the level of the individual child may have a substantial impact on the population as a whole if that factor occurs with high frequency. Bernard Weiss, a toxicologist at the University of Rochester (N.Y.) School of Medicine, has calculated that if lead decreases the mean IQ of a population of 100 million individuals by five points (*e.g.*, from 100, which is considered average, to 95), the number of people who score above 130 (a relatively high score) would decline from 2.3 million to 990,000. Similarly, the percentage who score below 70, significantly lower than average, would more than double, from 2.3 million to 4.8 million.

Screening: identifying youngsters at risk

Excess exposure to lead is generally silent. As a result, most children exposed to potentially hazardous levels are identified only if they participate in a screening program. The CDC recommends that all U.S. children between the ages of nine months and six years be screened for lead exposure as part of routine health care. Children at special risk should be screened frequently, perhaps every two to three months, and especially during the summer, when children's exposures tend to be greater. Groups warranting closer surveillance include younger children (aged 12 to 36 months), those living in older, dilapidated housing or near lead smelters, and those whose siblings or playmates have toxic blood lead levels.

The standard presently employed in most lead-screening programs is not the concentration of lead in a child's blood but the concentration of a metabolite (product of metabolism) that reflects lead's biochemical toxicity. Depending on the method used, this metabolite is either erythrocyte protoporphyrin (EP) or

The city of Boston was conducting a screening program for children at high risk of lead poisoning as early as 1975. The photo at right shows one young participant submitting—unhappily—to a blood test. Because of what is known today about the effects of clinically silent lead exposure on intellectual and nervous system functioning, screening of youngsters at risk is considered even more crucial.

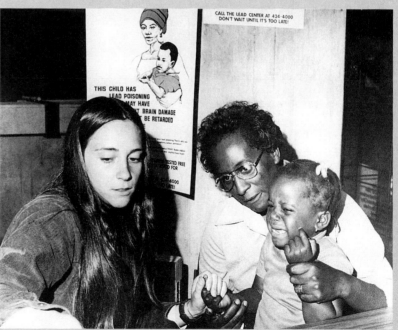

AP/Wide World

zinc protoporphyrin (ZPP). Both are indexes of the biosynthesis of a component of hemoglobin, which is the oxygen-carrying protein of red blood cells. An EP assay is less expensive than a blood lead assay and can be done with a small amount of capillary blood obtained by pricking the tip of a finger. However, lead poisoning is not the only condition that causes elevations in EP (iron deficiency is another), so a positive result must be followed up with an assay that yields information specifically about lead. For this purpose, blood is drawn by syringe from a vein and analyzed for lead content. Venous blood is used because lead on the skin of a child's finger can easily contaminate capillary blood.

Lead-screening practices will probably change considerably in the next few years. An EP assay will generally identify a child with a blood lead level above 25 µg/dL; if the criterion for an elevated lead level is lowered from the present standard of 25 µg/dL and identifying children with blood lead levels in this lower range becomes the goal of screening, EP will have to be replaced by a more sensitive biochemical marker or by direct assay of blood lead itself.

Currently, children who have a positive EP test (*i.e.,* above 35 µg/dL) and a blood lead concentration above 25 µg/dL undergo a diagnostic evaluation to assess the severity of the burden of lead in the body. This process usually includes a neurological examination focusing especially on symptoms of lead poisoning (*e.g.,* behavioral changes, loss of appetite, lethargy, constipation), a nutritional evaluation, additional blood lead and EP assessments to confirm the screening results, and a test for iron deficiency. X-rays of the abdomen may reveal whether the child recently ingested lead-containing materials. "Growth arrest" lines, revealed by X-rays of the long bones, reflect lead's interference with bone metabolism and provide information about the chronicity of exposure. The identification and elimination of the sources of lead exposure in the child's environment are a critical component of the evaluation.

Treatment of lead poisoning

In some cases, drug therapy is indicated. Substances called chelating agents (from the Greek *khele,* meaning "claw") bind lead and carry it from the body. The "lead mobilization" test, which assesses the amount of lead a child excretes in urine in response to a "challenge" dose of the chelating agent calcium disodium EDTA (CaNaEDTA), identifies children who may benefit from a full course of chelation therapy. Most chelation protocols require hospitalization and repeated injections of the chelating agent. The agents used most frequently are CaNaEDTA, BAL (British anti-lewisite, also called dimercaprol, a substance originally developed as an antidote for poison gas), and penicillamine. Another agent, dimercaptosuccinic acid (DMSA), is being evaluated in clinical trials. The initial results are promising,

and DMSA appears to have fewer side effects than other treatments. Another development on the near horizon is a noninvasive X-ray fluorescence method of assessing the amount of lead in a child's skeleton, the repository of a large fraction of the total burden of lead in an individual's body. This method may be useful in screening, identifying candidates for chelation therapy, and monitoring the course of therapy.

Outlook for the future: tempered optimism

Although lead has been recognized as a toxic substance for more than 2,000 years, substantial advances have recently been made in understanding the groups at greatest risk, the sources and routes of exposure, the various indications of toxic exposure, and the levels at which they occur. In many ways the story of the U.S. campaign against childhood lead poisoning is one of remarkable successes. In direct response to increasing evidence of the public health risks of lead exposure, specific steps were taken to limit exposure from those sources of lead having relatively centralized distribution systems; *i.e.,* lead in paint, gasoline, and food. These controls, along with more effective screening programs, led to significant reductions in the average blood lead levels of U.S. children. Satisfaction in these accomplishments has, however, been tempered by more recent evidence of adverse health effects at lower and lower levels of exposure.

For the most part, public health experts have until recently given higher priority to minimizing the impact of exposure that has already occurred than to preventing it outright. Just as miners once used canaries to warn them of falling oxygen levels in underground tunnels, children have, in a sense, been used as "biological monitors" to identify the presence in the environment of hazardous sources of lead. This approach is slowly changing. Primary prevention efforts must now focus on reducing exposure from less centralized, local sources such as soil, dust, water, and deteriorating leaded paint.

In one sense, eliminating childhood lead exposure should be a simple process—the sources and pathways of exposure are known, and the technologies needed to eliminate the hazards are relatively simple, although not inexpensive. It would cost billions of dollars to remove lead-contaminated soil outside of homes and leaded paint inside. Whether the anticipated benefits, including increased human productivity and reduced costs for health care and remedial education, are worth this investment is not a scientific issue. Money spent on lead abatement would not be available for addressing other social ills. On the other hand, achieving a permanent solution to childhood lead poisoning not only would improve the health of the nation's children but would demonstrate that with resolve and commitment environmental problems can be successfully addressed.

Environmental Health Special Report
Drinking Water: What's on Tap?

by Robert Keene McLellan, M.D., M.P.H.

The first glimmerings of life on Earth began in salty seawater. Today, some three billion years later, water remains the single most important life-sustaining nutrient. Water's unique properties as a universal solvent, however, also make it a medium capable of making people ill. Water contaminated by microbes, chemicals, and radioactive substances has carried disease to every civilization known to history. In the 20th century most developed countries have become so successful at providing clean water that their citizens tend to take plentiful, safe drinking water for granted. Recently, however, in the wake of revelations about the contamination of local water supplies by toxic chemicals, many Americans have begun to fear that their tap water is unhealthy. Some have installed water-treatment devices in their homes or will drink only bottled water. Such alternatives are expensive, perhaps costing the consumer 500 to 1,000 times more than the price of tap water; when adopted for health reasons, in many cases these actions are misguided. Nonetheless, the American public's concern about the quality of drinking water is justified, and those hazards that do exist need to be put into perspective.

Few people concerned about the quality of water think beyond the several glassfuls they drink every day. Other residential uses of water, however, involve much greater amounts and can involve exposure to toxins that are inhaled or absorbed through the skin. For example, minerals that are harmless when swallowed can become hazardous when they emerge from humidifiers as tiny particles and are inhaled deeply into the lungs. One research project showed that between 29 and 91% of the organic solvents people are exposed to daily could enter the body via the skin during a 15-minute bath—substantially more than from drinking two liters (a liter is slightly more than a quart) of water.

Setting and enforcing standards

The source of water inevitably affects its quality. Water—whether from the tap or from a bottle purchased in a store—is drawn from one of two sources: groundwater, which lies below ground, and surface water, such as lakes, rivers, and reservoirs. In general, microbial contamination threatens surface water more than groundwater, whereas groundwater is at greater risk of contamination by synthetic chemicals and naturally radioactive substances.

In the United States, since 1974, the Safe Drinking Water Act (SDWA) has regulated the more than 58,900 public water systems, which by definition have at least 15 or more service connections or regularly serve 25 or more people. The SDWA requires the Environmental Protection Agency (EPA) to set enforceable national standards for drinking water called maximum contaminant levels (MCLs); the EPA also sets maximum contaminant level goals (MCLGs), which represent targets for minimizing the health effects of contamination. MCLs have been established with the aim of protecting the most vulnerable members of society; for example,

The average U.S. household uses about 295 liters (78 gallons) of water per person per day for all indoor purposes, of which only a small fraction—about 2 liters (0.53 gallon) per person—is consumed as drinking water. About 102 liters (27 gallons) are used for toilet flushing, while another 83 liters (22 gallons) are used for baths and showers. Most people are not aware that bathing can expose them to water impurities that may be absorbed through the skin.

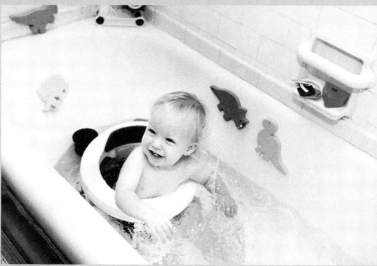

Robert F. Kusel

infants and people with the kind of high blood pressure that is affected by high levels of sodium. Usually, the MCL for a substance is higher than its MCLG because the former reflects the economic and technical feasibility of achieving a given level. Amendments to the SDWA, passed in 1986, require that by January 1991 an additional 60 substances be regulated, bringing to 83 the number of substances that have levels governed by national standards. An additional 25 substances will be regulated by June 1992. In addition to national primary drinking water standards set by the SDWA, secondary maximum contaminant levels have been established as nonenforceable guidelines for contaminants that adversely affect the aesthetic quality of drinking water.

The EPA also determines how often the water supply must be tested. The frequency of monitoring varies, depending on the contaminant in question and the type and size of the water-distribution system. The greater the number of people served by the system, the more closely the water is watched and the more assured consumers can be of its quality. For example, only systems serving more than 10,000 people are required to test for the carcinogens known as THMs (trihalomethanes). Systems serving more than 3,960,-000 people must perform at least 480 tests per month for bacteria, whereas those serving 25 to 1,000 people need test only one sample per month. Though in total they serve six million people, the majority (77%) of public water suppliers in the U.S. serve fewer than 1,000 people. These systems are barely regulated, and water treatment is often minimal. Some do not treat at all. It should also be noted that more than 40 million Americans draw their water from private wells; monitoring and treatment of this water is entirely the well owner's responsibility—making private well water potentially the most unfit to drink.

Bottled water: what's in it?

With sales increasing 400% in the last decade, today about one of every 15 U.S. households uses bottled drinking water. Americans drank about six billion liters of bottled water in 1988—a per capita consumption of 24.3 liters, almost all (97%) of which was domestic water. In the United States, bottled drinking water is considered a food and thus is regulated by the Food and Drug Administration (FDA) through its guidelines for good manufacturing practices and the same EPA standards as for tap water. Voluntary industry standards may in some cases exceed the EPA standards. The FDA defines bottled water as any water "sealed in bottles or other containers and intended for human consumption." Excluded from this category are mineral waters or soft drinks commonly known as soda or seltzer water and made by the dissolving of carbon dioxide in potable water. These beverages are regulated separately and less stringently.

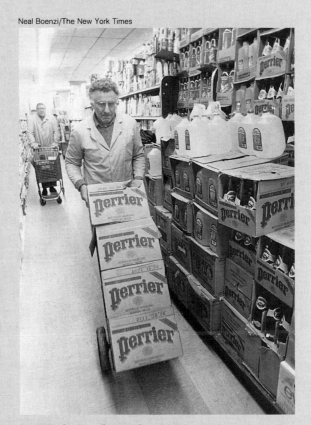

In 1990 the French manufacturer Perrier voluntarily recalled millions of bottles of its carbonated water because some were found to contain small amounts of the carcinogen benzene. Improperly maintained filters were to blame.

The International Bottled Water Association (IBWA), a trade association representing about 90% of bottled water suppliers in the U.S., is more specific in its descriptions of bottled water. The IBWA has its own set of standards and labeling requirements, but these are strictly voluntary. According to IBWA guidelines, bottled drinking water must be obtained from an approved source and must undergo minimum treatment consisting of filtration and ozonation (addition of ozone) or an equivalent disinfection process. Mineral water is described as containing at least 500 parts per million of dissolved solids. Natural water must come from an underground source not used for municipal purposes and may have no dissolved solids added or deleted. Spring water must flow naturally to the surface and meet the definition of natural water. Bottled well water is required to meet the definition of natural and, furthermore, must be extracted from an underground source through a man-made hole that taps the source. The IBWA also asks its members to label their products so as to differentiate between carbonation that comes from the same source as the water and that derived from another source. Many states enforce accurate labeling distinctions and other regulations similar to the IBWA's voluntary standards;

the FDA, however, does not define such terms as *natural* and *spring* water. Interested consumers are advised to contact state authorities to ascertain their state's regulations. Most bottled water companies, if requested, will send consumers an analysis of their water by an independent testing company.

The consumer cannot—and should not—assume that bottled water is pristine. Microorganisms and small amounts of many organic chemicals have been detected in bottled water. A survey of 22 bottled waters by New York state's Health Department in the early 1980s found that 15 contained one or more of 39 undesirable organic chemicals tested for. All of these chemicals were present in levels within EPA standards, however.

In 1990 Perrier, one of the most famous of bottled waters, recalled all of its water from store shelves in the U.S. and Canada because, in spot checking, benzene—an organic chemical known to be carcinogenic—was detected in several lots at levels ranging from 12 to 22 parts per billion, exceeding the EPA standard (5 parts per billion) in its finished product. According to the French manufacturer, its water and the carbon dioxide used for carbonation reside separately, though nearby, in the same geologic formation. The gas and water are piped individually to the bottling plant, where they are mixed. Perrier uses charcoal filters to remove naturally occurring benzene from the carbon dioxide. The problems apparently arose because these filters had not been properly maintained.

By definition, mineral waters have very high levels of minerals. In some cases these minerals have included potentially hazardous amounts of inorganic chemicals such as arsenic or fluoride. (At lower levels fluoride is considered beneficial.) The FDA requires that labeling warn the consumer that the water contains excessive amounts of chemical substances. To be safe, mineral waters are best consumed sparingly and should not be one's sole source of drinking water.

Water quality: major concerns

Truly "pure" water contains only hydrogen and oxygen. It is not available naturally and, except for special laboratory purposes, is never used. The water that is consumed is actually altered in a wide variety of ways— some harmful, some beneficial, and some affecting primarily taste and appearance. From this perspective, water quality is determined by several characteristics: aesthetic and physical factors, hazardous contaminants (microbiological, inorganic, organic, and radioactive), and purposeful additives.

Aesthetic considerations. Water's aesthetic and physical factors primarily affect utilitarian and sensory characteristics (taste, odor, and visual appearance). For example, excessive iron makes water a red-brown color, stains plumbing fixtures and clothing, and imparts a metallic taste, but it is not a health hazard. Excessive calcium and magnesium cause "hard water," leading to hard white deposits in pipes, steam irons, and teakettles. Drinking water with a high mineral content—greater than 500 mg of total dissolved minerals per liter—may have a laxative effect. Generally speaking, hard water is not considered to be a health hazard. Some research has even suggested that it can be beneficial. People who drink hard water may have less cardiovascular disease, for example, than those who drink softer water—perhaps because of the beneficial effects of magnesium and calcium. Corrosivity—a function of pH, inorganic carbonate, calcium, and total dissolved solids (TDS)—is another physical factor that in itself is not hazardous. It can have a leaching effect on metal pipes, however, causing toxic metals such

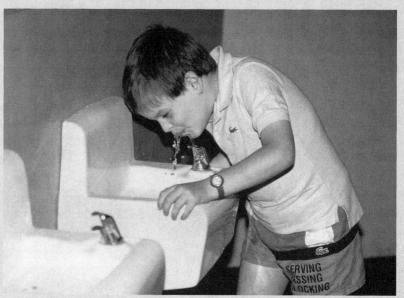

Lead in drinking water can be a serious health hazard, especially to young children. The most likely sources of the metallic contaminant are lead pipes in older buildings and lead solder used to join pipes in new construction. According to the Environmental Protection Agency, about one million U.S. schools have water fountains that contain lead components or lead-lined tanks.

as lead and cadmium to be released into the water.

Microbial contamination. Microbes cause more disease than any other single agent found in water. In the U.S. a measurement system has been formulated to screen for the variety of waterborne pathogenic microbes, some of which can be technically difficult to detect. As an indicator of contamination, the system measures total coliforms. (Coliforms are bacteria that grow naturally and in great quantities in mammalian intestinal tracts.) Because most of the pathogenic microorganisms found in water are a result of fecal contamination, the presence of coliforms has been used to assess the potential for other microbial contaminants. Although the use of the total coliform rule has greatly improved the safety of drinking water, it has pitfalls. For example, total coliforms is not an acceptable index for ruling out the presence of the parasites *Giardia* and *Cryptosporidium.* Between 1946 and 1980, close to 700 outbreaks of waterborne disease were reported in the U.S., affecting 150,000 persons using public water systems—and reported outbreaks are thought to be only the tip of the iceberg. Clearly, standards that rely solely on quantification of coliforms do not guarantee that treated water is safe water. For this reason, new standards of treatment, to be phased in over the next decade, have been promulgated.

Waterborne pathogens also get into building heating, air-conditioning, and humidifying systems and are ultimately inhaled with air treated by such systems. Epidemics of legionnaire's disease (an often fatal pneumonia), hypersensitivity pneumonitis (an allergic pneumonia), and humidifier fever (a flulike illness) serve to highlight the point that waterborne disease is transmitted not only by contaminated drinking water but also by air that has been conditioned by ventilation systems in which there is polluted water.

Inorganic substances. Numerous inorganic substances are found in drinking water. Lead, nitrates, asbestos, and pesticides serve as good examples because of their prevalence and recent publicity about the hazards they pose. Lead has received special attention because of its ubiquity in plumbing fixtures and solder and because recent research has shown that very low levels of lead are toxic to a child's developing brain. In the U.S. some 42 million people are thought to be at risk of excess lead ingestion through drinking water; more than 240,000 children may have suffered neurological damage from exposure to lead in drinking water. The June 1986 amendments to the SDWA banned from public water systems soldering materials containing more than 0.2% lead and pipes with a lead content greater than 8%. A testing program was recently instituted in schools throughout the U.S. to check for lead contamination of school drinking fountains and plumbing systems.

Nitrate contamination comes primarily from fertilizer runoff, with additions from human and animal fecal contamination. Over the last two decades, studies in agricultural states have shown that 27 to 80% of wells tested exceed EPA standards of 10 parts per billion for nitrate. Not surprisingly, shallow wells are at greatest risk. Nitrates are a particular health risk for infants less than six months old. In their immature digestive systems, nitrate is transformed into nitrite, which reacts with hemoglobin—the oxygen-carrying substance in the blood—to form methemoglobin. Methemoglobin binds oxygen, making it unavailable to the tissues. The result is a rare but potentially fatal syndrome called methemoglobinemia. Nitrites can react with other dietary substances to form nitrosamines, which are known animal carcinogens. Water sources, however, represent only about 10% of the average daily dietary consumption of nitrates.

Because asbestos cement water pipes were once widely used, asbestos contamination of water is common. The hazards to asbestos workers of inhaling fibers of the mineral are well known. There is, however, no firm evidence that swallowing asbestos is harmful. Some studies have confirmed that asbestos-laden water in showers and humidifiers might contaminate indoor air, but the levels and character of this contamination probably do not appreciably increase the risk of respiratory diseases. The fibers released into the air from water are primarily short ones, believed less dangerous than the longer fibers asbestos workers have been exposed to.

For many decades conventional wisdom held that groundwater would never become widely contaminated by pesticides because the chemical nature of these substances would inhibit their migration through soil and, furthermore, soil would act as a natural water purifier. Unfortunately, evidence is mounting that these assumptions were misguided. The EPA has reported that wells in 32 states have been contaminated by 45 different pesticides. The class of pesticides most commonly found in groundwater is nematocides (worm killers), which are designed to be mobile, persistent, and toxic. Contamination by the nematocides EDB (ethylene dibromide), DBCP (dibromochloropropane), and aldicarb has been widely recognized. In Florida alone more than 1,000 wells have been shut down because of EDB contamination. In California traces of DBCP have been found in 3,500 wells, and in New York more than 4,000 wells on Long Island are known to be tainted with aldicarb. EDB and DBCP are now banned. Aldicarb, however, remains in use.

Agriculture should not be singled out as the sole culprit in pesticide contamination of groundwater. Even pesticides used at home—about 7% of the total in the U.S.—contribute to the problem. In nonagricultural states such as Connecticut, household pesticides comprise about 61% of the total used; about half of these are applied outside, most intensively on lawns, and ultimately can end up in the groundwater.

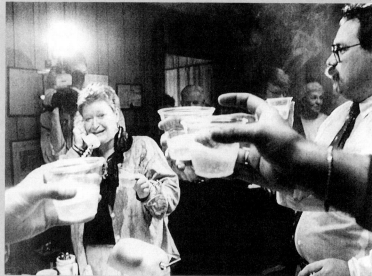
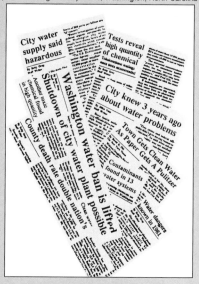

Reporters at the Washington *(North Carolina)* Daily News *toast the announcement that the paper has won a 1990 Pulitzer Prize for a series of articles revealing that the local water supply had for years been contaminated with the deadly chemicals known as trihalomethanes.*

Organic contaminants. Natural organic chemicals, in the form of vegetable and animal waste, have always contaminated the Earth's water. In the past 50 years, however, human industry has created thousands of new, synthetic organic chemicals, many of which have now begun to appear as contaminants of drinking water. One important group of carcinogenic organic contaminants is the THMs—chemical compounds resulting from the chlorination of water containing decaying vegetable matter. In 1983 the EPA published a survey of 34 volatile organic chemicals in U.S. groundwater. The survey covered about 1,000 large and small public water systems throughout the U.S., half chosen randomly and half chosen because they were at high risk of contamination because of proximity to a pollution source. Organic chemicals were detected in 17% of the randomly chosen small systems (serving fewer than 10,000 people) and in 28% of the larger systems. Of the high-risk small water supplies, 22% were contaminated; of the large systems, 37%.

Nationwide, thousands of private wells in both rural and suburban areas have been condemned because dangerous organic contaminants were identified—sometimes only after consumers' health was affected. In May 1979 the EPA found trichloroethylene, tetrachloroethylene, and chloroform in two of eight municipal wells in Woburn, Mass. Subsequently, epidemiologists determined that in the community in and around Woburn, 12 "excess" cases of leukemia (*i.e.,* 12 more than would normally be expected) had occurred. Of these 12 cases, they were able to link about half to the ingestion of contaminated water. Although this study was one of the most sophisticated of its kind, not all researchers agreed with the analysis; the key point

of contention is the enormous difficulty encountered in scientifically linking the development of cancer to water contaminants.

Waterborne radon. As water percolates through soil and rock, it is naturally contaminated by small quantities of radioactive, carcinogenic substances. In some cases man-made radioactive wastes can add to this contamination. Recently radon has achieved notoriety as the most important environmental carcinogen besides tobacco smoke. Radon does not seem to be hazardous when ingested; however, radon gas emitted from tap water becomes airborne and may be inhaled. The number of fatalities caused by the latter type of exposure—an estimated 30 to 600 deaths per year in the U.S.—exceeds the number caused by all other waterborne contaminants. Although radon is found in all waters, wells in New England are the most significantly contaminated. Large public water supplies are usually the least contaminated.

Chlorine and fluoride: benefits versus risks of additives. The chlorination and fluoridation of public water supplies have been among the most successful of all public health interventions to decrease disease. The chlorination process has greatly reduced the transmission of waterborne microbial diseases, and fluoridation has led to dramatic reductions in the incidence of tooth decay. Nonetheless, these interventions have not been without risks. Chlorination has been linked with increases in THMs, and fluoridation can lead to dental fluorosis, a discoloration of the teeth. Very high doses (20 mg a day over two decades) can result in skeletal fluorosis, which leads to brittle bones. The EPA has set standards for the amount of THMs and fluoride allowed in public water supplies.

Fluoride is naturally present at some level in all water supplies but is artificially added to water supplies reaching 121 million Americans in order to raise fluoride levels to about one milligram per liter—the optimal level for preventing tooth decay while avoiding side effects. Another 10 million people drink water naturally fluoridated at about optimal levels and, in some cases, at a level greater than four milligrams per liter, which is the MCL. In setting an MCL of four milligrams per liter, the EPA sought to minimize health risks without overburdening the technical and financial capabilities of community water suppliers. In fact, in 1990 the EPA estimated that about 300 community water systems exceed this MCL.

The controversy over the possible adverse effects of fluoridation was rekindled when it was reported that the results of a two-year animal study by the National Toxicology Program showed an association between the ingestion of sodium fluoride (the substance used to fluoridate public water supplies) and the development of a rare bone cancer (osteosarcoma). The report, which was officially released in May 1990, showed that some rats in the study had higher than expected rates of osteosarcoma. This was not seen in mice that ingested fluoride, however. Most scientists agreed that the data were insufficient to conclude that fluoridation threatens human health.

Chemical pollutants: risks uncertain

As increasingly sensitive measurement devices are developed, even more widespread synthetic chemical contamination is likely to be found. In the EPA's groundwater survey, only 1% of samples in randomly chosen water supplies were contaminated at levels higher than five parts per billion, whereas 4% of the large, high-risk systems were contaminated at levels above five parts per billion. What are the health implications of contamination at these levels? The diversity

of organic chemicals in the water supply raises the specter of a wide variety of health effects ranging from neurological damage to gastrointestinal disorders. Nonetheless, despite certain notable exceptions, contamination of water supplies by organic substances usually is not sufficient to cause any such illnesses.

Public concern about chemical pollutants has tended to center on the risks of birth defects and cancer. Although conservative policymakers currently assume that no safe level of exposure can be established for any known carcinogen, this does not mean that the slightest exposure to a carcinogenic substance causes cancer in everyone exposed to it. Rather it means that there is some risk—beginning at what is currently considered a negligible level—somewhere between one in 100,000 to one in one million. For example, if the risk associated with drinking water containing benzene at five parts per billion is an estimated lifetime risk of one in 400,000, it means that one in 400,000 similarly exposed people will contract cancer. In comparison, the risk of death from being struck by lightning is one in 30,000, in a motor vehicle accident one in 60, or from a lifetime in a house with four picocuries of radon (the level at which the EPA recommends remedial action) about one in 50.

Unfortunately, the actual human risks of exposure to pesticides and other chemicals in the water supply are not well understood and cannot really be accurately estimated. The EPA and other scientific groups base their estimates of the risks on the chemical nature of the contaminant in question, *in vitro* studies, animal studies, and studies of inadvertent human exposures. Not surprisingly, risk estimates often involve considerable uncertainty and are frequently the focus of scientific controversy. Even when epidemiologists have associated outbreaks of cancer with community water contamination, as in the well-documented case of Woburn, not all scientists can agree that the

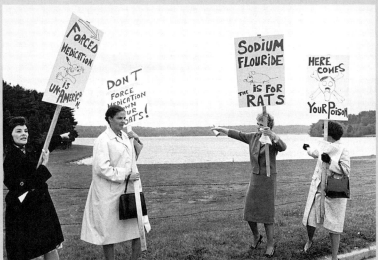

The possible risks of fluoridation have been a subject of controversy for years; the photo at left shows a 1965 protest at a New York City reservoir. A highly publicized report released in 1990 showing an association between sodium fluoride—which is added to water to prevent tooth decay—and the development of cancer in some laboratory animals reignited the dispute. Still, most scientists remain unconvinced that fluoridation poses a threat to human health.

link has been conclusively demonstrated. Nonetheless, enough credible evidence has been gathered in both the laboratory and the community to prompt the EPA to significantly increase the regulation and monitoring of water supplies for organic chemicals.

Ensuring safe water: what the consumer can do

Careful monitoring and appropriate treatment minimize the health risk of water consumption. There are three steps one can take to ascertain the safety of tap water:

1. Determine the source. Private well owners and consumers of water distributed by companies serving fewer than 500 people should be especially vigilant.

2. Be alert to any changes in taste, odor, or color. Consumers themselves are best equipped to judge the aesthetic qualities of their water. Some, but emphatically not all, hazardous contaminants can be identified by the senses. For example, a sharp chemical taste or odor or an oily consistency should warn of the need for immediate water testing.

3. Monitor the water. People who get their water from large municipal systems can obtain the results of the regular tests such systems are required by law to conduct. Those who drink bottled water can get the results of tests performed by the regulatory agencies responsible for monitoring these products. Some consumers, particularly those served by smaller public water systems, may want more comprehensive and frequent tests of their tap water than are performed by the local utility company. Of particular concern for all tap water users is lead, as household plumbing and old lead service pipes are the major sources of lead contamination. Private well owners are urged to establish a monitoring program for their wells. They may want to follow the EPA's testing guidelines for water systems serving fewer than 500 people. In general, a well should at least be tested for all primary and most secondary drinking water contaminants on commissioning (*i.e.*, before first use). Thereafter, testing for coliforms every year and comprehensive testing for other contaminants about every fifth year are warranted. Proximity to new construction sites or pollution sources warrants more frequent testing, focusing especially on indicator contaminants, such as benzene, which may signal an underground gasoline tank leak. Only an EPA-certified laboratory should be used. Consumers should beware of "free" tests provided by companies promoting water-treatment devices.

Home water treatment: wave of the future?

According to a 1986 survey, about 5% of all U.S. households elected to use home water-treatment devices. Many authorities denounce this trend; in their opinion, water treatment is a complex, potentially risky operation best left to professionals. Further, because some suppliers of water-treatment devices use unscrupulous tactics to convince consumers that the devices are necessary, some experts would prefer to see them banned entirely.

Other authorities, however, see home treatment as the wave of the future. They point out that since less than 1% of water in the home is actually used for cooking and drinking, it does not make sense that all of the water that is distributed meet the stringent criteria meant for culinary water. Another relevant consideration is that even after being centrally treated, water may be contaminated in the distribution system; thus, home treatment might be the only effective treatment. In addition, even the largest public water supplies are monitored only for a small percentage of all contaminants. The individual consumer may choose health or aesthetic criteria more stringent than those used by the water company. Thus, there seem to be some valid arguments both for and against the use of home water-treatment devices.

Two methods of improving water quality cost little and can be universally recommended. One method is to refrain from dumping household chemicals down the drain. Those who have a septic system and a well may unwittingly be contaminating their own water by such practices. Persons served by municipal systems are only adding to the contamination of groundwater. (The proper way to dispose of these products is to take them to the nearest household hazardous waste dump or to call the local health department or water company and ask for the schedule of days on which household hazardous waste is collected.) It is possible to effectively treat tap water contaminated with lead and other metals from household plumbing by using only cold water for culinary purposes and by letting the water run until it reaches its coldest temperature before using it.

No single water-treatment system is best for all homes. In selecting a system, the consumer should take into account environmental threats to the water, contaminants and aesthetic problems actually identified by water testing, and personal or family goals. The use of a device certified by the National Sanitation Foundation assures the consumer that the device will satisfy several requirements, not the least of which is that the device will meet the manufacturer's contaminant-reduction claims.

Finally, it should be noted that even when used as designed, some home water-treatment devices may actually degrade the safety of the water. As noted above, water softeners add sodium as they extract calcium and magnesium—possibly increasing the risk of cardiovascular disease. In addition, most treatment devices require regular maintenance to ensure their efficacy and to ensure that they do not add contaminants to the water. For example, if charcoal filters are not regularly flushed or changed, they may add microbial agents and return to the water the synthetic organic contaminants they were intended to remove.

Environmental Health Special Report
Electromagnetic Fields: Tempest in a Charged Teapot?
by Michael E. Newman

In 1894 engineers at General Electric's Niagara Falls, N.Y., electrical plant threw the switch on the world's first alternating current generator. At the end of a transmission line 42 km (26 mi) away, in Buffalo, lights began to hum, then suddenly shone. Accounts of the momentous event soon spread across the land, and newspapers nationwide hailed the day that the electrification of a nation began.

Nearly a century later, stories about alternating current, high-voltage transmission, and the U.S. electric power network are again big news. The focus now, however, is not what electricity is doing *for* people but what it may be doing *to* them. In question are the possible health risks from exposure to the electric and magnetic fields generated during the transmission, distribution, and use of standard household current. Public reaction has ranged from wary concern to outright fear, from heightened community interest to organized protests against a perceived health threat. In the scientific community, meanwhile, a stormy debate rages as to how the question of risk should be, whether it can be, or even if it needs to be answered.

The source of concern

What are the electromagnetic fields that have become such a source of concern? Unlike the direct current (DC) produced by batteries, the electric power that people use in their homes, offices, and schools depends on alternating current (AC). AC alternates back and forth 60 times each second; hence the term 60 hertz (Hz) power. Electric and magnetic fields created by this 60-Hz alternating current are commonly referred to together as extremely low-frequency (ELF) electromagnetic fields. Sixty-hertz ELF fields, as generated by high-voltage power lines, are at one end of the electromagnetic spectrum. They are quite a bit lower in energy than, for example, their cousin, AM radio waves (10^6 Hz), classified as very high-frequency, and considerably lower than their distant relative at the opposite end, X-rays (10^{18} Hz), classified as extremely high-frequency. In fact, even the naturally occurring fields along the Earth's surface are stronger than 60-Hz fields.

At low frequencies (*i.e.,* below 300 Hz), the electric and magnetic portions of electromagnetic fields act independently. The electric portion results from the strength of an electrical charge and is proportional to the amount of voltage present. Therefore, high-voltage sources such as transmission lines produce more intense fields than low-voltage household appliances. The magnetic portion, on the other hand, arises from a charged motion that creates a magnetic attraction and strengthens as current strength increases. A hair dryer operated on its "high" setting (which draws a lot of current) generates a greater magnetic field than it does when run at low heat. An electrical device that is plugged into a wall socket and activated generates both electric and magnetic fields. If the device is turned off and left plugged in, only the electric field remains (because no charges are in motion). Both fields are strongest at the socket; the greater the distance gets from the source, the weaker the fields.

The particular sources that have raised concern are overhead power lines near people's homes as well as such commonly used household appliances as electric stoves, refrigerators, televisions, computers and video display terminals, electrically heated water beds, and electric blankets. The latter have received much of the media's attention in the reporting about electromagnetic fields because electric blankets expose sleepers to a substantial ELF field over relatively long periods of time—*i.e.,* all night—and because the user has intimate contact with the source.

The start of a controversy

Before the late 1970s, the main public outcries heard about power lines were complaints about their ugliness or how their proximity to homes wreaked havoc with television or radio reception. Potential health hazards from associated ELF fields were generally dismissed by scientists and medical experts alike. Extremely low-frequency fields, it was believed, could not damage human cells because they did not possess enough energy to break molecular bonds (as can X-rays) or produce damaging heat (as can microwaves).

Then in 1979 an independent epidemiological study by psychologist Nancy Wertheimer and physicist Edward Leeper shattered the calm. Looking at reported deaths from childhood cancers in the Denver, Colo., area during the years 1950 to 1973, the pair determined that many young cancer victims resided in homes that were close to electrical transformers, distribution lines, and outside wiring that they classified as having a "high-current configuration." In their study

Wertheimer and Leeper reported that leukemias, lymphomas, and cancers of the central nervous system had occurred two to three times more often in children living in such "high-current" homes. Publication of this unprecedented finding brought immediate media attention, public concern, and scientific skepticism.

Chief among the complaints leveled against the researchers was the nature of their wire-coding system. They had not taken measurements of the ELF fields inside the homes where the cancer victims had lived. Rather, they measured outside wiring sources, rated as low, medium, or high current; these measures were then used as a "surrogate" measure of the field strengths inside residences.

Critical epidemiologists also found another problem with the study: it was not "blind." In other words, in deriving their measurements Wertheimer and Leeper knew which houses had been homes of leukemia patients, and that may have biased the assignments of the "high-current" label. Other researchers decried the lack of contact with relatives of leukemia victims. They suggested that interviews with parents and siblings might have turned up other causal factors, such as a family history of the disease, maternal X-rays during pregnancy, life-style factors, or chemical exposures.

Despite the obvious flaws in this initial investigation, ELF fields were firmly entrenched in the public's mind as "a suspected cancer agent." A major controversy over the real relationship of ELF fields to cancer—and to human health in general—had begun.

More research, more debate

The last decade has seen at least seven attempts to support or refute the correlation with childhood cancer shown by the Denver investigation. Two epidemiological studies, one in Rhode Island (1980) and the other in Yorkshire, England (1985), found no association between leukemia incidence and estimated exposure to ELF fields (however, Wertheimer and Leeper claim that their own analysis of the Rhode Island data "produced a statistically significant, though weak, association"). A Swedish study (1986), on the other hand, reported that cancer cases were twice as likely in homes where a higher "front-door measurement" of electric and magnetic fields had been recorded. Four other studies found a slight but not a statistically significant correlation, and one study gave ambiguous results.

Perhaps the most important and reliable of the post-Wertheimer and Leeper studies was the one completed in 1986 by a team headed by David Savitz, an epidemiologist from the University of North Carolina. Commissioned as part of the New York State Power Lines Project (a $5 million research program to look into the biological effects of power-line fields), the study again looked at childhood cancers in the Denver area, but Savitz sought to correct methodological flaws of earlier studies. The study replicated the wire

codes used in the Wertheimer and Leeper investigation, but those who did the coding were blind to the health status of exposed children. Family interviews and actual exposure measurements of magnetic fields were taken in about a third of the cases examined. The results showed a 1.4 to 2 times greater association between childhood leukemia and high-current homes. Savitz estimated that the cancer risk to a child exposed to such ELF levels might be 50% greater than in the normal population. Proponents of the ELF field-cancer link immediately hailed the work as vindication of Wertheimer and Leeper's conclusions. According to one researcher in the field, as a result of Savitz' findings "the interest of electric utility companies in ELF health effects went from very low to very high." Savitz himself, however, stressed that while his study appeared to show an association between higher childhood cancer risk and increasing exposure to ELF fields, it was only with wire codes (a "surrogate" measurement of ELF field intensity) and did not prove that electromagnetic fields cause cancer.

Many scientists refute even Savitz' evidence, saying it does not correlate with incidence (the actual numbers of cases diagnosed) of childhood leukemia. They contend that there has been an enormous increase in the consumption of electric power over the last 30 years but leukemia incidence rates have remained

Electric power travels to consumers from a generating plant via transmission and distribution lines. Typically, magnetic fields are strong in houses that are near (1) high-voltage transmission lines, (2) primary distribution wires conveying high current from substations, and (3) secondary distribution wires originating from a transformer and carrying current for more than a half dozen homes.

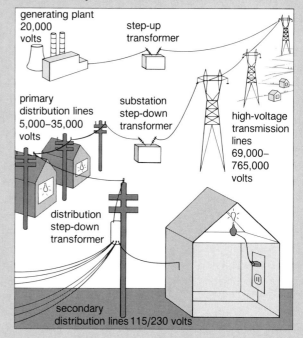

stable. This is not what one would be seeing if ELF field exposures were having a major effect.

While camps on both sides of the ELF field controversy continue battling for acceptance of their views, the U.S. Environmental Protection Agency (EPA) has joined the fray. In its June 1990 report, "An evaluation of the Potential Carcinogenicity of Electromagnetic Fields," the agency said that numerous epidemiological studies of children and workers exposed to ELF fields "show a consistent pattern of response which suggests, but does not prove, a causal link" with leukemias, lymphomas, and cancers of the central nervous system. The report's authors also determined that ELF fields could not yet be characterized as a carcinogen because "the interaction between ELF fields and biological processes leading to cancer is not understood."

A study that is presently being conducted may provide a better assessment of risk. The new study is a collaborative effort of the National Cancer Institute (NCI) and the Children's Cancer Study Group (CCSG) as part of the latter's large-scale investigation of all possible risk factors for childhood leukemia. The NCI-CCSG subjects will be registered soon after their disease has been diagnosed. This will permit extensive measuring of exposures to all risk factors, including ELF fields, within the actual environments of the children (their homes, play areas, schools, day-care centers, and so forth). Detailed family interviews will also be conducted. The NCI-CCSG epidemiological investigation will be carried out over five years and aims to study about 1,000 children who develop acute lymphocytic leukemia.

Adult health risks

In 1982 Wertheimer and Leeper were also the first to report an association between adult cancers and residential wiring configurations. They found a strong correlation between "high-current homes" and cancers of the nervous system, uterus, and breast. Again, however, as with their 1979 childhood leukemia study, their methodology came in for heavy criticism; other researchers pointed out that they did not look for potential confounding factors (life-style, exposure to chemicals, and so forth), nor were exposure levels assigned blindly.

In 1987 epidemiologist Richard Stevens at Battelle Pacific Northwest Laboratories in Richland, Wash., measured ELF fields in and around the homes of adult leukemia patients and then found similar levels in the residences of control subjects. This indicated that there was no association between field exposure and the cancer. An earlier English study (1983) of leukemia mortality in homes near power lines had reached the same conclusion. A study conducted by Susan Preston-Martin, an epidemiologist at the University of Southern California, looked at electric blanket

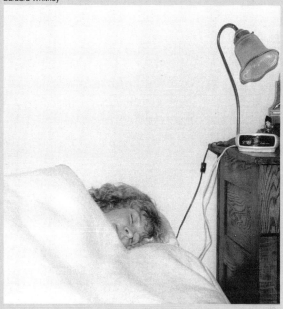

Several studies have linked electric blanket use to adverse health effects. Electric blankets have been a source of considerable concern because sleepers are in direct contact with a constant and substantial ELF field over a long period.

use and also found no connection between ELF fields and adult leukemias (1988).

Prior to 1989 about 20 studies had looked for a link between adult cancers—particularly leukemia and brain cancer—and occupational exposure to ELF fields. Most of the research efforts examined the cancer rates of electrical workers. Taken together, the results of the multiple studies indicated only a small positive association or no association.

In November 1989, however, epidemiologist Genevieve Matanoski of Johns Hopkins University, Baltimore, Md., reported a rate of cancer among 4,500 New York telephone cable splicers nearly two times greater than that in the general population. Her findings rocked the traditional scientific view of "harmless" ELF fields for at least two reasons: epidemiologists had already acknowledged the soundness of her experimental design and, perhaps more important, Matanoski had previously been a skeptic of the ELF field and cancer connection.

Possible ELF field health effects other than cancer have also been investigated. A 1986 Wertheimer and Leeper investigation indicated that expectant mothers who often used electric blankets or heated water beds had more miscarriages, longer gestations, and infants with lower birth weights than nonusers. Another study conducted by epidemiologist Michele Marcus of New York's Mount Sinai School of Medicine is currently looking at the health of 8,000 women who use video display terminals. Experiments with animals and human volunteers have suggested that ELF fields may affect learning ability, hormone regulation, bone growth, response to stress, and circadian rhythms (the internal mechanisms that synchronize daily functioning).

Laboratory investigations

Nonepidemiological findings, based on "bioelectromagnetic" experiments that look at ELF field effects on cells, have produced nearly as much controversy as epidemiological studies. W. Ross Adey, a physician-researcher at the Veterans Administration Medical Center in Loma Linda, Calif., is perhaps the chief proponent of this bioelectromagnetic form of experimentation. Adey has examined separately the effects of both cancer-promoting substances and ELF fields on cells and discovered certain common factors. For example, he has found that growth enzymes such as ornithine decarboxylase, which are seen at increased levels in tumor cells, also increase in cells receiving electrical stimulation. Adey and other bioelectromagnetic researchers contend that this indicates ELF fields may also be promoters of cancer. They hypothesize that ELF fields may be interfering with the way cellular instructions for coding amino acids and proteins are transmitted—*i.e.*, cells might mistakenly overproduce, underproduce, or eliminate enzymes (proteins that carry out cell functions), thereby affecting tumor growth.

Recent work by cell biologist Reba Goodman at Columbia University, New York City, appears to support the proposed mechanism of ELF fields disrupting the biological chain of command. She has shown that 60-Hz electric fields produce varying levels of proteins, different rates of protein production, and different molecular weights for proteins. Such findings, according to researcher Indira Nair at Carnegie Mellon University, Pittsburgh, Pa., suggest that the traditional reasoning—that ELF fields cannot break chemical bonds and therefore cannot cause genetic changes—now needs rethinking.

Another long-cherished argument minimizing the danger from ELF fields has also come under fire. Many scientists contend that natural heat disturbances within living cells are greater than any caused by low-level electromagnetic radiation; therefore, little harm can befall the cell from exposure to ELF fields. However, James Weaver of the Massachusetts Institute of Technology and R. Dean Astumian of the U.S. National Institute of Standards and Technology, Gaithersburg, Md., recently calculated that heat variations within cells do not always override the impact of ELF fields. Their study also found that enzymes and other molecules embedded in the outer membrane of cells were more vulnerable to weak fields than had been previously believed.

Others, including physicist Robert Adair of Yale University, remain critical of lab-induced ELF field effects. Adair has become one of the nation's most outspoken opponents of all ELF field research and has stated that "anyone who would believe that electromagnetic fields could promote cancer would believe in perpetual motion or cold fusion." Adair furthermore argues that bioelectromagnetic studies fall into what he calls "aberrant science"; *i.e.*, work involving difficult experiments that produce marginal data that are rarely reproducible. Moreover, argues Adair, the results do not increase proportionally when the factor under study increases. He says the effects being seen in the laboratory studies of ELF fields are at levels many times smaller than the natural electromagnetic fields already present in cells.

Critics of lab studies further contend that the effects being investigated can be so subtle that even slight alterations in the experimental conditions can alter findings. Another point stressed is that significant ELF field damage may occur only after years of cumulative dosage. Proponent Adey has suggested that ELF fields may produce "on-and-off effects" on various aspects of cell functioning that would result in long-term health problems not discernible in short-term laboratory-based experiments.

Public electrophobia?

While the scientists remain split on whether ELF fields pose a real threat to human health, the public is reacting more and more as if the danger has been proved. A number of examples in the past year can be pointed to as evidence. Two New Jersey housewives, for example, formed a citizen's action group to combat

After several disturbing reports about risks of ELF field exposure were released in June 1989, a Florida judge ruled that part of an elementary school's yard would be off limits to children because of its proximity to overhead cables.

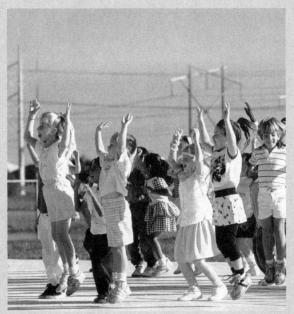

plans of the local utility company to run high-voltage transmission lines through their neighborhood, while in Florida a judge ruled that students at a Boca Raton-area elementary school could not play in a major portion of their school yard because of nearby power cables. In British Columbia a Canadian electric company attempted to quell public protests by offering to buy homes along a new 145-km (90-mi) power line under construction. The plan backfired, however, and the resulting outcry halted work on the line. In Fremont, Calif., the City Council passed a law requiring that potential buyers of homes adjacent to overhead power lines be warned of possible health hazards. By mid-1990 seven U.S. states had established "acceptable standards" for electric field strengths from transmission lines, and one state, Florida, also set limits for magnetic fields. Another indication of public alarm is that at least one enterprise now advertises and sells a product for testing home safety: its Safe Meter is designed "for people with children, pregnant women, house buyers, computer operators, or those living near power lines, or underground wiring." The device sells for "only" $145.

Why the sudden alarm? Although the research had been under way for over a decade, the public generally did not hear of it until June 1989, when the congressional Office of Technology Assessment (OTA) issued a background paper that had been prepared by a research team in the department of engineering and public policy at Carnegie Mellon University. The team reviewed the scientific literature on ELF fields and concluded that although the evidence of health effects was not clear-cut, Americans should practice "prudent avoidance" in dealing with fields in and around their homes. Among the panel's recommendations were that people avoid use of electric blankets (they recommended that those wanting a warm rest "preheat the bed, turn off the blanket, pull the plug, and store the blanket away before going to sleep"), that utility companies route new power lines away from residential areas, and that manufacturers design household appliances with greatly reduced ELF fields. The report also recommended that new research be carried out into whether electromagnetic fields affect the cellular interaction in the brain and nervous system—which normally utilize low-frequency fields for sending messages through the body.

Published almost concurrently with the OTA report, and probably the most provocative spur for alarm, was the first of three investigative articles in *The New Yorker* magazine by environmental writer Paul Brodeur. The series chronicled the "pioneering" studies of Wertheimer and Leeper, Savitz, Adey, and other ELF field scientists, strongly bemoaning the dearth of research funds available for their work. Brodeur pointedly accused governmental agencies and utility companies of cover-ups. His series was subsequently expanded into a best-selling book titled *Currents of Death: Power Lines, Computer Terminals, and the Attempt to Cover Up Their Threat to Your Health.*

The escalation of the public's "electrophobia" prompted Peter Huber of the Manhattan Institute to write, in an editorial published in the Sept. 4, 1989, issue of *Forbes*, that "a nation of hypochondriacs is now developing a phobia toward technology worthy of a primitive time."

Can it be said at present that extremely low-frequency electromagnetic fields are harmful to human health? Is the public's fear justified? An article on electromagnetic radiation in homes in the Dec. 16, 1989, issue of the *British Medical Journal* concluded: "There is no firm evidence that domestic exposure to electromagnetic fields harms health. But, on the other hand, neither is there any good evidence to calm public fears generated by scare stories in the press." Clearly the jury is still out—and it may be quite some time before a firm verdict comes in.

As with most scientific controversies, lack of adequate funding is the chief complaint among those attempting to study the missing link between ELF fields and health effects. Proponents of ELF field research claim that a concentrated, well-funded effort could erase much of the ambiguity and derive solid answers within five years. One group that believes that its current research efforts will resolve ambiguities is the Electric Power Research Institute (EPRI), Palo Alto, Calif., an organization that conducts technical studies and development programs for the U.S. electric utility industry. EPRI's stated goals are threefold: promoting more epidemiological research, improving the quality of exposure measurements, and intensifying basic science investigations, both cellular and animal. With a 1990 research budget of $6 million, EPRI supported nearly one-half of the world's electromagnetic field studies. Critics of the organization, however, say that any findings from EPRI-supported studies should be suspect because of the institute's ties to the electric power industry.

If, ultimately, a health hazard is proved, the economic and social impact will be devastating. Appliances will have to be discarded and new ones designed to replace them. Power lines will have to be moved or buried underground. In essence, the entire industrialized world will have to be rewired.

For now, until the ambiguities are resolved, what should people do? The March 1990 issue of the *Harvard Medical School Health Letter* suggested that "the very cautious may wish to unpack grandma's quilt, turn off the television, and curl up with a good novel or seed catalog." Most experts, however, would say that people should concentrate on *known* risks such as smoking, cholesterol, and stress—things they *can* do something about while they wait to learn the truth about ELF fields.

Genetics

In the past decade the development of powerful new analytic tools has quickened the pace of discovery in genetics and enabled biologists to undertake the herculean task of identifying every human gene and locating the position of each on the appropriate chromosome. An abundance of new strategies for combating hereditary disease has also begun to emerge. Some surprising recent findings have called into question long-accepted principles of genetics and will undoubtedly influence the future course of clinical experimentation.

In the meantime, teams of researchers in laboratories around the world are continuing to search for the genes responsible for specific hereditary diseases. The most notable recent success in this effort was announced in July 1990; two groups of scientists, one at the University of Michigan and the other at the University of Utah, independently identified the gene that causes neurofibromatosis, a potentially disfiguring nervous system disease. The discovery was the culmination of an intensive three-year search, which in 1987 had narrowed the site of the gene to chromosome 17. An interesting feature of the newly discovered gene is that it contains within it three smaller genes, which may or may not play a part in the development of the disease. Researchers were optimistic that the identification of the neurofibromatosis gene would lead to more accurate diagnosis of the disorder, which varies widely in clinical manifestations and severity.

The genome project

On Oct. 1, 1989, the Human Genome Initiative was officially inaugurated, with the expressed goal of identifying each of the approximately 100,000 human genes as well as the 3 billion pairs of nucleotides, or bases, that constitute DNA, the genetic material of a typical human cell. Scientists working on the project, a joint effort of the U.S. National Institutes of Health (NIH) and the Department of Energy, have devised strategies for creating the two types of maps, genetic and physical, needed to attain their goal. A genetic map is a relative one on which genes associated with diseases or physical traits are assigned to locations on chromosomes on the basis of how frequently they are inherited together; two genes are said to be one "centimorgan" apart if they are separated 1% of the time in each generation. A physical map displays the absolute distances between two genes in terms of the number of base pairs that lie between them. One centimorgan is estimated to be about one million base pairs.

To expedite genetic mapping, a steering committee decided to create an index map by identifying markers spaced 10 to 15 centimorgans apart. Their immediate goal is to complete the index map by 1992; known and newly discovered genes will be affixed to stations

between the markers. The committee expects to have a genetic map with markers spaced two centimorgans apart by the end of 1995.

Several recently developed techniques are expected to facilitate physical mapping. One of the most important is the use of unique stretches of DNA, which occur every few hundred base pairs, as physical signposts. The linear sequence of the bases in these DNA segments can be determined, and the sequence itself represented by an alphabetical designation such as AGTAGC (the letters stand for the names of the bases—adenine, guanine, thymine, and cytosine). These segments are known as sequence-tagged sites, or STSs. By identifying STSs within the markers on a genetic map, the researchers can create links between the genetic and physical maps. Other techniques being used to aid in physical mapping include polymerase chain reaction, or PCR, and harnessing yeast cells to replicate longer stretches of DNA than is possible with bacterial cells.

PCR: "copying machine" for the laboratory

The accelerating rate of genetic discovery owes much to the development of the technique known as polymerase chain reaction, a process for amplifying specific DNA sequences. Developed in the mid-1980s by scientists at Cetus Corp., a biotechnology firm in Emeryville, Calif., PCR essentially constitutes a biochemical equivalent of the office copying machine, having the capacity to create millions of identical copies of a given DNA sequence within a matter of hours.

Taking a cue from the natural DNA replication process, the Cetus researchers discovered a way to commandeer the cell's own duplicating equipment to reproduce genes at will. DNA is composed of two strands of nucleic acid molecules, intertwined in the distinctive ladderlike structure called the double helix. Central to DNA replication is an enzyme called a polymerase, which uses each strand of the double helix as a template upon which to construct a complementary DNA strand. Although the enzyme normally replicates an entire DNA molecule, and thus copies a cell's entire genetic complement, the PCR process restricts the duplicating activities to a particular region of interest. The enzyme is directed to a tiny segment of the chromosome by chemical primers—pieces of synthetic DNA that mimic the sequences at both ends of the target region and act as stop and start signals in the duplication process. When the primers and the polymerase are added to a sample of DNA in a closed container and subjected to alternate heating and cooling, two cycles, or rounds, of copying take place. In the first round, duplication proceeds from each primer to the end of the molecule. In the second round, only the region shared by the two copies created in the first round—the target region—is duplicated. From that point duplication proceeds exponentially, with each

Bruce Young

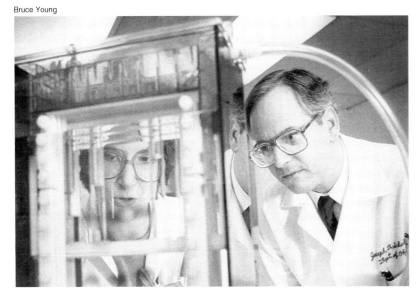

Doctors at the Genetics and IVF (In Vitro Fertilization) Institute in Fairfax, Virginia, observe a test that looks for the genetic defect responsible for most cases of cystic fibrosis (CF). The procedure was made possible by the identification in August 1989 of the mutation that causes about 75% of CF cases. Because the new test can identify only 75% of CF carriers—and fewer than half of the couples likely to have an affected child—many experts feel it should be offered only to those with a family history of the disease.

newly created DNA strand serving as a template in the next cycle. Within seconds, 8 strands become 16. In the blink of an eye, 16 are 32. By the end of 30 cycles, the DNA segment between the primers has been amplified a billionfold.

Because PCR makes it possible to locate a given gene in a sample as small as a single cell, it has myriad uses in human genetics. It has emerged as a valuable tool in prenatal diagnostics, enabling technicians to identify the defects responsible for hereditary disease in cell samples taken from chorionic villi, which are filamentous projections of the fetal membrane. PCR has also been used to amplify specific regions of chromosomes implicated in genetic diseases and in certain forms of cancer. Scientists studying the early stages of infection in AIDS have employed PCR to identify the human immunodeficiency virus in persons who, although infected, have not yet begun to produce antibodies to the virus.

Cystic fibrosis: to screen or not to screen?

Screening for carriers of cystic fibrosis (CF) emerged as a controversial issue in 1990. The identification in August 1989 of the gene mutation responsible for most cases of the disease enabled scientists to quickly develop a commercially available test capable of detecting the mutation in human blood cells. The test identifies a defect in the gene that encodes a protein called the cystic fibrosis transmembrane conductance regulator (CFTCR). In its normal version, this protein regulates the passage of chloride ions across the membranes of cells lining the lungs, pancreas, and intestines, thus diluting mucus secreted by these cells. Defects in the gene result in a protein that is incapable of regulating chloride transport, causing the production of mucus that is unusually thick and viscous. In people with CF this extremely heavy mucus

blocks passages in the airways and digestive organs, impeding breathing and metabolism. Because the mucus also harbors pathogens, CF patients are prone to infection and generally die in young adulthood.

People who inherit one copy of the normal gene and one copy of a defective gene are classified as carriers; they do not have the disease but are capable of transmitting the gene to their children. People who inherit two copies of the defective gene are inevitably affected.

Although within the Caucasian population one person in 20 has a mutation in the CFTCR gene, only 70–75% of those carrying mutations have the specific mutation that researchers identified in 1989. It is estimated that scores of other mutations (dozens of which have already been identified) account for the other 25–30% of defective CFTCR genes. Thus, the available screening test, which is based on the only known mutation, would identify only about 75% of CF carriers and fewer than half of the couples in the general Caucasian population who are likely to give birth to a child with CF. Many people who are carriers would have false-negative test results and would thus be falsely reassured that their offspring were safe from the disease. Because of this limitation in the effectiveness of available screening tests, a panel convened by the NIH in February 1990 advised against use of the screening test on people who have no family history of the disease, a recommendation that was also endorsed by the American Society of Human Genetics. Nonetheless, geneticists at several institutions agreed to offer the test, which costs from $150 to $200, to anyone who wanted it.

Gene therapy: first steps

In March 1990 researchers at the NIH applied for permission from the institute's Human Gene Therapy

Subcommittee to make the first attempt to correct a genetic deficiency by altering the genes of a human being. The researchers, W. French Anderson and R. Michael Blaese, sought permission to treat 10 children who have the congenital immune disease known as adenosine deaminase (ADA) deficiency. Because their white blood cells fail to produce ADA, an enzyme vital to the functioning of the immune system, individuals with the disorder usually die of infection in infancy or childhood. A Texas youngster with ADA known in the media as David, the "bubble boy," survived to the age of 12 but spent his entire life in a germ-free environment that was enclosed in plastic.

Under the research protocol presented to the NIH committee, the researchers plan first to remove some of the patients' circulating T lymphocytes (also called T cells), the white blood cells that mastermind the immune response, and infect them with retroviruses in which some of the viral genes have been replaced with the ADA gene. The virus will present no danger to the host cell, however, because the genes that enable it to reproduce will have been removed. The genetically altered virus will nonetheless be capable of integrating the ADA gene into the genome of the cell. Earlier experiments in nonhuman primates have indicated that lymphocytes treated in this way produce ADA in amounts large enough to improve immune function.

The next step in the proposal calls for growing these genetically altered T cells in a laboratory culture in the presence of a growth factor that would enable them to multiply rapidly. After the cells are tested to determine whether they are indeed producing ADA, they will be transfused back into the patients. Because T cells live only a few months, the procedure will have to be repeated several times a year.

This protocol represents a significant departure from the more ambitious gene therapy technique that Anderson and other researchers had once envisioned for treating ADA deficiency and other genetic disorders affecting the lymphocytes. The earlier proposals centered around inserting normal copies of the defective genes into stem cells—immature blood cells that differentiate into red cells and white cells. Patients would then undergo bone marrow transplants in which their stem cells would be replaced with genetically altered stem cells. Theoretically, the transplanted cells would repopulate the marrow, creating a self-sustaining supply of white blood cells bearing the normal gene. This technique, however, proved to be disappointing in the test tube as well as in animal experiments. Researchers found it hard to isolate stem cells, which are notoriously difficult to distinguish from other blood cells. Moreover, even when they succeeded in implanting the target gene in stem cells, the cells either did not produce the desired protein in cell cultures or could not sustain production of the protein once they were infused into animals.

Like Anderson and Blaese, other teams of researchers have also decided to pursue more limited approaches to gene therapy, narrowing their sites to the single organ or system most drastically affected by a specific disease. One such group is headed by Francis Collins of the University of Michigan, a member of the team that identified the CF gene. Collins has suggested that one way to treat the disease may be by disabling retroviruses, arming them with the normal gene, and suspending them in solutions that would be atomized into the lungs. He theorizes that the viruses would invade the epithelial cells lining the lungs, depositing the normal genes in the process; if the viruses were able to insert the gene into even a fraction of the lung cells, enough of the normal protein would be produced to alleviate the symptoms of the disease.

Another investigator, Ronald G. Crystal of the National Heart, Lung, and Blood Institute, has proposed a similar approach to the treatment of alpha-1 antitrypsin deficiency, another genetic disease affecting the lungs. The disorder is characterized by the absence of an enzyme that protects lung tissue from the effects of another natural enzyme, neutrophil elastase, which is excreted by white blood cells. People who have alpha-1 antitrypsin deficiency often develop emphysema when neutrophil elastase damages the alveoli, the small sacs in the lungs where gas exchange takes place. Crystal postulates that inserting the alpha-1 antitrypsin gene into alveolar cells could produce enough of the enzyme to arrest the progression of emphysema.

Mendel confounded: new forms of inheritance

Recent findings have shed new light on the inheritance of certain traits and disorders that scientists had not been able to explain by classical Mendelian principles of inheritance. Previously it had been believed that all of a cell's basic genetic material was contained within the nucleus of the cell. In the early 1980s, however, scientists discovered that the mitochondria, bodies within the cell that provide chemical energy for cellular functions, house a separate set of genes that regulate mitochondrial functions. A team of geneticists, led by Douglas Wallace of Emory University, Atlanta, Ga., has identified each of the mitochondrial genes and has associated them with disorders once assumed to be caused by defects in nuclear genes.

Diseases caused by mitochondrial DNA usually affect the muscular or nervous systems. Because mitochondria, like the X (female) chromosome, are inherited exclusively from the mother, diseases resulting from defects in mitochondrial DNA were originally thought to be X-linked disorders. Yet geneticists were unable to explain why, unlike typical X-linked disorders, which occur more frequently in males, certain apparently X-linked disorders were distributed evenly among males and females. Because many of these diseases involved malfunctions in nerve and muscle cells, both of which are rich in mitochondria, Wallace and his colleagues began to search the mitochondrial genome for probable causes. They were able to establish links between such diseases as Leber's hereditary optic neuropathy—a syndrome characterized by muscular deterioration and loss of vision—and MERRF (myoclonic epilepsy and ragged-red fiber disease—characterized by frequent seizures and degeneration of nerve tissues and heart and skeletal muscle) and defects in mitochondrial genes. They postulate that other neuromuscular disorders may be due to a combination of defects in both mitochondrial and nuclear genes.

Still other diseases with inheritance patterns that appeared to defy the rules of Mendelian genetics have been found to be explained by another recently discovered phenomenon—genetic imprinting. When genetic imprinting comes into play, a gene inherited from the mother may be expressed differently from an identical gene inherited from the father.

Evidence of imprinting was first reported in 1984 by M. Azim Surani of the AFRC (Agriculture and Food Research Council) Institute of Animal Physiology and Genetics Research, Cambridge, England, and Davor Solter of the Wistar Institute, Philadelphia. Using a just-fertilized mouse egg, in which the DNA from egg and sperm had not yet fused into a complete nucleus, the researchers replaced the nuclear material provided by the sperm with that from another egg, creating an embryo with a sole parent—a female. They repeated the procedure using another newly fertilized egg, this time replacing the egg's contribution to the nucleus with that of the sperm to create an embryo with a single, male parent. Both embryos were implanted in the uterus of a pregnant female mouse, but neither survived. The placenta of the first embryo failed to develop; in the second the placenta flourished, but the embryo failed to develop. On the basis of these experiments, the researchers concluded that the maternal and paternal genetic contributions are not functionally identical and that both are essential for normal growth and development.

Geneticists have since found evidence that a similar difference between maternal and paternal contributions comes into play in humans when a certain region of chromosome 15 is deleted. If the deletion occurs on the maternally inherited chromosome, the child will have Angelman's syndrome, which is characterized by muscle spasticity and uncontrollable bouts of laughter. However, when the same region of the paternally inherited chromosome 15 is deleted, the child will have Prader-Willi syndrome, a disorder in which the individual is lethargic and overeats compulsively. Some geneticists postulate that imprinting may play a part in other inherited disorders, such as Huntington's disease and, possibly, fragile-X syndrome, that vary in character or severity from one individual to another. The exact mechanism of imprinting has yet to be identified.

Role of genes in carcinogenesis

In 1989 and 1990 oncologists and geneticists alike continued to examine the mechanisms of genetic transformation involved in carcinogenesis, the process whereby a normal cell is transformed into a malignant one. As researchers identified an increasing number of genes as oncogenes (genes that cause cancer when inappropriately activated) and antioncogenes (genes that cause cancer when inappropriately deactivated), they also were becoming slightly uneasy with both of these terms. It was becoming increasingly apparent that the genes implicated in the multistage process of carcinogenesis are simply genes for normal cellular proteins that are somehow involved in regulating growth and differentiation and that mutations in these genes contribute to uncontrolled cell growth.

Recent discoveries have indicated that some of these genes are implicated in several forms of cancer, often in collusion with one another. For example, the gene for p53, an apparent growth-suppressor protein, has been found to be altered in nearly every form of lung cancer as well as in some colorectal and breast cancers. Another suppressor gene, named Rb because its deletion is associated with the development of retinoblastoma (a rare tumor of the eye), was discovered to be conspicuously absent from its normal position on chromosome 13 in tumors removed from patients with osteosarcoma (a bone cancer) and carcinoma of the bladder. A recently discovered gene on chromosome 18, named DCC for "deleted in colon cancer," is postulated to act as a suppressor gene that, when normally expressed, prevents the formation of colon tumors. The protein that the gene codes for is thought to affect intercellular reactions that govern cell proliferation. The expression of another gene, nm23, seems to keep breast cancer tumors from metastasizing; i.e., spreading to other sites in the body. Some studies have determined that tumors that are restricted to the breast have higher levels of the nm23 protein than do tumors that have spread to the lymph nodes.

In contrast, the overproduction of the protein products of other genes, most of which are involved in cell growth, have been implicated in the progress of several forms of cancer. Overproduction is usually a result of extra copies of the gene or failure of the cell to shut down protein production at the proper time. Although researchers have yet to find ways to halt production of these proteins, they have devised diagnostic tests based on identifying genes or their products. For example, the presence of extra copies of the HER-2/neu gene in breast tumors signals an advanced stage of disease and the need for aggressive treatment, as does the presence of the closely related neu protein in ovarian cancer. Moreover, an increase in the number of different oncogenes expressed in a tumor also indicates progression of the disease.

—Beverly Merz

Unraveling DNA: Knotty Issues

by Thomas H. Murray, Ph.D.

In almost every cell of everyone's body, a set of twisted molecular chains contains within its coils the instructions for building all the hormones and proteins necessary for life. The chain is DNA—the language of heredity. For most of the chain no function has yet been found. Pieces of it, though, are used by human bodies as templates on which crucial biological molecules are built.

These segments of the DNA chain, of course, are genes. Humans have an estimated 100,000 different genes. Each link in the chain must be one of only four possible shapes, yet long lengths of these four distinct shapes in varied combinations are sufficient to make 100,000 unique genes. The full chain with all segments combined is three billion links long. This chain, and the genes contained in it, is the human genome—the full complement of human genetic material.

In the past 15 years there have been stunning advances in medical scientists' ability to study—and on occasion manipulate—DNA. Scientists have begun to draw maps of the locations where particular genes fall on the DNA chains. They have found many of the genes themselves. In some instances they have been able to decipher the precise sequence of links in a gene. The gene that causes cystic fibrosis, for example, has recently had its sequence decoded.

The Human Genome Initiative: what's in store

Within the past two years the international scientific community has embarked on a loosely coordinated effort to draw ever more refined maps of the human genome and to determine the sequence of links in the full chain, beginning with the most interesting segments—genes. This project is known as the Human Genome Initiative. The U.S. effort is expected to last 15 years and cost $3 billion. Many Western European countries and Japan are also participating.

From very early in the planning for the Human Genome Initiative, ethics emerged as an important concern. The science of genetics was acquiring the power to make predictions and, at times, to alter human physiology. The genome effort enlarges those powers and raises the stakes. Thus, the question needed to be asked: How can it be assured that this knowledge and these powers will be used for good and not evil? Ethical matters were discussed at a congressional hearing on the genome project on April 27, 1988. By Oct. 1, 1988, James D. Watson had been appointed director of the genome initiative at the U.S.

National Institutes of Health (NIH), the agency chosen to play the largest role. (Watson, codiscoverer of the DNA double helix in 1953, shared a Nobel Prize for Physiology or Medicine with Francis H.C. Crick and Maurice Wilkins for that work in 1962.) Even before assuming the directorship, Watson announced his intention to commit 3 to 5% of the NIH's share of the genome budget to research and education on ethical issues. Early in 1990 the U.S. Department of Energy, also with a hefty budget for genome research, pledged to spend up to 3% of its share on ethical concerns.

A group of eminent scientists was formed to advise the government on the genome project. It quickly established several working groups, including one known officially as the Working Group on Ethical, Legal, and Social Issues (ELSI, for short). That group's role is to suggest general directions for research and education on the wide range of issues—ethical, legal, and social—the project touches.

Nonhuman genomes: important links to humanity

Although the project is officially the *Human* Genome Initiative, the genomes of many other organisms—plants, animals, and microbes—will also be studied. Much of what is known about how genes, including human genes, function comes from research on simpler forms of life, such as the weed *Arabidopsis* and the common yeast. There are intriguing differences in the way DNA is organized and translated into proteins between these humble organisms and humans, but there are also many similarities. Both the differences

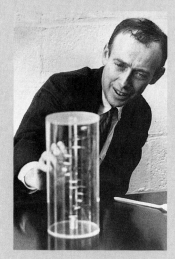

James Watson, codiscoverer of the DNA double helix—the "secret of life"—poses with his model in 1962, the year he shared a Nobel Prize. In 1988 Watson assumed the directorship of the Human Genome Initiative, at which time he pledged to commit at least 3% of the project's budget to ethical concerns.

UPI/Bettmann Newsphotos

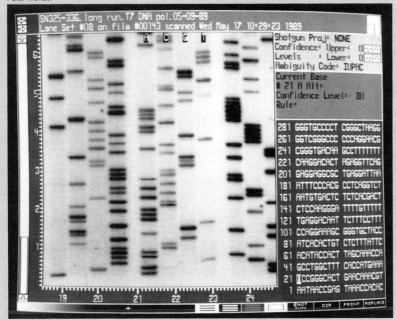

An automated sequencing machine developed at the California Institute of Technology is capable of reading out 7,000 "letters" of DNA in a day. The computer screen displays fragments of a single gene that have been separated and sequenced; the order of the fragments' chemical letters appears on the screen's right.

and the similarities reveal useful things about human genetics.

Nonhuman genetics research has led to dramatic changes in the breeding of new plants and animals. The genome initiative will accelerate those changes. For centuries breeders understood that by carefully choosing the parents, they could improve their chances of finding desirable traits in offspring. They applied this knowledge to create new varieties of crops and domestic animals. Genetic engineering confers new powers. Now, instead of relying on the chance that wanted traits will appear, genetic engineers are learning how to ensure that particular genes are incorporated into the organism. The gene need not come from the same species: bacteria, for example, have had the gene that produces human growth hormone, of which supplies are scarce, inserted into them; the bacteria then act like tiny factories churning out substantial quantities of the hormone. Chinese hamster ovary cells have been given the gene that makes human erythropoietin (EPO), a hormone that stimulates the bone marrow to make red blood cells. EPO has the potential for helping hundreds of thousands of people with chronic anemia. Like human growth hormone, however, it also has the potential of being misused.

The recently found ability to manipulate the genes of nonhuman organisms raises a host of questions. What effects will genetically engineered organisms have on the environment? Some scientists are developing new crop strains with increased resistance to pesticides that would allow larger amounts to be used; other scientists are creating crops with increased resistance to pests. Scientists now can develop more environmentally sensitive approaches to agriculture—or harsher

ones; which approaches are taken is society's choice. The genome project, even though its primary focus is on humans, will enhance general knowledge about plant and animal genetics as well as scientific skill at genetic manipulation. The human world will thus confront a series of ethical challenges in its relationship with the nonhuman world.

Genetic prediction

Many human diseases have at least some relationship to genetic makeup. Inheriting a defective form of a gene can mean quick and certain death. Tay Sachs disease, a fatal hereditary disorder of lipid metabolism affecting primarily Ashkenazi Jews, is an example; this degenerative condition begins to take its toll soon after birth and kills its victims in their first few years. A faulty gene can also mean a lifelong course of illness with death usually coming well before age 40; such is the case with cystic fibrosis. Another possibility is that a deadly gene can lie undetected for decades, afflicting its victims in their middle or late decades. Huntington's disease follows this pattern. Still other genes do not become lethal unless there is exposure to triggering environmental agents; those who are lucky (or wise) enough to avoid such exposures may escape without any manifestations of disease. The condition known as glucose-6-phosphate dehydrogenase (G-6-PD) deficiency works this way. People with G-6-PD deficiency have an abnormality that results in the disintegration of the walls of their red blood cells when they are exposed to certain chemicals. In ancient times the disease was known as favism; when people with the condition ate favas—a popular broad bean—they sickened or died. American soldiers sent to Korea in the

309

1950s were given an antimalarial drug that was similar to the active chemical in fava beans. GIs with G-6-PD deficiency suffered dangerous reactions to the drug. If those with this genetic predisposition knew they were sensitive to such chemicals, they could avoid them and live symptom free.

Matters of insurance. Perhaps the most important sets of genes are those associated with common disablers and killers—heart disease, stroke, lung disease, and cancer. A few rare genes such as the one causing familial hypercholesterolemia virtually guarantee that an individual will have the condition; the body produces an overabundance of low-density lipoprotein cholesterol, which it is not able to eliminate through normal processes. The person is thus at high risk of developing heart disease. However, there are likely to be a substantial number of other genes with very tentative links to disease. For example, it might be found that people with a particular gene are 10% more likely to suffer a heart attack by age 55 than are people without that gene. Insurance companies, for one, are very interested in genetic tests that can predict who is likely to become sick or die prematurely.

When genetic tests that help predict who will have an early heart attack become available and affordable, people will seek them. If people learn they are more likely than average to suffer a heart attack, they will also be more likely to buy more life and health insurance. Insurance companies, however, will not want to lose money. They will either raise their rates for everyone, or they will use the tests themselves in deciding whom to insure and how much to charge. If some companies use genetic tests, they will be able to offer lower rates to their low-risk applicants and will charge those with possible genetic risks higher rates. With the low-risk individuals siphoned off, the remaining companies will have to charge higher rates or use genetic tests themselves. People at increased risk for disease or early death may find it increasingly expensive or perhaps impossible to get life or health insurance.

Laws could be passed forbidding insurance companies to use genetic tests that improve their ability to predict who will become sick or die. Insurance companies, however, already do other forms of health screening—of blood pressure, family history, the applicant's medical history—intended to identify those at increased risk. Genetic tests strike many people as being different in crucial ways from the kind of risk screening currently used. People are not "responsible" for their genes, but they can, for example, modify blood pressure through careful diet, exercise, and medication. There is little reluctance to hold people accountable for things over which they have some control— where they can significantly alter their own chances of getting some diseases. There are, however, many afflictions that people can do little or nothing to avoid. Genetically caused disease can differ in many ways

from other disease in how much responsibility can be assigned to the individual. The debate over genetics and insurance is just beginning; the question of "responsibility" for disease is just one of many issues likely to be raised.

Huntington's disease: genetic death sentence? One of the most troubling aspects of the ever growing knowledge about human genetics is that the ability to predict is likely to run ahead of the ability to treat. Huntington's disease is one such case. As already indicated, people with Huntington's disease usually do not show their first symptoms until their thirties or forties. If one parent has Huntington's, there is a 50–50 chance that offspring will also have it. Until recently, that was the most accurate prediction anyone could make.

Researchers have now narrowed their search for the gene that causes Huntington's to a short length of one chromosome. By examining the similarities in that chromosome among family members who escaped Huntington's and those who developed it, scientists have developed a test that can predict with 99% accuracy whether a particular person has the fatal gene. Because there is no treatment for it yet, a positive test result is a virtual death sentence.

Not all genetic predictions will be as dire as Huntington's, but whenever there are no means of treating or preventing the disease, the availability of a genetic test that can determine an individual's very bleak destiny raises clear ethical questions. Not surprisingly, the Huntington's disease researchers found that once the test became available, many fewer people actually wanted it than had earlier indicated an interest.

Tay Sachs disease: valuable genetic screening. Other forms of genetic prediction are also likely to become more widely available. The Huntington's test is known as a presymptomatic test; it predicts disease before any symptoms appear. Another kind of prediction is carrier screening, which provides a way of learning whether a prospective parent has a type of a gene that causes disease when a child inherits copies of the gene from both parents. Carriers usually have no symptoms of the disease themselves. Prenatal genetic screening, as the name suggests, involves examining a fetus to see if it has a genetic disease.

In the case of one population at risk, carrier and prenatal screening have been used very successfully. Because Ashkenazi Jews are most at risk of having the Tay Sachs gene, a combination of carrier and prenatal screening has been used in that community to greatly reduce the number of children born with Tay Sachs. Although criticisms have been made, and some carriers of the gene may have experienced a degree of discrimination, most observers count the Tay Sachs program as an example of ethically sound genetic screening.

Sickle-cell screening: dangers and flaws. Early efforts to screen for carriers of the gene that causes sickle-cell disease, however, may have caused more harm than good. As in Tay Sachs, it takes two copies of the gene to cause sickle-cell disease. Those with a single copy are carriers and are said to have sickle-cell trait. Sickle-cell disease varies much more in its manifestations than Tay Sachs. When people were screened, they were often not given the counseling to help them understand that they did not have the disease itself. Some lived in the mistaken fear that the disease would erupt in them at any time. Others were treated as undesirable marriage partners.

Sickle-cell trait is most common among blacks and groups whose ancestors lived near the Mediterranean Sea. The early screening programs focused on American blacks. Some in the black community labeled the program a form of genocide designed to discourage black people from having children. This example of sickle-cell screening that began in the 1970s, with its many flaws, reveals the danger in ill-conceived genetic screening programs.

It is quite clear that the Human Genome Initiative will identify a host of genes that are in some way linked to disease and thus open the possibility for a myriad of genetic screening programs. It will be extremely important to heed the lessons of past mistakes as well as learn from past successes.

DNA fingerprinting: questions of genetic privacy

With three billion links in every individual's genetic chain, the odds are overwhelming that all but mono-zygotic (identical) twins are genetically distinct. Law-enforcement officials have lately tried to tap that enormous genetic diversity to identify criminals. If the police can find a sample of biological material—some blood, semen, skin underneath a victim's fingernail, or possibly even a hair bulb—they can amplify the DNA contained in the cells and create what is now known as a DNA or genetic fingerprint. DNA fingerprinting was used without challenge in hundreds of cases in the U.S. before lawyers in a New York case raised questions about its reliability. When a group of eminent scientists took a closer look at how it was being done, they found ambiguities in the way the findings were being interpreted as well as shaky estimates of the probability that the sample could have come from anyone other than the accused.

The essential idea behind DNA fingerprinting is recognized as sound. A variety of methods are being developed for it, without any clear consensus as to which is best. In the United States the National Academy of Sciences was commissioned to study DNA fingerprinting and make recommendations for its responsible use.

There are a number of potential uses for DNA fingerprinting beyond criminal investigations. It is already used to prove—or disprove—claims that one person is related to another. When immigration laws favor blood relations, or when a purported illegitimate offspring demands a share of an inheritance, knowing the genetic truth can be momentous.

In the future, ethicists and society will have to deal with proposals for wide-ranging genetic fingerprinting. A DNA fingerprint would make it much easier to prove that years earlier the "wrong" child was the one taken home by parents after its birth in a hospital, for example. In time, the technology might well permit DNA fingerprints to be automated, the results recorded by a bar code reader—like the ones used in supermarkets—and stored in a computer. The uses are relatively easy to imagine, the possible abuses perhaps less so. Nevertheless, the specter of a central data bank containing the genetic fingerprint of all residents of the U.S. frightens some people who worry about government intrusions on privacy.

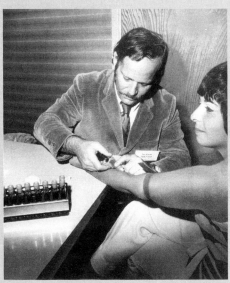 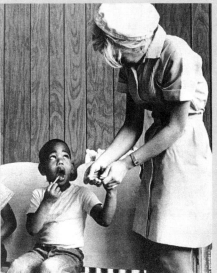

Screening for carriers of Tay Sachs disease (left) has been successful in greatly reducing the number of children born with that fatal hereditary disorder. Screening of newborns, schoolchildren, and marriage-license applicants for the gene that causes sickle-cell disease (right) has done considerable harm; without counseling, many black Americans with sickle-cell trait have mistakenly believed they have the disease.

(Left) Francis DiGennaro/Time Magazine; (right) UPI/Bettmann Newsphotos

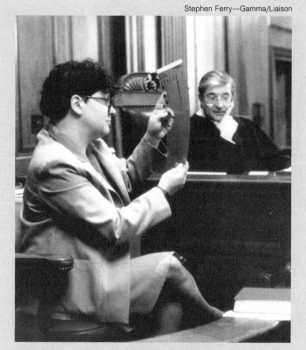

After a geneticist testified on whether DNA fingerprints from a bloodstain matched those of a murder suspect, the New York judge ruled against admitting the DNA test as evidence in the trial. This was the first time the reliability of such genetic fingerprints had been challenged in a court case.

Modifying humankind

The genome initiative will increase scientific ability to alter human physiology and sometimes genes themselves. Gene therapy has grabbed the public imagination, but other outgrowths of research on genetics have the potential for much broader impact on life in the next few decades.

The first approved experiment has begun in which a new gene is inserted into living human cells and those genetically transformed cells are returned to the person's body. Scientists studying a promising treatment for malignant melanoma, a very difficult cancer to treat, needed a way to follow the cells they had treated to enhance their cancer-fighting properties and then reinfused into the patient. They chose to insert a bacterial gene that confers resistance to the antibiotic neomycin. The gene acts like a flag, distinguishing the cancer-fighting cells with the new gene from other similar-looking cells. If this experiment proves successful, it may be possible to add other genes to living cells that actually will enhance the cells' cancer-fighting ability.

As with other experiments involving human beings, research that modifies human genetic material must meet strict ethical requirements. The experiment just described is no exception. It passed through 16 reviews before being approved by the director of the NIH. Research on gene therapy in the near future should continue to receive exacting ethical scrutiny. For all the attention it receives, gene therapy is likely to affect only a small number of persons in the next decade. Other fruits of modern genetics may not be so easily controlled.

As described previously, the human gene for erythropoietin has been cloned, inserted into cells that can be grown in vats, and the hormone isolated in substantial quantities. A boon to people suffering from chronic anemia, EPO is being used for other, ethically questionable purposes.

EPO increases the number of red blood cells that carry oxygen to the body's tissues and organs. Athletes who compete in events that test the limits of stamina might gain an advantage by a modest boost in the number of red cells in their blood. A major issue has been made in recent years of the widespread use by athletes of drugs (such as anabolic steroids) and other means (such as blood doping—also known as blood boosting, blood packing, and induced erythrocythemia—which involves transfusing additional red blood cells into an athlete's body in order to improve oxygen delivery) to gain a competitive edge. EPO is unlikely to be an exception. There are two moral problems associated with this use of EPO. First, it may be dangerous; it is possible to overshoot—to have too many red blood cells—resulting in a hindrance of blood flow that can cause pain, injury, or even death. Second, when the rules of sport prohibit performance-enhancing drugs, using EPO is unfair to the other competitors and therefore is cheating.

Sport is not usually a good metaphor for society. In this case, though, sport's stress on competition and victory provides a cautionary analogy for other social realms. Using that analogy, it can be said that the Human Genome Initiative is likely to accelerate the progress of genetics, which will give medical science new tools and new powers, including the power to alter human life in order to "get an edge" on "competitors." Ethical concerns might not be so great if the possible uses of human alteration were limited to sport, but they are not. Already there have been cases in which parents wanting to give their children the advantage of a few extra centimeters of height have had them injected with one fruit of the new genetics—human growth hormone. One can only guess what future temptations to "improve" human functioning will emerge, but it appears to be a virtual certainty that some will, and a few of these are likely to pose a powerful challenge to practical wisdom and to social and political institutions.

The Human Genome Initiative holds the potential of easing human suffering and saving human lives. As it evolves, it may or may not raise many ethical issues that are utterly novel, but it will surely accelerate and accentuate a large number of ethical quandaries that modern genetics has already posed.

312

Genetics Special Report

Of Mice and Maine

by Gail McBride, M.S.

Consider the dog or cat show. At such an eagerly anticipated gathering, devoted owners put meticulously groomed pets of diverse breeds through their paces, proudly exhibiting them for all (especially the judges) to admire. A not-so-dissimilar event occurs every summer at the Jackson Laboratory in Bar Harbor, Maine, where the "mutant mouse show" is part of the annual "Short Course" in genetics attended by scientists and physicians from around the world. There for the curious scientists and a coterie of science writers to observe are obese diabetic mice waddling alongside nonobese diabetic mice—animals that are studied to shed light on the two forms of human diabetes, adult-onset and juvenile-onset, respectively. Nearby are "twitcher" mice that cannot stay still; they have a disease similar to the genetic human illness Tay-Sachs disease, which affects primarily Jewish newborns of Ashkenazic heritage (one in every 2,500), causing, among other effects, severe degeneration of the nervous system, psychomotor deterioration, and uncontrollable seizures. The JAX mutant lineup (JAX derives from the laboratory's cable address) also includes highly prized immunologically deficient "nude" mice, "motheaten" mice, and "congenital goiter" mice—to mention just a few.

Like those who show their prize cats and dogs, Jackson Laboratory scientists who work with these strange breeds of mice—which have been inbred for their specific genetic traits so that all members of a strain are genetically identical—are rightfully proud of their animals and pleased to point out their breeds' divergent characteristics. Unlike the pet shows, though, the mutant "show" is not a competition. All Jackson Laboratory mice are considered invaluable for research on the many genetic diseases that afflict both mouse and man.

The Jackson Laboratory:
a renowned institution, a remote setting

The Jackson Laboratory is an unlikely place, an independent scientific laboratory devoted to the study of genetics in mammals. Supported by the sale of two million inbred mice for scientific research each year as well as by federal grants and private, foundation, and corporate donations, the lab is located near the small village of Bar Harbor, on Mt. Desert Island, along Maine's beautiful and rugged seacoast. The laboratory's placid, tree-surrounded exterior, however, belies the intense activity within. The institution is the largest

employer on Mt. Desert Island. Nearly half of the 550 full-time employees are engaged in raising mice, either for sale to other institutions or for research conducted at the laboratory by scientists on the staff. There are generally about 30 nonsalaried biomedical scientists carrying out their investigations at the laboratory. Their income and living expenses must be covered by the grant money they receive, which serves as a powerful incentive for them to do high-quality research. The Jackson Laboratory also acts as host to many visiting scientists and students and postdoctoral fellows. Often Ph.D. candidates will conduct their research at Bar Harbor but receive their degrees from their home universities.

The summer Short Courses for professionals have been held since 1960 as a joint venture with Johns Hopkins University, Baltimore, Md.; the courses have been largely supported by the March of Dimes Birth Defects Foundation. In addition, the laboratory holds an annual nine-week summer program for high school and college students. (Summers, of course, are an idyllic time to be on the coast of Maine.) Laboratory staffers are quick to point out that two alumni of the summer student program, both attending in the summer of 1955, were David Baltimore (then a high school student) and Howard Temin (a college student); the two went on to share the Nobel Prize for Physiology or Medicine in 1975.

Clarence Cook Little: a scientist with a dream and some generous friends

In the 1920s many of the country's most prominent and wealthy people spent summers at Bar Harbor. In 1922, at age 33, Clarence Cook Little, a Harvard-trained geneticist who had become president of the University of Maine at Orono, came in contact with some of these people when he started a summer field course and lectures in Bar Harbor for the university's biology students. Among those he met were Edsel Ford, who shared ownership of the Ford Motor Co. with his father and mother, Henry and Clara Ford; Roscoe B. Jackson, head of the Hudson Motorcar Co.; and fellow Harvard alumnus George B. Dorr, who was mainly responsible for aggregating sizeable gifts of land on the island into what is now Acadia National Park and who loaned the land for Little's field course. In 1925 Little accepted the presidency of the University of Michigan, where he continued to carry out investigations in the field of genetics; Little also continued

313

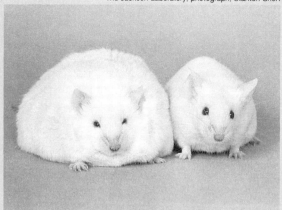

The mice above are from the same parents. The obese sibling—a Jackson mutant that has a severe form of diabetes—is from one of many mutant strains used by scientists for studying inherited metabolic disorders.

to take students to Bar Harbor every summer and to hold his annual field courses.

Then in 1929, having resigned from his Michigan post, Little set about realizing a long-held dream. With substantial donations from Ford, Jackson, and Jackson's brother-in-law, Richard Webber, head of the J.L. Hudson Co. Department Stores in Michigan, he was able to build and support a new laboratory in Bar Harbor for himself and a small staff, including eight of his colleagues from Michigan. With private donations to last five years and a yearly budget of under $50,-000, Little's great Bar Harbor adventure began. The laboratory was named for Roscoe B. Jackson, who died suddenly in March 1929.

Little was a creative, dynamic scientist who was far ahead of his time. He had raised mice as a young boy. In college he started doing research with mice, and he subsequently developed the first inbred strain (mice bred over many generations so that all have exactly the same genes). He later became interested in cancer as well as genetics. Noting that different strains of laboratory mice had inherent susceptibilities or resistances to cancer, he came to suspect that heredity might be an overriding factor in whether humans also succumb to cancers of various types. His notion was that because inbred mice were exactly the same genetically, it would be possible for many scientists, using the same mouse strain, to study the same problem; the results obtained by one group could then be compared with those of others with the knowledge that genetic differences among animals did not muddy the findings. Further, gene mutations occurring in some animals in a strain would be noticeable and more easily isolated for study because the animals were alike in all other ways. Such inbred mice were also convenient to work with because only three months were needed for raising a new generation.

Weathering hard times

As the Depression began to take its toll, contributions from the original donors dropped. In order to keep the enterprise alive, laboratory staffers and their families shared living quarters, took pay cuts, and even began fishing and starting vegetable gardens to cut food costs. Meanwhile, Little desperately sought money elsewhere. One helpful decision was to begin selling the specially bred mice to outside scientists. Thus began a long tradition.

In 1929 Clarence Cook Little, a Harvard-trained geneticist, realized his dream of establishing, in the small village of Bar Harbor on Mt. Desert Island, Maine, a private laboratory devoted to the study of mammalian genetics. Little, pictured in the center, served as the Jackson Laboratory's director until 1956. By that time the institution had long been attracting top scientists from around the world and had become internationally renowned for its breeding of special mouse strains that are invaluable to genetics research.

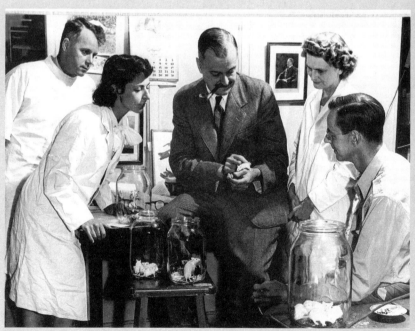

The spirit of the staffers enabled the institution to survive the hard times. The scientists' investigations into genetic and hormonal influences on specific types of cancer were expanding, and the institution's reputation grew. Outside scientists began to visit. In 1938 the Jackson Laboratory received a major grant for cancer research from the fledgling National Cancer Institute (NCI), which had just been established under the auspices of what was then the U.S. National Institute of Health. (Little himself, as the half-time managing director of what later became the American Cancer Society, had been instrumental in pushing for the NCI's establishment—a connection that certainly helped.) The laboratory's close relationship with the NCI has continued, and Jackson is now one of several NCI-supported Cancer Research Centers.

In the late 1930s and early '40s, the laboratory's mouse-breeding activities expanded, and during World War II large numbers of Jackson lab mice were sold to the federal government for investigations into preventive measures against the exotic diseases to which U.S. soldiers were being exposed overseas. In 1945 other laboratory animals entered the picture when Jackson received a substantial grant from the Rockefeller Foundation in New York City for a large study on genetic and environmental influences on behavior in dogs. This research was conducted in an outlying part of the laboratory called Hamilton Station, where two years later research on rabbits also began. The work on behavioral genetics in dogs lasted for two decades and attracted many psychologists as graduate students or visiting investigators. During that time Hamilton Station became a gathering place and national conference center for psychologists.

Then in 1947 disaster struck. A major forest fire broke out and was not contained before the enormous blaze destroyed much of the town of Bar Harbor and most of the laboratory's buildings, equipment, and library. Innumerable records of years of research were lost, and 60,000 mice were killed.

Little, however, resolved to rebuild the laboratory, and seemingly the whole country offered assistance. Scientists were given temporary work space in university laboratories and at other institutions; replacements for the mice were offered from genetic stocks of animals that had been developed from original Bar Harbor strains; individuals and institutions sent some 17,000 books and journals to reconstitute the library; war surplus materials were made available; and ultimately many donations, small and large, made rebuilding possible. Notably, the Jackson and Webber families were once again generous in their contributions.

In 1956, after 27 years of pursuing his dream, Little retired. There have been only four additional directors. The most recent, Kenneth Paigen, took the helm in 1989. Paigen had been chairman of the department of genetics at the University of California at Berke-

The Jackson Laboratory; photograph, Stanton Short

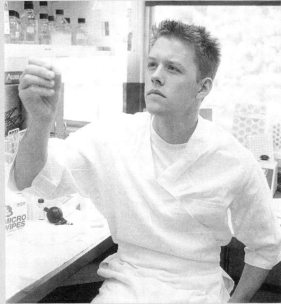

Every summer the Jackson Laboratory is host to many visiting scientists and students. Graduates of the nine-week course for high school and college students have gone on to become leading scientists and even Nobel Prize winners.

ley. Since 1969 he had been an investigator at the lab during the summers and a lecturer at the Short Courses. His wife, Beverly, is a senior staff scientist investigating the genetics of heart disease.

The mouse business

Approximately half the budget of the Jackson Laboratory comes from the sale of about two million mice per year, although only 20% of that is profit. The breeding is expensive, requiring stringently controlled environmental conditions and scrupulous handling by laboratory personnel. The air in the breeding labs must be filtered; those who work with the animals must don sterilized caps and gowns; and all the animals' food and water is sterilized. The aim in breeding experimental strains of mice is to avoid infection, which not only could cause illness in or death of the animals but could cause some of them to harbor microorganisms whose unsuspected presence might alter the animals' response to experimental investigations.

About 1,700 strains of mice are maintained at the laboratory; hundreds of strains are used commonly in widely varied types of research by scientists in many fields. Other highly specialized strains are used for research bearing specifically on rare human genetic diseases. For some of these there is no substitute; Jackson is the only laboratory in the world that produces such strains. The more common strains sell for under $5, while the rarer, more difficult-to-breed strains go for $25 or more per mouse. Mouse maintenance, on average, costs about 15 cents per mouse per day.

315

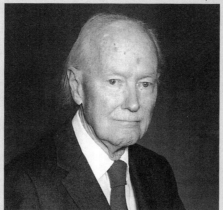
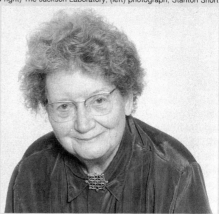

George Snell, who did pioneering work with tissue transplants in mice at the Jackson Laboratory from 1935 to 1973, won a Nobel Prize for his work in 1980. Elizabeth ("Tibby") Russell was on staff from 1937 to 1982; she was best known for her original research on hemoglobin and inherited anemias.

Some mice are coveted chiefly for their unique DNA. Genetic engineering techniques enable Jackson lab workers to harvest the mouse DNA, which is used in cellular-level research. It is also invaluable to scientists presently endeavoring to localize specific cloned genes on the mouse "gene map."

The 125 animal caretakers who tend the three million mutant mice raised each year are specially trained to notice animals that deviate from the norm for that strain. Their fur, for example, may be an unusual color, or their body shapes or behaviors unusual in some way. If through various tests such animals are found to actually carry new mutations, information about them is sent to scientists who may want to use them for research—*e.g.,* as mouse models of a specific human disease. All mouse strains are tested biochemically and immunologically from time to time to make sure that they are, genetically speaking, what they are supposed to be. Since mice tend to look alike, mutations could occur or mouse strains could get mixed up without anyone knowing, thereby confounding research results.

Major scientific contributions

Many advances in genetics have come from the Jackson Laboratory, and many outstanding scientists have conducted important work there. One such scientist is George Snell, who shared the Nobel Prize for Physiology or Medicine in 1980 with Baruj Benacerraf of Harvard Medical School and Jean Dausset of the University of Paris. All of them worked with genes of the major histocompatibility complex (known as MHC genes)—a group of genes that specifically codes for antigens on white blood cells and is the chief determinant of how the body recognizes "self" versus "foreign." Their discoveries underlie much of the present knowledge of the hereditary qualities that determine whether transplanted organs and tissues are accepted or rejected by the recipient's body. Equally important, histocompatibility genes control many immune cell reactions and are associated with susceptibility to some

diseases, such as certain types of arthritis (*e.g.,* systemic lupus erythematosus and rheumatoid arthritis).

Working with many generations of inbred mice to see whether they accepted tumor transplants from other mice, Snell, who joined the lab in 1935, elucidated the basic operation of MHC genes in mice. In years of breeding and grafting experiments, he developed 69 distinct inbred strains of mice, in which he found 11 distinct genetic loci associated with tissue compatibility. He found that mice would accept skin grafts only from mice of genetically identical strains. Scientists studying human immunology began to take notice when it became clear that MHC genes were similar in mice and humans and that Snell's work could be applied to transplantation of tissues in humans.

Another scientist whose work at the laboratory had far-reaching importance is Elizabeth Shull ("Tibby") Russell. From 1937 until 1982 her investigations focused on how red blood cells develop. She was also instrumental in describing and increasing the numbers of inbred and special mutant mice strains for use in biomedical research.

Among major advances that came from the work of scientists at the Jackson Laboratory was one of the first demonstrations of a link between cancer and viruses. It had been known that there were differences in the incidence of mammary (breast) cancer among mouse strains. In 1933 Jackson researchers reported in the journal *Science* that female mice were more likely to get mammary cancers if their mothers were from high-incidence rather than low-incidence strains and that the strain origin of the father seemed unimportant—a finding that did not follow the usual Mendelian rules of inheritance. This indicated that extrachromosomal forces possibly were at work.

These surprising findings led researcher John Bittner to take newborn mice from high-tumor-incidence mothers and place them for nursing with foster mothers from low-tumor-incidence strains. To his astonishment, female mice nursed by these foster mothers rarely developed mammary cancer, while female mice from low-incidence strains developed many such tumors when nursed by foster mothers from high-incidence strains. Reporting his findings in a now-famous paper, published in *Science* in 1936, Bittner referred to a mammary tumor "agent" or "inciter" passed in the milk by high-incidence-strain mothers to their offspring. Not until the 1940s was the agent acknowledged to be a virus.

Another early accomplishment at the Jackson Laboratory was the delicate manipulation of mouse eggs resulting in their fertilization outside the body. This work, among other things, helped set the stage for the first successful *in vitro* fertilization procedures in humans (in 1979). One of the scientists who conducted such embryo work, Peter Hoppe, also became involved in the research that led to "transgenic" technology. In this technology foreign genes, as well as additional DNA sequences that regulate their expression, are injected into fertilized eggs of mice or other mammals. The eggs are then transferred from the laboratory dish to the womb of a "pseudopregnant" female—one that has been primed to accept an embryo—and allowed to grow to term. Some offspring will integrate the foreign gene into their own genetic material, thus becoming so-called transgenic mice. This technique is now being used by many biologists and geneticists to study what factors control the expression of specific genes in living animals and how the genes regulate physiological processes.

Along similar lines, geneticist Eva Eicher is presently investigating how the Y chromosome functions in sex determination. Some genes on the Y chromosome appear to interact with genes of the autosomal (nonsex) chromosomes to steer the embryo toward maleness. How this occurs is not clear, but Eicher believes that the timing of gene action is crucial.

Yet another feather in the Jackson Laboratory's cap has been research that has helped clarify the genetic basis of human diabetes. Douglas Coleman and Edward Leiter have been carrying out extensive studies on diabetes by working with two mouse mutations, one that produces a disease similar to non-insulin-dependent diabetes, the type that can occur in obese adults, and another that is a model for the more severe insulin-dependent diabetes, which usually begins in childhood. One of their findings was that certain diets tend to accelerate the onset of diabetes in insulin-dependent mice.

In their quest to learn what genes do, Jackson Laboratory scientists have also pioneered in the science of gene mapping—determining the specific location of known mouse genes on the animal's 21 different chromosomes. Gene mapping relies on the fact that genes of unknown location can be more precisely located through study of their pattern of inheritance in association with other genes—or "markers"—whose locations are known. The genomes (*i.e.*, the total complement of genetic information) of mice and humans are similar, although humans have 22 pairs of nonsex chromosomes (or autosomes) plus one pair that determines sex (two X's for females or an X and a Y for males), making 46 chromosomes in all. Genes that are grouped together on a chromosome in mice are frequently also linked on chromosomes in humans, indicating that this group of genes has been conserved in evolution and probably plays an important role in the organism.

Once a mouse gene has been precisely located on its chromosome, it can be used to predict the location of a human gene that has a similar function. "Comparative mapping" can help in locating a disease-causing human gene on a human chromosome with respect

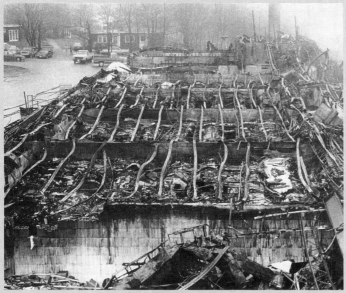

The Jackson Laboratory; photographs, Stanton Short

On May 10, 1989, the lab was devastated by a fire that swept through the main mouse-breeding facility, destroying some 500,000 mice. Many scientists around the world who were dependent on the exclusive JAX nude mice (below) had to delay or abandon their research.

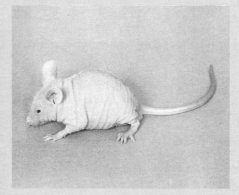

to its proximity to marker genes similar to the mouse marker genes. Mouse-gene mapping also enables researchers to use mice that serve as models of human diseases to learn what the basic defect in a genetic disorder is and what preventive methods or treatments may be possible.

In 1988 an achievement in which Stanford University and Jackson Laboratory researchers collaborated was hailed by the scientific community worldwide—the incorporation of a complete human immune system into a mouse with severe combined immunodeficiency (SCID). The SCID mouse—a mutant discovered at the University of Pennsylvania in 1983 that has no immune system of its own—was given a fetal thymus transplant from a human. Such a mouse model could prove enormously valuable in the study of AIDS, leukemia, hepatitis, diabetes, and other diseases affecting the immune system.

The fire of '89

On May 10, 1989, the Jackson Laboratory was devastated by another fire. This time an enormous blaze—the precise cause of which remains unclear—erupted in a section of the building that was undergoing renovation and swept through the laboratory's main mouse-production building. Half the laboratory's breeding space, the clean process facility (where cages are washed, water bottles sterilized, etc.), and the supplies warehouse were lost; employees who formed a "cage brigade" carried 100,000 mice out of the burning building, but another 400,000 perished. Luckily, because of their separate housing, none of the breeding stocks or frozen embryos were destroyed.

The laboratory's financial loss was estimated at about $40 million. The loss of research projects at Jackson and in the many scientific laboratories around the world that use JAX nude mice and other exclusive breeds was incalculable. Many scientists had to either cancel projects, delay or change them, or, if possible, turn to the few alternate sources of mice; generally, however, scientists are reluctant to change suppliers in the middle of an experiment.

Again, however, recovery was quick to start. The morning after the fire, a Bar Harbor businessman delivered a check for $1,000 to the laboratory. After that, insurance settlements brought in about $16.8 million and private donations close to $2 million. The Howard Hughes Medical Institute gave $750,000 to help rebuild the stocks of inbred mice, and a group of Japanese geneticists raised $175,000.

After a special NIH panel affirmed that Jackson was a "unique national resource," in August 1989 the U.S. Congress enacted a law that authorized up to $25 million for a "mouse production facility" to ease the shortage caused by the fire. The NIH subsequently announced that $10 million in federal funds would be made available on a competitive basis. Jackson applied for the funding and will likely seek more federal money in 1991.

Forging ahead

With the ever increasing importance of genetics in probing complex human disease problems and the extent to which mouse and human genetics have converged, the Jackson Laboratory is dedicated to forging ahead and has major plans for expansion of its basic research function. Although pushed back six months by the fire, the plans call for adding another 15 scientists to the staff over the next half decade. The lab will continue to focus on molecular and somatic cell genetics, developmental biology, immunology, cancer, and several common polygenic diseases (such as heart disease and diabetes).

With the mouse gene map, the laboratory also hopes to become one of the centers in the major international undertaking to sequence the entire human genome—*i.e.*, identify the precise order of the three billion chemical units that make up the 46 human chromosomes. Known as the Human Genome Initiative, the $3 billion effort is to be the largest single undertaking in the history of biology.

New director Paigen has emphasized that the laboratory will continue to offer resources unavailable anywhere else. His idea is to strengthen and expand the traditional and pivotal role that the Jackson Laboratory has played in mammalian genetics, both as a research institution and as a unique resource and preeminent mouse supplier for other institutions. Its role as a communications and information-exchange center for the worldwide community of mammalian geneticists will also grow. And, most certainly, each June there will be captivating new mutant mice for scientists attending the summer Short Course to marvel at.

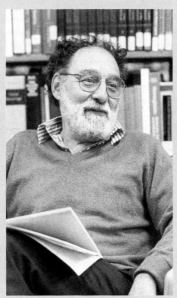

As the Jackson Laboratory recoups its losses after the recent fire, the new director, Kenneth Paigen, has big plans. These include expanding both staff and facilities. The lab will continue to be a major supplier of mice for research as well as a unique resource and information-exchange center for the international community of geneticists.

Gary Guisinger/ The New York Times

Headache

Headache is the most common complaint to which man—or, more frequently, woman—is heir. One recent study of a population of 1,000 persons in the U.K. found that between 79 and 83% of those surveyed had had a headache within the previous year—24% in the previous two weeks severe enough to require an analgesic—but only 1 or 2% consulted a doctor. Most headaches respond to one or two painkilling tablets, but when the pain is severe, persistent, or frequent, then help should be sought.

Because there are many causes of headache, and these are now significantly better understood than previously, the International Headache Society has recently produced a classification of headaches—representing the first major overhaul of categories since 1962. Headaches are now classified under 13 main headings. The first three are idiopathic; *i.e.,* the precise cause is unknown. The next nine are symptomatic of an underlying problem, and eliciting the cause may require special investigations. The 13th category is for headaches that are not classifiable. Diseases are classified for many reasons. For one, classification helps in determining diagnosis. It is also important in research; particularly if there is agreement between researchers as to nomenclature and definitions, a classification system facilitates obtaining meaningful results that can be communicated among international investigators.

The new classifications

The diagnosis of the cause of headache is usually made after a careful history is taken of the characteristics of the headache; then if there remain doubts about the cause, special investigations such as computed tomography (CT) scans or spinal tap (lumbar puncture) may be done.

1. Migraine. The most significant advances have come in the understanding of migraine. Long thought to have psychological origins, migraine is now viewed as a complex neurochemical disorder. Statistics vary, but migraine has been found to affect up to a quarter of any given population; thus, it is just as frequent in Tokyo as in Manhattan. It usually begins during childhood and is more common in females. Although the word *migraine* derives from *hemicrania* ("unilateral headache"), about a third of attacks affect both sides of the head. The headache is typically, but not invariably, throbbing or pulsating. There are two essential requirements. First, the headache must be episodic; *i.e.,* usually lasting a day or two. Any headache that goes on for more than a week cannot be solely due to migraine. Second, there is some accompanying gastric disturbance; *e.g.,* nausea or vomiting. Aversion to light (photophobia), noise (phonophobia), odor (osmophobia), and touch (haptophobia) are common and reflect the heightened sensitivity of the brain.

"Headache #1" by Heidi Tobler; photograph, Sandoz Pharmaceuticals

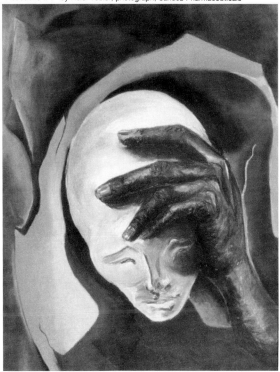

A compelling image by a patient with menstrual migraine was among more than 200 headache-inspired artworks exhibited in Boston during the American Association for the Study of Headache's 1989 scientific meeting.

The two main types of migraine are classical migraine, which has a warning aura, and common migraine, which does not. It is possible, particularly in older people, to have the aura without headache (acephalgic migraine).

Often there are factors that trigger attacks; if they can be avoided, then drug or other therapies may be obviated. The most common trigger is stress and, interestingly, the attacks may occur *after* the stress; *e.g.,* weekend migraine that afflicts the sufferer when a stressful workweek is over. While a quarter of migraine sufferers report that some dietary constituent (*e.g.,* cheese, chocolate, citrates, and caffeine—"the four C's") provokes migraine attacks, avoidance of these is not necessarily effective.

Menstrual migraine, *i.e.,* attacks confined to the first day of the monthly period (± one or two days), can be helped by hormonal therapy. Women who suffer from this type of migraine usually do not have attacks during pregnancy.

Migraine diagnosis is based on the headache's characteristics and a physical examination that rules out other conditions. Although there have been many attempts to find a biochemical, hematologic, or electrophysiological marker that could be identified through laboratory tests, this still remains elusive.

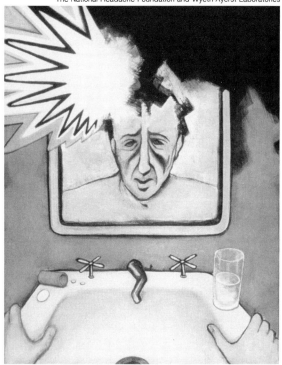

"Man with Migraine" by Peter Gachot; photograph,
The National Headache Foundation and Wyeth-Ayerst Laboratories

This award winner from the first U.S. "Migraine Masterpiece" Art Competition (1988) illustrates the intense visual aura experienced in a classical migraine attack, during which even the simplest task, such as taking medication, is taxing.

For half a century, the common explanation of a migraine attack—usually thought to have psychological origins—was that during the aura there was a constriction of blood vessels to the brain and that the subsequent head pain was due to a reflexive widening of the vessels. This vascular theory is now being questioned.

The aura. While it is inordinately difficult for the patient to carefully chart and time the progress of a visual aura, this has been done repeatedly by scientists and doctors. The very first indication is blurred vision in both eyes when looking ahead. After a minute or two, these blurred spots begin to shimmer and move to one side (the same side in each eye) to form a semicircle that is jagged, like a medieval fort when viewed from above, hence the term *fortification spectrum* or *teichopsia* (*teichos* is Greek for "wall"). Immediately within the semicircle there is a blind area (scotoma). The semicircular jagged edge appears to flash (scintillation), enlarges, and then spreads to one side, becoming larger and more irregular as it disappears.

The time from the first sign of visual difficulty to its disappearance is about 20 minutes. The evidence that this spreading, scintillating scotoma has a vascular cause is that some strokes produce a similar scotoma, and very occasionally scintillation, but never spread-

ing. Harold Wolff, an influential headache specialist, reported more than 40 years ago that if a vasodilator (a drug that induces the widening of blood vessels) was inhaled, the aura could be aborted, but this has not been repeatedly confirmed. Also arguing against this concept is the fact that the activity crosses different circulatory territories, both at the back of the brain (posterior, or vertebrobasilar) and at the front (anterior, or carotid).

Recent technology that is able to estimate cerebral blood flow accurately shows that there is diminished blood flow during the aura, starting at the back of the brain and spreading forward. The back of the brain (the occipital lobe) is affected initially; within this lobe is the visual cortex, which measures 6 cm (2.3 in). Since the visual aura lasts about 20 minutes, the activity in the brain proceeds across the visual cortex at the rate of three millimeters per minute. The reduction in blood flow is now thought to be secondary to neurochemical changes in the brain.

The headache. The evidence that the headache is due to vascular causes, *i.e.,* change in size of feeding blood vessels, is stronger than in the case of the aura. The pulsating, throbbing head pain is in time with the pulse and is relieved by compression of the artery at its origin (in the neck); both the pulsation and headache are lessened by drugs that constrict blood vessels, *e.g.,* ergotamine, but since vasoconstricting drugs have other actions, one of these actions could be responsible for headache relief. Because the size of the blood vessels on the pain-free side is not different from that on the painful side, the vasodilation itself cannot be the cause of the pain. Cerebral blood-flow studies also show no change in blood vessel size during the headache phase. It is more likely that the chemicals (neurotransmitters) released around the blood vessels transmit pain and the pulsating vessels act on these to produce the throbbing headache.

Established approaches to treatment and prevention. Because the stomach essentially does not function during an acute attack (gastric stasis), drugs given by mouth—which are absorbed beyond the stomach in the small intestine—are not absorbed. Therefore, painkillers and antivomiting drugs are best given by suppository; ergotamine, an antimigraine drug, can also be given by nasal spray or in formulations that dissolve under the tongue. The drugs metoclopramide and domperidone promote normal activity of the stomach, however, and thus aid absorption. While aspirin and acetaminophen (paracetamol in the U.K.) are the most common painkillers used, the former can cause gastric irritation, and chronic usage can produce habituation and analgesic rebound headaches.

If attacks are frequent—more than twice monthly—preventive drugs are recommended. The most commonly used are beta blockers, which affect the nerves that supply blood vessels. The first to be used was pro-

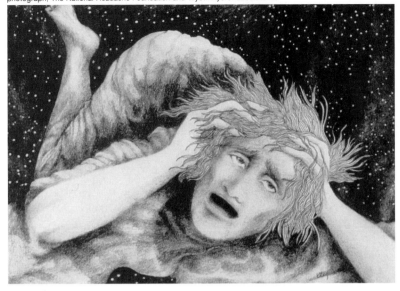

A sufferer portrayed her feeling of confinement during a five-day bout of migraine. The peripheral lights (white dots) are a symptom experienced during the visual aura, at the onset of the attack.

pranolol, which had been given to cardiac and hypertensive patients, and those who were also migraine sufferers found, unexpectedly, that their migraine was better. Since not all beta blockers are effective, they cannot be working solely because of their beta-blocking action. The next most commonly used preventive drugs are antiserotonergic drugs (methysergide and pizotifen) and the calcium-channel blockers (flunarizine and verapamil). The latter are considered to work because of their action on blood vessels.

Treatment breakthrough. Of all the biological sciences, the most rapidly expanding is neuroscience. This is largely due to breakthroughs in two areas: neuroimaging, *e.g.,* estimating cerebral blood flow, and knowledge of neurotransmitters, chemicals that transmit messages from one nerve cell (neuron) to another.

It has been known for about 30 years that one particular neurotransmitter—serotonin, or 5-hydroxytryptamine—is involved in migraine attack. There is an increase in its breakdown product (5-HIAA) in the urine following an attack. Nearly all the serotonin in the blood resides in the platelet, a cellular constituent that aggregates and breaks down (platelet-release reaction) during a migraine attack. Because of this, one theory for migraine was that it was primarily a platelet disorder, a view not widely accepted. It was these alterations in serotonin during an attack that seemed to explain the efficacy of antiserotonergic drugs.

The recent exciting advance involves serotonin, or 5-HT, which consists of three main types—$5HT_1$, $5HT_2$, and $5HT_3$—each of which has subtypes. There are now drugs, designed molecules, that can be targeted at these receptor subtypes. They can dramatically abort the headache and sickness of an acute migraine attack. They are the greatest advance in migraine therapy in many years, and some of these drugs should

be generally available after 1991. Precisely how they work is still a subject of intense investigation, but they are likely not only to relieve the sufferer's pain but also to help unravel the enigma of migraine.

2. Tension-type headache. Tension headaches are generalized headaches of mild to moderate intensity that may be episodic or chronic. They do not have gastrointestinal symptoms, but photophobia and phonophobia may occur. Tension headache and migraine often coexist. Contraction, or tension, causing tenderness in the pericranial muscles occurs with some but not all tension headaches. The term *tension* more accurately describes the underlying psychological tension. Nearly anyone who experiences stress can have this type of headache, but the more chronic of such headaches may be due to an underlying depression

Cerebral blood flow monitoring during the migraine aura typically reveals a diminished flow, starting at the back of the head and spreading forward, which is presumed to be caused by neurochemical changes in the brain.

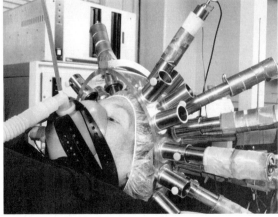

Headache

and are often cured by amitriptyline or similar antidepressant drugs of the tricyclic variety.

3. Cluster headache. One of the most severe headache types known, cluster headache affects mainly men over the age of 30. The pain is around the eye, is always on the same side, and lasts about an hour or two, and with it the eye on the same side is often reddened and weepy; the nostril of that side can feel stuffy or may run. The attacks occur about once daily, typically waking the patient, for about 6 to 12 weeks once a year or less often (hence the term *cluster*). Cluster headache usually responds to drug therapy, but many of the drugs used have major side effects and thus must be monitored closely. For short cluster periods ergotamine can be used, but for chronic cases lithium, which works by acting on the surfaces (membranes) of nerve cells, has been one of the most effective agents. Other drugs that are often tried are methysergide and corticosteroids, and oxygen treatment is sometimes given during the attack.

4. Miscellaneous headaches. Headache can be produced by exercise, cough, or even sexual intercourse (benign orgasmic dephalalgia). Usually these do not signify any serious underlying disorder. They tend to occur in migraine patients and may be prevented by migraine prophylactics.

5. Head injury. Headache often follows head trauma but is usually temporary. More persistent headache as a result of trauma can occur if there are complications—*e.g.,* accumulation of blood clots (subdural hematoma), which requires surgical removal. Psychological factors—*e.g.,* litigation following injury—also may prolong the headache.

6. Vascular disorder headache. Stroke, which produces brain damage due to interruption of blood supply, especially when the cause is a hemorrhage rather than a clot, is one example of a vascular disorder that causes head pain. Another occurs in persons over the age of 60 years; a very persistent headache with tenderness—on combing hair, for example—and thickened pulseless blood vessels may be due to temporal arteritis. Sufferers may have a warning of generalized aches and pains (polymyalgia) with loss of weight. An increase in the sedimentation of red blood cells (the erythrocyte sedimentation rate) and biopsy of the temporal artery showing so-called giant cells in the vessel wall will confirm diagnosis. Rapid diagnosis is important because a complication—blindness in one eye, or sometimes in both—can be prevented by steroid treatment. Steroids—*e.g.,* prednisolone—work by means of anti-inflammatory and immunosuppressive action.

7. Intracranial pressure. Because intracranial pressure is often a symptom of a brain tumor, intracranial causes of headache are the most feared. Tumors of the brain, which can be benign or malignant, are among the most commonly occurring tumors (after

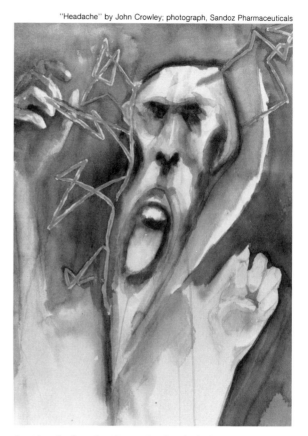

"Headache" by John Crowley; photograph, Sandoz Pharmaceuticals

A patient in the grip of a tension headache has suggested an aversion to light and sound. Although often stress induced, tension headaches may be caused by an underlying depression; some sufferers respond well to antidepressants.

tumors of the lung, breast, uterus, and stomach). A headache caused by increased intracranial pressure is worse in the morning and is aggravated by bending or coughing, which increases the pressure even more; accompanying nausea is also worse in the morning. A CT scan of the brain is mandatory for this type of headache. Treatment, when needed, is usually surgical, particularly for benign tumors.

Low intracranial pressure, which occurs after spinal tap and can last up to a week, is also a cause of headache. The headaches are due to the stretching of the blood vessels and meninges (the coverings of the brain); the brain itself is insensitive to pain.

8. Drug-induced headaches. Drug-related headaches are more frequent than is generally realized. The most common form is the hangover following excessive consumption of alcohol. Alcohol causes dilation of cranial blood vessels, producing throbbing pain that is exacerbated by movement of the head. Because alcohol has a diuretic effect—it increases the secretion of urine and depletes the body of fluids—the most effective remedy is to drink several glasses of water; if done before the alcohol is consumed, water consumption may minimize headache—depending, of course, on the amount of alcohol consumed. Less recognized is the fact that painkillers—*e.g.,* narcotics such as codeine and antimigraine remedies—can, if taken on a daily basis, produce rebound headaches. Prolonged use interferes with tissues the drugs act upon; larger and larger doses are then needed; and a drug-induced dependence begins a vicious cycle. Because withdrawal from medication can be difficult, hospitalization may be necessary.

Caffeine withdrawal will also produce headache. Estrogens and birth control pills, too, are known to cause headaches, although the mechanism of action is unknown.

Related to drug-induced headaches are those due to specific chemicals; *e.g.,* "hot-dog headache," in which nitrates used to even out the color of prepared meats act as vasodilators. Another example is "Chinese restaurant syndrome," in which headache and flushing are blamed on monosodium glutamate, a flavor enhancer.

9. Infections. Headache can be associated with both viral and bacterial infections. Infections such as influenza will produce headache, which disappears when the illness resolves. The headache is usually overshadowed by other symptoms and does not require specific treatment. More serious are specific infections of the nervous system, such as meningitis or encephalitis. Examination of the cerebrospinal fluid, obtained by spinal tap, will usually reveal the organism responsible.

10. Metabolic headache. At high altitudes mountain sickness causes such symptoms as headache, nausea, and disorientation as a result of poor oxygenation of red blood cells (hypoxia) due to low barometric pressure. Gradual acclimatization can prevent the condition, but when it occurs, acetazolamide, a carbonic anhydrase inhibitor that acts as a diuretic, has proved useful in treatment. Hypoglycemia, an abnormal decrease in blood sugar, and sleep apnea, in which abnormal breathing interferes with sleep and produces hypoxia, are other, though infrequent, metabolically related causes of headache.

11. Cranial headaches. Headaches or facial pain can be associated with disorders of the cranium, neck (*e.g.,* disorders of the cervical spine), eyes (*e.g.,* acute glaucoma and refractive errors), ears, teeth and jaws, and the nose and sinuses. Perhaps most common is the pain from sinusitis. Such pain is easily recognized since it often follows a cold or flu, settles over the cheek or forehead, and is worse in the afternoon. X-ray of the sinuses reveals an opaque sinus due to accumulation of fluid. The condition is cured by antibiotics, but sometimes interventional drainage may be needed.

12. Neuralgia. The word *neuralgia* means "pain in a nerve," and the most common nerve affected is the trigeminal (or fifth cranial) nerve, which governs sensation of the face. Trigeminal neuralgia usually occurs

	migraine	cluster
pain quality	throbbing, pulsating, aggravated by physical activity	steady, intense, piercing, boring, or burning
duration	8 to 36 hours	15 minutes to 3 hours
site	temple	in the eye, forehead, and temple; radiating into neck; around the eye, radiating behind the eye socket or into the jaw
sufferers	more common in women; heredity a factor	more common in men over age 30; heredity not a factor
pattern of attacks	attacks may occur any time; pain often present on awakening	typically, two or more times a day for weeks or months, usually followed by pain-free intervals of months or years; attacks often occur early in the morning or two to three hours after retiring
warning symptoms	classic type with aura: visual, neurological, or mental symptoms, lasting about 20 minutes; *e.g.,* blurred vision, seeing flashing lights	none
other common symptoms	nausea and vomiting, photophobia and phonophobia	sinus congestion, runny or stuffy nose, tearing, eyelid swelling or drooping, facial sweating

Migraine versus cluster headache

after the age of 50 and is recognized by its sharp shooting pains, usually in the jaw, cheek, or both but sometimes involving the eye. It is nearly always confined to one side and is provoked by washing, talking, chewing, or cold drafts. The pain lasts only a few seconds but is so intense that the face tends to contract, or screw up, hence the alternative name of tic douloureux (*tic* means "spasm"; *douloureux* means "painful"). Involuntary repetition of the painful paroxysms can be set off by a touch to certain "trigger" areas on the face. Sufferers are usually helped by carbamazepine (Tegretol), which need not be taken permanently, as the pain often disappears for months or even years. This drug is used mostly in epilepsy; it reduces the likelihood of seizures caused by abnormal nerve signals in the brain. In rare cases of neuralgia, surgery is performed to sever the nerve.

It is expected that the new classification of headache disorders will benefit sufferers by enabling improved and more expedient diagnoses. Jes Olesen, professor of neurology at the University of Copenhagen, who served as the chairman of the classification committee of the International Headache Society, has recommended that patients keep "headache diaries"—careful records of the occurrence and nature of their headaches; such records, in conjunction with the new classifications, should help physicians modify or change treatments so patients receive optimal therapy.

—*F. Clifford Rose, M.D.*

323

Heart and Blood Vessels

Cardiovascular disease (CVD), the great modern plague, continues to be the leading cause of untimely mortality in most economically developed nations of the world. CVD causes nearly a million deaths a year in the United States alone and costs the nation an estimated $136 billion. Many victims and would-be victims are now benefiting from important recent advances in the field of cardiology; these have come in the areas of understanding, diagnosis, treatment, and prevention. Brief reports below suggest the range of advances.

One problem whose prevention continues to pose a major challenge is sudden cardiac death. Another subject, cholesterol, continues to spark controversy: How should the lay public interpret the conflicting and confusing published reports? These topics are addressed in more detail.

Advances: in brief

Small inflatable balloons placed at the tip of cardiac catheters are now commonly introduced through arm or leg blood vessels to dilate narrowed segments of arteries. Although they are frequently used to open arteries of the lower limbs in patients whose vessels are narrowed by atherosclerosis and who develop leg pain due to inadequate blood flow, their most frequent use is to improve the blood supply to the heart. Percutaneous transluminal coronary angioplasty (PTCA) is cost-effective, involves relatively little discomfort to the patient, and often makes open-heart surgery unnecessary. Approximately 250,000 of these procedures will be performed in the United States alone this year.

There have been notable advances in the design of the balloon catheters and catheter delivery systems. Consequently, many coronary blockages or narrowings (stenoses) can now be treated by this method. More recently a number of other catheter-based techniques have evolved, in conjunction with coronary angioplasty, to open up certain coronary artery stenoses. These include lasers; atherectomy devices that make use of mechanical rotating surfaces to cut or pulverize, and then remove, the material that is responsible for the narrowing of the blood vessel; and coronary artery stents. Stents are composed of a flexible, expandable metal support mesh that is introduced into the coronary artery by the balloon catheter. After the narrowed artery is dilated by the inflated balloon, the stent is introduced into the dilated segment, expanded by inflation of the balloon, and left in place to ensure that the coronary artery stays open.

Specially designed inflatable catheter balloons, larger than those used for PTCA, are also being used in the cardiac-catheterization laboratory to open narrowed heart valves (mitral, pulmonary, and aortic valve stenosis) and blood vessels (coarctation of the aorta). Results have been particularly good in young patients with mitral stenosis or with pulmonary stenosis; the procedure has not proved as effective in patients with aortic valve disease.

Cardiac surgery has become established as a treatment of an increasing number of congenital and acquired cardiac abnormalities. Specifically, there have been recent advances in the ability to prevent rejection of transplanted organs by judicious use of medications that inhibit the immune response causing graft rejection. This has resulted in the establishment of cardiac transplantation as an effective long-term treatment in patients who are severely limited and do not respond to conventional therapeutic measures. Increasing success with combined heart and lung transplantations has also allowed many complex congenital cardiac malformations to be treated effectively in children and young adults.

There have been important advances in the management of disorders of heart rhythm. Pacemakers were initially developed to prevent dangerous slowing of the heart rate with resultant loss of consciousness. Advances in microchip electronic technology and battery design have allowed for marked reductions in the size of pacemakers and in the increased longevity and programmability of the devices. Modern physiological pacemakers mimic closely the natural rhythm of the heart and allow for proper sequence of cardiac-chamber activation and for increases in heart rate in response to physical exercise. These modifications improve the efficacy of the heart as a pump in patients with various slow heart rate problems and allow for substantial improvement in exercise performance.

Sudden cardiac death:
identifying and managing those at risk

Sudden unexpected cardiac death claims an estimated 450,000 lives annually in the United States

Remote monitors track the progress of a PTCA, or balloon angioplasty, procedure to open blocked coronary arteries. Advances in the design of PTCA catheters and systems have steadily reduced the need for open-heart surgery.

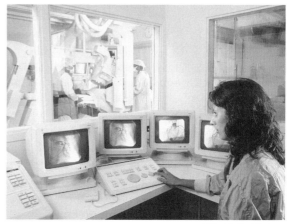

alone and occurs most commonly in the industrial nations of Europe and North America. Although major advances have been made in understanding its underlying mechanisms, prevention continues to pose a major challenge.

Sudden cardiac death can occur as a result of many conditions. Among the known causes are the following:

Heart attacks. Coronary artery disease, characterized by narrowing of the vessels that supply blood to the heart muscle, or myocardium, by fibrous and fatty deposits within the vessel wall (atherosclerosis), is the most common cause of sudden cardiac death. There are basically two major circumstances in which sudden cardiac death may strike people who have coronary artery disease: during a heart attack (myocardial infarction) and after a heart attack that has left the heart electrically unstable.

Myocardial infarction usually results from sudden blockage of a coronary artery by a clot that has formed at the site of atherosclerotic disease. Sudden cardiac death may then follow from acute failure of the heart's pumping action, rupture of the heart, or abnormalities of the heart rhythm (cardiac arrhythmias). Importantly, most deaths from arrhythmia happen within the first few minutes or hours of the heart attack. The risk of sudden cardiac death can therefore be reduced if persons who experience prolonged or frequently recurring chest discomfort are transferred rapidly to coronary care units, where heart rhythm can be monitored. Early administration of drugs that can dissolve the clot (thrombolytic therapy) and thus reduce the extent of myocardial damage and of drugs that prevent further buildup or recurrence of clots (aspirin and heparin) also reduces the risk of subsequent sudden cardiac death.

Several thrombolytic agents are now available (streptokinase, tissue plasminogen activator [t-PA], urokinase, anistreplase), although controversy still abounds as to which is the most effective. Thrombolytic therapy reduces mortality in the weeks following a myocardial infarction by about 25%. The main beneficiaries are patients treated in the first few hours after the heart attack begins, although benefits have been reported for patients whose treatment began as long as 12 hours after onset of symptoms.

The use of clot-dissolving agents represents a major advance in treating heart attacks. Another breakthrough occurred when it was shown that taking aspirin shortly after the onset of a heart attack produces an equally dramatic decrease (about 25%) in mortality. The effectiveness of aspirin probably arises from the fact that the drug inhibits the activity of platelets, a component of the blood essential to the formation of clots. Of note, the beneficial effects of streptokinase and those achieved with aspirin appear to work together, as combined therapy reduces mortality associated with myocardial infarction by more than 40%.

A medical team demonstrates delivery of a clot-dissolving agent directly to the site of arterial blockage in a heart attack victim. Primary beneficiaries of this therapy are those treated within hours after the attack begins.

Although many who survive a heart attack recover virtually normal cardiac function, other, less fortunate people are left with a damaged, scarred left ventricle (the major pumping chamber of the heart) and impaired pumping function. Sudden death among the latter group may be caused by another myocardial infarction. However, most sudden deaths in this group occur because the scarred heart is often electrically irritable. In such circumstances the heart may experience ventricular tachycardia, an abnormally rapid regular rhythm arising from an area near the scarred muscle. Frequently, ventricular tachycardia degenerates into ventricular fibrillation, a chaotic rhythm that invariably results in death unless a satisfactory rhythm is restored within a few minutes by application of a direct-current shock to the chest.

Patients who survived a heart attack and who are at increased risk of sudden cardiac death include: (1) those with extensive myocardial damage; (2) those whose ventricular arrhythmias could trigger more life-threatening arrhythmias (not all arrhythmias are inherently dangerous); and (3) those with an abnormal signal-averaged electrocardiogram, a special electrical recording of the heart that can identify patients having an electrical irritability that can lead to ventricular arrhythmias.

Cardiomyopathy. Cardiomyopathies are primary diseases of the heart muscle. They are frequently associated with ventricular arrhythmias that can result in sudden cardiac death.

Wolff-Parkinson-White (WPW) syndrome. Normally, the electrical impulses that control heart-muscle contraction are generated in the right atrium (one of the two reservoir chambers sitting on top of the ventricles, the pumping chambers of the heart) and conducted to the ventricles by a single pathway of specialized muscle tissue. This pathway normally transmits the electrical impulses slowly. Extra, or accessory, pathways between the atria and ventricles, however, sometimes exist, and when they do, they often conduct faster than the normal pathway. Their presence thus may result in very rapid heart rates if the heart experiences atrial arrhythmias that, in the absence of such pathways, would be much slower and better tolerated. Because of the very rapid rates, otherwise nonserious arrhythmias may degenerate into ventricular fibrillation and consequent sudden cardiac death.

Syndromes associated with a prolonged "Q-T interval." The so-called Q-T interval is the particular interval on an electrocardiogram that represents the time during which the ventricles of the heart contract. An abnormally long Q-T interval is associated with occurrence of a form of rapid ventricular arrhythmia termed *torsades de pointes,* which can result in sudden cardiac death. Q-T prolongation may result from certain electrolyte (potassium, magnesium) deficiencies, drugs (tricyclic antidepressants and antiarrhythmic drugs), and nutritional states (liquid-protein–modified-fat diets). Additionally, two hereditary syndromes—Jervell and Lange-Nielsen, and Romano-Ward—and a similar but noninherited disorder are associated with abnormal Q-T prolongation and sudden cardiac death. These conditions are typically discovered in childhood or early adulthood when their victims suffer from recurrent syncope (fainting) or have convulsive seizures precipitated by emotional or physical stress.

Valvular heart disease. Severe narrowing of the aortic valve of the heart (the outflow valve of the left ventricle) may result in syncope and, if unrelieved, in sudden cardiac death.

Primary ventricular electrical instability. Finally, occasionally otherwise healthy people experience ventricular fibrillation. In these cases sudden cardiac death may occur in the absence of any known cardiac disease.

Public education programs and increased availability of rapidly deployable paramedic teams allow the delivery of lifesaving emergency medical care to many individuals who suffer cardiac arrest. Survivors, however, are at high risk of a potentially fatal recurrent episode. A careful history, clinical examination, and series of tests are necessary to determine potentially reversible causes of the cardiac arrest and to prevent

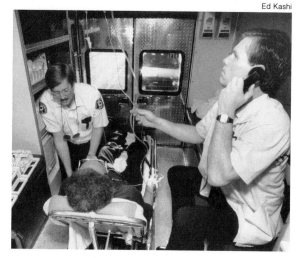

Ed Kashi

Increased availability of quick-response paramedic teams and sophisticated mobile equipment has given many victims of cardiac arrest a second chance. These survivors, however, remain at high risk of another, potentially fatal episode.

subsequent sudden death. This kind of comprehensive evaluation is also necessary for the patient who has not had a cardiac arrest but who has been identified as having one of the disorders discussed above. If, by means of these studies, the patient is judged to be at increased risk, an electrophysiological (EP) study is usually performed.

An EP study involves insertion of several catheters into the heart (through blood vessels in the arm or groin) for recording cardiac electrical activity and for electrically stimulating the heart. These studies identify persons with sinus node disease (the sinus node, a mass of specialized heart muscle, is the source of the electrical stimulus that initiates the natural heart rhythm) and those with abnormalities of electrical conduction across the atrioventricular node, another source of electrical stimulus that lies between the upper (atrial) and lower (ventricular) chambers of the heart. Patients with sinus node disease or conduction disorders may be prone to sudden slowing of the heart rate and thus suffer loss of consciousness or, if the slowing is profound and prolonged, sudden cardiac death.

The EP study also identifies those who are prone to atrial and ventricular arrhythmias. The perpetuating mechanism of most ventricular arrhythmias is believed to involve a process termed *reentry.* Reentry is dependent on the presence of an impulse-carrying pathway of heart muscle that acts abnormally by allowing part of the impulse to reverse its travel and then enter the pathway a second time. This reentry, or feedback, of the electrical impulse may become continuous, thus perpetuating the arrhythmia. Consequently, for tachycardia to occur, both a source of initiating impulses and a pathway that allows impulse reentry must exist.

Initiating mechanisms are usually extra heartbeats, which occur more often (but not exclusively) in persons with diseased heart muscle. These extra beats can be detected by electrocardiographic monitoring. On the other hand, the existence of a reentry pathway capable of sustaining an arrhythmia can be detected in an EP study. If a patient does have the necessary reentry pathway, ventricular tachycardia can be started and stopped reliably during the EP study by delivery of critically timed electrical stimuli via a catheter placed near the pathway. Such a demonstration implies that the patient has the necessary pathway to sustain an arrhythmia spontaneously if initiating mechanisms occur. It also allows its properties and its effect on the patient's blood pressure to be evaluated.

In many patients antiarrhythmic drugs are effective; they eliminate occurrence of the initiating extra heartbeats or favorably modify the reentry pathway. In some patients, however, the same drugs show little effect or are actually proarrhythmic; *i.e.,* they encourage the arrhythmia.

If antiarrhythmic drugs suppress ventricular tachycardia induced during the EP study, it is likely that the patient will benefit from their long-term use. If, however, they fail to control the arrhythmia or result in serious side effects, nonpharmacological therapeutic methods are employed. These include attempts to destroy the arrhythmia (by surgery or by catheter-delivered laser beams or electrical energy) or surgical implantation of a defibrillator device. The latter continuously monitors the heart rhythm and delivers an electric shock directly to the heart if its sensing mechanism detects the start of a potentially lethal ventricular arrhythmia.

This diagnostic and therapeutic approach to patients at high risk of dying suddenly because of a ventricular arrhythmia has been extremely successful. Ordinarily, the chances that a patient who has been resuscitated from a cardiac arrest will die of a subsequent one is about 30% after one year and about 45% after two years. The use of EP studies to guide therapy in this subgroup of patients changes these statistics quite remarkably. If a drug is identified that suppresses induction of ventricular arrhythmia (found in about a third of the patients), incidence of sudden cardiac death is reduced to 6% at one year and to 15% at three years. Patients who continue to have an inducible ventricular arrhythmia remain at high risk for sudden cardiac death—30% at three years—unless they receive an implantable defibrillator. First introduced in 1984, the device has been implanted in several thousand patients worldwide, in whom it has reduced incidence of sudden cardiac death to less than 1% per year.

The problem of sudden cardiac death caused by coronary artery disease represents the consequences of a disease that often takes years or even decades to advance to the point that it can cause sudden death. A broader approach to coronary artery disease is to pre-vent its development or progression entirely. Although several preventive measures have been advocated, perhaps the one that has been most publicized, and at the same time most embroiled in controversy, is advocacy of reducing cholesterol levels in the blood.

Cholesterol update: review of the evidence

In the past year, several questions have been raised about the scientific basis for lowering high blood cholesterol to reduce the risk of coronary heart disease (CHD). The controversy has focused on three major issues. First, is elevated blood cholesterol an important risk factor for CHD? And is it a risk factor in women and the elderly as well as in middle-aged men? Second, does lowering high blood cholesterol reduce illness and death from CHD? And does it prolong life? And third, is diet a significant factor in determining the level of blood cholesterol and the risk of CHD? To answer these questions, it is worthwhile to review the scientific evidence from major studies and clinical trials linking cholesterol to CHD. (*See* Table on page 329 for summary of studies cited.)

Elevated blood cholesterol and CHD. There is compelling evidence implicating elevated levels of blood cholesterol as a risk factor for CHD. The Framingham Heart Study, which has been evaluating the coronary risk profiles of men and women in Framingham, Mass., for nearly half a century, has shown that the risk of CHD rises steadily as the blood cholesterol level rises and that elevated blood cholesterol is one of the three major modifiable CHD risk factors, together with smoking and high blood pressure. Follow-up of the more than 360,000 men aged 35–57 who were screened for the Multiple Risk Factor Intervention Trial (MRFIT) has clearly demonstrated the relationship between increasing serum cholesterol levels and increasing risk

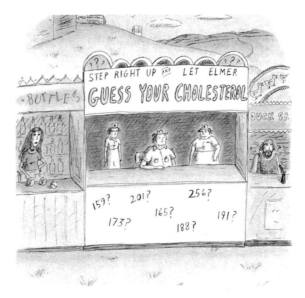

Drawing by R. Chast; © 1989 The New Yorker Magazine, Inc.

of CHD death. The risk is relatively low below 180–200 milligrams per deciliter (mg/dl) and increases more rapidly as the cholesterol level rises past 200 mg/dl. At a serum cholesterol level of 240 mg/dl, the risk of CHD is about double that at 200 mg/dl, and it rises still more steeply above 240 mg/dl. These observed risk relationships are an important part of the reason that the Adult Treatment Panel of the National Cholesterol Education Program (NCEP) established the current classification of total cholesterol levels: less than 200 mg/dl is desirable, 200–239 mg/dl is borderline-high, and 240 mg/dl or above is high blood cholesterol. Together, the evidence from animal, biochemical, genetic, epidemiological, and clinical studies shows that elevated blood cholesterol is a cause of CHD.

High blood cholesterol is a risk factor for CHD not only in middle-aged men but also in women and the elderly. Although women generally develop CHD at later ages than men, it is the number one killer of women (as well as men), accounting for the deaths of nearly 250,000 women a year. Survey and epidemiological data show that the rates of CHD in women rise rapidly after menopause and catch up to those of men. Framingham and other studies have shown that elevated blood cholesterol is an important factor in this rise.

The elderly have high rates of CHD, and elevated blood cholesterol is common in this age group. Framingham has shown that a high level of low-density lipoprotein (LDL)-cholesterol ("bad" cholesterol) is a predictor of coronary heart disease in older persons; an elevated level of total serum cholesterol is also a predictor of coronary heart disease, but it is weaker than at younger ages. Nonetheless, the elderly have such high absolute rates of CHD that the number of cases of CHD associated with a rise in total cholesterol is actually greater than in younger individuals.

Lowering blood cholesterol: clearly established benefits. Clinical trials have proved that lowering high blood cholesterol levels will reduce the risk of CHD. In the Coronary Primary Prevention Trial (CPPT), a 9% reduction in total cholesterol levels produced a 19% reduction in CHD deaths and nonfatal myocardial infarctions. In the Helsinki (Finland) Heart Study, an 8% reduction in total and LDL-cholesterol, together with a 10% rise in high-density lipoprotein (HDL)-cholesterol ("good" cholesterol), yielded a 34% reduction in CHD risk. This study confirmed the benefits of lowering total and LDL-cholesterol and suggested that additional benefit was gained by raising HDL-cholesterol. The benefit of raising HDL-cholesterol in individuals with high serum cholesterol has also been seen in several other studies.

HDL is thought to play a significant role in transporting cholesterol away from tissues. In epidemiological studies such as Framingham, low levels of HDL-cholesterol predict an increased risk of CHD, whereas high levels appear to be protective. However, accurate measurement of HDL-cholesterol is difficult to accomplish in the standard clinical laboratory, and the benefit of raising a low HDL-cholesterol where this is the only cholesterol problem has not been proved in a clinical trial. Because of these considerations, the Adult Treatment Panel of NCEP did not recommend universal screening for HDL-cholesterol and recommended that hygienic measures (such as weight loss to correct obesity, smoking cessation, and exercise) rather than drug treatment be used to raise an isolated low HDL level.

A question that has been raised about the CPPT and Helsinki trials is whether the magnitude of the absolute reduction in CHD rates (as contrasted with the percentage of reduction) is substantial enough to justify cholesterol-lowering treatment. Thus, the Helsinki Heart Study, although it achieved a 34% reduction in CHD, also showed that the absolute reduction in CHD that would result from treating 1,000 hypothetical men for five years is only 14 cases (27 cases of CHD if the 1,000 men were treated versus 41 cases if they were not). The problem with this critique is that it bases a judgment about the absolute reduction in CHD on the data from the limited five-year period of the trial. In actual clinical practice, patients with high blood cholesterol levels would be treated for a lifetime, not for five years alone.

What is the risk of CHD over a lifetime? Framingham data show that a 40-year-old man has about a 50% chance of developing CHD over his remaining lifetime. In other words, 500 out of 1,000 middle-aged men will develop CHD if no cholesterol-lowering treatment is carried out. With treatment, if blood cholesterol levels were lowered 10–15% (which is likely to be attainable in light of the reductions seen in the clinical trials with diet, drugs, or both), the CHD risk would be reduced about 25%. That means that out of 1,000 men only 375 would develop CHD, instead of 500—an absolute reduction of 125 cases of CHD per 1,000 men. This is clearly a substantial reduction in the absolute number of CHD cases, but it can be appreciated only in view of the lifetime incidence of CHD, not the incidence over the necessarily short duration of the clinical trials.

Clinical trials have also provided clear X-ray evidence of the beneficial effects of cholesterol reduction on the rate of progression of coronary artery disease as determined by investigations that studied the coronary arteries (coronary angiography). Thus, the Cholesterol Lowering Atherosclerosis Study (CLAS) showed that substantial cholesterol lowering produces slowed progression and even regression of atherosclerotic plaques in the coronary arteries. The patients in the study had recently undergone coronary artery bypass surgery; the results, therefore, indicate that cholesterol lowering can be beneficial even in advanced CHD. The recently released early results of the Familial Atherosclerosis Treatment Study (FATS) provide

Cholesterol: cited studies and clinical trials

name of study	focus of study	study population	name of study	focus of study	study population
I. epidemiological studies			Helsinki Heart Study	randomized, double-blind, placebo-controlled study of changes in blood lipids and CHD rates in men treated with gemfibrozil	4,081 men, aged 40–55
Framingham Heart Study	long-term study of risk factors for CVD	5,209 men and women, aged 30–60 at entry (1948)			
MRFIT Screenees	follow-up of men screened for the Multiple Risk Factor Intervention Trial to determine cause of death	361,662 men, aged 35–57	Cholesterol Lowering Atherosclerosis Study (CLAS)	randomized, placebo-controlled angiographic study of changes in coronary atherosclerotic plaque in men who had previously undergone coronary artery bypass surgery and who were treated with combined colestipol-nicotinic acid therapy and diet	162 men, aged 40–59
Seven Countries Study	study to examine the effects of culture, differences in diet, and other health habits on risk factors and CHD	11,579 men, aged 40–59			
Ni-Hon-San Study	comparison of diet, blood cholesterol levels, and CVD rates in Japanese living in Japan with those in people originally from same regions who were living in Hawaii or California	12,485 men, aged 45–69	Familial Atherosclerosis Treatment Study (FATS)	randomized, double-blind, quantitative arteriographic comparison of changes in coronary atherosclerosis and lipid alterations with nicotinic acid + colestipol, lovastatin + colestipol, or placebo (± colestipol) in patients with existing CHD and familial lipoprotein disorders	165 subjects
Honolulu Heart Program	prospective study of diet, blood cholesterol levels, and CVD among men living in Hawaii	8,006 men, aged 45–64			
Zutphen Study	investigation into relationship between diet, blood cholesterol and other risk characteristics, and CVD incidence	871 men, aged 40–59	Coronary Drug Project	assessment of the efficacy and safety of several lipid-influencing drugs, including nicotinic acid, in men with previous myocardial infarction	8,341 men, aged 30–64
Ireland-Boston Study	comparison of diet, blood cholesterol, and CHD in men of Irish descent in Ireland and Boston	1,001 men, aged 29–70	Oslo Study Diet and Antismoking Trial	assessment of the effect of diet and antismoking interventions on CHD and risk factors	1,232 men, aged 40–49
Western Electric Study	investigation of diet, blood cholesterol, and other variables in relation to the subsequent development of CVD	1,900 men, aged 40–55	Stockholm Ischemic Heart Disease Study	study of mortality rates in survivors of myocardial infarction treated with clofibrate and nicotinic acid	555 subjects (men and women)
II. clinical trials			Los Angeles Veterans Administration Domiciliary Study	randomized double-blind study of men assigned to a control or cholesterol-lowering diet	846 men, aged 55–89
Lipid Research Clinics-Coronary Primary Prevention Trial (LRC-CPPT)	randomized, double-blind, placebo-controlled study of changes in blood cholesterol levels and CHD rates in hypercholesterolemic men treated with cholestyramine and a moderate cholesterol-lowering diet	3,806 men, aged 35–59	Finnish Mental Hospital Study	comparison of usual diet with a diet reduced in saturated fats, in which there was partial replacement with unsaturated fats	4,178 men, 6,434 women, aged 15+

Compiled with the assistance of Nancy Ernst, Nutrition Coordinator, National Heart, Lung, and Blood Institute

additional X-ray evidence that cholesterol lowering can lead to actual regression of coronary atherosclerotic plaques.

Most of the cholesterol-lowering clinical trials have been conducted in middle-aged men with high cholesterol levels because their high rates of CHD allow the trials to be carried out as efficiently as possible. However, the total body of evidence, including animal, metabolic, and epidemiological studies, suggests that the results can be extended to women and the elderly. As already indicated, elevated blood cholesterol is a CHD risk factor in women and the elderly; the atherosclerotic process itself does not appear to be different in these groups; and advanced disease responds to cholesterol lowering. All in all, the evidence suggests that women and the elderly can reap the same benefits from cholesterol reduction as middle-aged men.

Despite a clear reduction in CHD, the CPPT and Helsinki studies did not show a reduction in overall death rates from lowered cholesterol. These trials, however, were of too short duration to show reductions in total mortality. Epidemiological studies such as Framingham and the Seven Countries Study suggest that individuals with the lowest cholesterol levels have the greatest life expectancy, while those with more elevated levels do not live as long. In addition, three clinical trials (the nicotinic-acid arm of the Coronary Drug Project, the Oslo [Norway] Study Diet and Antismoking Trial, and the Stockholm Ischemic Heart Disease Study) have reported reductions in total mortality. More evidence is needed to establish definitively the effect of cholesterol lowering on total death rates. The currently available evidence shows conclusively that lowering high blood cholesterol will reduce illness and death from CHD, thereby leading to improved quality of life, and suggests that cholesterol lowering may well lead to prolongation of life as well.

Diet. Findings from metabolic, epidemiological, and clinical studies show that diet is an important determinant of blood cholesterol levels and CHD risk. The evidence for these relationships has been carefully reviewed in two recent reports, that of the NCEP Population Panel and the National Research Council's report, *Diet and Health.* These two reviews have concluded that high intakes of saturated fatty acids, cholesterol, and calories leading to obesity raise blood cholesterol levels and increase the risk of CHD.

The scientific basis for these conclusions comes from a variety of types of studies: (1) from epidemiological studies of the relationships between dietary components, blood cholesterol levels, and CHD rates, in particular the Seven Countries Study, the Ni-Hon-San Study, the Honolulu Heart Program, the Zutphen (Neth.) Study, the Ireland-Boston Study, and the Western Electric Study; (2) from studies conducted on metabolic wards showing that dietary saturated fatty acids raise total and LDL-cholesterol levels, that substitution of carbohydrates, monounsaturated, or polyunsaturated fatty acids for saturated fatty acids reduces blood cholesterol levels, and that diet alone can produce 15–25% reductions in blood cholesterol; and (3) from clinical trials, such as the Oslo Study, the Los Angeles Veterans Administration Domiciliary Study, and the Finnish Mental Hospital Study, which

have shown that diet alone can produce 10–15% reductions in blood cholesterol in free-living patients who are making their own dietary choices.

The strong evidence linking diet to blood cholesterol and CHD has led many major health and medical organizations (including the NCEP Population Panel, the National Research Council, and the American Heart Association) to recommend that Americans adopt an eating pattern that is low in saturated fatty acids and dietary cholesterol and that they avoid excess calories. Adopting such dietary habits can lower blood cholesterol levels by about 10%, which should translate into a 20% reduction in CHD. The evidence has also led the NCEP Adult Treatment Panel to recommend that a diet low in saturated fatty acids and dietary cholesterol be the mainstay of clinical treatment for individuals with high blood cholesterol.

What is needed to lower blood cholesterol through diet is a habitual pattern of heart-healthy eating. Despite the fact that fish oil and soluble fiber (such as oat bran) have been promoted in some quarters as "magic bullets," no single food or supplement is the key to reducing blood cholesterol. Fish oil supplements do not generally lower blood cholesterol levels and are not recommended. On the other hand, fish is a good source of protein, is low in saturated fatty acids, and has an important role to play in a health-promoting dietary pattern. Oat bran has been found in a few studies to add modestly to the degree of blood cholesterol lowering, but dietary fiber supplements are not a panacea. However, foods rich in soluble fiber (such as oats and oat bran) are a useful component of an overall eating pattern that is low in saturated fatty acids, total fat, and cholesterol.

Reasonable conclusions: the current consensus. The strength of the scientific evidence has produced a consensus among most informed scientists that elevated blood cholesterol is an important risk factor for CHD, that lowering elevated blood cholesterol levels

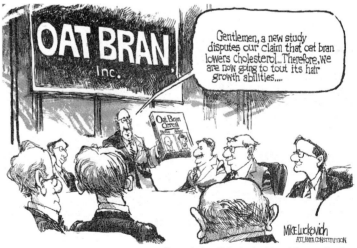

By permission of Mike Luckovich and Creators Syndicate

will reduce CHD rates, and that diet is the cornerstone for lowering blood cholesterol levels. Over 6 million Americans have symptomatic CHD, and there are about 1,250,000 myocardial infarctions annually. Despite impressive declines in CHD death rates over the past 20 years, CHD remains the leading killer of men and of women, accounting for over 500,000 deaths a year. The economic burden imposed by CHD exceeds $50 billion annually. Approximately 60 million American adults have blood cholesterol levels that, either alone or in combination with other risk factors, raise their risk of CHD sufficiently to require medical advice and treatment, with a diet low in saturated fatty acids and cholesterol being the primary therapy. The data also show that tens of millions more would benefit from reducing cholesterol on their own by adopting a diet that is low in saturated fat and cholesterol.

—*James I. Cleeman, M.D.,*
Stephen E. Epstein, M.D.,
Lameh Fananapazir, M.D.,
and Claude Lenfant, M.D.

Hypertension

High blood pressure, affecting about one of every five Americans, is associated with increased risks of premature death due to stroke, heart attack, or kidney failure. In the black population severe hypertension is particularly prevalent—five times more common than in whites. Insidious, generally without symptoms until irreversible damage has been done, the disorder deserves its sobriquet, "the silent killer." Virtually every primary physician deals with the problem every day, pursuing the evidence that timely detection and control of high blood pressure can significantly improve the longevity of affected patients.

Past ignorance giving way to new insights

However, victory in this field is celebrated only in broad and frequently ambiguous statistics. Until very recently, no one has been able to reliably predict or explain the success or failure of treatment or even, except for the more extreme types of hypertension, define the degree of risk in individual patients. Fortunately, that is changing now as modern medicine begins to recognize and characterize hypertension's biological heterogeneity.

That is not to say that the past was without discrimination or understanding. Some hypertensions were known to be the result of an adrenal tumor causing runaway production of a salt-retaining hormone, aldosterone. Another type of hypertension resulted from tumors causing excessive production of the vasoconstrictive hormones epinephrine and norepinephrine. Both tumorous types could be corrected by surgery. Surgery could also cure some forms of hypertension resulting from blockage of renal arteries. Hypertension

Because hypertension can lead to irreversible damage to the heart, brain, or kidneys without any symptoms at all, it is very properly called a "silent killer." Early detection of the problem, quite simply, saves lives.

was known to be the outcome of certain congenital cardiovascular defects and such hormonally turbulent disorders as Cushing's syndrome (overproduction of steroids). Most of these hypertensions with recognizable causes were characterized by dramatically soaring blood pressure readings, as was the irreversible, mysterious, and lethal form given the name of "malignant hypertension."

These extreme manifestations of high blood pressure, however, continue to account for only about 15% of the hypertensive population. The remaining 85% have chronic hypertension, blanketed under the label "essential hypertension." The term, however, to a great extent has been an admission of ignorance, for the precise causes are unknown, and there has been considerable debate in the medical community concerning its treatment and even the risks that chronic hypertension imposes. There has been an unfortunate tendency to consider essential hypertension—indeed, most hypertension—to be a single disorder traceable to a common aberrant mechanism. This was so despite the daily practical evidence that more than one abnormal process was involved. Some patients responded to available drugs; some did not. Some patients with only relatively mild elevations of blood pressure died early of what appeared to be hypertension-related

331

cardiovascular disease despite treatment, while others with huge elevations of blood pressure seemed to be unaffected even without treatment. From such evidence it would seem to be obvious that different mechanisms were at work.

Nevertheless, until fairly recently most physicians treated hypertension with a trial-and-error protocol called "stepped care." Under the broad assumption that the major cause of essential hypertension was excessive retention of sodium, therapy was begun with a trial of diuretics, agents that stimulate the kidney to excrete more sodium. The practice was not unreasonable since for a long time diuretics were the only antihypertensive drugs available. Weight loss and reduced consumption of salt were also stressed. If this failed to control the high blood pressure, other drugs were substituted or added to the regimen; some of these drugs acted by interfering with nervous system signals in such a way as to cause arteries to dilate.

The stepped care formula worked fairly successfully in about half of the patients with essential hypertension, at least to the extent of proving that blood pressure could be brought under control in these patients and that blood pressure control had a salutary effect on the incidence of stroke. However, the record is flawed by the failure so far to show that such treatment can significantly lower the cardiac-related consequences of hypertension (in particular, heart attack), which constitute the major burden of the disorder.

The good news is that in recent years technological and pharmacological advances have brought fresh concepts and increased understanding of the pathophysiology and variety of essential hypertension, as well as of the more extreme forms. The single-disease concept of essential hypertension is giving way to the evidence that it more likely comprises a heterogenous group of disorders that have in common an elevated blood pressure. This way of viewing hypertension means that it, like fever, is a biophysical sign for which several causes are possible and for which no single treatment is appropriate.

The renin system

A seminal recent accomplishment was the verification of the central role of the renin system in normal physiology and in hypertensive states. The renin-angiotensin-aldosterone system is now acknowledged to be the central physiological agency for maintaining blood pressure within normal bounds. The kidneys function as the control center for this hormonal system.

When special detector cells in the kidneys perceive a fall in arterial blood pressure or a decrease in the blood's component of sodium, signals are sent to other kidney cells to produce and release into the blood a hormonal substance called renin. Renin acts as an enzyme to set off a series of events in the bloodstream that ultimately produces the hormone angiotensin II.

Angiotensin II has three immediate and powerful direct pressure-raising actions: (1) it causes the small arteries of the arterial tree to constrict; (2) it directly influences the kidney to reabsorb and retain more of its filtered sodium; and (3) it further stimulates the reclamation of sodium by an indirect effect, signaling the adrenal cortex to release a hormone called aldosterone, which causes the kidney to reabsorb sodium and release potassium in exchange. The sum effect of these actions is a rise in blood pressure to the point where the renal detector cells, sensing a return to normal pressure and flow, shut off the secretion of renin. The renin-angiotensin-aldosterone system thus functions as what is known as a hormonal feedback-servocontrol system for blood pressure.

A fall in blood pressure can occur for a number of natural reasons. A simple change in posture, from lying down to standing up, can shift blood to the legs, causing blood pressure to fall—a stimulus for release of renin. The most common reason for a fall in blood pressure is a reduction in the intake of dietary salt. Normally, increased consumption of salt will cause renin production to decrease, and lowered consumption of salt causes renin production to rise. This reciprocal, see-saw effect has been well documented in persons with normal blood pressure; it is now known that the measurement of renin in the blood can be considered normal or abnormal *only* when related to the intake of dietary sodium. Salt—sodium chloride—is the most common source of sodium; it attracts and holds water in the bloodstream and body tissues, as well as exerting its own vasoconstrictive effect on arteries. If the blood loses its volume (*i.e.,* "dries out") because of reduced sodium in the diet, renin, with its vasoconstrictive and sodium-reclaiming effects, will be released to maintain blood pressure.

ACE inhibitors: new pharmacological probes

While evidence for the renin system's activities has accumulated for 20 years or more, considerable debate has swirled around the central importance of its functions and its relevance to the maintenance and treatment of hypertension. Two recent scientific advances have changed all that.

One of these advances, in the field of laboratory science, was the development of more standardized and reliable assays for measuring the levels of renin activity in the blood. Much of the earlier controversy was doubtless a product of nonuniform laboratory techniques and methods, along with a failure to appreciate the importance of indexing renin values to the current state of salt intake.

The other advance was the recent discovery of a new class of drugs called ACE (angiotensin converting enzyme) inhibitors. ACE inhibitors have a clear-cut, specific action: they prevent the conversion of angiotensin I, released by renin, to angiotensin II, the

Drugs for treating hypertension			
category	action; patient suitability	possible side effects (vary with specific drug)	examples
ACE inhibitors	act in bloodstream to block conversion of angiotensin I to angiotensin II, the active blood vessel constrictor of renin system	skin rash, loss of taste, weakness, cough, kidney problems (rare)	captopril, enalapril, lisinopril
	most effective in patients with high or moderate blood renin levels; drugs of choice		
calcium-channel blockers	act primarily on small arterial blood vessels (arterioles) to prevent sodium-imposed flow of calcium into arterial smooth muscle and consequent vessel constriction	headache, palpitations, rapid heart rate, edema, constipation, dizziness	verapamil, nifedipine, diltiazem
	most effective in patients with low blood renin levels (excessive sodium retention); drugs of choice		
diuretics	act on kidneys to stimulate elimination of sodium, which lowers water retention and consequently blood volume	thickened blood and slowed blood flow, weakened blood vessels, depression, confusion, weakness, potassium depletion, raised cholesterol levels, impotence in men	thiazides, bumetanide, amiloride
	primarily effective in patients with low blood renin levels; no longer drugs of choice		
beta-adrenergic blockers	act on kidneys to curb secretion of renin and so interfere with renin system	insomnia, nightmares, slowed heart rate, muscle cramps, depression, decreased exercise tolerance	propanolol, metoprolol, atenolol
	primarily effective in patients with high or moderate renin levels		
alpha-adrenergic blockers	act on smooth muscle of arteriole walls to relax them and increase vessel diameter	vertigo, dizziness, palpitations, headache, edema, drowsiness, weakness	prazosin, terazosin
	primarily effective in patients with low blood renin levels		

active vasoconstrictor component of the renin system. By what amounts to pharmacological surgery—in effect an excision of the final, active product of the renin system—these agents can dramatically demonstrate the system's involvement for good or ill. In normal individuals blockade of the renin system by ACE inhibitors lowers systemic and renal arterial pressure. This results in a marked rise in sodium retention and increased, although blocked, renin secretion as the system attempts to compensate the blood pressure.

Thus, in hypertensive patients with high serum renin values, ACE inhibitors (*e.g.,* captopril, enalapril, lisinopril) reduce blood pressure impressively but have little or no depressor effect in patients with low or absent renin levels. By also achieving corrections of blood pressure in many hypertensive patients with medium renin levels, they verify a renin-mediated component in these patients as well. So specific are these drugs in their action that their positive depressor effect virtually identifies a form of hypertension mediated by excessive renin production, while a negative effect suggests instead a form mediated by excessive sodium retention.

Vasoconstriction: two forms

The experimental and clinical employment of ACE inhibitors has sharpened perception of the reciprocal interplay between renin and sodium in maintaining normal blood pressure and of the nature of the failed reciprocity that sustains chronic hypertension. Clearly, the common factor in all diastolic hypertension, whether renin-mediated or sodium-mediated, is increased total resistance to blood flow in the smaller arteries, most often due to the narrowing of blood vessels (vasoconstriction) but sometimes complicated by secondary structural changes.

Two forms of vasoconstriction are now being proposed. The form mediated by renin—actually by renin's active agent angiotensin II—is readily apparent and can be demonstrated even in the test tube. Angiotensin II acts directly on arterial vessels; it is the most powerful circulating vasoconstrictor chemical known. The blood vessel narrowing imposed by sodium, however, is more circuitous and less easily demonstrated. The most recent research suggests that sodium may act within arteriolar tissue cells to

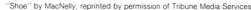

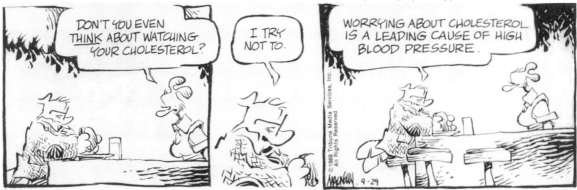

cause an abnormal influx of calcium, activating vaso-constriction. Increased intracellular calcium is known to stimulate smooth muscle; indeed, this is the reason why drugs called calcium-channel blockers are pre-scribed for certain cardiac patients. A new benefit of calcium-channel blockers, only recently realized, is that they have antihypertensive actions parallel to those of diuretics. Like diuretics, calcium-channel blockers (*e.g.,* verapamil, nifedipine, diltiazem) are antihypertensive primarily in patients with low serum renin values; *i.e.,* those whose hypertension is presumed to be related to abnormal sodium retention.

The more widespread ability to do accurate renin assays and the availability of a more varied spectrum of antihypertensive drugs have at last brought a wel-come specificity to the diagnosis and treatment of hypertension. Large-scale renin studies show a wide disparity among patients with essential hypertension; about 30% have low renin levels, about 20% have high levels, and about 50% have intermediate or "normal" renin levels in the range seen in persons without high blood pressure. Moreover, it is the low-renin patients who respond best to diuretics or calcium antagonists, demonstrating that their hypertension is a product of the sodium-related form of vasoconstriction. Generally, they do not respond to antirenin drugs. Recently, cal-cium antagonists and alpha-adrenergic blocking drugs have superseded diuretics as first-line therapy in these patients.

Conversely, patients with medium or high renin lev-els respond poorly to the latter drugs but favorably to drugs that block the release or activity of renin (*e.g.,* beta-adrenergic blockers and ACE inhibitors). Some patients whose renin levels are in the intermediate range turn out to be a mixed bag; that is, they respond to one or the other or to a combination of antirenin and antisodium agents.

Angiotensin converting enzyme inhibitors and cal-cium antagonists now are the leading hypertension drugs prescribed. Their use is followed by that of beta blockers (*e.g.,* propanolol, metoprolol, atenolol), diuret-ics (*e.g.,* thiazides, bumetanide, amiloride), and alpha blockers (*e.g.,* prazosin, terazosin).

Diuretics reassessed

One important outcome of the above developments is a radical change in treatment policy. With the availabil-ity of new treatment alternatives, the role of diuretics in the treatment of hypertension is being sharply reevalu-ated. A flurry of studies just this past year, widely reported in the medical and lay media, suggest that diuretics are not as innocuous as they seemed in the days when they were the only effective agents avail-able. In accelerating the elimination of sodium from the body—and along with sodium, water—diuretics tend to make the bloodstream thicker, turgid, and more prone to coagulation and clotting of blood. Because of the poor blood flow, delicate blood vessels become undernourished, fragile, and vulnerable to rupture and decay. Side effects of diminished blood flow include lack of energy, depression, clouded thinking, and im-potence; such side effects are largely responsible for the failure of many patients to take diuretic drugs as prescribed. Potassium depletion (an inevitable conse-quence of diuretic usage), hyperlipidemia, and impaired glucose tolerance are the other negative effects of long-term diuretic therapy.

Diuretics are no longer the antihypertensive drug of choice except in circumstances where it is clear that sodium retention is the principal factor and cannot be countered with better alternatives. Calcium-chan-nel blockers are now considered a better alternative by many physicians because they counter the vaso-constrictive effects of sodium without a companion reduction in blood volume and flow and because they also promote the elimination of excess sodium. An-other alternative to diuretics may be one of the newer alpha-1-adrenergic blockers (*e.g.,* prazosin, terazosin), which help relax vasoconstricted arterioles without some of the distressing neural side effects induced by older vasorelaxant drugs (*e.g.,* hydralazine, minoxidil).

Risk factors reevaluated

The importance of maintaining good blood flow, what-ever the level of blood pressure, is highlighted by the growing realization that patients with low renin levels tend to live longer, with less cardiovascular damage.

Retaining sodium and water, low-renin hypertensive patients appear to have better blood flow and nourishment to tissues. Patients with high renin levels, on the other hand, are more intensely vasoconstricted; their blood volume and flow are diminished, and their vascular tissues are less well nourished. A rigorously controlled and important new study has confirmed clinical impressions that a high serum renin level is an independent risk factor for heart attack in treated patients with mild hypertension. For such reasons, the new trend in the management of essential hypertension is toward treating the renin factor first, using an antirenin drug by itself.

The salt factor. The search for risk factors for hypertension inevitably turns to the role of dietary salt. Past concepts had so linked salt retention and diuretic therapy to a monolithic view of hypertension that dietary salt became mythicized by some as the popular enemy for all hypertensives and even for normotensive individuals. Reduced salt intake is undoubtedly advisable for that subgroup of hypertensive patients whose hypertension is improved or corrected by it; however, sodium depletion is not indicated or necessary for that majority of patients in whom it has no significant value.

Furthermore, there is no real evidence that reduced salt intake prevents the development of hypertension in normal individuals. In them, as in hypertensive patients who are not salt-sensitive, the question remains whether it is really healthy, in the absence of hypertension or a demonstrable antihypertensive effect, to dry out the blood. With dehydration, renin production rises reactively in order to protect the blood pressure level, generating its own form of vasoconstriction. Indeed, several recent studies show that sodium deprivation in a significant percentage of hypertensive patients results paradoxically in a blood pressure *rise*. In the majority of hypertensive patients, reduction of salt intake has no effect on blood pressure.

In 1988 a major investigation known as the Intersalt Study, which had correlated dietary habits with blood pressure studies involving over 10,000 people at 52 medical centers in 32 countries, reported a small reduction in blood pressure in populations that consume less salt. Closer inspection of the data, however, raises doubts that the reduced incidence of hypertension in those persons can be attributed to their low-salt diets. In fact, in a majority of subjects higher dietary salt intake correlates with slightly lower blood pressures! For many observers the predominant conclusion from the study is that salt intake is little related to blood pressure on a population-wide basis. By far the more important factors related to hypertension in this as in most other studies are body weight and use of alcohol.

Insulin as a factor? Another new study that has elicited considerable interest concerns the finding of high blood insulin levels in obese persons—specifically in diabetics and hypertensive patients. From this it was suggested that insulin might be the link between these states, explaining why so many diabetics become hypertensive. However, problems with this concept arise from the observation that infusions of insulin can actually reduce blood pressure and that at least half of obese persons with hyperinsulinemia are not hypertensive. A more basic link between hypertension, obesity, and diabetes, it has recently been suggested, is the common abnormal intracellular mineral contents of calcium and magnesium found in each of these diseases.

Potassium link. A hopeful finding, from a recent epidemiological study, is that dietary intake of potassium may be protective; subjects with higher intakes of potassium appeared to have a lower incidence of stroke. This is in keeping with an even more recent study, reported in 1990, showing that feeding stroke-prone hypertensive animals potassium protects them from stroke and markedly improves their survival. The benefits of potassium supplementation may occur because potassium suppresses plasma renin levels in the protected animals.

Enlightened patterns of treatment

The most important question in the diagnosis and treatment of hypertension is the determination of risk. A solid contribution to the assessment of risk was recently made by the demonstration that the blood pressure level itself is far less an indicator of risk than is the measurement of left ventricular mass (the thickness of the heart muscle), which is easily measured by echocardiography. This supports the growing view that not all hypertension is alike. Indeed, 99% of mild hypertensives will never have a stroke or heart attack. The challenge for the physician is to identify that 1% at appreciable risk rather than submit all to lifetime therapies that carry their own—or possibly greater—risk.

With the availability of a broader antihypertensive armamentarium, a growth of understanding of hypertensive mechanisms, and a realization that hypertension may be various not only in form but in risk, a more conservative approach to the treatment of hypertension appears to be evolving. This is particularly true in Europe, where hypertension is now studied more intensively than in the United States. The European levels considered to be low, normal, and high blood pressures are about five millimeters of mercury (mm Hg) higher than in the U.S.

In the U.S. normal blood pressure is generally defined as a diastolic pressure (the heart at peak relaxation) equal to or below 90 mm Hg. A "borderline" state is defined at diastolic readings from 90 to 95 mm Hg. Within this range the patient is watched but not treated, although a regimen of weight reduction, regular exercise (exercise is generally hypotensive), and withdrawal from alcohol and tobacco is usually recommended. While some physicians may recommend a blanket reduction in salt intake, newer thinking about

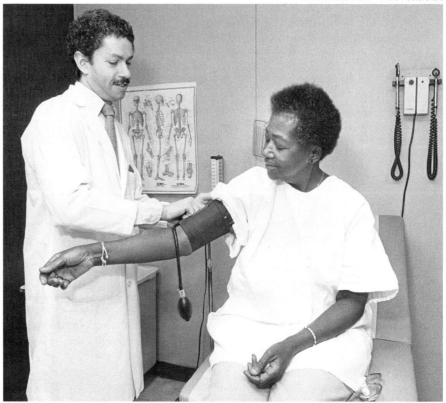

A phenomenon that occurs more commonly in older than younger people is so-called white-coat hypertension: the office blood pressure is deceptively elevated, presumably a stress reaction to the nurse or doctor who takes the reading or to the office setting itself. Therefore, pressure may need to be more accurately determined over a 24-hour period with an ambulatory monitor before a diagnosis is confirmed and a therapeutic regimen established.

the role of salt and fluid management counsels salt reduction only as a trial, to be abandoned if it does not bring blood pressure down. At mildly hypertensive ranges (between 95 and 104 mm Hg), U.S. physicians generally begin to employ pharmacological therapy, but with restraint if there does not appear to be cardiovascular damage. More aggressive pharmacological therapy is instituted at the moderately hypertensive range of 104–115 mm Hg, beyond which a "severe hypertension" state is said to exist. It should be recognized that the measurement of blood pressure is not highly precise and that the transition points of these stages represent gray areas.

How low to lower blood pressure? The question as to how much blood pressure should be lowered is particularly relevant in the range of severe hypertension. The most recent thinking, based on studies conducted in the U.S., Sweden, and England and reported within the past year or so, is that too aggressive a reduction of blood pressure, by whatever means, can be harmful, resulting in reduced blood flow and decreased perfusion of the heart, which in turn may lead to increased incidences of heart attack and stroke. One of these studies counsels a reduction of no more than 17 mm Hg even in patients with the most severe hypertension; in no case should blood pressure be reduced below 86 mm Hg.

In some patients an extra component of suspicion

is indicated before a diagnosis of hypertension is concluded and a commitment to long-term drug therapy is made. This has been made particularly clear by the new technology of portable blood pressure monitors that can be worn for 24 hours. These devices have shown that many patients who register impressive blood pressure elevations in the doctor's office lose their hypertension as soon as they go home. The phenomenon, now dubbed "white-coat hypertension," is clearly a consequence of a psychological reaction to the doctor or other medical personnel; it appears to be especially common among elderly patients. In one investigation of the white-coat phenomenon, 40% of elderly persons seen at the hypertension clinic of the Robert Wood Johnson Medical School, Piscataway, N.J., were found to have it.

Distinctions in the elderly and children. In fact, new onset of diastolic hypertension requiring control in the elderly is very rare. Most hypertension in the elderly is systolic, occurring at the peak of the heart's contraction. This is a biologically different form of hypertension—the outcome of vascular disease of the large arteries, which increases their stiffness. There are no data from any controlled trials showing benefit from pharmacological therapy in patients with systolic hypertension, although a few ongoing studies in the U.S. and Europe suggest that certain drugs may offer protection against stroke but not against heart attack.

In recent years there has also been some stir about so-called hypertension in children and whether it merits treatment. Essential hypertension probably does not occur in children. There is no convincing evidence that youngsters with *relatively* higher blood pressures develop hypertension as adults. These children tend to be ones with faster growth rates. Children with bona fide high blood pressure resulting in retinopathy (a noninflammatory disorder of the retina, often leading to blindness) and renal failure usually prove to have known causes of hypertension, such as renovascular disease; primary aldosteronism, a condition characterized by excessive production and excretion of aldosterone, potassium loss, and muscular weakness; or pheochromocytoma, a usually benign tumor of chromoffin cells.

Current research directions

One active area of hypertension research today concerns the possibility of another hormonal system, originating in the atria of the heart, exerting important corrective effects against both sodium-mediated and renin-mediated hypertension. A peptide hormone recently identified in atrial tissue has been found experimentally to stimulate sodium excretion by the kidney and to counter the vasoconstrictive properties of angiotensin II. As these findings are pursued, investigators believe they may be on the verge of revealing a new cardiovascular regulatory system operating in tandem with, or opposition to, the renin system. If so, the search has great implications for enlarging the understanding of the mechanisms of hypertension and of natural and pharmacological defenses against it.

With accelerated research in hypertension and increased public awareness of it, regrettably, the findings of many studies reach the popular media and excite public interest before the findings can be fully validated or evaluated. For example, a recent report generating considerable excitement claimed that the agent interleukin-2, most often used as an anticancer treatment, permanently corrects the hypertension of spontaneously hypertensive rats. Interleukin-2's major action stems from its role in the immune system. While to some this raises the possibility of a whole new avenue of therapy for human hypertension, it may, on the other hand, simply mean that the experimental animals studied suffer from an immune disorder that is very different from essential hypertension. Whether the dramatic antihypertensive effect observed in experimental animals will occur in human hypertension is uncertain. Serious research continues on this question, but conclusions must be considered extremely premature until the relationship is examined in humans.

Advances: already paying off

In the clinical arena, however, there is little question that the ranks of patients are being whittled down; an important segment of patients with hypertension may have curable renovascular hypertension. It is characteristic of renovascular hypertension that the blockage results in greatly increased production of renin and angiotensin. ACE inhibitors are so specific against the activity of angiotensin II that results are seen promptly after administration of captopril, the first orally administered version of this class of drugs. Captopril, because of its ability to wipe out angiotensin II, usually results in an impressive reactive rise in renin production that is accompanied by a dramatic fall in blood pressure. Where renovascular hypertension is suspected, it can now be verified by studies that have become available in recent years—for example, digital subtraction angiography and reliable renin assays.

All the efforts described here represent a heartening growth of the capacity for separating and stratifying the phenomenon of hypertension according to its particular biological elements. This salubrious movement is indicative of an ever growing ability of medical science to accomplish the objectives of specific, safe, and rational individualized therapy for human patients who have hypertension.

—John H. Laragh, M.D.

Mental Health and Illness

Among the most important recent developments in the areas of mental health and illness have been large-scale studies showing that mental disorders such as panic disorder and depression are very common, and that they can be as disabling as major physical disorders. For example, one large study conducted by the Rand Corporation showed that the functioning of depressed patients was comparable to (and often worse than) that of patients with chronic medical conditions such as heart disease, diabetes, and arthritis. Such studies highlight the importance of identifying and treating these disorders, particularly since several types of effective treatment—including medications and psychotherapies—have been established. Another area of considerable interest is the search for connections between mental states and physical functions, perhaps modulated by immune processes that are not yet understood.

The recent developments in the field of mental health and illness that are addressed in some detail below are the publication of a new guide for the treatment of psychiatric disorders and two notable advances in the understanding and treatment of the disorder schizophrenia.

Treatment guide: first of its kind

Publication of an influential book often serves as a landmark in the history of an area of human endeavor. This occurred in 1989 in the field of psychiatry with the American Psychiatric Association's (APA's) publication

From Emil Kraepelin, *Psychiatrie*, 5th edition (Leipzig: Verlag von Johann Ambrosius Barth, 1896)

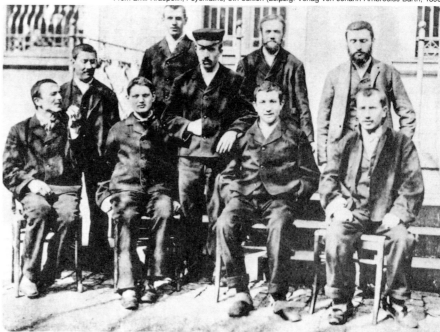

This photograph is from the fifth edition of Emil Kraepelin's Textbook of Psychiatry *(published in Leipzig, Germany, in 1896), one of a handful of truly monumental books in the history of psychiatry. Pictured are patients with "dementia praecox" (what is now known as schizophrenia); the author classified their disorder on the basis of its characteristic symptoms and its typical course over time—a course he viewed as inexorably downhill.*

of *Treatments of Psychiatric Disorders.* Before consideration of this volume's importance, several precedents that serve to highlight the history of psychiatry are worth looking at.

Precedent-setting publications. Benjamin Rush (1746–1813), famous both as a physician and as a signer of the Declaration of Independence, published *Medical Inquiries and Observations upon the Diseases of the Mind* in 1812. Subsequently regarded as the father of American psychiatry, Rush was noteworthy for advocating humane hospital conditions for the mentally ill; however, he also advocated bloodletting as treatment for mental disorders on the basis of his erroneous belief that such disorders were caused by irregular actions of blood vessels in the brain due to "vascular congestion."

In the late 19th and early 20th century, the German psychiatrist Emil Kraepelin (1856–1926) published eight editions of his influential *Textbook of Psychiatry.* From careful observations of patients, Kraepelin proposed classifications of mental disorders based on characteristic symptoms and typical courses of illness over time, including the distinction between manic-depressive psychosis (now called bipolar disorder) and dementia praecox (now called schizophrenia). Because he viewed the major mental disorders as following characteristic, inexorable courses, Kraepelin was not optimistic about treatment.

Sigmund Freud (1856–1939) published *The Interpretation of Dreams* in 1899 (dated 1900), in which he described the two fundamental concepts of psychoanalysis: psychic determinism and unconscious motivation. The former holds that mental phenomena are not random but are determined by the individual's previous thoughts and emotions, while the latter affirms that conscious thoughts, emotions, and behaviors can be caused by mental events outside the individual's conscious awareness. These ideas led to the development of psychoanalysis as a "talking treatment," in which the unconscious origins of patients' symptoms are uncovered and interpreted.

A landmark event in psychiatric publishing occurring just over a decade ago (1980) was the issuance of the third edition of the APA's *Diagnostic and Statistical Manual of Mental Disorders,* often referred to as *DSM-III.* It embodied a consequential new emphasis on attempts to diagnose mental disorders through the use of reliable, specific criteria that are supported by empirical data and free of unproven assumptions about causes.

The first *DSM* had appeared in 1952 as the first official manual of mental disorders that contained a glossary of descriptions of diagnostic categories. The term *reaction* throughout the classification reflected the psychobiological view that psychiatric disorders were individuals' reactions to psychological, social, and biological factors. *DSM-II* was published in 1968, dropping the term *reaction* and basing mental disorder classifications on the *International Classification of Diseases.* The impact of *DSM-III,* however, was considerably greater than that of its predecessors. The manual is used internationally and has been translated into Chinese, Danish, Dutch, Finnish, French, German, Greek, Italian, Japanese, Norwegian, Portuguese, Spanish, and Swedish.

DSM-III was followed in 1987 by a major revision

338

(*DSM-III-R*). The latter incorporated the latest information about psychiatric disorders, including refinements of the new approach to psychiatric diagnosis, changes in criteria for certain diagnostic categories, inclusion of some entirely new categories (*e.g.,* sleep disorders), and elimination of some previous categories (*e.g.,* ego-dystonic homosexuality).

Rationale for new guide. The new publication in question, the APA's *Treatments of Psychiatric Disorders,* does for psychiatric treatment what *DSM-III* did for diagnosis. The historical significance of this work can be viewed as the convergence of two major trends, one in psychiatry and one in medicine as a whole.

Until about the mid-1970s, the history of psychiatry was characterized by various competing "schools" of treatment. The treatments advocated by each group were based on its view of the causes of mental illness, and each group considered its particular form of treatment to be appropriate for virtually all types of mental disorders. Thus, the treatment a patient received often depended more on the theoretical allegiance of the treating clinician than on the characteristics of the patient's disorder. The main treatment orientations were (1) psychodynamic, viewing psychological conflicts as central and psychotherapy as the appropriate treatment; (2) biological, viewing brain biology as central and medications as the appropriate treatment; (3) behavioral, viewing maladaptive learning as central and behavioral deconditioning as appropriate treatment; and (4) social systems, viewing interpersonal conflicts and distortions as central and family or group therapy as appropriate treatment. Not surprisingly, many patients felt they needed to "shop around" until they found the right treatment for their problem.

While there are still remnants of the former competing orthodoxies, the more current and increasingly accepted approach in psychiatry is centered on the performance of a careful diagnostic assessment, which then leads to therapeutic recommendations that are based on the known effectiveness of available treatments for the individual patient's problems. For some disorders, combinations of treatments (for example, a tricyclic antidepressant medication in addition to individual psychodynamic psychotherapy for major depression) may be optimal. Reflecting this important shift in the approach to psychiatric therapeutics, *Treatments of Psychiatric Disorders* summarizes the available information on the effectiveness of a wide range of treatments for each of 26 major categories of mental disorders that were classified in *DSM-III-R.*

Controversies. The new APA publication also reflects an important trend affecting all aspects of health care in the United States—increasing pressure from cost-conscious governmental agencies and other third-party payers for quality assurance and accountability. One manifestation of this has been vigorous, sometimes divisive, debate about the development of written guidelines for diagnosis and treatment of various disorders. Such guidelines, now often called "practice parameters," are usually conceived as being more specific than the patient care recommendations in medical textbooks and journals; they also differ in carrying some official stamp of approval, usually from a specialty society. Proponents of such guidelines argue that they assist physicians in rendering safe and effective care in this new era of accountability; opponents protest that such official guidelines constitute "cookbook medicine," restricting the latitude of physi-

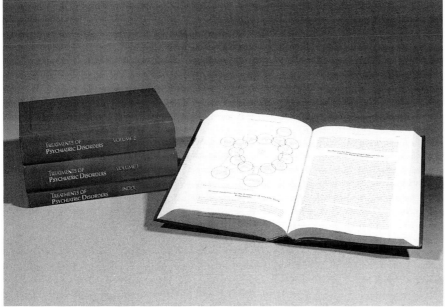

The publication of Treatments of Psychiatric Disorders *in 1989 represented a new direction for the discipline of psychiatry. Over seven years in the making, the three volumes plus detailed index summarize present knowledge about the range and effectiveness of treatments for 26 categories of mental disorders.* Treatments *is not meant to impose rigid therapeutic methods; the editors scrupulously emphasized that clinical judgment on the part of the psychiatrist using the information is always required.*

cian judgment required for responding to the variability of illnesses in individual patients.

The development of *Treatments of Psychiatric Disorders* was marked by just this kind of debate. The leadership of the American Psychiatric Association pursued the task because it felt a careful summary of current knowledge about psychiatric treatments would benefit both the profession and its patients. However, some psychiatrists vigorously protested the idea of the APA publishing a "manual" on treatment, fearing that it would stifle creative therapists and be used against psychiatrists by insurance companies and malpractice lawyers. In this atmosphere of controversy, development of the volumes took seven years.

Format. The massive project was directed by T. Byram Karasu of the Albert Einstein College of Medicine of Yeshiva University, Bronx, N.Y., and involved consensus reports from 26 panels utilizing over 400 consultants as expert reviewers. The publication itself is also massive; the four-volume set, comprising over 3,000 pages, includes extensive references and a detailed index. Karasu's introduction begins with the epigram "Science provides only interim knowledge." It stresses that the document is not intended to impose rigid treatment methods, since effective treatment requires clinical judgment, and that knowledge about treatments will continue to evolve. As an additional precaution against misuse, each of the volumes carries the following "Cautionary Statement":

This report does not represent the official policy of the American Psychiatric Association. It is an APA task force report, signifying that members of the APA have contributed to its development, but it has not been passed through those official channels required to make it an APA policy document. THIS REPORT IS NOT INTENDED TO BE CONSTRUED AS OR TO SERVE AS A STANDARD FOR PSYCHIATRIC CARE.

As an example of its content, the section on schizophrenia covers 122 pages in volume 2. The section's introduction stresses that it "cannot be definitive" because "there is no textbook in which an individual patient can be looked up to find treatment directions." Despite individual variability and incomplete knowledge, "the clinician must treat patients now and cannot merely wait until all questions are resolved at a level of scientific certainty."

The section on schizophrenia then briefly reviews the diagnosis of the disorder, which is a chronic and often devastating form of mental illness affecting approximately 1% of the population (about 2.8 million Americans), which is characterized by impairments in social and goal-oriented functioning as well as delusions (false beliefs) and unusual perceptual experiences, including hallucinations.

As in other sections of the book, the main content consists of a comprehensive review of the available treatments, with careful assessment of how the treatments are performed, evidence for their efficacy, and positive and negative effects. For schizophrenia the reviewed treatments include (1) antipsychotic drugs, considered extremely helpful for many patients in controlling "positive" psychotic symptoms such as delusions and hallucinations but less effective for the "negative" symptoms of blunted motivation and social withdrawal; (2) individual psychotherapy, viewed as important by many psychiatrists, although with less definite evidence for efficacy than is true for drug treatment; (3) group therapy, now often focused on providing practical help in social functioning; (4) family therapy, now usually centered on helping the family cope with the many problems of having a relative with schizophrenia; and (5) rehabilitation, the provision of skills and techniques to enhance the patient's long-term functioning.

That no book can provide completely up-to-date coverage in areas marked by continuing research and development is illustrated by two important new developments concerning the disorder schizophrenia. Both were too recent to be covered in *Treatments of Psychiatric Disorders.*

Biological factor in schizophrenia

An important study from the U.S. National Institute of Mental Health (NIMH) published in March 1990 provided some of the most persuasive evidence to date that schizophrenia has a biological component. In many previous studies comparing schizophrenic patients with controls (individuals without schizophrenia but similar to the patients in other ways such as age, race, sex, and education), concerns have been raised that results might be contaminated by differences between patients and controls other than the presence of a schizophrenic disorder. The new NIMH study circumvented this problem by studying 15 pairs of identical (monozygotic) twins in which one twin had schizophrenia and one did not. Since monozygotic twins share the same genetic endowment and usually share very similar socioeconomic, developmental, and psychological influences, the sources of variability between patients and their identical twin controls are markedly reduced.

Using magnetic resonance imaging (MRI) to evaluate brain structure, the new study found that in 14 of the 15 pairs of twins, the twin with schizophrenia had reduced total brain volume and reduction in the size of specific brain areas—the left temporal lobe and the anterior hippocampus. The investigators could not completely rule out the possibility that these findings were secondary effects of the schizophrenia rather than a primary aspect of the illness itself. However, they thought the secondary effect possibility unlikely because the brain findings were correlated with neither the duration of illness nor the extent of exposure to antipsychotic drugs.

Daniel R. Weinberger, National Institute of Mental Health, NIH

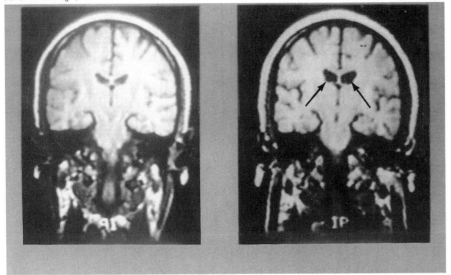

MRI scans compare the brains of male identical twins. The twin on the left does not have schizophrenia; the one on the right does. Arrows pointing to the large fluid-filled cavities in the brain image on the right reveal an overall reduced brain volume. This pattern was seen in 14 of 15 identical twin pairs in which one had schizophrenia, providing persuasive evidence of a structural brain deficit that is nongenetic in origin.

The NIMH twin study, particularly when considered along with the results of other recent studies, strongly supports the existence of brain abnormalities that may cause schizophrenia. Furthermore, since genetically identical twins did not share those abnormalities, there must be nongenetic factors operative in the development of schizophrenia in addition to any genetic predisposition or vulnerability. What such factors might be is presently unknown. They could range from neurotoxins or viruses to particular developmental experiences, all of which are areas of considerable importance for further research.

Medication for hard-to-treat schizophrenia

Another highly significant recent development in the area of schizophrenia is the availability of a new drug treatment, clozapine (Clozaril), which holds considerable hope for many patients who have not responded well to previously available antipsychotic drugs. There had been great interest in clozapine when it was first used in Europe in the 1970s because, unlike other antipsychotic drugs, it did not cause acute neurological side effects (such as muscle stiffness or spasms). Of even greater importance, it did not cause tardive dyskinesia, a syndrome of abnormal and sometimes irreversible involuntary movements of the face, mouth, trunk, or extremities that occurs in about 20% of persons who take antipsychotic drugs for long periods. Unfortunately, it was discovered that clozapine causes agranulocytosis (destruction of infection-fighting white blood cells) in about 1–2% of the patients who take it. Clozapine can also cause seizures, but it was the occurrence of fatal infections from agranulocytosis that led to an interruption of its development for clinical use.

Because of the needs of treatment-resistant schizophrenic patients, however, clinical research on clozapine resumed, and in a large-scale multicenter trial, 30% of patients who had failed to respond to several courses of standard antipsychotic drugs showed marked improvement with clozapine. Improvement occurred in negative symptoms (*e.g.,* blunted motivation) as well as positive symptoms (*e.g.,* delusions). After this demonstration of its usefulness, clozapine was approved by the U.S. Food and Drug Administration for use in treatment-resistant schizophrenia and was released for clinical use in the U.S. by Sandoz Pharmaceuticals in February 1990.

In a unique system of drug marketing, it is available only through a special patient management system, rather than through drug stores or hospital pharmacies. This system involves weekly visits by a home health care worker, who dispenses the medication by prescription and also obtains a blood sample for a white blood cell count in order to detect early evidence of agranulocytosis before any symptoms develop and, importantly, while it is still reversible. If the white blood cell count drops, clozapine is discontinued and the prescribing physician is notified.

The human costs of schizophrenia for patients and their families are enormous, but so are the strictly economic costs of hospitalization and other treatments, lost income from inability to work, subsidies for housing and food, and hours of care by family members. An effective treatment could reduce those costs, but clozapine treatment itself costs about $9,000 per year owing to the Sandoz requirement for a patient management system. This high cost has become a matter of considerable controversy. For eligible patients who are not covered by insurance, a scholarship program for clozapine treatment has been developed by Sandoz in cooperation with the National Alliance for the Mentally Ill (NAMI). A toll-free number (1-800-332-NAMI) is available for inquiries about the program.

—*Richard M. Glass, M.D.*

Shopping Out of Control

by Carole Lieberman, M.D., M.P.H.

"Born to shop."
"Shop till you drop."
"When the going gets tough, the tough go shopping."

Common as they are, these jokes about committed shoppers only mask a deeper reality—one that is no laughing matter. Compulsive shopping, also called pathological shopping and shopping addiction, is actually a serious disorder that, if unresolved, can have devastating consequences for the individual: financial ruin, destroyed relationships, and personal chaos.

A recent article in the *Wall Street Journal* pointed out that the average American adult spends about six hours a week shopping—that is more than most people devote to reading, exercising, or playing with their children. Shopping malls are visited at least once a week by more than two-thirds of the adult population. Of course, many people shop more often than this, and for many teens, going to the mall may be a daily recreational activity.

Typical pattern

One dictionary definition of *shopping* is: "visiting shops in order to look at, price, or buy things that are for sale." Compulsive shoppers may vary in their approach to the looking, pricing, or buying phases of shopping, but they almost always end up buying at least one item on each shopping excursion. Moreover, the compulsive shopper indulges beyond the occasional shopping spree, although there is no specific number of sprees that defines the disorder. Rather, the sprees represent a continuous pattern of reacting to certain stimuli that trigger the compulsive shopper to answer a conscious or unconscious psychological need by shopping.

Compulsive shopping is, then, the repeated and continuous loss of control over the impulse to buy more than one needs or can afford. Typically it leaves the individual feeling disillusioned because the purchases do not fill up inner emptiness, and the shopping behavior brings on some form of self-punishment.

A compulsion is an uncontrollable impulse to perform some behavior repeatedly. In this sense, compulsive shopping can be classified in current psychological terms as a disorder of impulse control. (The official diagnostic terminology is further discussed below.) Control—and the loss of it—is a major issue for compulsive shoppers, not just as it pertains to the purchase of items but in how they, as individuals, relate to the world. They feel perpetually out of control and, by shopping, attempt ineffectually to regain it.

Buying more than they need or can afford is a key characteristic that distinguishes compulsive shoppers from those who shop only for items they truly, objectively need and that their budget can accommodate. Compulsive shoppers rationalize, convincing themselves that they really do need whatever item they want to buy. Any honest examination of need becomes distorted by the psychological urgency that compels them to buy something, especially something they hope will impress others. Determining what they can realistically afford becomes distorted by the existence of easy credit, the many methods of delaying payment, their fantasies about being rescued from their overwhelming indebtedness, and fantasies that they are entitled to have the things they want. Compulsive shoppers allow themselves to be only vaguely aware of the true state of their finances because, if acknowledged, these realities would dampen the elation of the spending mood.

Disillusionment usually follows a buying spree. Upon leaving the store, after having found the magical item that was supposed to make them feel good, compulsive shoppers realize that their lives have not really changed the way it seemed that they would while they were shopping. Their inner pain then becomes even more unbearable. The hardest, cruelest lesson for compulsive shoppers to learn is that they cannot fill up the emptiness they feel inside by surrounding themselves with their purchases. Self-punishment is sought, as self-hate, guilt, and shame unconsciously drive compulsive shoppers toward ruin, both financial and emotional. They get perverse pleasure out of punishing themselves for real or imagined faults, which signify to them that they do not deserve the things they have bought.

According to the current *Diagnostic and Statistical Manual of Mental Disorders,* third edition, revised (*DSM-III-R*), the standard handbook used by a majority of psychiatrists and psychotherapists to classify various mental and emotional disorders, compulsive shopping best fits under "Impulse control disorders not elsewhere classified," a category that includes, among other things, pathological gambling and kleptomania. The essential features of disorders of impulse control are: (1) failure to resist an impulse or temptation to perform some act (in this case, shopping) that is harmful to the individual or others; (2) an increasing tension before committing the act (on the way to the store or cash register); and (3) pleasure or release at the time of committing the act (upon walking into the store or at the cash register), with regret or guilt usually following the act (some time after the purchase has been made).

Compulsive spending is a term sometimes used interchangeably with *compulsive shopping*. More precisely, however, the former would include not only compulsive shopping but other means of pathological spending, such as compulsive gambling. (Pathological shopping is being considered for inclusion as a specific subcategory of impulse control disorders in the next revision of the *DSM*.)

Parallels with substance abuse

There is a fine line between compulsive shopping and "normal" shopping or even the occasional shopping spree. One of the key determinants is the concept of "need." People may think they are shopping because they need a particular tangible object, such as a sweater or a tennis racket, when what they really need is something intangible—good feelings about themselves. Sometimes the purchased object may be symbolic. For example, through the sweater or tennis racket what they are really seeking is warmth in a human relationship or the motivation to exercise and take better care of their body. Like people with other kinds of addictions, compulsive shoppers look to a substance—in this case material possessions—outside of themselves instead of looking within to solve their problems. They lose the ability to make rational judgments about what things they really have a need for, just as compulsive overeaters have trouble interpreting their hunger and deciding when they have eaten enough.

Just like other addicts, compulsive shoppers invariably deny that they have a "problem." Most say that they could cut down on shopping any time they choose. Even in the face of stacks of unpaid bills and collapsing personal relationships, they continue to deny that their shopping "habit" is out of control. As in other addictions, there is a "high," a feeling of omnipotence experienced while buying things. This illusive and all-too-transient sensation—that all is possible now that they will be more attractive and looked upon more favorably by others—is desperately and repeatedly sought after, with increasing levels of tolerance. That is, as with a drug, there is a need to increase the "dose" of shopping to produce the same "high." There is also withdrawal; deprivation from shopping causes distress and an irresistible urge for another shopping "fix."

Other signs of trouble

There are many additional warning signals that indicate that a person's shopping behavior has become pathological. These include:

- lying to oneself and others about the extent of one's shopping and going to such lengths as hiding purchases and charge account statements
- experiencing serious conflicts in relationships with spouses, parents, and children
- feeling out of touch with reality when shopping
- choosing designer clothes or other status symbol products as a means of courting acceptance and envy
- becoming aroused by the word *sale* and basking in the attention paid by salespeople
- making irrational choices in the rush to buy something, such as purchasing the wrong size or buying a duplicate of something one already owns
- living with the constant frenzy of trying to meet the monthly payments on credit cards and charge accounts
- spending money on shopping instead of more vital expenses such as rent, food, or the pediatrician
- resorting to illegal maneuvers, such as writing bad checks, dodging creditors, or shoplifting
- promising to stop but being unable to do so

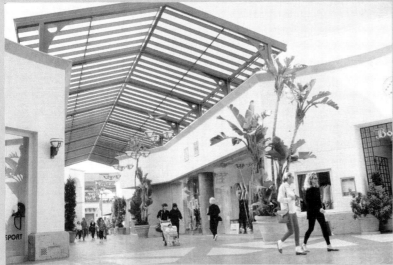

Bart Bartholomew—Black Star

The lure of the shopping mall can be virtually irresistible to the shopper who is buying to assuage inner pain or fill emotional emptiness. Retailers—along with advertisers, banks, and credit agencies—contribute to the "cultural seduction" of the compulsive shopper, filling stores with perfumed air and upbeat music designed to make buying a sensually pleasurable experience.

Triggers to buying

A compulsive shopping spree can be triggered by something good happening (for example, getting a promotion) or something bad happening (having an argument with a spouse). These situations arouse turbulent, fearful emotions by evoking unconscious memories of infancy and childhood. Compulsive shoppers immediately try to resolve this anxiety by automatically heading to the store, just as an alcoholic would reach for a drink. Feelings of sexual frustration, rejection, depression, anger, inadequacy, or being unloved are examples of typical trigger emotions. Another common example is powerlessness a woman might feel toward an overly controlling husband; in retaliation she runs up exorbitant bills to make him "pay" for the hurts he has inflicted upon her.

These disturbing situations and emotions trigger the thought of going shopping as a means of resolving the problem. For compulsive shoppers this thought becomes an obsession—that is, a persistent, recurrent thought that cannot be eliminated from their consciousness by logic or reasoning. The obsession, in turn, fuels the craving for the shopping high and compels them to seek instant gratification, excitement, comfort, and power in the most accessible and appealing shopping environment. A vicious cycle develops: compulsive shoppers shop because they feel bad—and then they feel bad because they shop.

Who are the vulnerable?

Estimates of the number of compulsive shoppers in the United States today range from 25 million to 60 million, and the number is rapidly rising. Of course, the true number can only be approximated, as many people cling, as a form of denial, to the notion that they are merely pursing the "American dream" of material success and do not have a problem.

Clinical data indicate that women make up about 65–70% of compulsive shoppers. They generally shop for clothes, cosmetics, jewelry, and other traditionally "feminine" products. Male compulsive shoppers buy traditionally "masculine" products—cars, sports equipment, luxury office supplies, and expensive tools and gadgets. Women, because they traditionally have the responsibility of shopping for food and other family necessities, are more vulnerable than men to becoming compulsive shoppers. Furthermore, women are raised to be fashion consumers, often beginning as little girls, for example, dressing their Barbie dolls in elaborate wardrobes with every conceivable accessory.

When a national U.S. women's magazine invited readers who considered themselves to be compulsive shoppers to write in, within weeks more than 1,600 had responded. Some had already suffered bankruptcy or foreclosure on their homes or had made desperate attempts to steal money from friends, relatives, or employers.

All socioeconomic classes are represented among the ranks of compulsive shoppers. The behavior is diagnosed on the basis of what the person can afford to spend, not the absolute amount of money spent. Thus, someone who buys 10 lipsticks at the drugstore may have just as serious a problem as someone who spends thousands of dollars on designer dresses. Compulsive shopping crosses ethnic and geographical boundaries, occurring in most developed countries. Cosmopolitan cities, where there is an atmosphere of competitiveness and where people depend largely on external appearances for quick information about others, have relatively higher populations of compulsive shoppers. Although most compulsive shoppers are between 20 and 50 years old, teenagers and even younger children are fast joining the ranks; parents feel guilty about not spending more time with them

"Shopping has just replaced baseball as the national pastime. Pass it on."

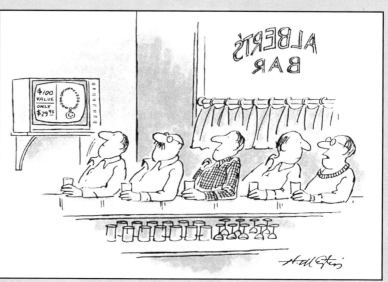

Drawing by H. Martin; © 1989 The New Yorker Magazine, Inc.

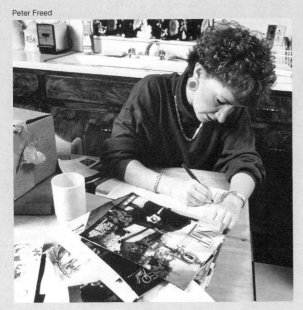

With the unprecedented boom in the international mail order sales business, everything from panty hose to patio furniture can be purchased from a catalog. The compulsive shopper can go on a buying spree without ever leaving home.

and hand over cash or credit cards and encourage them to go to the mall.

Studies have found that a third to a half of U.S. adults have at least one addiction, and most have more than one. "Shopaholics" often have or have had other compulsive disorders or addictions. This is because all addictive behaviors—from cocaine abuse to "workaholism"—have some psychological roots in common.

Early disappointments, fears of inadequacy

The psychological roots of compulsive shopping are laid down in infancy, during the first 18 months of life, or what Sigmund Freud called the oral phase of psychological development. When a parent does not satisfy the infant's need to be fed, changed, or cuddled in a timely or adequate way, the infant will grow up to be extremely sensitive to any hints of deprivation and will unconsciously come to feel that the world cannot be relied upon to meet his or her needs. This individual may then become overindulgent of his or her own needs, especially when experiencing feelings of anxiety or unhappiness in a way that evokes unconscious memories of early disappointments in the interaction with the parent.

Mothers (or other primary care givers) of future compulsive shoppers play a crucial role when they fail to "mirror" their infants and young children appropriately—that is, when they fail to reflect unconditional love and admiration back to the infant. The child then suffers from a sense of not being "seen"—of not being important enough—and these feelings foster the low self-esteem that persists into adulthood.

The sense of inner emptiness experienced by the compulsive shopper also originates in childhood, in a situation where parents have unreasonably high expectations of the child, which usually grow out of their need for the child to make up for their own failures. Such parents cause their children to feel that they can never "measure up," regardless of their actual qualities and abilities. Later, as adults, these individuals seek in the objects of their shopping compulsions what they feel is missing to make them whole or "good enough" to please the "unpleasable" parent.

Inner emptiness may also originate from the period in which an obsessive-compulsive pattern may be developing as the child's personality structure is forming. This theoretically occurs around age two (or during what Freud called the anal phase) if parents struggle too hard over issues of control in toilet training. Obsessive-compulsive people are afraid of being overwhelmed by their feelings, so they push all feelings away—the good and the bad. This leaves a gaping emptiness, which they then seek to fill with their purchases.

The oedipal phase of childhood development, as Freud called the period from ages two to six, plays an especially significant role in fostering compulsive shopping later on—and in causing it to predominate in an individual over other potential addictions. During this phase the child seeks special love, admiration, and attention from the opposite-sex parent. If a little girl, for example, feels rejected or unnoticed by her father, she will begin to think that she is unattractive and unlovable. This causes her to become excessively preoccupied with her appearance, with which she is then destined to be eternally dissatisfied. She may try to resolve these unconscious conflicts by desperately trying to buy something that will magically cause her father and, by extension, other men to love her. Of course, no purchase can ever resolve these early childhood traumas, and she finds herself on a never-ending quest.

Finally, a significant percentage of female compulsive shoppers are victims of childhood sexual abuse. These women have conflicts over making themselves more attractive because they fear having been responsible for the early episodes of abuse. In fact, the connection between sex and shopping goes further, since compulsive shoppers are usually unfulfilled sexually and may turn to shopping sprees for "orgasmic" release and satisfaction.

The cultural seduction

It is only in the past decade that compulsive shopping has been recognized as a syndrome. Its burgeoning is most likely due to a synergistic effect of psychological predisposition and sociocultural influences. The limits of what society considers shopping excess have been greatly extended in recent times, as reflected in pop culture—from Dagwood Bumstead's wife buying a new hat to Imelda Marcos' well-publicized ownership of thousands of pairs of shoes. In the days before credit cards, shoppers were obliged to stay within their means. When shopkeepers did extend credit, it was only to customers they knew, and these face-to-face dealings did not allow shoppers to run up the enormous bills made possible by computerized credit systems.

Credit experts say that to owe 20% of one's take-home pay (not including mortgage payments) is to incur a dangerous level of installment debt. Nevertheless, many compulsive shoppers with incomes of $20,000–25,000 a year owe more than $10,000 on their credit cards. Clearly, a person whose installment debt is 50% of his or her income is on the brink of financial disaster. Automatic teller machines, "gold cards," and other marketing strategies lure consumers into borrowing and spending more and more money. Credit cards make it easy for compulsive shoppers to pretend to themselves that they are not spending "real" money.

Of course, banks and credit agencies are not the only institutions that encourage the development of compulsive shopping in susceptible individuals. The federal government's habitual practice of deficit financing is cited by many people as a way to rationalize spending money they do not have. The pervasive influence of advertising is another cultural factor that cannot be underestimated. In appealing to people's desire to be loved, admired, accepted, and envied, they unfailingly target the most vulnerable shoppers, those who are not simply buying objects but are attempting to assuage emotional pain. Finally, there is the part played by store owners and managers. Retailers hire teams of experts to create an environment that is conducive to spending. They make shopping a sensually pleasurable experience, filling stores with perfumed air and upbeat music.

Ultimately, for the person who feels deeply inadequate and unloved, no car, clothes, makeup, or jewelry will suffice. In what appears to be a growing trend, some of these desperate individuals are now falling victim to yet another addiction—cosmetic surgery. As with compulsive shopping, one purchase—or, in this case, one face-lift or "tummy tuck"—fails to produce lasting self-confidence and contentment, but the individual becomes convinced that a subsequent procedure will magically solve his or her problems.

Getting help

Self-help techniques may alleviate the symptoms of an emotional problem, but they usually do not correct the underlying causes. With that caveat in mind, the following techniques may be of some use in helping compulsive shoppers to control their habit. Compulsive shoppers should:

● keep a diary of their shopping habits, writing down what was bought in a given day, how much it cost, what triggered the desire to shop, and how they felt before, during, and after shopping

● find alternate, longer-lasting ways to improve their appearance or bolster self-esteem—for example, getting additional education to advance their career goals or committing to a long-term weight-loss and exercise program—instead of choosing the immediate gratification of shopping

● organize their closets to find creative ways of using clothes and accessories they have forgotten they owned

● destroy or return credit cards until all the balances have been paid and the problem is under control

● make any remaining credit cards less accessible by putting them in a difficult-to-reach place, such as a safe-deposit box

● keep relatively little money in a checking account and more money in less-accessible savings or similar accounts

● resist watching TV home-shopping shows and perusing mail-order catalogs

● join a self-help group: the support of others who are coping with the same problem can be enormously beneficial (Debtors Anonymous is one such group. It uses a program patterned after the original 12-step approach of Alcoholics Anonymous [AA]. Other self-help groups, such as Gamblers Anonymous, Overeaters Anonymous, or AA, can be useful for the person who cannot find a nearby group specifically targeted to compulsive shoppers or for the compulsive shopper who has one of these other addictions.)

● consider financial counseling; the guidance of a private consultant or a counselor with a governmental agency can help the individual to objectively tackle what may seem to be an overwhelming problem

As noted above, self-help techniques are useful in controlling compulsions and addictions; however, the individual who is seeking both to understand and to change the feelings that lead to compulsive behavior would be wise to consider psychotherapy. A psychiatrist or other mental health professional can diagnose and treat compulsive shopping in a way that helps the individual understand the basis of the problem, a step necessary to resolve the underlying conflicts. In addition to individual psychotherapy, couple or family psychotherapy may also be necessary, as compulsive shopping typically disrupts all of the individual's close relationships. Group psychotherapy is often valuable for support and feedback and may be especially helpful in altering compulsive shoppers' distorted images of their physical appearance. In a small percentage of cases, compulsive shopping can be a manifestation of some other psychiatric disorder, such as bipolar disorder (manic-depression). In these cases a psychiatrist can determine the appropriate diagnosis and treat the person with medication as well as psychotherapy.

Anniversary Reactions: Not Just Coincidence

by Charles-Gene McDaniel, M.S.J.

On a bright, sunny day, a widow from a prominent Chicago family drove her car into the side of a suburban commuter train and was killed. Although in her seventies, she was in apparent good health, and her car had no mechanical problems. Her death was deemed an accident. Her newspaper obituary, however, provided a clue that something else may have been involved. Her accident took place one year to the day after her husband's death.

On the surface, her death by "accident" was face-saving for her family's reputation. Mental health professionals would suggest, however, that this woman's death was the result of suicide—either deliberate or subconscious—and represented what is known as an anniversary reaction, albeit an extreme manifestation.

Remembering sad or traumatic events on their anniversaries is natural, and the intensity of these memories usually diminishes over time. For some people, however, the complicated workings of the human psyche on these occasions may result in emotional disturbances, such as depression, or a variety of physical illnesses, including heart attack.

Even though anniversary reactions are said to be quite common in clinical practice, given their very nature, the incidence cannot be determined. There are no reliable estimates of how frequently psychotherapists see patients suffering from problems growing out of these reactions. What may appear to the therapist to be an endogenous depression may reflect a response to previous situations in which mourning failed to occur or was abnormal or incomplete.

It is not unusual, and perhaps is even common, for people to imagine that they will not live beyond the age of, say, a parent. Ordinarily, these anniversaries pass without incident, except for the normal sadness of remembering the loss of the loved one. In vulnerable individuals, though, these anniversaries take on a more insidious meaning.

Unresolved mourning

Anniversary reaction may be defined as "unresolved mourning" following not only the loss through death of a loved one but other types of loss, such as of a job or of a partner through divorce or other separation, as well. The reaction represents an unconscious effort by the individual to master or control the trauma by reliving the experience without being consciously aware of the anniversary. This effort may express itself in symptoms, dreams, or overt behavior.

The loss may leave an emotional lesion in much the same way as a wound to the body leaves a scar, and this lesion may flare up many years after bereavement. Just as not all bodily wounds result in infection, not all emotional traumas result in pathological reactions. However, there is no way to predict with any certainty who might be susceptible because an emotionally vulnerable person may show unexpected resilience in the face of loss.

Those who experience the often tragic anniversary reactions are said to feel a sense of hopelessness about life events, keeping to themselves their problems and their efforts to deal with them. Like a malignancy, the destructive forces continue to work within these individuals, waiting only for the subconscious time clock to trigger them. These people are able to repress their intrapsychic conflict—that is, until the anniversary sets off the trigger.

Mourning begins with an acute stage wherein the bereaved individual begins the process of what is called decathexis (the divestment of psychic energy from the lost loved one) so that the energy may be freed for attachment to others. The acute stage consists of the immediate phases of shock, grief, pain, reaction to separation, and the beginning of decathexis as the loss becomes recognized internally. The reaction of separation may involve anxiety and anger.

The chronic stage of mourning gradually takes over as the acute stage abates. The psyche uses adaptive mechanisms in trying to integrate the loss with reality so that life can go on. Here the ego begins its repair as part of the more lasting adaptation. This chronic stage is what Sigmund Freud, the father of psychoanalysis, called the "mourning work," a continuation of the process that began during the acute phase. If for any reason the process is interrupted and the individual denies the death of the loved one, mourning is incomplete and pathological reactions may result.

Although he did not use the term *anniversary reaction,* Freud first described such a phenomenon in 1895 in the case of "Freulein Elisabeth von R," who had nursed three of her four loved ones until they died. Later, "this lady celebrated annual festivals of remembrance at the period of her various catastrophes, and on these occasions her vivid visual reproduction and expressions of feeling kept to the date precisely," Freud wrote.

Virtually all of the research into anniversary reactions has grown out of psychoanalysis, although non-

347

analytic psychiatrists, psychologists, physicians, social workers, and other therapists accept the validity of the reaction and use this knowledge in therapy when it is appropriate. Psychoanalytic theories hold that childhood trauma and repression are important predecessors of these reactions, which may result from suppression of the immune response. Another theory, that of psychobiologists, holds that Pavlovian conditioning is key to the formation. The theories are not incompatible. Indeed, some other mammals and birds (but not reptiles, amphibians, or fish) are known to experience depression after removal of a meaningful figure, indicating that reaction to loss is an adaptational process. The event that triggers the reaction, regardless of its origin, usually remains beyond conscious recall of the person, who suffers as a result.

The age at which children are capable of full-fledged mourning is not agreed upon. One theory holds that the ego functions that are necessary for mourning are not firmly established before adolescence. One researcher, for example, cites the case of a 15-year-old girl who developed lymphedema of the hand as a reaction on the first anniversary of her grandmother's death.

Anniversary reactions among the famous

History is replete with instances in which famous people have experienced what may appear to be curious coincidences but which psychiatrists would likely consider anniversary reactions. These reactions may occur on the very day or within a few days of the anniversary of an important event.

Thomas Jefferson, terminally ill, hoped to live to observe the 50th anniversary of the Declaration of Independence. On that very day, July 4, 1826, he died, nearly 83 years old. Mark Twain had noted that he came into the world with Halley's Comet in 1835 and would go out with it. He did—at age 75 in 1910. Sir Winston Churchill died on the anniversary of his father's death 70 years earlier. And the legendary American frontierswoman Martha Jane Burke, known as Calamity Jane, died of pneumonia one day before the 27th anniversary of the death of Wild Bill Hickok; her last words were, "Bury me next to Bill."

The singer Elvis Presley was very attached to his mother. When she died on Aug. 14, 1958, at age 42, Presley said, "My life has ended!" Then, 19 years later, within a few days of the anniversary of her death, he, too, died at age 42.

W. Horsley Gantt, an American disciple, friend, and associate of Ivan Petrovich Pavlov, the well-known Russian physiologist and pioneer behavioral psychologist, died at age 86 in Baltimore, Md., at the end of February 1980. Pavlov had died at age 86 on Feb. 27, 1936.

Nikolay Gogol, the Russian writer, was one of 5 surviving children of the 12 his parents bore. A sensitive boy, he was confronted with a seemingly endless succession of deaths in his family. His 43-year-old father became fatally ill when Gogol was 16 and died two years later. At the time, Gogol had suicidal thoughts but repressed his sadness. Then when he was 43, on the verge of semimadness, Gogol died of self-inflicted starvation, having commented shortly before that his father "died at the same age of the same disease."

The rock singer Janis Joplin died of a drug overdose a few weeks after purchasing a tombstone for Bessie Smith, her idol. Joplin's death came within a matter of days of the anniversary of Smith's death 33 years earlier.

Not only suicide but homicide may occur as an anniversary reaction. Sirhan Sirhan, a Jerusalem-born Jordanian, assassinated Robert F. Kennedy on June 6, 1968, almost one year to the day after the Israeli defeat of the Arabs in the Six-Day War.

Triggers and manifestations

While the phenomenon is referred to as *anniversary* reaction, implying yearly, reactions may also be related to a specific time of day, day of the week, day of

Thomas Jefferson yearned to live to observe the 50th anniversary of the Declaration of Independence; it may not be coincidence that he lived until precisely that day—July 4, 1826.

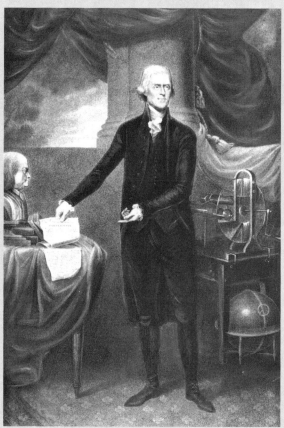

The Granger Collection

348

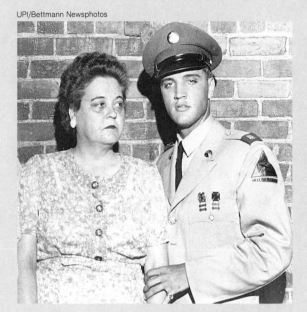

Elvis Presley had a special attachment to his mother and was devastated when she died at age 42. Nineteen years later, when he was 42, he died within just a few days of the anniversary of her death.

the month, season of the year, festival, birthday, or holiday.

One mother reported awakening every year on the same day at 5:30 AM—the day and time her daughter had telephoned from a distant city to report that she had been raped. A man in his mid-thirties became depressed and anxious each Thursday afternoon. His therapist helped him associate this with his having found his mother dead when, at age 14, he returned home from school on a Thursday afternoon. In Freud's classic case of "The Wolf Man," the patient repeatedly experienced a five o'clock depression. That was the hour when, as a young child, he awoke lying on his cot in his parents' bedroom and witnessed what analysts call "the primal scene," his parents having sexual intercourse. Other patients in analysis have experienced headache, depression, gastrointestinal upset, and oversleeping on Sundays and vacations at key "anniversaries."

Closely related to so-called anniversary reactions are symptoms tied to holidays—sometimes called holiday neurosis. For many people, the period between Thanksgiving and Christmas and lasting until after New Year's Day is marked particularly by anxiety and depression; feelings of helplessness, possessiveness, and increased irritability; nostalgia or bitter remembrances about youthful holiday experiences; and a wish for magical resolution of problems.

Although the psychodynamics differ, other holidays that are fraught with meaning and may occasion illness include Easter, Passover, Armistice Day, the Fourth of July, Good Friday, and All Souls Day. So too may

anniversaries of deaths, weddings, births, divorce, and sibling pregnancies. The trigger occasions are as varied as human experience. One woman, for example, was found to lactate on the anniversary of the delivery of a stillborn child.

Posttraumatic stress disorder is, in effect, a form of anniversary reaction in that the individual relives an awful event, such as the horrors of combat, a serious accident, or a natural disaster. Jews, homosexuals, and other survivors of the Holocaust are known to experience such traumatic recalling of the enormities they suffered.

Just as the trigger event varies with the individual, so too does the nature of the reaction. Researchers have noted such physical manifestations as chest pain, headache, back pain, abdominal pain, weight gain, relapse of ulcerative colitis, rheumatoid arthritis, skin diseases, cancer, coronary disease, and glaucoma and other eye conditions, as well as psychological symptoms such as depression, anxiety, and insomnia.

"Anniversary" suicide

The most extreme manifestation, although not an uncommon one, is suicide. One woman jumped to her death from a 14th-story window on Good Friday on the 14th anniversary of her mother's death. In another instance a 43-year-old lawyer killed himself with poison the day after his son reached the age of 12. Some 32 years earlier, the day after the lawyer's own 12th birthday, his brilliant, scholastically successful brother had died suddenly and unexpectedly of encephalitis. The victim, a successful criminal lawyer, had harbored throughout his life a deep sense of guilt about his brother's death, saying that his own success had come about as a result of that loss. He felt that he, like his brother, would have to remove himself through death in order for his son to have an opportunity to develop to his full potential.

Suicide may, of course, be the result of any number of psychological disturbances and can occur even when the individual is considered to be "normal." As a manifestation of the anniversary reaction, however, suicide and suicidal fantasies that are not acted upon are viewed as the result of incomplete mourning that involves pathological identification with a deceased person.

Death rituals

Reactions to death are not unique to any one culture or cultures. One study showed that in 78 societies in America, Europe, Japan, Africa, and the Pacific islands, reactions to death are similar. Archaeological evidence shows that ceremonial rituals have been used to commemorate the dead for nearly 60,000 years. While these rituals vary from the highly emotional high-pitched keening and wailing that are common in Arab, Greek, and Gaelic funeral ceremonies to the more se-

349

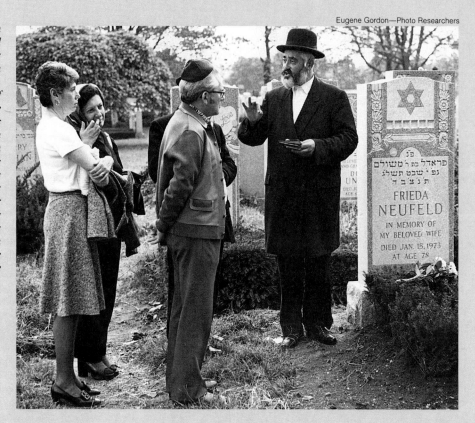

Mourning is an important psychological process that enables people to deal with the reality of death. Each anniversary of the death of someone close is a time for people to go through a "minimourning." In Judaism the unveiling of the tombstone is a ceremony that is usually held one year after a death, enabling relatives and loved ones to gather and share in the remembrance of the deceased and to hear the rabbi's eulogy.

date practices surrounding contemporary Protestant funerals and memorial services, they all serve to help the bereaved separate from their loved ones.

Likewise, Jewish and Catholic anniversary rituals provide a way for relatives and friends to deal with the reality of death and an opportunity to do some of the further work of mourning. Each anniversary of the death offers a time for people to go through a "minimourning."

Treatment and prevention

Although most of the research involving anniversary reactions has been done by psychoanalysts and is based on their therapeutic work with analysands (analytic patients), such long, intense therapy is not always necessary to uncover the deeply buried source of an anniversary reaction. Other types of therapy, such as brief insight-oriented therapy offered by a psychologist or psychiatric social worker, may resolve the problem. Explanation and support are sometimes sufficient when the alert therapist is able to help the individual connect disturbing events with something in the past. When the therapist is not certain why the individual is reacting pathologically, medications such as antidepressants may help the patient through the difficult period, although this may interfere with the patient's ability to get at the root of the problem; thus, the problem may recur—for example, manifested in a manic-depressive reaction.

Awareness seems to be the key to prevention of anniversary reactions. Awareness of the possibility also is essential for the therapist dealing with problems that seemingly are unrelated to any known event, relationship, or memory in the patient's life. Psychoanalytic research has shown that when a child loses a parent, certain factors do serve to mediate in preventing the revived anniversary trauma of the death. These factors are: an intact home, with the surviving parent assuming a dual paternal and maternal role so that the child develops a strong ego; support outside the home, with the parent being able to use this support; a meaningful relationship between the parent and child before that parent's death; separation tolerance to the emergency created by death; and appropriate grief and mourning that immediately follow the loss.

From the above factors may also be deduced other preventive strategies relating not only to loss of a parent but to other traumas. It is important for the individual to recognize that any loss may have pathological consequences and to acknowledge the loss and do the mourning work necessary for coming to grips with it psychologically. This may thereby prevent recurrence of the overwhelming emotions that Henry Wadsworth Longfellow described in his poem *Holidays*:

The holiest of all holidays are those
Kept by ourselves in silence and apart;
The secret anniversaries of the heart,
When the full river of feeling overflows.

350

Obesity

Concern about body weight is an ongoing national obsession in the United States, and a vast industry, the weight-loss business, reaps huge profits each year selling diets and weight-loss products to an ever willing population of people wishing to reduce. Indeed, a great many people think they are overweight. But how do they know? Furthermore, should it matter? And if they are overweight and want to do something about it, what should they do? What about the widely publicized very low-calorie liquid diets? What about drugs or any of the other currently used treatments?

"Good weights" for adults

Before deciding whether they ought to do anything about their weight, those who think they are overweight need to have some objective measures for determining if in fact they are right. There are two important components of this evaluation. The first is the individual's weight relative to his or her height. For individuals who are not regular and strenuous exercisers and who are not pregnant, any increase in body weight after age 25 is almost certainly due to extra body fat. So the question becomes not only what one's weight is in relation to height but also whether one has too much body fat for age as well as height.

In the past decade, three major studies have provided a basis for making recommendations about what are currently accepted as "good weights" for most adults. These three major studies included one from the life insurance industry (conducted by the Society of Actuaries and the Association of Life Insurance Medical Directors of America, 1980), one of the Norwegian population (conducted by Hans T. Waaler, 1984), and a third large study carried out by the American Cancer Society in 1979. All three studies found that for women the body weight associated with the lowest risk of early death increased with age; thus, it is normal for women to get heavier as they get older. The striking similarity of the optimal weight ranges provided guidelines for establishing new recommendations for good weights for women. These weights, calculated as "body mass index units," were published in 1989 by the U.S. National Academy of Sciences. Converted into pounds and related to height and age, these numbers are shown in Table 1.

There is an easy biological explanation for this healthy increase in weight with age in women. It is related to their biological equipment for childbearing. The female hormones that equip women for childbearing and are associated with pregnancy cause fat to be deposited on their hips and thighs. This fat is intended for lactation and carries less risk to health than fat located elsewhere. For men, however, a different relationship of good weights for age exists. Above age 30 there is no benefit in gaining weight. Table 2 provides what are presently considered good weights for men.

Health risks of being too fat or too thin

For individuals who are above the upper limits of the good weight range for their height, the risks of a variety of illnesses will increase as the degree of excess weight increases. The diseases associated with this increase in weight are heart disease, high blood pressure, gallbladder disease, diabetes mellitus, and some forms of cancer (including those of the breast and uterus). It is also clear that weights below the lower limits for these weight ranges are associated with increased risks to health, but they are different from those in the overweight category. For individuals who are significantly underweight, there is an increased risk of lung disease, particularly tuberculosis and lung cancer, and of some forms of digestive disease.

| | *Table 1:* **Good weights for women (in pounds)** | | | | | |
| | | | age | | | |
height (inches)	19–24	25–34	35–44	45–54	55–64	65+
58	91–115	96–119	100–124	105–129	110–134	115–138
59	94–119	99–124	104–128	109–133	114–138	119–143
60	97–123	102–128	107–133	112–138	118–143	123–148
61	100–127	106–132	111–137	116–143	122–148	127–153
62	104–131	109–136	115–142	120–147	126–153	131–158
63	107–135	113–141	118–146	124–152	130–158	135–163
64	110–140	116–145	122–151	128–157	134–163	140–169
65	114–144	120–150	126–156	132–162	138–168	144–174
66	117–148	124–155	130–161	136–167	142–173	148–179
67	121–153	127–159	134–166	140–172	146–178	153–185
68	125–158	131–164	138–171	144–177	151–184	158–190
69	128–162	135–169	142–176	149–182	155–189	162–196
70	132–167	139–174	146–181	153–189	160–195	167–202
71	136–172	143–179	150–186	157–193	166–200	172–208
72	140–177	147–184	154–191	162–199	169–206	177–213

Diet and Health, 1989, U.S. National Academy of Sciences

Table 2: **Good weights for men** (in pounds)		
	age	
height (inches)	19–24	25–65+
60	91–115	96–119
61	94–119	99–124
62	97–123	102–128
63	100–127	106–132
64	104–131	109–136
65	107–135	113–141
66	110–140	116–145
67	114–144	120–150
68	117–148	124–155
69	121–153	127–159
70	125–158	131–164
71	128–162	135–169
72	132–167	139–174
73	136–172	143–179
74	140–177	147–184
75	144–182	151–189
76	148–186	155–194

Source: *Diet and Health*, 1989, U.S. National Academy of Sciences

However, recent studies of health risks associated with obesity have found that it is not only how fat people are but where the fat is located that determines their risk. For both men and women, carrying a larger than normal amount of fat on the abdomen is associated with an increase in the same risks that are identified with excess body fat. That is, the risks for heart disease, high blood pressure, stroke, diabetes mellitus, gallbladder disease, and probably some forms of cancer increase with the extent of abdominal (or upper-body) fat. Consequently, guidelines for high-risk categories of men and women have been determined on the basis of the ratio of the circumference obtained at the waist (defined as the smallest circumference below the ribs and above the hip bones) divided by the circumference of the hips (defined as the line parallel to the floor at the widest posterior extension of the buttocks). For women a ratio greater than 0.85 puts them in the high-risk category, while men with a ratio above 0.95 are considered at high risk. As a general rule, it can be said that for people whose body weight is 20% or more above the upper limits for the good weight range for their age, the health risks associated with being overweight are significant.

Today's liquid very low-calorie diets

In recent years the use of prepared liquid-formula very low-calorie diets has become widespread and popular. This form of treatment was arrived at from two different perspectives. More than 20 years ago it was realized that a major problem with liquid diets then on the market was that the patient also lost protein. This problem could be largely but not completely overcome by adding small amounts of protein as a meal replacement. The total daily calorie intake from these so-called fasting programs tends to be between 240 and 400 cal per day. Thus, very low-calorie diets have been defined as those above 200 and below 600 cal a day. The alternative approach for arriving at a low-calorie formulation was derived by determining what the optimal protein intake would be and then adding sufficient amounts of carbohydrate to minimize ketosis (an abnormal metabolic state that occurs with reduced carbohydrate metabolism) and a sufficient amount of fat to provide the necessary amounts of essential fatty acids. With this approach, obesity experts reached the conclusion that a diet below 600 cal per day was not satisfactory.

Optifast, Medifast, and Health Management Resources (HMR) are among the most commonly used of today's medically supervised formula diets, but there are many others. The major differences in the products are in the amounts of protein, carbohydrates, and fats that are present. In addition, there are minor differences in the amounts of most of the micronutrients. In some supervised very low-calorie diet programs, micronutrients are given as capsules, and in others they are added directly to the formula diets. The preference of many hospital-based programs and physicians who are specialists in obesity treatment is for the latter approach.

Some weight-loss programs use powders that can be mixed with water as the total source of food (usually in five portions per day), while others use them as meal replacements for two of three meals per day. For any weight-loss program containing less than 600 total calories per day, adequate supervision is required

Participants in an Optifast program who have lost significant amounts of weight on liquid-formula very low-calorie diets proudly display the fact that they have become too small for their britches.

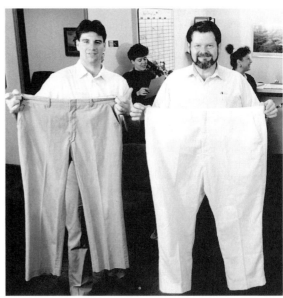

Michael L. Abramson

since some individuals can develop undesirable side effects such as low serum potassium, episodes of gout, or cardiac irregularities. When higher levels of calories are in the diet, less supervision is needed. Generally no supervision is required for diets over 1,000 cal per day, and in the range between 800 and 1,000 cal, there is usually little need for supervision. However, since the magnitude of caloric restriction varies as a function of the degree of weight to be lost, for some individuals an 800-cal diet can be as restrictive as a 400-cal diet is for others. Thus, for most individuals consuming less than 800 cal per day, some level of supervision is desirable. The very low-calorie diets are not meant for those who need to lose moderate amounts of weight. To enter these programs individuals should usually be about 30% above their "good weight" range (usually 18 kg [40 lb] overweight).

The very low-calorie diets have been particularly useful because they provide an easy meal replacement schedule. It is clear, however, that the major component of treatment programs should be a modular one that teaches dieters to live at their goal weight. These learning techniques, commonly called behavior modification, should address both nutritional and energy-expenditure needs. They should also provide practical solutions to such life situations as dining out, going to parties, food selection, and food preparation. With this behavior modification as a base, very low-calorie diets can be an important adjunct of treatment for properly selected and motivated obese individuals. The success of the individual in maintaining a lower weight after completing a program that uses very low-calorie liquid-formula diets—people usually stay on the diets for 12 to 16 weeks—appears to be related to the degree to which they have learned to change their food selection and food preparation and whether they have become more physically active in their everyday lives.

Potentially effective new drugs

Recently, two prescription medications have been introduced that may be helpful in the treatment of overweight individuals. The first of these is dexfenfluramine (Isomeride), a drug made in France. The results of a clinical trial conducted in nine European countries comparing this drug with a placebo were quite promising. The drug, used in conjunction with diet programs, appears to be effective in helping individuals lose more weight than they would by appropriate behavioral and nutritional intervention alone. Moreover, the available data on this medication suggest that it can be useful for a long time and that its effectiveness persists as long as it is used. Dexfenfluramine acts by releasing serotonin, an important neurotransmitter, from its storage granules in nerve endings in the brain. Serotonin apparently affects the appetite-control center of the brain, which controls satiety; the higher level of serotonin therefore reduces food intake.

A second drug, fluoxetine (Prozac), has recently been approved for use in the U.S. in the treatment of depression. This drug, like dexfenfluramine, works by increasing the concentrations of serotonin. It does this by preventing the movement of serotonin back into the nerve endings. The data available on fluoxetine show that it too can reduce food intake and body weight of overweight and normal-weight subjects. As yet clinical trials have not been carried out in the U.S. on either dexfenfluramine or fluoxetine for weight loss.

Prevalence of obesity in the U.S.

In a country so obsessed with weight, how common is obesity? The answer depends on how *overweight* is defined. The U.S. government has recently published figures that place in the overweight category anyone whose body mass index is in the top 15% of weights for heights of women or men in their twenties. On the basis of these figures, 24% of the adult American population are overweight. In recent surveys applying the same criteria to Americans of Hispanic origin in Florida, Texas, Arizona, New York, and California, the prevalence of overweight has been shown to be significantly higher than in the rest of the population. Approximately 30% of Mexican-American men, 29% of Cuban-American men, and 25% of Puerto Rican men were overweight. The corresponding overweight figures were 39% of Mexican-American, 34% of Cuban-American, and 37% of Puerto Rican women. Other recent surveys have found that the prevalence of obesity is significantly higher among black women and women below the poverty level than it is in white women above the poverty level.

A recent survey conducted by the Centers for Disease Control found that obesity in the U.S. is highest among Hispanic Americans. Mexican-Americans were the most overweight, followed by Cuban-Americans, then Puerto Ricans.

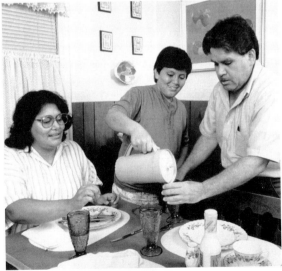

Bob Daemmrich—Stock, Boston

Data based on the criteria proposed in the aforementioned good weights for women and men, however, have not yet been applied in the evaluation of overall prevalence of overweight in the American population. If the criteria for optimal weight differ by age, as appears to be the case for women, then the prevalence of overweight will likely be lower than indicated by the U.S. government figures cited above. Since the optimal weights for men do not appear to change with age, applying the newer criteria will probably not change their prevalence rate.

Genetics and body weight: new insights

A number of factors contribute to the development of obesity. One of these is surely diet. Another is the interaction of diet with genetic makeup. Several recent studies of twins and their relatives have highlighted the importance of genetic factors in obesity. If the genetic component is factored out, it appears to contribute between 25 and 35% of the risk of overweight. This is important to everyone with a weight problem because it indicates that most of the influence is from environmental factors, which people may be able to control.

These important factors were examined in a follow-up of a group of children who were initially examined in Sweden 40 years ago. A total of 504 obese children were followed. Obesity in the family, particularly the mother, increased the likelihood that these children would remain obese as adults. Those who were more than 35% overweight as children experienced the highest proportion of complications due to their excess weight in adult life.

Unanswered questions

The fact that obesity as a human problem and a significant health risk continues indicates that there are still key questions to be answered. The first of these is why the human body does not regulate its fat stores better. This question is being investigated through examinations of both human and animal types of obesity. It is known that there are glandular problems that can be related to obesity and also that genetic factors are important. Attempting to answer the questions about the fundamental basis for the control of food intake and its relation to energy stores is key to developing rational approaches to treatment of obesity.

The situation of treatment for overweight problems is now similar to the status of treatment for hypertension (high blood pressure) over 30 years ago. It was in 1958 that the first important and well-tolerated drug for treatment of high blood pressure was introduced. Since that time medical science's understanding of the factors that cause high blood pressure has expanded, and the variety of mechanisms that can contribute to its development has come to be recognized. Those advances have led to important therapeutic approaches. Likewise, in the 1990s it is highly probable that a more advanced understanding of the mechanisms that control fat stores and fat distribution will enable the development of a number of new and novel approaches to the treatment of obesity.

—*George O. Bray, M.D.*

Obstetrics and Gynecology

Proper care for the pregnant woman is presently a major area of focus in the specialty of obstetrics and gynecology. New attention is being directed toward determining what constitutes adequate prenatal care, reducing infant mortality rates, explaining the high incidence of cesarean sections performed in the United States and reassessing the indications for these procedures, utilizing newer and safer methods of pain relief during labor and delivery, and determining the relative safety of nonhospital deliveries. Abortion issues continue to spark controversy and action on many fronts in the U.S. and in many other nations. Another matter of growing importance concerns women beyond their childbearing years; as the population ages, new attention is being directed, very appropriately, toward the health and well-being of women after menopause.

The high infant mortality rate in the U.S. has become a critical national problem. Premature, low-birth-weight infants are between 40 and 200 times more likely to die in their first month than normal-weight babies.

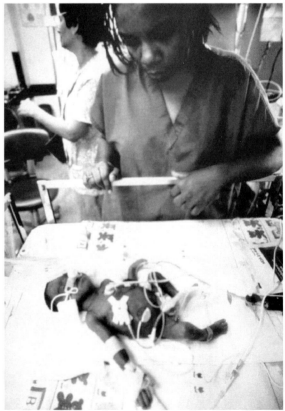

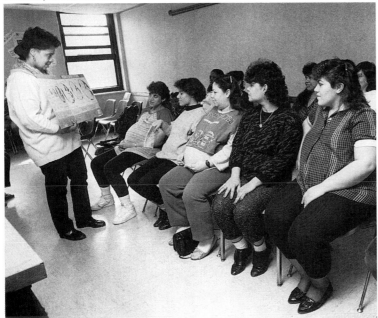

Pregnant women get instruction on fetal development at a maternity clinic in Brooklyn, New York. To curtail high infant mortality rates, there is an urgent need for high-level prenatal care, especially for those in low socioeconomic groups, teenage mothers, and drug abusers.

Prenatal care

For many years the infant mortality rate in the United States has been notably high. Currently the U.S. ranks 18th in the world, far behind other developed nations such as Japan, Sweden, Switzerland, Denmark, Norway, The Netherlands, and Canada. Nearly 40,000 U.S. babies per year die before their first birthday; this translates to 10.4 deaths for every 1,000 live births. More than 75% of U.S. perinatal deaths occur in premature, low-birth-weight infants, who are between 40 and 200 times more likely to die in their first month than normal-weight babies.

During the Jimmy Carter administration (1977–81), the stated federal goal was to reduce infant mortality to nine deaths per 1,000 live births by 1990. However, little attention was subsequently paid to this particular goal by succeeding administrations. As a result, the ability of the health care system to provide improved care, particularly for women in rural areas and lower socioeconomic groups, has simply not materialized. A number of legislative bills are currently being introduced to deal with the infant mortality problem, but to date, no major impact has been made on this very critical national problem.

The three situations that contribute most heavily to the high infant mortality picture are: (1) an increasing number of pregnancies in teenage girls, (2) a growing epidemic of sexually transmitted diseases (STD), and (3) a rapidly escalating incidence of substance abuse among childbearing women. Women who are at high risk need not only routine visits for prenatal monitoring but also instruction in proper nutrition and counseling regarding the adverse effects of STD, alcohol, cigarettes, and street drugs on their own physical health as well as that of their unborn infants. Women in the high-risk group also need evaluation for psychological problems that may make them inadequate mothers and potential child abusers.

While the urgency of providing high-level prenatal care for women whose babies are at high risk is irrefutable, especially for those from low socioeconomic groups who lack medical care, at the other end of the spectrum, less prenatal care is now being recommended for women who are basically in good health at the time that they become pregnant. About 1.6 million women in the U.S. each year are in this low-risk group. It is currently believed that low-risk women need fewer prenatal medical visits than have been advised until now. In a report issued by the U.S. Public Health Service in October 1989, a panel of experts recommended that these women have 7 or 8 prenatal visits rather than the usual 13. Also, the number of pelvic exams and laboratory tests could be cut back for those women who consistently remain at low risk. If this approach is adopted, it will have considerable economic implications and could be of great importance in redirecting services and funds to those who need them most.

New attention to cesarean delivery

For a number of years there has been growing concern about the steadily increasing rate of cesarean sections (c-sections) carried out in the United States. Twenty years ago only about 5% of obstetrical deliveries were by this method; they were performed when it appeared that the mother, the baby, or both were unlikely to be able to survive a vaginal delivery or that the delivery would result in excessive damage to one or both of them. By 1989 the c-section rate had increased to approximately 24% of all deliveries; only Brazil, with 26%, was higher. By contrast, Canada's rate was estimated to be approximately 19%, Denmark's 13%, Norway's 12%, and Japan's 7%, leaving the U.S. the highest of all of the developed countries surveyed.

A certain number of cesarean deliveries are necessary for the proper medical management of specific abnormalities of pregnancy, both maternal and fetal. Primary among the maternal indications have been the failure of a woman to progress in labor, a previous cesarean section, a disproportion between the size of the baby and that of the mother's pelvis, or a breech presentation (feet or buttocks first). Other less common indications include chronic illness in the mother, presence of an active STD, a pregnancy that is postterm (*i.e.*, beyond 42 weeks), premature rupture of the fetal membranes, an abnormal position of the placenta, as in a placenta previa (a condition in which the placenta precedes the child at birth, potentially causing severe maternal hemorrhage), and a medical need to avoid stretching the pelvic muscles. The imminent delivery of a low-birth-weight baby and evident fetal distress, detected by fetal monitoring, are the two most common fetal indications. As will be noted later, several maternal and fetal indications are now under intense scrutiny.

Medical indications alone cannot account for the staggeringly high U.S. c-section rates. Surveys also show wide geographic variation. For example, it was recently reported that 30% of all births in the District of Columbia ended in c-sections, whereas only 18% did so in Alabama. The same study looked at the rates in 2,388 hospitals in 30 states and found that they ranged from 0 to 53%.

One of the more recent and provocative reports that attempted to explain the wide variations in rates indicated that levels of affluence were directly correlated with c-section rates. Women with a median family income under $11,000 had only a 13% rate, whereas those with median family incomes of more than $30,000 had a 23% rate. These differences were consistent regardless of maternal age, number of previous births, race, ethnicity, fetal birth weight, or medical complications.

	Affluence and c-sections*			
	income less than $11,000		income greater than $30,000	
mother's age	no. of women	c-section rate	no. of women	c-section rate
under 18	1,926	12.7	241	14.1
18–34	18,563	12.8	13,824	22.5
over 34	1,407	19.0	2,491	26.0
all ages	21,896	13.2	16,556	22.9

*numbers of c-sections per 100 births in Los Angeles county 1982–83

Adapted from Jeffrey B. Gould *et al.*, "Socioeconomic Differences in Rates of Cesarean Section," *New England Journal of Medicine*, vol. 321, no. 4 (July 27, 1989), pp. 233–239

Another observation has been that obstetricians schedule cesarean operations for cost-efficiency reasons and to accommodate their own work schedules. A c-section alleviates the unpredictability of labor and enables doctors to avoid middle-of-the-night deliveries.

Many evaluations have concluded that one of the major reasons for the rising cesarean rates is the current litigious climate in which all physicians are being forced to practice. This situation is now viewed as insurmountable by many doctors; many obstetricians are simply no longer delivering babies. This ongoing loss has been documented in annual surveys by the American College of Obstetricians and Gynecologists (ACOG). The national average is currently one in eight physicians discontinuing the practice of obstetrics; in Florida the rate is one in four. It has recently been estimated that about 60% of American obstetricians are sued at least once during their years of practice and that a young obstetrician starting out can expect to be sued eight times during his or her next 35 years of practice. The threat to practicing obstetricians is considerably exacerbated by the fact that they may be held liable for the support of a child up to the age of majority if the child is found to have some physical abnormality that is blamed on the delivery per se. Because of the fear of lawsuits, many physicians feel that any indication of fetal distress, no matter how slight, mandates the immediate performance of a c-section; it is rare for a physician to be sued for doing a cesarean section even if a vaginal delivery would have been feasible and possibly better.

Clearly, there is no single fully satisfactory explanation for the unprecedented high rates of cesareans. When the trend had been noted over many years, the question was asked whether they were all truly necessary. Many evaluations concluded that almost half of these procedures were not medically indicated and actually posed additional risks to the mother's life or health without at the same time offering a corresponding increase in the benefits to her offspring. A cesarean delivery performed by a skilled physician in a good medical facility carries a very low level of risk, currently estimated to be about one death per 2,500 procedures. This figure, however, is two- to fourfold higher than that for deliveries carried out by the vaginal route. Even in the best of hands, with surgical delivery there will inevitably be instances of hemorrhage, infection, and surgical damage to the bladder or intestines as well as problems related to anesthesia.

It is also believed that some babies are being subjected to increased and unnecessary risks. This is particularly true when the procedure is carried out on a woman whose baby is thought to be full-term but is actually premature. There are additional concerns that babies born by c-section are deprived of the stimulus of labor and vaginal delivery and do not have the opportunity to absorb certain chemical substances

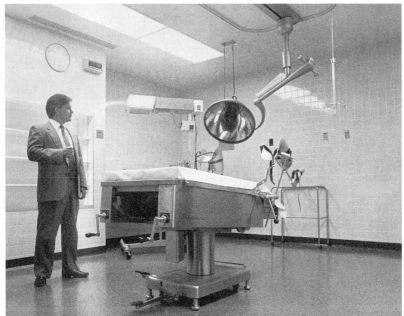

There has been a concerted effort to account for the steadily increasing rate of cesarean sections done in the U.S. Many evaluations have pointed to the intensely litigious climate in which obstetricians are now forced to practice. The rate of malpractice suits has become so high that performing cesareans is one way of practicing defensive medicine. Many other obstetricians are now discontinuing practice altogether because they cannot afford insurance. At this medical center in Missouri, the delivery room is empty and the obstetrics ward has been closed.

produced by the mother only during labor. For example, there are data suggesting that the mother's body releases certain substances during labor that may help to clear the lungs of the newborn. There is also evidence that infants who are surgically delivered after a trial of labor are in better condition than those who are delivered prior to the onset of labor.

In 1916 a New York obstetrician declared before a medical society meeting: "Once a cesarean, always a cesarean"—a dictum that became entrenched in obstetrical practice. Today there is a concerted effort to have more women attempt vaginal deliveries following a previous c-section. Recent studies from the U.S., Israel, and Sweden have all shown that vaginal delivery can be achieved in women who formerly had cesareans. The primary concern about vaginal delivery had been that the strain of labor could rupture the scar from a cesarean, causing a bleeding risk for both mother and baby. The "classical" incision for a c-section until about a decade ago was a vertical cut in the uterine wall. It has now become standard for cesareans to be performed with a low, horizontal incision—sometimes called a "bikini cut"—which is considerably less likely to rupture during vaginal delivery.

ACOG has urged that it become routine for a woman to have a trial of labor and, if possible, a vaginal birth. Where no additional risk is involved, a trial of labor is indicated even when more than one c-section has been performed in the past. When this has been done, 50–80% of properly selected patients have had successful vaginal deliveries. Unfortunately, however, the medicolegal climate has intervened; the fear of lawsuits has led to a less than enthusiastic adoption of this recommendation in obstetrical practice. When

ACOG last surveyed 538 hospitals, it was found that 54% of practicing obstetricians had yet to attempt a vaginal delivery in women who had previously had a cesarean.

As already mentioned, several indications for performing cesareans have recently been reevaluated. In three instances the indications have been determined not to be universally valid. First, it has been conventional obstetrical wisdom that low-birth-weight babies are better delivered abdominally than vaginally and, indeed, the survival rates of these infants during their first 24 hours of life appeared to justify this conclusion. However, recent studies have found that cesarean babies observed throughout the first week of life have had a higher death rate than those delivered vaginally; by the end of the first week, there was no statistically significant difference in outcome between the two groups.

Second, when infections due to the herpes simplex virus (HSV) were first recognized to be growing in incidence and importance, it was believed that women with genital herpes should be delivered by c-section so that their babies would not be exposed to the virus during the delivery process. Although it has been well documented that the herpesvirus may be transmitted from the mother to the baby during labor and delivery, more recently it has been demonstrated that HSV can also be transmitted to the fetus during pregnancy. Thus, it is now believed that the babies of women who are infected with genital herpes but who do not have active lesions at the time that they go into labor are at greater overall risk by having a c-section delivery than they would be with a vaginal delivery.

Finally, a third and urgent problem at the present

time is how best to handle women who are either infected with the human immunodeficiency virus (HIV) or who have clinical AIDS. Again, the earlier tendency was to deliver their babies by c-section to avoid infecting the baby during delivery. Recent studies, however, suggest that there is no clear indication for universal c-section, as many of these babies are already infected prior to the onset of labor.

In January 1989 New York became the first state in the U.S. to institute a formal program to curb cesareans; hospitals are now required to keep records accounting for all c-section operations. Likewise, attempts are now being made around the country to try to identify how many c-sections are being done, for what indications, and how many of them may be unnecessary. The goal of these efforts is to reduce the rates to a level that will ensure or even improve the safety of childbirth for both mothers and infants.

Natural childbirth redefined

Another notable development in the management of labor and delivery today has to do with the concept of natural childbirth. Formerly this approach called for no medical intervention whatsoever, but gradually this had changed. The early impetus for natural childbirth arose primarily from fears about the effects of anesthesia—particularly those that could be damaging to the fetus. In 1942 Grantly Dick Read, a British obstetrician, published the book *Childbirth Without Fear,* which was translated into 10 languages and had a major international impact on the practice of obstetrics. At a time when anesthetized childbirth was very much in vogue, he proposed that women could instead use relaxation techniques during labor and thereby obviate the need for sedating drugs. In 1951 the French obstetrician Fernand Lamaze introduced a form of natural childbirth that eliminated anesthesia and instead used a regimen of breathing exercises and other distraction techniques to minimize pain during labor and delivery—a regimen he had observed to be highly effective in the Soviet Union. His system was widely adopted in childbirth practices in many parts of the world.

In addition to having fears about anesthesia's effects, women were becoming more eager to be active participants in the labor and delivery process, in many cases in conjunction with their husbands. At first, natural childbirth techniques were utilized most often by women of the middle classes who were, in general, well educated and often considered themselves feminists. Over the years, however, the techniques employed have altered considerably, and they are now used by a much wider range of women.

Although there were many benefits for mother and baby associated with these new approaches, they were not always an unmitigated blessing. Recent studies that have reevaluated the risks associated with anesthesia in childbirth have revealed that properly administered pain relief can actually expedite the process of labor and delivery, reducing the trauma to both mothers and babies. Consequently, the term *natural childbirth* is now much more broadly interpreted; basically it means the vaginal delivery of a baby with the active participation of the mother.

Advances in the understanding and safety of treating pain have meant the growing use of small amounts of medication for pain relief in childbirth. Nowadays a variety of pain-relief options can ease the process and still allow the mother to participate fully in the delivery. Moreover, she need not feel like a "failure" if she accepts one of the pain-relief methods, which offer intermittent administration of small doses of a drug. Among the options are the epidural block, in which a local anesthetic lasting one to two hours is given through a catheter that is inserted into the epidural space (comprising the membranes that cover the spinal nerves). The epidural block provides quick pain relief from the waist to the knees. The paracervical block—local anesthesia injected in either side of the cervix—is another method used during active labor; it helps during the transition from labor to delivery without affecting the mother's ability to push. The pudendal block, also using local anesthesia, lasts about an hour. It numbs the area around the vagina and eliminates pain from vaginal stretching and episiotomy during the actual delivery.

Alternatives to hospital delivery

Since the mid-1970s at least 250 nonhospital facilities offering family-centered maternity for women judged to be at low risk for complications have been established in the U.S. (Some of the centers subsequently closed because of the liability risk.) As this option became increasingly popular, questions about the safety of the facilities were raised by the American Academy of Pediatrics and the ACOG. Consequently, a formal study, known as the National Birth Center Study, was organized.

The conclusions of the study were released late in 1989. Data on the outcomes of almost 12,000 deliveries conducted in 84 free-standing birth centers were assessed. The American Public Health Association has defined *birth center* as "any health facility, place or institution which is not a hospital or in a hospital and where births are planned to occur away from the mother's usual residence following normal, uncomplicated pregnancy." Regulations in most states are based on this definition.

The women who were studied were considered to be at low risk for complications during labor and delivery and thus were deemed to be appropriate for childbirth outside the conventional hospital setting. The overall risk to these mothers and their infants was found to be essentially the same as that found for similar women in large studies conducted in hospitals.

The National Birth Center Study thus concluded that deliveries in birth centers were a reasonable and acceptable alternative, particularly for women who had already had a previous child.

Nevertheless, many obstetricians and pediatricians point out that a woman may suddenly, without warning, develop a major complication such as a massive hemorrhage from a placental abruption or prolapse of the umbilical cord. Although rare, these potential occurrences could place both mothers and babies at high risk when no backup critical care medical help is available. Further, birth centers that were not included in the study might have a higher incidence of adverse outcomes. An option that many specialists favor is the location of birth centers offering homelike settings that would accommodate mothers and their families in hospitals, which could then handle rare complications if need be.

Alternative positions for childbirth

In addition to the changes in natural childbirth techniques and in settings for delivery, the optimal position for labor and delivery is being reevaluated. Several different types of chairs and cushions have been developed, including some that allow a woman to deliver in a squatting position. There are data suggesting that this position results in a less traumatic and often safer delivery. Since it allows greater opening of the pelvis and utilizes gravity as part of the delivery process, it is considered more physiologically natural than the semirecumbent position most frequently used. Birth cushions have been introduced in a few dozen medical centers in the United States and Europe. Their use, in essence, represents an interesting throwback to the days when women working in the fields squatted to have their babies and returned directly to work after delivery.

Abortion update

The last few years have seen ever increasing political activity surrounding the issue of abortion in many countries around the world. In the U.S., following the Supreme Court ruling in the case of *Webster* v. *Reproductive Health Services* on July 3, 1989, which gave greater control over abortion to the states, a number of antiabortion, right-to-life groups, such as Operation Rescue, have been increasingly aggressive in their attempts to prevent abortions and to encourage the Supreme Court to overturn its 1973 decision in the *Roe* v. *Wade* case, which legalized abortion. At the same time, equal or perhaps even greater levels of activity on the part of pro-choice groups have been directed toward ensuring that this does not happen and that women will not be returned to the days of illegal, dangerous, and often fatal abortions. Abortion also has become the focal point of many local, state, and national elections.

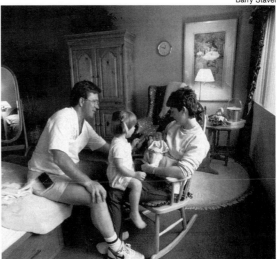

A recent study found that birth centers offering family-centered maternity in homelike settings are a safe and acceptable alternative to hospital childbirth for mothers at low risk for complications during labor and delivery.

Amid the heated controversy surrounding the abortion issue, it is of interest that a study prepared for former president Ronald Reagan and reported in 1989 by then U.S. surgeon general C. Everett Koop found that there were no sufficient data that proved that women suffer long-term adverse effects—either physical or psychological—following abortion procedures. A more recent assessment of the psychological consequences of abortion, commissioned by the American Psychological Association, found even more conclusively that "severe negative reactions after abortions are rare." One study found that 76% of women who seek abortions reported feeling relief afterward; only 17% reported feeling guilt or remorse. Such conclusions are of particular importance, given the data that had been collected previously by the U.S. Centers for Disease Control (CDC) showing that the maternal death rate from abortion had dropped from 4 per 100,000 procedures in 1972 (pre-*Roe* v. *Wade*) to 0.5 in 1985. Furthermore, the level of risk associated with abortion is seven times lower than that associated with a full-term pregnancy and delivery.

Demographers and economists have begun to assess the potential impact of the partial or complete restriction of legal abortion. Estimates are being made of the possible increase in births, with one study recently concluding that in just the category of teenagers giving birth, the number could rise by 75,000 per year. Another report calculated that 1.2 million unwanted pregnancies could cost the U.S. public $1.8 billion each year.

Another development has occurred among women themselves, who are now voicing their refusal to return to the days of humiliating and dangerous back-alley abortions or to coat hangers or douching with Lysol to induce their own abortions if they are not able to get safe, legal abortions. Many feminists are now focusing their attention on two methods for future abortions. One is RU-486 (mifepristone), the highly effective "abortion pill" introduced in France in 1988 but whose introduction in the United States has so far been blocked by intense antiabortion activities. Barring that, some women are looking to the use of menstrual extraction instruments to carry out their own abortions. Menstrual extraction is a vacuum aspiration method used at the time menstruation should occur. A plastic tube is inserted into the uterus, and a syringe is used to extract the uterine contents. This method has drawn adverse criticism from the medical community. The dangers in doing menstrual extraction procedures, particularly when the operator is relatively untrained, include injury to the uterus, hemorrhage, and infection, and in some cases the method may fail to terminate the pregnancy.

At the moment, abortion is of major concern in the United States, but issues related to abortion have also led to debate in numerous other countries. In Great Britain the first survey of consultant gynecologists' attitudes toward abortion was conducted in 1989. It found that 76% felt the 1967 Abortion Act, which enabled women to obtain legal abortions through the National Health Service if two doctors sign approval papers, had worked successfully. However, it was also found that 73% were in favor of a woman's right to decide, in consultation with her physician, whether abortion was an appropriate option for her. This led the authors of the survey to conclude that Britain should enact legislation to make it easier than it presently is for women to obtain abortions. The survey's findings were of particular interest, given the fact that a challenge to abortion rights was expected to be made in Parliament during 1990. This challenge has been fueled, at least in part, by events in the U.S. and directly aided by American antiabortion groups such as Operation Rescue.

The country in which the greatest number of abortions are performed is the Soviet Union, where in 1987, 6.5 million were done. However, in the Soviet Union abortion is the main method of family planning, and the operations themselves are often painful and degrading. Most methods of contraception are not widely available and are primarily used by women of greater financial means.

Overall, about 40% of women worldwide have access to legal first-trimester abortions upon request. The remaining 60% of women live in countries with limited or no availability of safe, legal procedures—the most restrictive laws being in Muslim countries of Asia, two-thirds of the Latin-American countries, about half of the African nations, Belgium, Ireland, and Malta. Regardless of the illegality, however, women in all parts of the world continue to use abortion to prevent unwanted births, often with serious illness or death as the result.

Health care for older women

Women's health care is now being recognized as extending considerably beyond the more traditional areas of obstetrics and gynecology that are geared to younger women; *e.g.*, contraception, pregnancy and childbirth, infertility, and regular Pap tests. Whereas the number of American woman aged 65 or older was

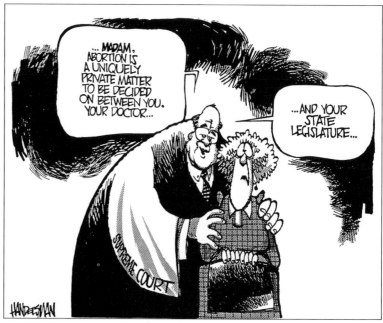

Walt Handelsman; reprinted by permission of Tribune Media Services

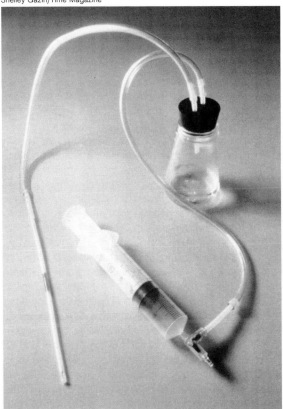

An alarming outcome of the increasing restrictions on legal abortions is that some women are opting to use a menstrual extraction kit that sells for $90 to carry out their own abortions.

one in 25 in 1990, it is estimated that one in 5 will be in the older population group by the year 2050. As women's life expectancy increases and postmenopausal women constitute an ever larger percentage of the population, it is appropriate and inevitable that health care be increasingly oriented to meeting their needs.

In the past few years, there has been a growing impetus for the increased use of hormone replacement therapy (HRT); this practice comes from the realization that the postmenopausal woman is in a state of chronic hormone deficiency. The short-term problems related to the loss of estrogen once the ovaries have become inactive include hot flushes, vaginal and urinary tract changes, mood changes, and sometimes headaches, insomnia, and fatigue. Most of these unpleasant, though not serious, symptoms are alleviated by the replacement of hormones. However, the main reason for the increased prescription of HRT is that the risk of more serious long-term effects of estrogen loss can be reduced. There is now substantial evidence that when this therapy is instituted around the time of or shortly after menopause and is continued for the remainder of a woman's life, there is significant prevention of osteoporosis; women treated with

HRT have about a 70% lower risk of fracture than those who are not treated for estrogen loss. Whereas women rarely suffer heart attacks before menopause, after menopause cardiovascular disease becomes the leading cause of death in American women. The evidence is growing that estrogen helps lower levels of low-density lipoprotein ("bad" cholesterol) and raise levels of high-density lipoprotein ("good" cholesterol), providing protection against cardiovascular disease.

A number of years ago, when estrogen was commonly used alone, an increased incidence of cancer of the endometrium, the lining of the uterus, was found. However, with the coadministration of a progestogen, which is the common practice today, this increased cancer risk is no longer a matter of concern. The major controversy surrounding HRT presently is whether the use of these agents is linked to breast cancer. Various studies over the past few years have come to diametrically opposite conclusions. Nonetheless, the majority consensus at the present time, drawn from the larger and better controlled studies, is that for most women HRT does not pose an added risk of cancer of the breast. In fact, a recent study by the CDC failed to show an increased breast cancer rate even among women receiving HRT who are typically classified at high risk for breast cancer—*i.e.,* those with breast cancer in their families, those who have benign breast disease, and those who have delayed childbearing or have never given birth.

The residual question is whether there are specific subgroups in the population who may be at increased cancer risk with the utilization of hormonal agents. Multiple studies are in the process of evaluating this question; firmer data should emerge within the next few years. In the meantime, it is generally agreed that the benefits of HRT in the prevention of osteoporosis and heart disease considerably outweigh the uncertain risks related to breast or any other form of cancer for the vast majority of postmenopausal women.

—Elizabeth B. Connell, M.D.

Osteoporosis

The realization of the importance of osteoporosis as a public health problem has prompted worldwide investigation into this disorder, which in the United States alone causes over one million fractures each year and affects millions of people, a significant proportion of them postmenopausal women. Osteoporosis is the thinning and increased porosity of the bones that occurs with aging. As the population in the developed countries ages, the number of individuals at risk can only be expected to increase. Thus, the magnitude of the problem is expected to grow as well. For this reason, osteoporosis has been the topic of a series of consensus conferences held in the U.S. and Europe during the past several years.

Bone remodeling: a cyclical process

Bone is a tissue that, in adults, is continually under-going remodeling, a process designed to fulfill at least two functions. The first is a kind of "preventive main-tenance," in which old, worn-out parts of the skeleton are replaced with young, resilient bone. The second function of remodeling is to ensure that an adequate level of calcium will be maintained in the blood should there be insufficient dietary sources. Remodeling oc-curs in cycles. The physiology and control of these cycles are still not completely understood, but for the former function it seems logical that control is ex-erted at the local level, while for the latter a more general regulation by the endocrine system can be conjectured. Loss of bone tissue occurs when there is an imbalance in the remodeling process such that the amount of bone formed at any remodeling site is less than the amount that has been resorbed (broken down and reassimilated) at that same site. The rate of net loss of bone tissue is dependent on the difference between resorption and formation, as well as the rate at which new remodeling sites are activated—on av-erage, one new remodeling cycle is activated every 10 seconds somewhere in the skeleton of a healthy adult.

Activation is a complex and little-understood pro-cess in which the cells covering the surface of bone retract and appear to resorb a small amount of bone, possibly releasing compounds that attract osteoclasts (the bone-resorbing cells) to the site. Osteoclasts at-tach to the bone surface and release acid that dis-solves the mineral of the bone. Enzymes then digest the collagenous matrix of the bone. After resorbing a certain set amount of bone, the osteoclasts disappear and are replaced by bone-forming cells, or osteoblasts. These cells form new nonmineralized bone (osteoid), which after about 20 days gradually mineralizes. A single complete remodeling cycle may take from four months to two years in normal individuals.

Bone loss is a universal phenomenon of aging, pro-ducing osteoporosis and predisposing elderly people to fractures. In a relatively sedentary person, there is more rapid activation of remodeling cycles and a shift at each remodeling site in favor of resorption. With disuse, therefore, bone loss proceeds rapidly. In a woman's body after menopause, there is a general-ized increase in activation that is not as great as that seen during disuse; however, it is also coupled with a shift in favor of resorption. The result is accelerated loss of bone. Remodeling is a surface process and, consequently, bone loss is greater in bone with the maximum surface area—the spongy, or cancellous, bone that makes up the bodies of the vertebrae and to a lesser extent the ends of the long bones. The result of this excessive loss is an increased incidence of fractures of the vertebral bodies (crush fractures), the distal radius (the bone on the thumb side of the forearm; Colles' fracture), and, eventually, the hip. Be-cause bone loss is generalized, however, and occurs in cortical bone also (the shafts of the long bones), fracture of any bone can occur.

Intriguing findings in the laboratory

Both local and systemic factors control the activation of remodeling sites and the cellular activity of osteoblasts and osteoclasts. The actions and interactions of the various cells involved are complex. One area of signifi-cant interest at present is the discovery that there is in-creased production of interleukin-1 by circulating white blood cells in women with osteoporosis. Interleukin-1 is one of a family of immune system proteins produced by many cell types but principally by the white blood cells known as monocytes. Interleukin-1 is a potent stimulator of the bone-destroying osteoclasts, while it inhibits osteoblast (bone-building) function. Monocytes are found in bone marrow, and often groups of mono-cytes are located close to the bone during at least part of the remodeling cycle. In the past few years, researchers have demonstrated not only increased production of interleukin-1 by monocytes immediately after the menopause but also the suppression of interleukin-1 production in these circulating cells af-ter treatment with estrogen. Increased bone loss in women after menopause and the preventive effect of estrogen on this bone loss have long been known and have been confirmed by many clinical studies. Further research is clearly required for confirmation of the role of interleukin in bone loss.

Recent studies have demonstrated that osteoblasts or osteoblast-like cells appear to have estrogen re-ceptors and may respond physiologically to low doses of the hormone. When human osteoblasts grown in laboratory culture are incubated with concentrations of estrogen, the concentration of another growth factor (called transforming growth factor beta, or TGF-β) is apparently increased. TGF-β is a recognized inhibitor of bone resorption. For the first time, therefore, med-ical scientists are now beginning to achieve some in-sight into the control of bone remodeling at the cellular level, which may eventually allow the development of new therapeutic approaches to osteoporosis.

Despite these findings, which have been observed only *in vitro* (outside the living body), the clinical ef-fects of estrogen are known to be compatible with reduced osteoclast function—something that cannot be demonstrated *in vitro*—i.e., by adding appropri-ate and physiological concentrations of estrogen to cultured osteoclasts. Thus, not only are estrogen re-ceptors present on the "wrong" cell type (osteoblasts) but the physiological response to estrogen by these cells, *in vitro*, is not what would be predicted from knowledge of clinical response to treatment, as the activity of both osteoblasts and osteoclasts declines during estrogen treatment.

It is tempting to speculate that when menopause

occurs, and estrogen levels fall, there is increased production and secretion of interleukin-1 by monocytes within bone marrow, thereby stimulating osteoclast activity, and that the reverse occurs when estrogens are given as therapy. However, monocytes do not appear to have estrogen receptors, suggesting that if this hypothesis is correct a further step would be required. An alternative scenario might be that decreased production of TGF-β (which inhibits bone resorption) by osteoblasts after menopause leads to increased activity of osteoclasts and, therefore, to bone loss. It remains to be seen if either, both, or neither one of these processes is indeed responsible for bone loss. Further, there are other "chemical messengers," for example, the insulin-like growth factors, that may also play a role in control of bone remodeling.

Estrogen: mainstay of preventive therapy

Estrogen currently remains the main therapeutic agent used in prevention of osteoporosis. Further assessment of the risks and benefits of estrogen therapy is ongoing, supported in the U.S. primarily by the National Institutes of Health (NIH). Estrogens are potent hormones that have wide-ranging effects in the body beyond their effects on bone; it is, therefore, important that estrogen therapy in postmenopausal women be studied prospectively in a large population of healthy women.

Now that most estrogen replacement therapy regimens almost routinely have a progestogen component to reduce the risk of endometrial cancer, it has become necessary to closely monitor the effects of the therapy on the risk of cardiovascular disease. Estrogen therapy prescribed by itself has been associated with a reduced risk of coronary heart disease; the addition of progestogens could potentially reduce or negate this beneficial effect. Estrogens improve the lipid profile of the blood, raising the level of high-density lipoproteins (HDL) and lowering low-density lipoproteins (LDL), and may thereby reduce the risk of atherosclerosis. Progestogens, depending on dose, tend to negate these effects. If, however, estrogen reduces cardiovascular risk by direct effects through estrogen receptors in blood vessels, then progestogens would not be expected to negate these effects. Further study is required, as the cardioprotective effects clearly outweigh all other benefits and risks of estrogen therapy.

The possible effects of estrogen therapy on the risk of breast malignancy are still under debate. There is much equivocal information in this area. Still, if treatment with hormones does indeed alter the risk, the effect cannot be too great, or the epidemiological studies would have been expected to find more evidence of it. A Swedish study published in 1989 only added to the already existing confusion. While demonstrating a small increase in breast cancer risk associated with

the potent estrogens used in Europe, the investigators failed to find any change in risk associated with the use of conjugated equine estrogen, the more common therapy in the U.S. The researchers attributed the latter finding to the small number of patients receiving the conjugated estrogen treatment. They suggested, however, that the addition of progestogens would not prevent estrogen's effects on breast tissue. While this speculation is also borne out by other studies of cellular response, much further work is needed before the effects of combined estrogen-progestogen therapy can be completely understood.

New strategies for prevention

The development of a nasal-spray mode of delivery for calcitonin, a peptide hormone normally synthesized in the thyroid gland, may shortly give U.S. physicians an alternative to estrogen for prevention of bone loss. Calcitonin delivered by this route has not yet been given Food and Drug Administration (FDA) approval for use in osteoporosis, although it has been used for many years for the treatment of Paget's disease (another bone disease associated with local increases in remodeling) and to treat high blood calcium levels (hypercalcemia) when caused by excessive bone resorption produced by some cancers. In the past, however, it was necessary to administer calcitonin by daily injection. Preliminary data indicate that when

This magazine ad powerfully conveys the extent and seriousness of the health problem posed by osteoporosis—especially for the growing number of older women who constitute the population at greatest risk.

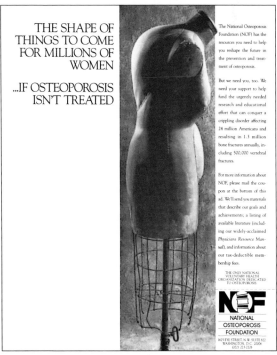

National Osteoporosis Foundation

Osteoporosis

Adapted from Tommy Storm et al., "Effect of Intermittent Cyclical Etidronate Therapy. . .," New England Journal of Medicine, vol. 322, no. 18 (May 3, 1990), pp. 1265–71

given by nasal spray this peptide hormone specifically reduces bone loss without causing the other wide-ranging effects of estrogens. It remains to be seen if the beneficial effect can be substantiated in long-term studies. It must also be determined whether compliance with intranasal administration will become a problem in the long term, since the treatment would have to be continued over a period of several years to significantly reduce fractures. Further in the future, it is hoped, will be a method to administer such proteins by mouth, protecting them from destruction by digestive enzymes and acid in the stomach but allowing their absorption via the intestine.

More recent developments in the area of prevention and treatment of osteoporosis include the use of bisphosphonates, chemical compounds that were originally by-products of soap manufacture. Bisphosphonates resemble the naturally occurring biphosphates but have a carbon atom instead of an oxygen atom between two phosphorus atoms as the "backbone" of the molecule. The molecule then becomes resistant to the action of alkaline phosphatase, the enzyme that splits biphosphates produced in the body. Bisphosphonates (sometimes called diphosphonates) adhere to bone and are thought to be devoured by osteoclasts as they resorb bone mineral. Once inside the osteoclast, these compounds act as cell inhibitors or poisons and thus slow the rate of bone resorption. Preliminary data suggest that bisphosphonates may be useful oral agents in prevention of bone loss and could provide another alternative therapy in the future. One bisphosphonate, etidronate, or EHDP (Didronel), is currently marketed for the treatment of Paget's disease and hypercalcemia in the same way as calcitonin and has recently been shown to prevent bone loss in patients with osteoporosis.

Stimulating bone formation

Treatment of osteoporosis once fractures of the spine or hip have begun remains problematic. Destruction of the basic architecture of the skeleton is often so extensive that the therapies now available do not work well. Antiresorptive agents, estrogen, calcitonin, and possibly bisphosphonates remain the first choice for both prevention and treatment, but none of these is capable of rebuilding the skeleton or repairing the damaged architecture. Considerable attention is currently being focused on agents that show some promise of stimulating new bone formation. The most advanced of these is sodium fluoride, which has been available for many years and is used in low doses during pregnancy and early childhood to prevent tooth decay. In much larger doses, fluoride stimulates bone formation, principally in the spongy bone of the central skeleton. If administered in large doses or for long periods of time, fluoride produces a bone disorder known as fluorosis, which is endemic in some parts of India

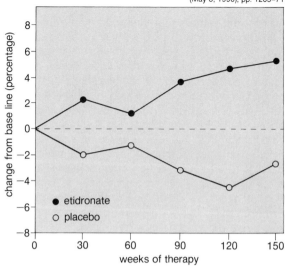

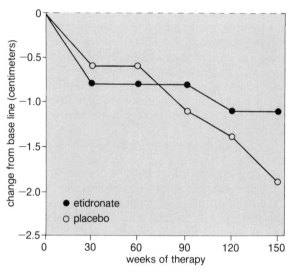

In a three-year study of treatment for postmenopausal osteoporosis, Swedish researchers found that vertebral bone mineral content increased significantly in women who received the bisphosphonate drug etidronate but decreased in the placebo group (top). The height of those in the treatment group remained relatively stable, while there was marked decline among those taking placebo (above).

because of environmental pollution with fluoride and which causes excessive abnormal bone growth and calcification of tendons and ligaments. Patients with fluorosis experience considerable pain, are relatively immobile, and easily develop fractures.

Clearly, fluoride must be used carefully. Even in doses now being used clinically at some centers, there have been reports of considerable side effects from fluoride treatment, including gastric irritation and, occasionally, bleeding, as well as pains around the joints of the lower limbs thought to be caused by tiny fractures in the spongy bone that forms the ends of the long bones. A new slow-release form of sodium fluoride, which passes through the stomach without causing side effects and then releases fluoride slowly in the intestine, is being studied in clinical trials at several medical centers. According to one recent report on the new treatment, while this form of fluoride appears to have fewer gastric side effects than traditional fluoride therapy, the increases in bone mass do not appear to be as great as those achieved previously. The study suggests a reduction in fractures with treatment, but the lack of control data (*i.e.,* data comparing the progress of treated and untreated individuals) limits the conclusions that can be drawn.

The results of two well-controlled studies, both sponsored by the NIH, were even less promising. While the expected increases in bone mass of the spine were seen in the fluoride-treated groups, there were no reductions in the incidence of spinal fractures in these groups. Indeed, one of these studies showed an insignificant increase in peripheral fractures, especially fractures of the hip. Previous uncontrolled studies suggested the same outcome. For the present time, at least, sodium fluoride should not be used for routine treatment of individuals with spinal osteoporosis, and fluoride use in the U.S. should be limited to clinical trial settings. Fluoride remains a therapy used in other countries (principally in Europe), where physicians are more confident of the outcome and where it is felt that the dose of fluoride used and perhaps the study design were responsible for the negative findings of U.S. studies.

Parathyroid hormone is an endocrine agent that may prove useful in stimulating bone formation in people with osteoporosis. This may seem paradoxical, as the primary effect of parathyroid hormone is to stimulate osteoclastic bone resorption. However, this increase in resorption is apparently coupled with an increase in bone formation. Studies of the bone tissue of patients with primary hyperparathyroidism (a condition characterized by excessive secretion of parathyroid hormone) have revealed maintenance of and, in a significant proportion of cases, an increase in cancellous bone mass. Preliminary studies of the treatment of osteoporotic men with parathyroid hormone have yielded encouraging results. Now that large quantities of synthetic human parathyroid hormone are available—produced through genetic engineering techniques—it will be possible to assess the efficacy of this agent in the treatment of osteoporosis. A related peptide produced as a by-product of some cancers may be another possible protein that could be used in therapy.

There is one other experimental treatment being tried that is based on the theory that the process of bone remodeling can be controlled and exploited in such a way as to produce bone formation. It has been hypothesized that if a large number of remodeling sites could be activated at the same time, the process could

then be modified by therapeutic agents. Because all remodeling cycles would be in the resorption phase at the same time, antiresorptive agents could be used during the expected duration of this portion of the cycle. The theory is that the osteoclasts would then resorb less bone, and the resorption cavities they create in the bone would be correspondingly shallower. Therapy would then be stopped, and the second portion of the cycle, the formation period, would begin; in this phase the osteoblasts would lay down their preprogrammed amount of bone. Since less bone would have been resorbed but a normal amount of bone synthesized, the bone balance at each remodeling site would be positive. The whole process—synchronous activation of remodeling cycles, depression of the resorption phase, and overfilling of the resorption cavities—could be repeated as often as necessary to rebuild the skeleton.

Several studies of this treatment in patients with osteoporosis have been initiated. It is not yet clear, however, if remodeling cycles can be activated synchronously; nor is it known whether once the antiresorptive agent has been discontinued, the osteoclasts will increase their activity in order to complete a cavity of normal depth. In addition, there is no evidence that osteoblasts are indeed preprogrammed; they may have the ability to adjust their production to the reduced size of the cavity. In other words, the amount of bone synthesized may not be as great as proponents of this theory expect. Indeed, there are so many unknowns about this form of treatment that actual clinical studies may be premature.

Future developments

It is clear that significant advances are now being made in the understanding of bone physiology and the underlying processes in osteoporosis. At the current rate of progress, it seems likely that novel therapeutic approaches to the treatment of osteoporosis will be in development throughout the 1990s. It is important to remember that most hip fractures occur as the result of falls and that the incidence of falls increases with age. Measures to prevent elderly persons from falling and suffering consequent injury may therefore be a practical and reasonable approach to this public health problem. Improvements in nutrition, increases in physical activity, and reductions in alcohol and drug use—including some prescription drugs that cause dizziness or impair balance—might be expected to reduce the likelihood of falls. Attention to the older person's eyesight, hearing, and balance and to his or her home environment (eliminating hazards such as loose rugs, trailing electrical cords, poor lighting, and sharp corners on furniture) is also a measure that might be expected to help reduce the impact of osteoporosis on the aging population.

—Robert Lindsay, M.D., Ph.D.

Computer Consultants: The Future of Medical Decision Making?

by Diana Brahams, Barrister-at-Law, and Jeremy Wyatt, M.A.

The autonomy that doctors have previously enjoyed is being challenged. The wide-ranging reasons include the explosion of medical knowledge that has occurred in the past decade and doctors' sheer inability to keep up with it, the sharply escalating costs of medical care and the crucial need to contain them, the unrestrained use of diagnostic testing, and the malpractice "crisis," reflected by excessive litigation. In addition, evidence that medical opinions can vary widely, even over major issues, has focused attention on how doctors make decisions and how those decisions can be improved. One possible solution being investigated is the computer as an aid for medical decision making. Already this solution is being employed successfully—albeit on a limited basis.

Computers of various sorts have been widely used in health care for many years, but traditionally their role has been to store and process administrative rather than clinical data; in hospitals, for example, they are widely used in patient billing, accounting, and medical records departments. Now, however, increasing numbers of medical centers and clinics are computerizing their clinical data. These medical data bases do not themselves advise medical practitioners about individual diagnostic or management problems of patients, but they have been used as the basis for a number of computer decision aids that do.

The following scenario will help clarify the distinction between the use of computers for data storage and as decision aids.

A doctor at a hospital-based clinic has a desk-top computer that is linked up to the hospital's information system. When Tom C., a patient with diabetes, goes to his doctor's office, the doctor types in an identity number for him, and the system uses its data base to display previously stored information on Tom C.: complete medical history, including earlier diagnoses and conditions he has been treated for as well as any complications. Because Tom C.'s diabetes is poorly controlled, the doctor decides to adjust his insulin dosage. He enters the proposed regimen; the computer then utilizes a mathematical model that takes into account such data as the patient's weight, the type of diabetes he has, and its duration, along with the proposed insulin dosage and timing of dosages, to predict Tom C.'s blood sugar levels at six key times during the day. The decision aid then assesses these predictions against standard clinical data for this kind of patient, in this case an insulin-dependent male with diabetes, overweight, age 39—and reports its findings: "Predicted blood glucose levels all within the correct range." The system also informs the doctor of the advisability of annual screenings for ophthalmic and renal disease for diabetic patients of Tom's age whose condition has been present for as long as Tom's has. The doctor chooses to wait to order tests until the next appointment, when the adjusted insulin regimen will be assessed.

Here the computer has used its stored medical knowledge and data on an individual patient to act as a helpful colleague—an endocrinologist with expertise in diabetes management—assisting the practitioner in making crucial decisions about an optimal treatment approach for Tom C.

Medical expertise computerized

To build a decision aid, one starts either with a source of expertise—a textbook or a live expert—or with data gathered from patients. A third approach that is gaining ground with the highly sophisticated programming techniques that are now available is to combine expert knowledge and patient data.

One of the first medical decision aids was built by a group of doctors from LDS (Latter-day Saints) Hospital, in Salt Lake City, Utah, who added programs to a hospital-wide information system geared to alert doctors to abnormal laboratory results and potential adverse drug reactions, advise on the management of fluid balance in patients in the intensive care unit, and assist in diagnosis. This "HELP" system is now disseminated to four other medical centers in Utah. Evaluations have shown that it improves both the process and the outcome of patient care—for example, by providing early warnings of about 50 adverse drug reactions per month. This system remains one of the most extensive and best-evaluated medical decision aids.

Another type of decision aid in current use is based on clinical algorithms, or protocols, which can be computerized. These are step-by-step flow charts that evaluate individual symptoms, usually composed of a series of boxes that pose yes-or-no questions and lead in an orderly progression along one of various paths, ultimately arriving at a terminal box that provides a medical diagnosis or an appropriate treatment. Paper versions of such algorithms are particularly appropriate for use by "barefoot doctors" (health care providers with limited training) in less developed countries; their use has enabled such paraprofessional workers to be as much as five times more efficient in evaluating and treating patients. Algorithms, however, can cover only a limited range of diseases and can be overly simplistic in their analyses.

Knowledge-based, or "expert," systems are an alternative way of encoding expertise. Most of the early expert systems addressed medical problems, but nowadays they are used in fields ranging from archaeology to aerospace science. To create such a system, an expert, e.g., a medical specialist, works with a "knowledge engineer" to record his or her knowledge in a program that can then be accessed by, say, a junior doctor or paramedic for use in solving a specific problem concerning a specific patient. Because the knowledge is recorded in an explicit form, the system can explain to the user how it arrived at a certain answer, how this might differ if the details of the case varied, and why any particular item of data is needed for arriving at the answer. The expert's knowledge thus may take a form such as: "IF the patient has recent onset abdominal pain AND the pain has begun in the small of the back AND the pain moved to the groin, THEN a possible diagnosis is urinary tract infection." In medical centers where knowledge-based systems of this kind are in use, they have been shown to improve the quality of patient data collected and of decisions made. Examples of medical expert systems include ONCOCIN, which helps doctors to administer complex chemotherapy regimens to patients at the Stanford Oncology Center; QMR and DXplain, which assist physicians with diagnoses by producing ranked lists of possible diseases based on patient findings; and HT-Advisor, which assists in the ambulatory care of patients with high blood pressure. A disadvantage of any expertise-derived system, however, is that it can be difficult to harvest the knowledge of experts; moreover, one expert's knowledge may not reflect the experience of doctors elsewhere.

An alternative is to build decision aids that, instead of relying on experts' opinions, are based on facts derived from sample cases. This approach has been used in the building of many medical decision aids. First, data are collected from, say, patients seeking treatment for abdominal pain, who are all followed up to find out the true cause of their pain. A statistical technique such as Bayes theorem is then used to identify which symptoms and signs are associated with each diagnosis. (Bayes theorem relates the probability that an individual patient has a particular diagnosis [e.g., urinary tract infection], given the presence of certain attributes [e.g., the patient is a male, and the pain started in the small of the back and then moved to the groin], to the established finding that male patients with urinary tract infections typically manifest that type and course of pain.) Providing that enough accurate data are available and that certain assumptions are not violated, such a decision aid can correctly classify a large proportion of patients.

One of the best established of these is an abdominal pain diagnosis system developed in Leeds, England, through the use of data from nearly 50,000 cases collected over 20 years. This Bayesian system assists junior surgeons in diagnosing emergency patients with abdominal pain and was recently subjected to a trial in 11 British hospitals. While the system was in use, many fewer incorrect diagnoses were made than had been prior to the system's use. For example, the number of perforated appendixes resulting from doctors' not recognizing appendicitis fell by half, as did the number of unnecessary operations for misdiagnosed appendicitis, and patients experienced shorter hospital stays. Some of these changes may have been due to the fact that the junior doctors, who were using a printed questionnaire to collate information for the system, took more time and trouble than usual over their diagnoses in order to collect more complete data (the so-called checklist effect). However, the decision aid itself was deemed to be responsible for most of the improvements seen, and it is now in use in 20 hospitals across the U.K. and, in a modified form, in U.S.-owned nuclear submarines. Other similar systems, based on fewer cases, have met with only limited success.

Another statistical system, GLADYS, helps doctors to distinguish between the causes of indigestion. In this case the patients interact directly with the computer; they are interviewed by a computer and input their symptoms by means of a relatively simple keyboard. These data are then transformed into various "weights of evidence," which are totaled to give a probability for each possible diagnosis. Studies on the data collected by this system revealed that patients were more open about their alcohol intake—an important factor that is often *not* revealed—to the computer than to their doctors. This increased honesty with computers has been confirmed in other studies.

The Glasgow Coma System uses another analysis technique to estimate patient survival probability following severe head trauma. In studies involving thousands of patients from several countries, the system's predictions were remarkably accurate, and it is now routinely used by neurosurgeons to help them to plan their strategies for managing head-injured patients and to counsel relatives on likely outcomes. A system developed at the Mayo Clinic in Rochester, Minn., provides survival odds for patients with serious liver disease; it is expected to help in the allocation of the scarce supply of donated organs for transplantation by determining those patients most likely to benefit.

A number of other classification or "pattern-recognition" techniques, such as computer simulations of the neural networks found in human brains, are being investigated as medical decision aids. These, however, may gain only limited acceptance because the systems, as presently formulated, cannot explain their conclusions. This is a significant failing, as doctors need to know the justification for any particular advice, as well as what information the system has used in its analysis, in order to assess its applicability to individual patients.

Limitations and prospects

Patients nowadays may be quite used to doctors' consulting other sources of information—seeking advice from the medical literature or from colleagues. The idea of seeking advice from computers, however, is new. Certain doubts and questions about this new method of deriving medical information naturally arise: What problems might these systems cause? What evidence is there that they actually help patients? And what legal implications might their use have on hospitals and doctors?

The developers of medical decision aids may feel that their system is sure to help doctors and patients. However, like drugs, decision aids can have side effects; among those that have been cited are that doctors may become too reliant on them, thus losing some of their skills, and that their use will result in patients having more tests done—many of which are unnecessary and costly. Decision aids thus need to be subjected to randomized controlled trials, just as other new medical procedures and technologies are. However, unlike other technologies, decision aids can affect patients only indirectly—*i.e.*, by influencing decision makers. This makes the design of such trials quite complex, as certain factors that could have a bearing, such as the checklist effect mentioned above, need to be taken into account.

In studies that have evaluated these methods thus far, the benefits of decision aids have usually outweighed their disadvantages. For example, the QMR system, developed at the University of Pittsburgh, Pa., was recently evaluated at the Veterans Administration Medical Center in Pittsburgh. It was concluded that "the system provided reasonable diagnostic suggestions not previously considered by the ward teams and these suggestions were valued sufficiently to cause alteration of the original differential diagnoses."

However, decision aids require large resources to develop and test—up to 20 man-years, even for a system that assists with only a limited range of decisions—thus, only a few are yet commercial prospects. Other limitations include their lack of common sense, instinct, and flair and the fact that their recommendations may be too cautious to be useful. Although expert systems incorporate a fair amount of flexibility and are capable of using symbolic reasoning to explain their conclusions, most systems thus far have not been of practical value, perhaps because in the designing of many of the programs, the inherent difficulty of mastering medical knowledge has been underestimated.

Various developments may improve matters, though. For example, new techniques will allow experts to load their knowledge directly into an expert system, without the intervention of a "knowledge engineer," and systems may soon begin to reason by analogy and to fine-tune their reasoning from recent experiences. The poor performance of these systems outside specific specialty areas and the rigidity of their explanations should to some extent be alleviated by the incorporation of more detailed knowledge about human physiology and anatomy and drug mechanisms and by new programming that will enable the systems to "reason" about symptom or disease changes over periods of time—facets upon which doctors rely extensively. Additionally, large systems tend to operate slowly and are prone to making errors, but developments in programming and in the automatic validation of knowledge bases are expected to minimize some of these difficulties.

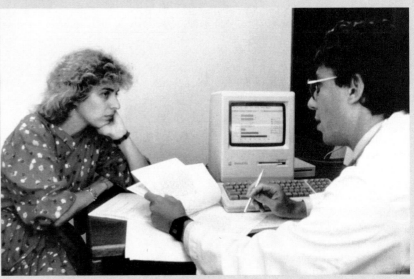

Here a physician has consulted a computer decision aid to assist him in a potential cancer diagnosis. Some proponents predict that as a new tool in medicine such aids may eventually become as necessary to doctors as the stethoscope. If so, the important question arises: Who will be liable if the advice provided is wrong?

A further obstacle to wider use of decision aids thus far has been the reluctance of physicians to give up some of their autonomy; moreover, few have had adequate training in the use of computers in their daily practices. However, the acceptability of these systems may ultimately depend on a different issue entirely: Who will be liable if the wrong advice is given?

Litigious medical climate

The law does not expect medical treatment to guarantee success or a perfect result, so unless a health care provider or a manufacturer of medical equipment is unwise enough to warrant this, an unsuccessful or less than perfect outcome will not in itself provide the basis for a claim in damages. Nonetheless, many patients' expectations about their cases are unrealistically high and, perhaps ironically, as medical techniques improve, litigation against doctors and manufacturers of medical products increases. This has been particularly so in the United States, where many health care providers and, in turn, many consumers of health care services now feel the situation is out of hand. For example, the cost of medical malpractice insurance for a surgeon or an obstetrician for one year can run to $130,000 or more—a cost that is passed on to patients in fees charged. In some cases doctors have stopped providing certain services altogether. Many U.S. obstetricians, to avoid the high risk of malpractice suits, have stopped delivering babies. Additionally, product liability suits have forced pharmaceutical companies and manufacturers of medical devices to curtail development of valuable drugs and products, resulting in vastly limited options for consumers—for example, in availability of contraceptives.

As a result of the rising tide of litigation, there is concern with regard to the legal implications arising from the design and use of computer programs intended to assist with the process of medical decision making. The speed and extent of the development of this new technology on a commercial basis will likely be affected by its legal status.

Product or service?

One key question is whether a decision-aid program and any advice it provides—be it on disk, on screen, or on a printed page—should be regarded (primarily) as a product or as a service. The legal and commercial consequences of such a distinction may be very important in the future. This may be more true in the United States than in some other countries because of the strictness of the U.S. product-licensing laws and of legal liability for "products." (In Britain and other European countries, licensing laws tend to be more relaxed.) So far, however, the U.S. Food and Drug Administration (FDA), the federal agency charged with the regulation of medicines and medical devices, has not deemed decision aids to be within its scope. The FDA has stated that its control extends only to software that "enables a computing machine to control, monitor, or otherwise interact with a medical device." As products that allow competent human interaction, decision aids in the U.S. do not now require approval, nor are they subject to government regulation.

Technically, the mechanism within the computer that enables it to calculate is a product—as is the disk that houses it—whereas its output or advice may be regarded as a service. It is, however, uncertain whether the courts in Britain or the U.S. would define any advice provided or printed out of a computerized decision aid in itself as a product. However, indications are that the U.S. courts would be more likely to do this than the British courts and that they would also be more inclined than their British counterparts to find the manufacturers of the decision aid liable if the advice proved to be incorrect or in some way harmful to a patient.

In the U.S., if the program and any advice it offers are held to be products rather than part of the medical services provided by the doctor or hospital, liability may be proved more readily and legal retribution may be greater than they would be in a case of professional negligence. Frequently when U.S. juries have found medical products defective, they not only have awarded generous compensatory damages to the plaintiff but also have levied massive punitive damages against manufacturers if it was deemed that a company had been irresponsible in marketing faulty merchandise.

In the U.K., too, there may be stricter liability for a "defective" product than for a service that fails to satisfy the consumer, but punitive damages are not allowed; judges assess awards for personal injuries on a purely compensatory basis. Further, the stricter liability for defective products has been much watered down by the "development-risks" defense (sometimes called the "state of the art" defense). This allows the developers and manufacturers, particularly of new and innovative technologies and medicines—which may cause unforeseeable injury—to avoid liability if the defect was not one they could reasonably have determined or discovered in advance. The defense was included in the new legislation concerning defective products (the U.K. Consumer Protection Act, which commenced on March 1, 1988)—in order not to discourage innovation, invention, technological advance, and commercial investment. (A defective product in Britain is defined as one that is not as safe as might *reasonably* have been expected.)

In a program designed to assist medical decision making, there is generally not a distinct line that can be drawn between the elements of advice and product, either pragmatically, as a matter of strict principle, or by way of analogy. In cases that come before the law, decisions regarding advice versus product are likely to vary according to the circumstances and the nature of the claims that are being made. For instance, some years ago the English Court of Appeal debated the question of whether badly fitting false teeth were goods or a service. Unfortunately, the point was never finally decided, as it was not material to the issue of whether any payment was due to the dentist for the teeth. It could be argued, however, that the teeth were both a product and a service that the dentist had contracted to provide. The product element would be relevant if the dentures were made of a material that caused harm, whereas the design and fit constituted the advice, or service, element—i.e., the dental expertise (allegedly lacking in this case).

Many legal experts believe that the most logical approach to adopt with regard to computer programs aimed at assisting in the process of medical decision making is to view the advice extracted from such a program, which is then utilized by a doctor in deciding on a particular patient's treatment, as a service or an opinion—just as it would be if the doctor had taken it from a manual of treatment or medical textbook or received it from a colleague; this should include the calculations made in order to tailor the information derived to the therapeutic regimen established by the doctor for the individual patient.

Poor advice: who is responsible?

Physicians who use decision aids must satisfy themselves that the advice seems reasonable and appropriate, and they must exercise reasonable skill and care when assessing and applying it, just as they would with advice obtained and given in other circumstances. It is uncertain whether any error (involving negligence or not) would in itself be actionable against the supplier or writer of the program if the alleged faulty information caused injury and the patient chose to sue.

In what may be viewed as precedents, in the 1950s the English Court of Appeal postulated that a marine hydrographer would not be liable for the omission of a reef in his charting of a body of water that caused the wreck of an ocean liner. However, in the case of the shipwreck of the Australian vessel *The Willemstad* (1976), 227 producers of a navigation plotting chart were held liable at first instance. In *Brocklesby* v. *U.S.* (1955) the publisher of an inaccurate instrument approach chart for aircraft was held liable for a crash on strict product liability and negligence theory. Likewise, in cases concerning medical decision aids, experts and producers of computer programs that are designed to aid doctors or hospitals—and indeed their patients—would be an identifiable class that the courts could include or exclude for the purposes of liability.

Once it can be established that computer decision aids can improve the quality of medical services, it may become standard for practitioners to have them at hand, and their use may be required when an occasion warrants it. Failure to use equipment that is available and that in a specific instance could have improved a patient's condition—or even saved a life—could in itself constitute negligence. This occurred recently in the U.S. when an obstetrician was held negligent because he failed to use fetal monitoring and X-ray pelvimetry equipment that would have indicated the need to perform a cesarean section; his injudicious use of forceps during a vaginal delivery led to the baby's suffering trauma and brain damage. Similarly, in a British case a coroner presented evidence that a dental anesthetist neglected to use some of the resuscitation equipment that he had available—the result being that the patient died.

If and when computerized medical decision aids are accepted as necessary equipment for patient care, failure to use one, to use it competently or appropriately, to maintain it properly, or to ensure that its advice complies with current medical thinking could lead to a suit in negligence. Whether incorrect advice or information offered by a computer program will be actionable will depend on many variables, including the state of the art of medicine at the time as well as the physician's expected or notional level of professional expertise. The indications so far are that the consumer-oriented juries and powerful consumer lobbies in the U.S. will make the American courts more ready and willing to hold professionals and manufacturers liable than would be the case in the British courts. Whether this new ripple in the medicolegal arena is a desirable one for progress as a whole is another question.

The future

Despite doubts over their legal status, the use of medical decision aids seems likely to grow in the years to come. This is especially true in areas of medicine in which vast sums of detailed knowledge must be accessed—e.g., for the interpretation of complex test results or in the classification of genetic anomalies. On the other hand, clinical areas involving more wide-ranging problems such as general practice or very urgent problems such as emergency medicine will prove more difficult niches for the relatively narrow, generally slow systems that can currently be built.

With around two dozen medical decision aids already of proven effectiveness and in use, one may expect to see problems emerge, such as overreliance on the advice given. However, more sophisticated systems that complement rather than replace users' own abilities may avoid this. Advances that are rapidly being made in technology and in the designing of statistical and knowledge-based systems will make it easier to build, maintain, and upgrade medical decision aids. Systems that are currently being developed in academic centers will be distributed more widely. Eventually, such systems may even become as necessary to medical practice as the stethoscope and X-ray equipment.

Pediatrics

Important studies published in the past year contributed to better understanding of a number of pediatric issues, among them the long-term effects of the antiepileptic drug phenobarbital, the importance of vision testing in preschool children, and the potential for spontaneous abortion in susceptible pregnant women exposed to youngsters with the childhood infection known as fifth disease. Researchers around the world continued to work toward developing an improved vaccine against pertussis (whooping cough), but recent studies—and a reevaluation of earlier data—indicated that the concern over neurological complications attributed to the current vaccine may not be valid. An alarming increase in the number of measles cases in the United States in 1989 and a study of measles immunization in Haiti underlined the importance of a worldwide effort to vaccinate children against this common, but sometimes deadly, childhood disease. Finally, a pediatrician, Antonia Novello, was appointed surgeon general in the U.S., replacing C. Everett Koop, a pediatric surgeon.

Phenobarbital: new concerns

The drug phenobarbital (Belladenal; Bellergal; Donnatal; Mudrane) has been used for many generations in the treatment of children with epilepsy. It has also been prescribed for some young children who have had febrile seizures, or fever convulsions—seizures associated with a rise in body temperature to over 38° C (100.4° F). While febrile seizures do recur in a certain percentage of children, they are not usually regarded as a convulsive disorder. Until very recently, however, phenobarbital has been used prophylactically, to prevent recurrence of seizures, in both children with epilepsy and those who have had a febrile seizure.

Doctors do not know why some youngsters have convulsions when fever develops while others do not; genetic susceptibility appears to play a part in some cases. Children who have a single febrile seizure may never have a recurrence, even during high fever. Early age of onset of febrile seizures (under 12 months of age) suggests that the convulsions may recur. When seizures do recur during subsequent fevers, some physicians prescribe anticonvulsive medication to be taken daily until the child is about five years old.

Since the advent of phenobarbital, many other antiepileptic drugs have become available: primidone (Mysoline), phenytoin (Dilantin, Diphenylan), carbamazepine (Tegretol), valproate (Depakene). Because of this choice of antiepileptics, it has been possible for researchers to conduct studies comparing them not only for their anticonvulsive properties but also for their long-term effects on children's intelligence (cognition), behavior, and mood. In 1987 investigators at Johns Hopkins University Hospital, Baltimore, Md., compared

children taking valproate and those on phenobarbital. This study showed that behavior and cognitive function were superior in children taking valproate. Another more recent study focused on phenobarbital treatment in children with a history of febrile seizures. Half of the children studied took phenobarbital daily; the other half took a placebo. After two years the youngsters on phenobarbital scored an average of 8.4 points lower on an IQ test than did children in the placebo group. The researchers, who were from the University of Washington School of Medicine and the National Institute of Neurological Disorders and Stroke, Bethesda, Md., concluded that the adverse effects of phenobarbital were not offset by the benefit of seizure prevention. (The proportion of children having seizure recurrences was approximately the same in both treated and untreated groups.) These findings are likely to discourage the use of phenobarbital for prevention of febrile seizures and may ultimately result in a reevaluation of its place in anticonvulsive therapy.

Vitamins and neural tube defects: controversy rekindled

In early prenatal life, when the embryo is about 20 days old, the nervous system consists of a neural groove, which then closes to form what is called the neural tube. Failure of the groove to close at one end causes a defect in the skull of the developing fetus, absence of part of the brain, or both; the most severe form of this particular defect is called anencephaly. Newborns with this condition have no cerebrum and, if not stillborn, inevitably die within a few days. More commonly, the neural tube fails to close at the other end, causing spinal defects such as spina bifida (exposure of the spinal cord through an opening anywhere from the lower back to the neck) or meningomyelocele, a condition in which the spinal cord and the membranes that normally enclose the brain protrude through an opening in the back. Depending on the location along the length of the spine and the extent of the defect, the child's eventual disability will be more or less severe. Fortunately, neurosurgery—especially if done soon after birth—can repair some of these defects and prevent the development of hydrocephalus (fluid collecting in the brain). All of these malformations are known collectively as neural tube defects (NTDs).

Although the cause of NTDs is not fully understood, there is a genetic component. Women who have had one child with a neural tube defect have a higher than average risk of bearing another with the condition. Other factors may be involved in the development of NTDs—it is known that at least one drug, aminopterin (an anticancer drug), if it is taken in early pregnancy, can cause spina bifida. (For this reason, the drug is not available for therapeutic use in the U.S.) In addition, for reasons not understood, NTDs occur more frequently in certain geographic areas. Because of the higher rate of NTDs in the United Kingdom, many studies of these conditions have been conducted there.

Data collected in Europe after World War II showed that dietary deficiencies, caused by wartime food shortages, were associated with an increased incidence of NTDs. A deficiency in one nutrient in particular, folic acid, was implicated in the development of NTDs. Because of evidence showing that women who take multivitamin-folic acid supplements before and during pregnancy are less likely to have children with NTDs, numerous studies have been undertaken over the past 30 or 40 years to conclusively prove or disprove the efficacy of such supplements in preventing NTDs.

In the past year alone there were a number of well-designed studies of this issue, which, interestingly, came to conflicting conclusions. In 1989 a British study of women in the Yorkshire area found that dietary supplementation with vitamins and folic acid protected against the development of NTDs. The National Institute of Child Health and Human Development of the U.S. National Institutes of Health (NIH), and other participating institutions, also published research on NTDs in 1989. This showed that women who took vitamins and folic acid around the time of conception did not decrease their risk of having an infant with an NTD. A still more recent U.S. study supported the use of vitamin supplements. This investigation, conducted in the Boston area by researchers from several cooperating institutions, showed that among women who took a folic acid-containing multivitamin preparation before and during the first six weeks of pregnancy, the prevalence of NTDs decreased by more than 50%. The difference was most striking among women with a family history of NTDs. One of the Boston researchers felt that the negative results in the NIH study could have been a result of memory bias; because the women had been interviewed as much as five months after they

gave birth, those whose infants had been diagnosed with an NTD might have been more likely to remember their failure to take the supplements faithfully. A large-scale study now under way in the U.K. may resolve these discrepant findings.

Several aspects of this issue remain to be studied and clarified—among them, whether supplements are useful or effective only when taken prior to conception and during the first six weeks of pregnancy, providing no further protection against NTDs when taken throughout the course of the pregnancy. Also not yet clear is whether multivitamin supplements lacking folic acid have a preventive effect. Finally, physicians do not agree on the question of prescribing supplements for pregnant women who have no prior history of giving birth to a child with an NTD.

Benefits of early vision testing

In 1945, in the first edition of his *Common Sense Book of Baby and Child Care,* Benjamin Spock recommended that children have their vision tested, either at school or in the doctor's office, each year after age six. Current recommendations, however, call for starting vision testing much earlier—at two to three years of age. Newborns who are at special risk for eye problems such as retinopathy of prematurity (formerly called retrolental fibroplasia—a form of damage to the retina that occurs almost exclusively in premature infants) or those with a family history of congenital cataracts or retinoblastoma (a rare malignant eye tumor that occurs in very young children) should be examined in the hospital nursery.

A Canadian task force on periodic health examination recently reviewed medical evidence for the usefulness of screening preschoolers for vision and hearing problems. The study involved two groups of children, one given vision and hearing tests, the other

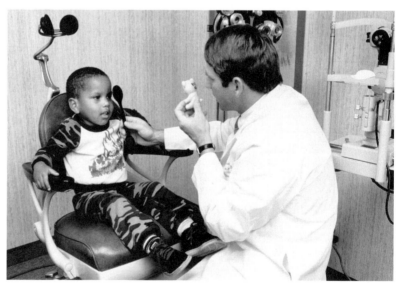

A Canadian study of the benefits of regular vision exams for preschool youngsters concluded that such tests are valuable because they help to reveal problems that, if uncorrected, could later interfere with academic progress. In the United States, unfortunately, many children under age five do not receive any sort of vision screening during regular pediatric exams.

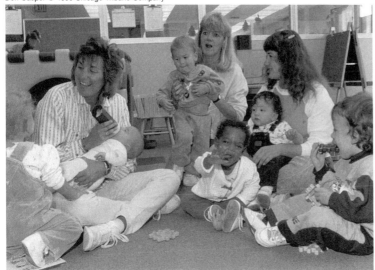

Although some women who work in schools and day-care centers may be at increased risk of miscarriage if exposed to youngsters with the common childhood infection called fifth disease, the American Academy of Pediatrics has concluded that pregnant women should not be routinely excluded from these occupational settings. When there are better tests to detect antibody to the virus that causes fifth disease— making it possible to identify women who are susceptible—such women, when pregnant, may choose to avoid jobs that involve exposure to the disease.

untested. In follow-up tests conducted six months to a year later, those who had been given visual screening had 50% fewer visual problems than their unscreened counterparts, as a result of correction of problems found previously. Surprisingly, prior hearing screening did not diminish the number of problems found 6–12 months later. The Canadian investigators concluded that the vision but not the hearing of preschool children should be tested.

A recent U.S. survey sponsored by the American Academy of Pediatrics found that of more than 8,000 children, one-third of 3–5-year-olds had *not* been visually screened when examined by pediatricians. A child who cannot see well will have difficulty reading and, inevitably, problems in learning. There are many office tests to evaluate the preschooler's visual acuity, including the familiar Snellen "E" chart (which consists of letters and numbers diminishing in size from the top of the chart to the bottom; it depends, of course, on the child's knowing and recognizing these symbols) and tests that use picture cards. Binocular screening equipment, which is used in testing adult vision for driving, is also available. These various tests detect hyperopia (farsightedness) and problems of acuity and muscle balance (*i.e.*, relative strength of the muscles that control eye movement). Simple tests that assess range of visual field and ocular mobility involve observation of eye movements, sometimes while one of the child's eyes is covered and the child is asked to watch a moving object. Such tests are also used to detect amblyopia ("lazy eye"). The fundus, or back of the eye—site of the retina and the optic disk, where the optic nerve enters the orbit (eye socket)—is examined with an ophthalmoscope; this instrument also allows the physician to evaluate the clarity of the fluids in the anterior and posterior orbit.

By the time children attain full growth, nearly 20%

have errors of refraction that require the use of corrective lenses. Although early vision testing does not prevent the eventual need for glasses or contact lenses, the timely correction of visual defects enables youngsters to make uninterrupted progress in learning.

Fifth disease—risk to pregnant women?

In 1988 a large study in West Germany found that pregnant women exposed to children with fifth disease, or erythema infectiosum, a common childhood infection, sometimes spontaneously aborted (miscarried). Several of the women studied had worked in kindergartens during an outbreak of the illness.

Early in the 20th century, the common childhood diseases that are accompanied by a skin rash (*e.g.*, measles, rubella, scarlet fever) were assigned numbers; the numbers gradually fell out of use and were replaced by the common names. Only erythema infectiosum continued to be called by number rather than by name, perhaps because the name is so daunting to one encountering it for the first time. Fifth disease is caused by a virus known as parvovirus B19. In preschool- and school-age children, the B19 virus causes a mild illness with low fever and a characteristic rash that starts on the face and is usually described as having a "slapped cheek" appearance. Subsequently, a rash appears on the child's trunk and limbs in a symmetrical lacelike pattern. The infection spreads by respiratory droplets and is highly contagious.

In a recent outbreak in Connecticut, most adults— nearly 60%—were found to have serological evidence of past infection, probably in their childhood. However, people who never had the infection in childhood, and therefore have no antibody to the virus, are susceptible; if they become infected, they may develop arthritis involving joints in the hands, feet, and knees. Pregnant women who are susceptible are at additional risk of spontaneous abortion. According to data from a British panel on fifth disease and from the Connecticut researchers, the risk of parvovirus-related fetal death in women infected during the first 20 weeks of pregnancy is relatively low, 3 to 9%. (The risk after 20 weeks of pregnancy is not known.)

The virus, once in the body, enters bone marrow cells and multiplies. After a variable incubation period of 4–18 days, it produces fever and a drop in red blood cell production that is usually transient and unimportant. However, if children with chronic hemolytic anemia become infected with the virus, they may develop an aplastic anemia crisis. Such children are extremely sick and highly infectious; for this reason, pregnant hospital personnel should not care for these patients. Because fifth disease is most contagious *before* the onset of symptoms, it is unreasonable to exclude children who have symptomatic infections from school if they feel well. Nor does it make sense to routinely exclude pregnant women from employment in places where they might be exposed to infection; *e.g.,* daycare centers and school classrooms and cafeterias. This was the policy adopted by the American Academy of Pediatrics' committee on infectious diseases early in 1990.

When a test for antibody to parvovirus B19 becomes widely available, it will be possible to identify adults who have been previously infected and are, therefore, not susceptible. At that time pregnant women who are shown to be susceptible may choose to avoid employment that exposes them to the risk of infection.

Reevaluation of pertussis vaccine

The pertussis (whooping cough) vaccine, which has been under attack for some years because of its putative potential to cause brain damage and sudden infant death syndrome (SIDS), has recently been vindicated by data from new studies and reevaluation of old ones. A great deal depends on these new findings: the cost and availability of future vaccines and the future of the U.S. National Childhood Vaccine Injury Compensation Act of 1982, which provides for compensation of children who are injured as a result of being vaccinated against various childhood diseases.

The controversy over the pertussis vaccine currently in use in the U.S. stems from the nature of the vaccine itself and the serious neurological reactions that have been reported in children in association with, if not as a result of, the vaccine. Pertussis is caused by a small bacterium, *Bordetella pertussis,* which is gram negative (*i.e.,* turns a pink color upon contact with a stain called Gram's solution). For technical reasons, it is difficult to make a vaccine from gram-negative bacteria. The vaccine now used in the U.S. is a "whole-cell" vaccine—made from inactivated whole cells of the *B. pertussis* organism. It is generally acknowledged to be relatively crude compared with so-called acellular

Westminster Hospital, University of London

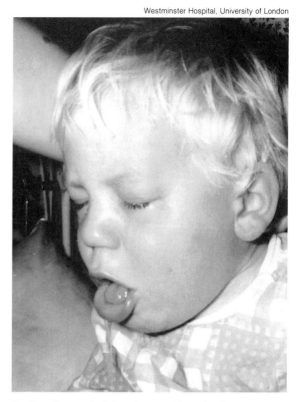

Studies of pertussis (whooping cough) vaccine have cast doubt on earlier findings of rare instances of severe immunization-related side effects. Work continues, however, on developing an effective but more refined vaccine.

vaccines, which are made from bacterial extracts. The whole-cell pertussis vaccine, although it is at least 90% effective in preventing infection, has been under attack in several countries because of side effects, both mild (local pain and swelling, fever, drowsiness, excessive crying) and severe (shocklike episodes, convulsions, inflammation of the brain, and, in some cases, brain damage). Moreover, under the provisions of the National Vaccine Injury Compensation Program, encephalopathy (inflammation of the brain) following pertussis vaccine immunization is a compensable event; the law itself thus lends credence to the belief that encephalopathy can be caused by the vaccine. The vaccine has also been implicated as a cause of SIDS, although sudden death following immunization is not mentioned in the compensation legislation.

Researchers have had difficulty ascertaining the frequency of severe reactions to the pertussis vaccine. One three-year British study, the National Childhood Encephalopathy Study (1976–79), provided data that were used to calculate the generally accepted risk of acute encephalopathy with brain damage due to pertussis vaccine at one in 310,000 doses. But more recent studies and continued analysis of the British data from the '70s have cast serious doubts on the assumption that whole-cell pertussis vaccine causes either brain damage or SIDS. A study by investigators at Vanderbilt University School of Medicine, Nashville, Tenn., published in the *Journal of the American Medical Association* in March 1990 was one of three recent epidemiological studies that found no evidence of permanent neurological illness after hundreds of thousands of doses of DTP (diphtheria-tetanus-pertussis) vaccine. The Vanderbilt team examined the risk of neurological complications in more than 35,000 Tennessee children who had a total of nearly 107,000 DTP shots. An accompanying editorial in the journal stated, "It is time for the myth of pertussis vaccine encephalopathy to end."

This reassurance about the vaccine is good news for parents concerned about possible adverse effects of pertussis immunization. Nevertheless, it should not, and undoubtedly will not, discourage the efforts of vaccine manufacturers to produce an equally effective but more refined, acellular product. Acellular vaccines are now in use in Japan and have been found to cause fewer local side effects (soreness, swelling). It is still not known whether these vaccines are as effective as the one used in the U.S. or whether they cause severe neurological side effects. In Japan the vaccine is given at a later age, when there is less chance of confusing vaccine reactions with neurological diseases that are common in early infancy.

A final note: the U.S. Centers for Disease Control (CDC) documented a sharp rise in pertussis cases in 1986 compared with both previous and subsequent years. In the course of that year, up to 1% of the children with pertussis developed encephalopathy from the infection itself, the highest percentages being found for children under six months of age. This finding emphasizes the importance of immunizing infants at the currently recommended times: at 2, 4, 6, and 18 months.

Measles vaccine: costly but crucial

There was an extremely sharp increase—more than 400%—in the number of measles cases in the U.S. in 1989, and at least 40 measles-associated deaths were reported. Concern about these increases has caused both the CDC and the American Academy of Pediatrics to recommend a second dose of measles vaccine. The CDC recommends the second dose at four to six years of age; the academy recommends it at entry to middle or junior high school (at about age 12).

Measles is an important cause of childhood death in Third World countries. It is usually difficult to show the beneficial effects of the measles vaccine in population studies in these countries because of the many other factors that contribute to their high infant and child mortality rates. However, a study published in *Pediatrics* in 1990 did demonstrate a highly significant improvement of survival in children who were vaccinated against measles. The study was conducted in Haiti in a slum area with high mortality rates. In their conclusions the researchers—from Johns Hopkins University and Tulane University, New Orleans, La., and the Centers for Health and Development in Haiti—urged that efforts be stepped up to eliminate this potentially deadly disease from all countries.

—*Jean D. Lockhart, M.D.*

Physical Fitness

Over the past decade it has become increasingly apparent that life-style changes can profoundly affect health status and disease risk. It is now evident that sedentary living is alone probably to blame for as many as 200,000 preventable cardiovascular deaths in the United States each year. This is independent of the death tolls attributable to such well-established heart disease risk factors as hypertension, smoking, and

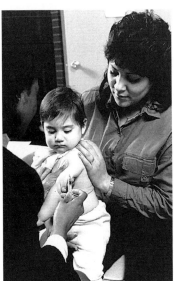

Paul Howell—Gamma-Liaison

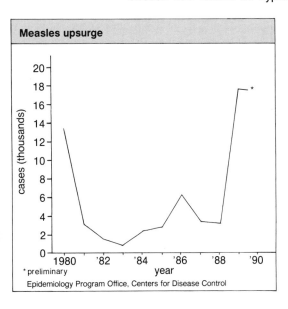

Measles upsurge

cases (thousands) / year

*preliminary

Epidemiology Program Office, Centers for Disease Control

At the Westend Clinic in Houston, Texas, a youngster receives a shot of measles vaccine. The number of cases of measles in the U.S. soared in 1989; the most concentrated outbreaks occurred among unvaccinated preschoolers in inner-city black and Hispanic neighborhoods.

diabetes, which together kill at least 300,000 Americans per year. In response to such statistics, many Americans have altered their health-related behaviors: changing their diets to reduce salt, cholesterol, and saturated fats while increasing their intake of poultry, fish, and high-fiber foods; reducing their consumption of hard liquor; treating their high blood pressure; quitting smoking; and apparently increasing their level of daily physical activity.

But to what extent have Americans truly given up their sedentary ways? Consumer research indicates that the American public spends more than $1 billion annually on exercise equipment, and sales of fitness products will reach $2.1 billion in 1991. And given the number of people jogging, joining health clubs, or working out at the local gym, one might conclude that Americans are indeed quite active. That, however, is the illusion. In fact, when one takes a closer look at the evidence, one finds that while many may begin an exercise program, few actually stick with it. Available data indicate that generally about half of those who start exercising have given it up within the first six months.

U.S. adults: how active?

While it is difficult to obtain precise estimates of physical activity in large populations—more than 30 different methods have been applied in various assessments—most objective evidence indicates that the current status of exercise participation among American adults is not very encouraging. According to the latest data from the U.S. National Center for Health Statistics, only about 8% of men and 7% of women regularly engage in vigorous exercise. When less intense physical activity is added, a total of 44% of males and 39% of females engage in some regular physical activity, which means well over half *do not.* Other surveys have found that about 40% of the adult national population can be classified as being predominantly sedentary.

A recent large-scale study based on interviews conducted by investigators from the University of Michigan assessed the exercise participation of more than 15,000 adults who ranged in age from 19 to 64 years. As a total group, almost 53% participated at least once during the year in moderate-to-high levels of physical activity, but only about 18% were this active on more than 60 days, with men being only slightly more active than women. With increasing age there was a predictable and progressive decline in fitness-activity participation, such that in the 55–64-year-old group only about 6% were physically active on 60 or more days per year. Such findings are complemented by another recent report that revealed that only 14% of the adults studied expended more than 1,600 cal per week in leisure-time activities, and only 10% participated in vigorous physical activity on a regular basis.

All in all, from the cumulative evidence available, it is fair to say that at best no more than 20%, and possibly fewer than 10%, of American adults obtain sufficient physical activity to impart discernible health and fitness benefits. At least 40% are completely sedentary, and 40% exercise below recommended levels.

Clearly, there is a real need to improve the physical-activity profile of the population as a whole. This is especially important in light of the steady decline in the physical requirements at work and in the home resulting from increased automation and use of labor-saving aids. Moreover, surveys indicate that even the rate of increase in leisure-time physical activity observed over the last two decades—the "exercise boom"—now appears to be leveling off. For example, the drop-out rate for most health clubs is now estimated at about 70%!

Because the health-related benefits of regular exercise were well established and because the daily energy expenditure of the majority of the adult population was relatively low, in 1980 the U.S. Public Health

"Aerobic dancing could prolong our lives up to seven years."

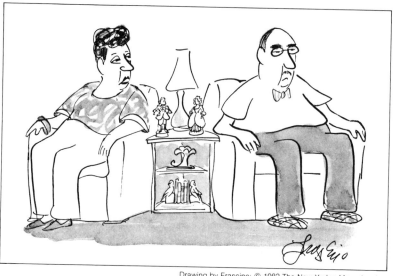

Drawing by Frascino; © 1982 The New Yorker Magazine, Inc.

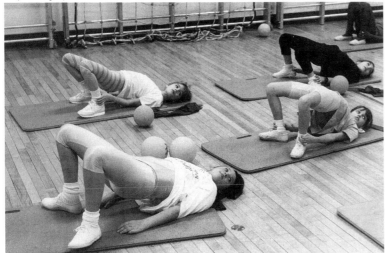

A recent Chrysler Fund-Amateur Athletic Union study that evaluated the physical fitness of U.S. children aged 6–17 each year from 1980 through 1989 showed distinctly declining endurance levels and steadily increasing body weights. While some gain was seen in strength, the overall findings were summarized as "ominous"—confirming what numerous other surveys had found and suggesting that American youth are at increased risk for heart disease and the complications associated with obesity in later life. Experts agree that children need to learn early the important health-related aspects of physical fitness and that the quality of school physical education programs must be improved.

Service established national objectives for health promotion and disease prevention for the year 1990. One of the main objectives was to increase to over 60% the proportion of adults who participate regularly in vigorous physical activity. A review of the progress toward the objectives, published in August 1989, found that that goal was unlikely to be met. Given the population's current level of exercise participation and the high drop-out rates, the achievement of such an ambitious goal by the year 2000 will require the application of new strategies to encourage the broad spectrum of American adults to adopt increased physical activity as a way of life.

Children: declining fitness profile

Over the past 25 years the overall physical fitness and exercise performance of American children have decreased. This has been seen in measures of body fat, in cardiovascular fitness, and, to some extent, in muscular strength. A fairly large percentage of children also show abnormally high levels of blood lipids, which puts them at high risk for subsequent cardiovascular disease.

In the most recent nationwide youth fitness assessment, sponsored by the Chrysler Fund and the Amateur Athletic Union, 12,000 children aged 6 to 17 were evaluated each year from 1980 through 1989. Physical-fitness assessment was based mainly on level of performance in four events: (1) an endurance run for cardiovascular fitness, (2) pull-ups (boys) and flexed-arm hang (girls) for strength and endurance of the arms and shoulder girdle, (3) the "sit-and-reach" test for lower back and hamstring flexibility, and (4) bent-knee sit-ups for abdominal muscular strength and endurance. Over the 10-year period, endurance running performance slowed about 10%, with the proportion of students scoring "satisfactory" decreasing from 43 to 32%. In addition, body weight increased steadily over

the decade without a corresponding height increase, thus supporting evidence of the trend toward obesity among children noted in other studies. On the bright side, children of the latter 1980s seemed stronger than their counterparts at the beginning of the decade, at least as reflected by a higher performance level in sit-ups. In general, however, the director of the project called the increase in body weight and slower run times "ominous" in that they reflected a decline in cardiovascular fitness and possible increased risk for obesity and heart disease in later life.

Experts generally agree that the best approach to assuring greater involvement in regular exercise among youth is to improve the quality of required school physical education programs. School phys ed classes should emphasize the development of fundamental motor skills as well as the important health-related aspects of physical fitness. One approach that is beneficial to both children and parents is family participation in exercise. This has been supported by research showing that when parents and children exercise together, the children tend to be leaner than the children of less active parents.

Senior citizen fitness

The elderly represent the fastest-growing segment of the American population, with the life expectancy for both men and women rapidly approaching 80 years. Sadly, the elderly represent a group who might benefit the most from exercising, yet they are doing so the least. In fact, there are an alarmingly large number of older citizens with such poor functional capacity that they cannot do relatively simple physical tasks without assistance. This is indeed unfortunate, for it is now clear that the elderly adapt to regular physical activity in a manner that not only improves their level of fitness but also imparts positive health benefits.

According to the 1985 National Health Interview

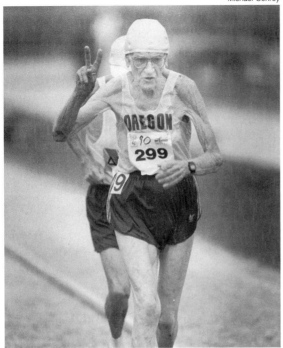

A growing body of evidence indicates that seniors who exercise retain levels of physiological function equivalent to those of much younger individuals. This would come as no surprise to Paul Spangler, 91, who in August 1990 won the men's 5,000-meter race at the Athletic Congress Master Track Meet.

Survey, regular activity of the magnitude required for inducing fitness benefits is uncommon among men and women over 65 years of age. Only about 8% were physically active on a regular basis; almost 70% were active irregularly or totally sedentary. The remainder who exercised did not do so at an intensity sufficient to improve their aerobic fitness. To change these trends a Surgeon General's Workshop on Health Promotion and Aging in 1988 made the following recommendations: (1) Physicians and other health care providers should receive more training in the area of exercise and its related health benefits and provide assessment, prescription, and follow-up to increase physical activity among the elderly. (2) All levels of government should provide leadership and support for developing and coordinating physical activity promotion for older citizens in both urban and rural settings. (3) Physical activity assessment should be incorporated into regular medical visits and exams, and older patients should be educated as to the methods and benefits of appropriate physical activity. (4) Research should be focused on expanding understanding of the various factors that affect participation in and maintenance of a physical activity program as well as an understanding of the appropriate exercise to achieve the optimal health and fitness benefits for the elderly.

Regular exercise: a fountain of youth?

It is not completely clear whether or to what extent changes that occur in physiological function are a direct result of the aging process per se or are the result of a lack of habitual physical activity. In fact, sedentary living may bring about losses in functional capacity that are as great as the effects of aging itself! Results from training studies show that regular exercise consistently enables older individuals to retain levels of cardiovascular function much above those of an age-paired sedentary group. When middle-aged men followed a regular endurance exercise program over a 10-year period, the usual 9 to 15% decline seen in exercise capacity and aerobic fitness was quite clearly forestalled. Many of these active men had maintained the same values for blood pressure and body weight that they had had at the start of the study.

While exercise may not necessarily be a "fountain of youth," researchers are finding that regular physical activity not only retards the loss in functional capacity associated with aging and disuse but often reverses the loss regardless of when in life a person becomes active. With both low- and high-intensity exercise, large improvements in physiological function take place in the healthy elderly, often at the rate and magnitude recorded for much younger individuals. Some researchers maintain that a 30-minute program of rapid walking performed by an older person three or four times a week can turn back the biological clock some 10 years. Improvements have also been noted in body composition, joint flexibility (stiff joints are often the result of disuse, not arthritis), pulmonary and neural functions, heart disease risk profile, and mental outlook. Evidence is also accumulating that regular exercise can conserve and actually retard the loss of bone mass in the elderly, thus staving off the ravages of osteoporosis that afflict both women and men.

In terms of muscle structure and function, habitual physical activity facilitates the retention of muscle protein and can delay the decrements of lean body mass and strength that come with aging. In a recent study healthy men between the ages of 60 and 72 years were trained for 12 weeks with a standard resistance-training program. The results were dramatic. Muscular strength increased progressively throughout the program. By week 12, knee-flexion strength had more than doubled and knee-extension strength increased by 22%. This rate of strength increase (about 5% per training session) was similar to increases previously reported for young adults. In addition, these improvements were accompanied by a significant enlargement of existing muscle fibers. Such findings clearly indicate an impressive plasticity in physiological, structural, and performance characteristics and demonstrate that marked and rapid improvement can be achieved at least into the seventh decade of life. Moreover, improvement in muscular strength with resistance training may be the best way to reduce the incidence of injury among older individuals; *e.g.,* from falls.

Can exercise extend life?

It is now apparent that regular and present participation rather than past participation in physical activity is of major health importance. When the findings of 43 different studies of the relationship between physical inactivity and coronary heart disease were reviewed, it was evident that lack of regular activity contributes to the heart disease process in a cause-and-effect manner, with the sedentary person being almost twice as likely to develop heart disease as the most active individuals. The strength of this association was essentially the same as the associations for hypertension, cigarette smoking, and high serum cholesterol. The researchers who reviewed the evidence felt that this determination placed physical inactivity as the greatest heart disease risk factor, considering that more people lead sedentary lives than possess one or more of the other risk factors.

The most notable study to date concerning life extension through exercise followed more than 16,000 Harvard University alumni who entered college between 1916 and 1950. The study provided strong evidence that moderate aerobic exercise promotes good health and may actually add years to life. Men who expended about 2,000 cal through exercise on a weekly basis had death rates one-quarter to one-third lower than those of classmates who got little or no exercise, and they lived about two years longer. Expenditure of 2,000 cal in weekly exercise could be achieved by a daily brisk 30-minute walk; jogging nearly 10 km (about 6 mi) three or four times a week; or cycling, swimming, or participating in an aerobic dance class for one hour several times a week. Regular exercise was also found to counter the life-shortening effects of cigarette smoking, hypertension, and excess body weight. Moreover, genetic tendencies toward an early death were blunted by regular exercise; if individuals who had one or both parents die before age 65 had a life-style that included physical activity, their risk of dying by 65 was reduced by about 25%.

The life expectancy of Harvard alumni increased steadily from a weekly exercise energy expenditure of 500 cal to 3,500 cal, the equivalent of six to eight hours of strenuous exercise. There were no additional health or longevity benefits in weekly exercise expending more than 3,500 cal. In fact, when exercise was carried to extremes, the men had higher death rates than their more moderately active fellow alumni. Thus, within limits, individuals who exercised more had an improved health profile. For example, the mortality rates were 21% lower for men who walked 15 km (9 mi) or more a week than for men who walked about 2 km or less. Exercising in light sport activities increased life expectancy 24% over men who remained sedentary.

Improved fitness: a little goes a long way

Heroic levels of physical fitness are prerequisite for running in marathons but not for reaping the health benefits of physical activity. Exercise physiologists now hold that the "no pain, no gain" approach to exercise is not the key; rather, moderation is favored—thus making injury- and risk-free exercise more appealing and accessible to the general population.

A recent study of the physical fitness of 13,344 men and women followed for an average of eight years indicated that even modest amounts of exercise substantially reduce the risk of dying from heart disease, cancer, or other causes. This was one of the few studies that looked directly at fitness performance as measured on a treadmill rather than less accurate verbal or written reports of personal physical activity habits. The study also considered such factors as smoking, cholesterol and blood sugar levels, blood pressure, and family history of heart disease in order to isolate the influence of physical fitness per se. Each individual was ranked in one of five fitness categories, ranging from low to high, according to treadmill scores. Death

Older people who engage in 30 minutes of rapid walking three or four times a week reap many benefits: joints gain flexibility; body composition alters; cardiac, neural, and pulmonary functions improve; and mental outlook is enhanced. In fact, the biological clock may be turned back by as much as 10 years!

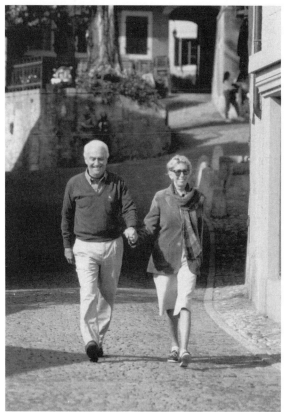

Dick Boyer—Nawrocki Stock Photo

James Ketelsen, chairman of Tenneco Inc., runs on the indoor track—part of an $11 million complex—at his company's Houston headquarters. Loraine Binion takes advantage of the workout equipment that her company, Levi Strauss of San Francisco, has installed. While it is a positive sign that employers are encouraging fitness among employees, too often "wellness programs" are aimed only at the executive hierarchy. The "fitness movement" needs to encompass a much broader population—particularly those in lower socioeconomic groups who bear the burden of disease associated with sedentary life-styles.

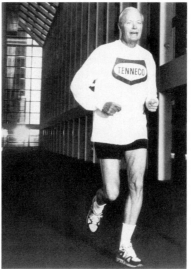 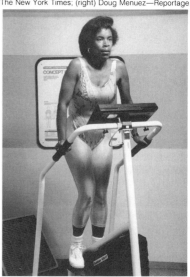

rates of the least fit group were 3.4 times higher than those of the most fit for men and for the least fit women 4.6 times higher than for the most fit women. Even in the presence of other risk factors, higher levels of physical fitness proved beneficial to health. In fact, those people who had no risk factors but were judged unfit had higher death rates than fit people with other risk factors. The most striking finding was that the greatest health benefit occurred in the group rated just above those in the most sedentary category.

In other words, just a modest improvement in fitness among the least fit (easily brought about with lower intensity activities such as walking) conferred substantial health benefits. Commenting on the findings of this research in an accompanying editorial in the *Journal of the American Medical Association* (Nov. 3, 1989), public health specialists from the U.S. Centers for Disease Control recommend that health professionals promote participation in "an activity that is pleasurable (or at least not abhorrent) for the patient and emphasizing that it should be done regularly (at least 3 days per week) and long enough (about 20 minutes) to strengthen cardiorespiratory capacity. In so doing, we can advocate physical activity that will improve the fitness and health of a large portion of the American population."

The exercise message: reaching only the affluent?

While many Americans have adopted a life-style that includes exercise and provides the dividends of improved cardiovascular and overall health, many who could benefit most from life-style changes appear to be the least likely to alter their risky behavioral patterns. Recent surveys indicate that the switch to healthful pursuits is occurring primarily among the educated, wealthy, and, for the most part, white Americans. According to a Lou Harris and Associates poll, the

socioeconomically disadvantaged bear a disproportionately large burden of chronic disease and health risk. Obesity, cigarette smoking, and high consumption of dietary fat and cholesterol combined with a sedentary life-style are most prevalent among this group.

The actual reasons for this notable disparity are complex and poorly understood. To some extent the exercise boom of the past decades was as much a commercial movement as a health movement. Manufacturers of exercise equipment, owners of health clubs and spas, and other organizations that push physical fitness as a commodity generally target the economically advantaged, and these are generally the white population and the better educated. Nowadays more than half of American companies with 750 or more employees offer some sort of physical-fitness program. Many larger corporations have in-house fitness facilities, often staffed by highly trained exercise specialists. In most instances, however, the group having access to such "corporate fitness" programs is the executive hierarchy of the company.

From the perspective of national fitness, it is now clear that if the objective of 60% participation in regular and vigorous activity is to be achieved, the fitness movement must broaden its horizon to encompass the diverse segments of the population. To accomplish this, health professionals emphasize that programs to upgrade physical fitness must recognize and respect cultural values. Rigidly formulated exercise programs that are acceptable to middle- and upper-class groups may be ineffective for other segments of the population. When exercise programs consider socially meaningful approaches—people's means and the facilities they have access to, for example—the likelihood that the population group in question will view exercise as desirable and adopt a program that fosters lasting behavior change will be enhanced.

Activities Americans like best

There are many routes to fitness. Presently the following approaches appear to be most favored by the exercise-prone American populace.

Walking. The U.S. Census Bureau estimates that about 100 million Americans walk for heath, fitness, weight loss, and pleasure. Walking is the most basic form of exercise. No special equipment is required except supportive and well-cushioned shoes to absorb shock and control the angle of the foot as it strikes the ground. Walking, even at a rapid pace, is relatively gentle on the bones and joints; this is because there is no airborne phase as there is with running. Because intensity can be geared down to very low levels, it is an accessible, safe, and easily regulated way for previously sedentary men and women and those who are obese to ease into exercise; this also makes it ideal for people recovering from a heart attack. Even those who want to maintain a high level of fitness can increase walking intensity by using hand-held and ankle weights or adding weight to the torso—such as walking with a backpack.

Jogging or running. Slow jogging requires no complex skill. As with walking, large muscle groups of the body are exercised in rhythmic, continuous movement, and there is usually little localized muscle fatigue or cramping. Because the body weight is transported while walking or running, as opposed to swimming or stationary bicycling, in which the body weight is supported, the number of calories burned is relatively high, especially for the overweight. Running or jogging, however, can place an unnecessary strain on the knees, hips, and ankle joints. Uneven and varying terrains (*i.e.,* potholes, curbs, soft grass, asphalt, and hills) create strains on joints, muscles, ligaments, and tendons, increasing the chances of being injured. It is estimated that during running the impact force when the foot hits the ground with each stride is equal to two to three times the runner's body weight. Several studies have reported that from 70 to 90% of road runners experience at least one musculoskeletal problem directly attributed to running.

Outdoor exercise enthusiasts also run at the mercy of the weather. Extremes of temperature and humidity place added strain on the body's regulatory mechanisms, and episodes of heat exhaustion and dehydration as well as cold injury are not uncommon. Certainly rain, snow, and heavy wind restrict the frequency of training and make it difficult to gauge exercise intensity.

Treadmills. Treadmills have been a traditional means used by exercise physiologists and cardiologists to evaluate the aerobic and cardiovascular fitness of individuals. Now, however, many health clubs have treadmills for workouts, and increasingly people are buying them for home use. The motorized treadmill provides a means of finely regulating exercise intensity during each workout and on a day-to-day basis, making it ideal for those who require a controlled and closely monitored exercise environment.

One begins by walking, but intensity can be increased to a jog. The tread belt absorbs the shock of strides, minimizing strain on shins, knees, and leg joints that are encountered on a hard roadway. On some models the exerciser can regulate intensity by adjusting the speed of the motor-driven belt or altering the slope of the platform. More advanced computer-regulated models enable programming of an exercise routine, calculation of caloric expenditure, and monitoring of heart rate.

Exercise bicycles. Stationary cycling offers a means of well-regulated indoor exercise in the privacy of one's home. The retail cost of a dependable exercise bike ranges between $200 and $2,500. The top-of-the-line models come equipped with monitors for heart rate and computerized packages to visually display caloric expenditure and continually adjust exercise level in accordance with the preprogrammed exercise prescrip-

According to a 1989 survey, the fastest-growing American fitness trend is exercising on stair-climbing machines. Although one can derive the same aerobic benefits from climbing real stairs, there are now at least a dozen electronic stair machines on the market, with some costing upwards of $3,000.

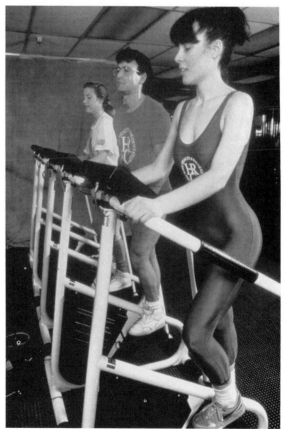

James Keyser/Time Magazine

tion. Some even have software packages that provide visual effects to simulate scenic touring. Because body weight is supported in bicycling, the exercise is ideal for the overweight, who may have compromised mobility and are susceptible to orthopedic problems that can result from weight-bearing exercise. A major complaint is that stationary cycling becomes boring. This can be circumvented, however, by scheduling exercise during a favorite television program, or one can purchase an attachment to hold reading material during cycling. Dual-action air-resistance models have moving handlebars that enable the rider to exercise upper body and legs at the same time.

Other aerobic exercise machines. In addition to treadmills and stationary cycles, today's health clubs provide a multitude of exercise devices, including rowing ergometers, laddermills, stair climbers, and cross-country skiing machines, each of which involves continuous exercise of large muscle groups for effective aerobic training. More and more these devices, too, are being purchased for use at home. The selection of such equipment for training should be made on the basis of individual preference and comfort. It is important to keep in mind that there is nothing magical about each new machine that comes on the market (although their promoters might lead one to believe otherwise). With any such equipment, if large muscle groups are exercised in a rhythmic and continuous manner for 20 to 30 minutes several times a week, the cardiovascular system will be conditioned and aerobic fitness improved. However, the various types of equipment may emphasize only certain muscle groups, such as the legs on laddermills and stair climbers or the upper body with rowing machines. Therefore, for a complete aerobic workout one should include several exercise devices with appropriate time allocated to each.

Although the computer-enhanced exercise equipment often dominates the exercise marketplace, the basic "old standby" exercises such as rope skipping, bench stepping, running in place, and calisthenics, if done regularly, are still an effective and inexpensive means of achieving and maintaining aerobic fitness.

Water exercise. Swimming and other forms of exercise in water have shown a rapid increase in popularity in the last several years. In the water environment body weight is supported by the buoyant force of the water. Consequently, there is essentially no strain on bones and joints while exercising. Because the legs and arms are used in the rhythmic swimming movement, major muscles of the body are exercised. In addition, the cool water is a pleasant environment in which to dissipate the metabolic heat generated by exercise. This makes water exercise especially attractive for the overfat and pregnant exerciser.

Aquatic aerobics and simulated walking and jogging in water have recently become quite popular with senior citizens. Simply walking in water at thigh level

almost doubles the calories burned compared with walking at the same speed on level ground. Additional conditioning can be gained by vigorous arm movements against the resistance of the water.

Aerobic dancing. Over the past decade aerobic dance has emerged as one of the fastest-growing forms of exercise, especially among females. Concurrently, research has verified that rhythmic and vigorous exercise choreographed to music is effective for burning significant calories and improving cardiovascular fitness. For many participants, however, nagging injuries have resulted from aerobic dancing. These have been attributed mainly to the shock resulting from the rapid jogging in place and jumping movements associated with this high-impact form of dance. To reduce risk of injury, the present trend is toward an alternative low-impact dance form. This approach requires the dancer to keep one foot on the ground at all times during the routine. Available research indicates that low-impact dance exercise, if performed at a fairly high intensity, can be very effective in conditioning the body.

Exercise videos. The Aerobics and Fitness Association of America estimates that there are more than

Low-impact aerobic dance, in which one foot is always on the ground, provides the cardiovascular benefits and significant caloric expenditure of the higher-impact style but reduces the risk of injury.

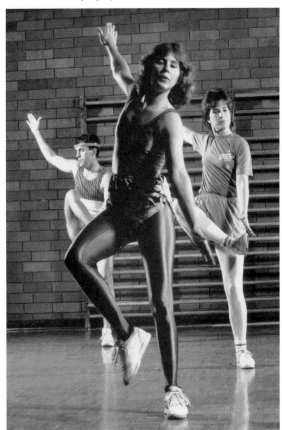

Richard Hamilton Smith

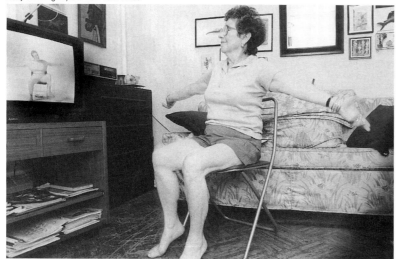

Exercise videos are a convenient choice for fitness buffs who are self-motivated and like the privacy of exercising at home. Belle Joseph, 72, helped produce "Fit After 50"; the 45-minute workout routine starts with gentle stretching movements while sitting in a chair, working up to energetic skipping around the chair. As the developers say, the program's goal is not to provide a "Jane Fonda wipeout" but to help the older person who has been sedentary gain flexibility, strengthen muscles, and learn relaxation techniques.

220 exercise videos on the market today. Estimates of "good" or "safe and scientifically sound" tapes range from 20 to 60%. This form of highly structured exercise is a convenient choice for those who are on a tight time schedule and desire to supplement a regular exercise program or to exercise in the privacy of their own home. There are videos that focus on firming and toning specific body areas, that provide yoga instructions, that lead the viewer through aerobic and low-impact dance workouts, and that even guide women through routines during the various phases of pregnancy. Programs are also geared for beginners and those at intermediate and advanced levels. In addition to the varying quality of the programs, other drawbacks of video exercise include the possibility that a home exerciser may not get help should an injury occur, the likelihood that an improper technique will not be corrected, and the lack of reinforcement and group camaraderie that can be important motivators to many individuals who enroll in classes when beginning an exercise program. As the exercise-video market continues to expand, more of the programs are paying attention to such important factors as appropriate warm-up, cool down, stretching techniques, and exercise progression.

—*William D. McArdle, Ph.D., and Michael M. Toner, Ph.D.*

Sickle-Cell Disease

Sickle-cell disease is a chronic genetic blood disorder for which there is no cure. In the United States as well as in many other parts of the world, sickle-cell disease (also called sickle-cell anemia) is a major public health issue. Sudden, unexpected medical complications leading to significant illness characterize its clinical course. Recent advances in early diagnosis and treatment, however, have significantly improved the quality of life and prolonged the life-span of afflicted individuals.

In the U.S. approximately one in 400 blacks of African descent is born with sickle-cell disease, while one in 12 has sickle-cell trait—the carrier state for the disease. The disease, however, is not restricted to blacks but is found in many races throughout the world. The greatest frequency is in populations in which malaria is endemic. This includes people of Mediterranean, Indian, and Middle Eastern descent. The relationship to malaria is the result of a random genetic mutation of the hemoglobin molecule that afforded a protective effect against fatal malaria infections; once the parasite infects the red blood cell that contains sickle hemoglobin, the cell becomes sickled and the parasite is destroyed, along with the cell itself, by the body's immune system. The genetic advantage, however, has been offset by the major disadvantage: the serious illness that is sickle-cell disease.

Distinguishing the trait from the disease

Hemoglobin is the protein inside the red cell that carries oxygen to and carbon dioxide from tissues of the body. The type of hemoglobin a person makes is determined by inherited hemoglobin genes; one hemoglobin gene is inherited from each parent. *In utero* the normal fetus makes fetal hemoglobin (hemoglobin F). Normally the baby stops making fetal hemoglobin after birth and then produces hemoglobin A, which he or she is able to do because of the inheritance of one hemoglobin A gene from the mother and one hemoglobin A gene from the father.

In sickle-cell trait one of the two genes inherited for hemoglobin A is altered so that it produces sickle hemoglobin (hemoglobin S). Sickle hemoglobin differs from normal hemoglobin by one amino acid—specifically, valine substituted for glutamic acid. The hemoglobin in these cells is roughly 60% hemoglobin A

A five-year-old sickle-cell patient has his regular checkup in the pediatric clinic at the University of Illinois in Chicago while his eight-month-old sister, who also has the disease, awaits her turn. An Illinois screening program, begun in 1989, enabled the children to be diagnosed and to begin penicillin therapy to help prevent the kind of infections that could seriously jeopardize their health. Neither of the parents has the disease but both are asymptomatic carriers; the mother's brother had the disease and died at age 25 of heart failure.

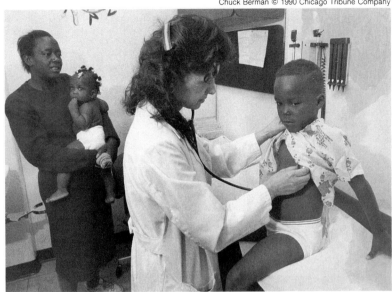

and 40% hemoglobin S. At this relatively low concentration of hemoglobin S, cells generally function and survive normally. Individuals with sickle-cell trait are healthy and have normal morbidity and mortality rates. A recent study conducted by the Walter Reed Army Institute of Research, Washington, D.C., found an increased risk of sudden, unexpected death in military recruits with sickle-cell trait exposed to extreme physical conditions. However, previous studies of athletes with sickle-cell trait have not revealed any increased medical problems. At the present time there is no consensus among investigators as to whether there is an increased risk of sudden death during extreme exercise among individuals with sickle-cell trait. The results of the military recruits study should be viewed in perspective; for the majority of people with sickle-cell trait, the condition is benign, and no restrictions in physical activity are necessary.

However, when patients have sickle-cell disease, they have inherited a sickle gene from both parents and thus produce no normal hemoglobin A. At this high concentration of hemoglobin S, the red cell's basic properties are severely altered. With deoxygenation the hemoglobin S molecules form rigid rods that change the shape of the red cell from a bioconcave disk to an elongated or crescent (sickle) configuration. The extremely rigid sickle cells are inflexible and are very fragile. These properties of the sickle red cells cause two cardinal problems: chronic hemolytic anemia and tissue injury as a result of ischemia (lack of oxygen).

Each time the sickle cell travels from an artery to a vein and back to an artery, it sickles and unsickles often, losing pieces of its membrane. Repeated episodes of such sickling and unsickling, induced by changes in the blood oxygen content, permanently damage the

red cell membranes. The average sickle red cell life-span is only about 20 days, compared with over 100 days for a normal red cell. This excessive destruction of red blood cells results in the marked deficiency of red cells that causes the patient's anemic state.

Tissue injury is usually produced by the obstruction of blood vessels caused by an accumulation of sickle cells. Sickled cells markedly increase blood viscosity (*i.e.,* its resistance to flow through the blood vessels). This highly viscous blood flows slowly through the microcirculation and produces progressive sickling. In the circulatory system, normal red cells that have a diameter of seven micrometers (a micrometer equals one-millionth of a meter) must squeeze through tiny nutrient vessels with a diameter of two micrometers. Sickle cells are often not capable of such a task and get permanently trapped at these points. This results in blood vessel obstruction, which in turn causes small areas of tissue injury (microinfarcts). Such small areas may not be felt by a patient but can lead to progressive damage to vital organs. When a large tissue area is injured, nerve endings are stimulated and the patient experiences sudden and severe pain.

Fundamentals of diagnosis

Sickle-cell disease can now be identified in the prenatal, neonatal, and postnatal periods. Intrauterine diagnosis within the first trimester of pregnancy enables couples at risk of having children with sickle-cell disease to make informed reproductive decisions. The sickle gene can be detected in the genetic material (DNA) from fetal cells obtained by amniocentesis. Amniocentesis can be safely performed at the 12th week of gestation. In most cases, gene mapping of fetal fibroblasts—undifferentiated cells that are harvested from the amniotic fluid—can directly determine if the sickle gene is present in the fetal DNA samples.

Diagnosis of sickle-cell disease in the newborn (neonatal) period—within the first month of life—permits adequate counseling of the parents and initiation of preventive treatment before the onset of clinical manifestations. Newborn diagnosis can be made by a technique called hemoglobin electrophoresis, which uses small amounts of the newborn's blood. This technique separates sickle hemoglobin from normal hemoglobin. Most states in the U.S. have for some time had newborn screening programs for serious congenital diseases such as hypothyroidism, phenylketonuria, and galactosemia but not for sickle-cell disease; only recently have approximately 30 states begun screening programs for sickle-cell disease. Preliminary indications from these screenings show a marked decrease in the mortality rates of affected patients, largely because of the prevention of life-threatening infections.

Normal red blood cells containing oxygen-binding hemoglobin (below) are disk shaped with a depression in the middle. Sickle cells (bottom) are characterized by an abnormal hemoglobin S molecule that becomes rigid at low oxygen concentrations, reducing the cells' flexibility and increasing their fragility.

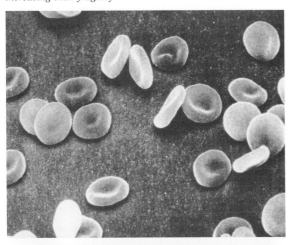

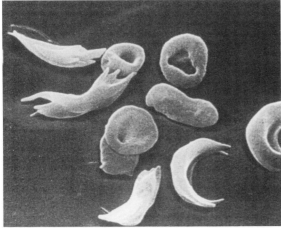

Photographs, Science Source/Photo Researchers; (top) K.R. Porter and (above) Nigel Calder

After the newborn period, diagnosis through routine laboratory tests generally shows significant abnormalities. By six months of age, those who have inherited the disease already have a moderately severe anemia; a blood test shows evident sickle forms and small red cell fragments.

Widely varied clinical manifestations

There is marked variation in the clinical features of sickle-cell disease. In a large group of patients who have the same type of sickle-cell disease, some will die early in infancy, others will suffer recurrent episodes of ischemic tissue damage, and a few will remain asymptomatic. This variation in the clinical course causes it to be very difficult to make a prognosis. There are many factors that play a significant role in determining the clinical variability of sickle-cell disease, but only a few are well understood.

All newborns continue to make variable levels of fetal blood (hemoglobin F) after birth. While the fetal blood level normally drops down to a small amount, individual sickle-cell patients vary in the amounts they continue to produce. Fetal blood appears to inhibit sickling. Variations in fetal hemoglobin levels, therefore, have been used to explain the differences in the severity of sickle-cell disease among different ethnic groups. For example, it has been known that patients from the Middle East and Far East have a relatively mild course of sickle-cell disease; close study of these individuals has shown they have unusually high levels of fetal blood.

Another factor found to modify the course of sickle-cell disease positively is the concomitant inheritance of alpha thalassemia trait. Alpha thalassemia trait is a benign blood condition characterized by production of small red cells. Recent studies have shown that when patients with sickle-cell disease also inherit the alpha thalassemia trait, they are less anemic.

There are many other factors that modulate the course of sickle-cell disease, including the degree of stickiness that causes the sickle-cell membrane to adhere to the blood vessel membrane. However, less is known about this and other possible modifiers.

Painful episodes

What are known as vasoocclusive crises are painful episodes of ischemic damage, typically lasting five or six days. Infection, dehydration, extreme cold, or possibly emotional stress may precipitate a crisis, although the majority of cases have no definite trigger.

Infants with sickle-cell disease usually remain asymptomatic until approximately four months of age, when their protected fetal hemoglobin levels fall and the sickle level predominates. The majority of sickle-cell anemia patients experience a painful episode within the first year of life, and virtually all experience pain by the age of five.

Musculoskeletal pain is the most common complaint. So-called hand-foot syndrome (dactylitis) is the first manifestation of sickle-cell disease in a majority of patients. This complication results from the occlusion (blockage) of small blood vessels that supply the bones of the hands and feet, causing painful swelling. This swelling of the hands and feet, which is often symmetrical, is a distinctive characteristic of sickle-cell disease in children. In contrast to the young patient with hand-foot syndrome, older patients experience asymmetric pain in the extremities and back, which is not associated with swelling.

Compromised immunity and serious infections

Unfortunately, the first manifestation of sickle-cell disease may be an overwhelming and potentially fatal infection. The high frequency of fatal infections in sickle-cell disease results from a loss of function of the spleen in early infancy. The spleen is a large lymph node in the abdomen that is essential for fighting infections. It filters bacteria out of the blood, destroys the bacteria, and then makes antibodies or chemicals to circulate in the blood and kill bacteria. The loss of a functioning spleen renders children with sickle-cell disease extremely susceptible to life-threatening pneumococcal and *Hemophilus influenzae* infections. In addition, these patients have a marked increase in frequency of salmonella osteomyelitis (a life-threatening inflammatory infection of bone), a form of pneumonia caused by the *Mycoplasmataceae* microorganism, and *Escherichia coli* pyelonephritis (a kidney infection). As a result of the generalized immune deficiency state, infections are the number one cause of death in children with sickle-cell disease.

Anemic crises

A chronic, stable anemia characterizes sickle-cell disease; however, two types of anemic complications can cause a rapid fall in the red blood cell level. The first and most serious anemic crisis is known as a splenic sequestration crisis. The typical patient suddenly develops weakness and pallor with a rapidly enlarging spleen. The pooling of a large amount of blood in the spleen results in shock and death unless the victim receives a prompt transfusion. After a single episode of splenic sequestration, splenectomy (an operation to remove the spleen) is often recommended. After the age of five years, crises involving the spleen usually do not occur because the spleen has been scarred from recurrent tissue-damaging episodes.

The second type of anemic crisis typically follows a viral infection and may affect patients of any age. A transient cessation of red cell production causes a dangerous drop in the patient's blood level due to the short life-span of sickle cells. (Such a fall in the number of red cells does not occur after a viral infection in a healthy person.) This second crisis is called an aplastic episode.

Complications involving diverse systems

Among the many systems in which complications can occur in patients with sickle-cell disease are the vascular, nervous, respiratory, musculoskeletal, hepatic, and genitourinary systems. Neurological complications have been reported in 25% of patients with sickle-cell disease. Strokes—cerebrovascular accidents caused by an occlusion of a major artery in the brain—are the most common and serious of these complications. In contrast to strokes caused by atherosclerosis or hypertension, strokes in sickle-cell disease occur in young children.

Approximately one-half of patients with sickle-cell disease develop acute pulmonary disease, characterized by pneumonia, fever, and chest pain. Such episodes account for approximately 15% of deaths in sickle-cell patients and cause significant illness for

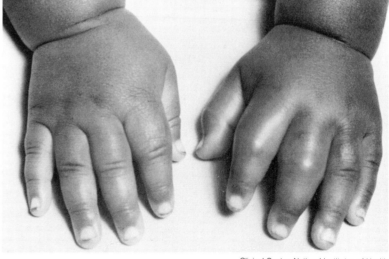

Dactylitis, or hand-foot syndrome, is a common early manifestation of sickle-cell disease. Small blood vessels that supply the bones of the hands and feet become blocked, producing severe swelling in young patients. Here a baby's left hand (shown at right in the picture) is affected, while the right hand is normal-sized and unaffected.

Clinical Center, National Institutes of Health

all patients. In childhood these lung complications are often due to infection, while in older patients they are more often due to sickling in the lung. These recurrent episodes of lung damage result in a chronic reduction in the oxygen level of older patients.

Orthopedic abnormalities develop in approximately 50% of patients. Severe damage to the head of the femoral bone (thighbone) due to sickling of the blood supply is the most serious skeletal complication. This results in a limp and hip pain. Osteomyelitis, or infection of the bone, occurs in 10% of patients.

Patients with sickle-cell disease have a very high frequency of what are known as pigment gallstones, with the majority of older patients being affected. The sickle-cell disease patients' gallstones are formed as a result of the precipitation of bilirubin (a reddish-yellow pigment characteristic of jaundice) in the gallbladder. (In other patients gallstones generally form as a result of insoluble masses of cholesterol within the gallbladder.) Pigment gallstones may cause pain for the sickle-cell patient, sometimes necessitating surgery.

Abnormalities in the genitourinary tract develop early in children with sickle-cell disease. The most frequent abnormalities develop from sickling in the middle of the kidney (the renal medulla). Sickling in this area results in the inability to concentrate urine. This complication frequently causes bed-wetting. In older patients sickling in the kidney may lead to end-stage renal failure.

Priapism, a persistent erection that is caused by an obstruction of the venous blood supply to the penis, occurs in 5% of the male patients. Priapism can produce severe pain, urinary retention, impotence, and severe psychological problems.

As the care of patients with sickle-cell disease has improved, most patients live to middle and late adulthood. Many of these patients are living normal lives. Therefore, problems related to pregnancy in women are becoming more important. Women with sickle-cell disease can have normal pregnancies and healthy children. However, most of these women experience more complications during pregnancy and a high frequency of miscarriage. These complications generally can be managed by early prenatal care and close monitoring throughout the pregnancy. Some specialists involved in the care of these patients recommend prophylactic transfusions during pregnancy. Others believe transfusions are necessary only if indicated clinically in the individual patient.

These are the major but by no means the only complications that can arise in sickle-cell disease. Other problems include obstruction of blood vessels in the eye, skin ulcers in the lower leg, and—in children— growth failure that is secondary to anemia.

Maximizing health

Advances in the medical treatment of complications have dramatically increased the life expectancy of patients with sickle-cell disease. Comprehensive care early in life maximizes the individual's opportunity for a productive future. Such care includes regular immunizations, auditory and visual screening, and counseling. At the time of diagnosis, likely problems such as fever, pain, and anemia need to be discussed with families of children with sickle-cell disease, and guidelines for the management of these problems should be reviewed. The serious psychological effects of chronic pain need to be addressed; special tutorial programs for school children may be needed to help the patient make up for time lost from school. Older patients may need vocational counseling or rehabilitation when illness interferes with work.

Patients with sickle-cell disease have a markedly increased caloric requirement because of their need to constantly produce blood, which can result in delays in growth and sexual maturation. For example, a child with sickle-cell anemia requires approximately 2,400 cal per day in contrast to 1,500 cal per day for a normal 20-kg (44-lb) child. Such characteristic delays can be partially corrected by a well-balanced, high-calorie diet.

Prevention of infection is a major goal of health care maintenance. It has recently been proved that daily prophylactic penicillin can produce an 85% reduction in life-threatening infections in young patients. Therefore, the present goal of care should be the diagnosis of sickle-cell disease in the newborn period before the clinical symptoms develop and the immediate initiation of daily prophylactic penicillin. Penicillin should be continued to at least the age of five years. With this kind of care, up to a sixfold decrease in deaths in young children has been seen.

Vasoocculusive crises produce great anxiety for families and patients. Because dehydration tends to increase sickling within each red cell, large amounts of fluids are given during a painful crisis, and liberal fluid intake on a regular basis may prevent such episodes. Many patients can be managed with nonnarcotic analgesics such as acetaminophen or aspirin. However, it is common that during these painful episodes individuals will require narcotics such as morphine.

Need for transfusions

Red blood cell transfusions are commonly used to treat many complications of sickle-cell disease. The use of transfusions is based on theoretical benefits of: (1) increasing the blood's ability to carry oxygen and (2) improving blood flow in the circulation. It has been proved that red cell transfusions can prevent patients who have experienced a stroke from having a recurrence. Transfusions are also used to treat other life-threatening complications. The risks of transfusions, however, are significant and include infection, hepatitis, destruction of transfused cells, allergic reaction, fever, and progressive iron overload.

New and future therapies

There has been an explosion of new therapeutic approaches to sickle-cell disease. Increasing the level of fetal blood in patients has become a major focus of experimental treatment. As noted previously, the fetus with sickle-cell disease is totally asymptomatic because the predominant form of blood is fetal blood, which does not sickle. After birth, the body stops making fetal blood and begins to make sickle blood. Once the sickle blood has risen to a significant level, symptoms begin. The affected infant has the genetic material to continue to make large amounts of fetal blood; these controlling genes, however, become dormant.

Chemotherapy is now available that may reactivate dormant genes and increase the sickle-cell patient's level of fetal blood. The production of increased fetal blood would improve the anemia and decrease sickling. Preliminary data suggest that such a treatment approach may be of major clinical benefit. Unfortunately, the experimental drugs now available that can accomplish this are mainly cytotoxic agents used in cancer treatment, which have significant side effects. Hydroxyurea is the safest and most widely used experimental cytotoxic drug available to increase sickle-cell patients' fetal blood level. However, there are side

A 27-year-old who suffers from sickle-cell disease and has had several potentially fatal crises undergoes a transfusion. After blood is removed with a syringe, he is rehydrated with saline solution and packed red blood cells.

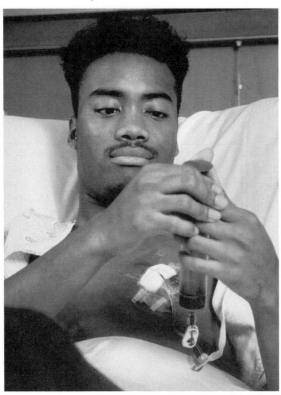

Rich Frishman

effects with this medication, which is taken orally; these include lowering of the patient's blood counts, potential liver damage, and a small but increased risk of malignancy. Research is now under way to develop new drugs that can increase the fetal blood level without the serious side effects associated with cytotoxic agents.

Bone marrow transplantation may be a therapeutic treatment for sickle-cell patients in the future. A few children with sickle-cell anemia have been cured of their disease as a result of bone marrow transplantation. However, this form of treatment is unlikely to become a major therapeutic option until its safety improves significantly.

Another therapeutic approach aims to decrease the sickling of red blood cells by increasing the amount of water within the sickle cell, which dilutes the effects of sickle hemoglobin and improves the red cell's life-span. One way of accomplishing this has been to make the red cell membrane more permeable to water by giving patients a drug of the calcium-channel-blocking class known as Cetiedil. This agent has been used in Europe as a local anesthetic. Preliminary research suggests that it may have a role in improving the clinical course of sickle-cell disease.

Another research initiative in which there has been recent progress is in the development of an animal model for sickle-cell disease. Genetically engineered mice are being bred with clinical profiles closely resembling the human disease; the hybrid mice may prove useful in tests of new antisickling drugs and genetic therapies.

Perhaps the greatest hope for the future treatment of sickle-cell disease is gene therapy. In gene therapy the genetic defect is corrected by insertion of a normal gene into the patient's tissue. Linking the gene that is to be transplanted to benign viruses (accomplished by genetic engineering techniques) enables the normal gene to be carried into the DNA of the affected tissue. Presently, such gene transfers are being done in animal models. A serious hurdle that must be overcome before gene therapy can be a viable option for patients is ensuring that the transferred gene is integrated into the correct genetic material and expresses its product—normal hemoglobin—appropriately. Gene therapy presently raises numerous ethical and safety questions that must be addressed before the treatment is undertaken to cure sickle-cell disease in human patients.

—*Elliott P. Vichinsky, M.D.*

Sleep Disorders

The field of sleep disorders is a rapidly growing, multidisciplinary, specialized area of patient care. Prior to 1979 the various forms of sleep difficulties that occur had not been well defined, nor were there recognized guidelines for their treatment. Within the decade that followed, a whole new clinical field was defined, and specialized centers for patient evaluation and treatment were established in most major hospitals. Disorders are evaluated in sleep laboratories, where it is possible to monitor patients' sleep states. In a test called a polysomnogram, electrodes are attached to various parts of the body to produce records of the patient's heart activity, breathing effort, airflow through the nose and mouth, blood oxygen saturation, electrical activity in the brain, leg movements, and eye movements. Such recordings are taken while the patient is asleep for six to eight hours in a setting that is as nearly normal as possible.

Sleep disorders themselves, of course, are not new. Gilbert and Sullivan described the horrors of insomnia in the patter song from *Iolanthe:* "When you're lying awake with a dismal headache, and repose is taboo'd by anxiety. . ."; Charles Dickens described another kind of problem, sleep apnea, in his portrayal of the sleepy fat boy, Joe, in the *The Pickwick Papers;* Shakespeare created the sleepwalker Lady Macbeth; and many an author has produced a fear-inspiring tale based on his or her own real-life nightmares—Mary Wollstonecraft Shelley, for example, created *Frankenstein.*

Once the public learned of the existence of the specialized sleep centers, the demand for the services they can provide rose sharply—in fact, faster than there were trained professionals able to diagnose and treat them. Fortunately, this problem is now being remedied by the development of training programs for physicians and clinical psychologists who specialize in the care of sleep disorders.

The range of sleep problems

The disorders themselves are classed into four major groups: (1) disorders of initiating and maintaining sleep (the insomnias); (2) disorders of excessive somnolence (the inability to maintain daytime wakefulness); (3) disorders of the sleep–wake cycle (problems of sleep timing due to shift work, long-distance air travel, etc.); and (4) the dyssomnias (behaviors intruding into sleep, such as sleepwalking). Within each of these four broad descriptive categories are a number of specific disorders with varying underlying causes. Some of these are physical in nature, such as pain that can disrupt a night's sleep; some are psychological; and many are a mixture of the two.

Sleep is a time of profound change from normal waking life, both physiologically and psychologically. Further, within sleep itself there are regular cycles of change: periods of low activity alternating with periods of high activity. Periods of the peaceful-looking rest of deep sleep, called non-rapid eye movement (NREM) sleep, which last from 70 to 90 minutes, change to periods of muscle paralysis and hallucinatory activity of dreaming sleep, known as REM, or rapid eye move-

ment, sleep, which last from 5 to 15 minutes. What is more, sleep is a time when Murphy's Law holds: anything that can go wrong will.

What goes wrong may be in the sleep mechanism itself. It may fail to turn on when the individual wants to sleep, or it may fail to stay on long enough for a good night of rest. The wrong stage of sleep may occur at the beginning of the night or it may occur at the end of the night. There may be a problem of switching between the two main types of sleep, from NREM to REM sleep, resulting in partial arousals during which some abnormal behaviors can take place (*e.g.,* sleepwalking or night terrors). Sometimes the problem is specific to one stage of sleep. For example, recently a new disorder has been described that occurs within the REM-sleep stage when the muscle paralysis that ordinarily accompanies dreaming is not complete. When this occurs it is possible for sleepers to get up and act out their dreams, sometimes with disturbing consequences.

Sleep disorders can be caused by physiological changes brought about by sleep itself. When the muscles that hold the upper airway open relax too much,

Brain waves and eye movements are monitored in a study investigating the connection between depression and dreaming. The microphone is used to record the subject's dreams when she is awakened during REM sleep.

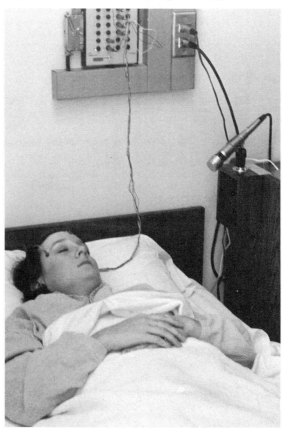

Rush-Presbyterian-St. Luke's Medical Center

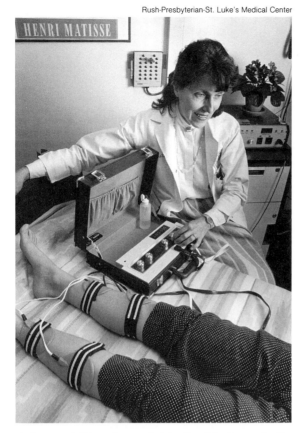

A sleep specialist applies an electric stimulator to a patient's leg muscles to ease leg twitching. People who suffer from periodic movements of sleep, which can cause multiple arousals during the night, often are prevented from getting the restful, sound sleep they need.

they can cause obstruction that interrupts breathing. Sleep is not beneficial when one cannot breathe as a result.

Sometimes sleep problems are a consequence of not letting go of waking-life troubles. It is well established that those persons who have not dealt adequately with the daytime dilemmas and difficulties that beset them find that their anxieties linger into the night, and frequently they are unable to get a restful night of sleep.

Presently there are over 60 distinct sleep disorders that affect all age groups, ranging from the sleep-related head banging of the young child to the fragmentation of sleep and confusional nocturnal episodes of those with senile psychoses. Understanding what causes these difficulties has proved to be complex.

Snoring and apnea: new insights

Snoring, which seems as if it should be one of the simplest of sleep problems, illustrates just how complex these problems can be. In fact, a key question is: Who is the patient? Is it the wife who complains *she* cannot sleep because of her husband's noisy breathing or the husband whose respiration is partially compromised in sleep? Sleeping arrangements of couples are usually close, and this physical proximity that fosters intimacy is important for the preservation of the marriage. When one spouse snores—most often it is the husband—this frequently leads to sleeping in separate bedrooms, which in turn brings on other feelings of dissatisfaction with the relationship. The wife may insist that the husband's sleep troubles be treated before she returns to the marriage bed, while he may deny he has any difficulty at all. He claims that he sleeps very well and that it is her light, easily fragmented sleep that is the problem that needs to be addressed. Snoring, then, is a physical problem, a marital problem, and may be also the cause of a second sleep disorder—the spouse's insomnia.

Snoring, as indicated above, is most commonly a male disorder; it can begin in early childhood. It has been estimated that 20% of men under 40 and 70% of men over 40 snore heavily. Women are usually not snorers until they pass through menopause in their late forties or early fifties. The reasons women start snoring at this time in life are not well understood; there is, however, speculation that the female hormones (in particular, progesterone) have a preventive effect on snoring. Thus, the marked decline of hormone levels at menopause may contribute to snoring's onset. Weight gain, which is known to increase the likelihood of snoring, is also common in women after menopause.

Snoring is sometimes due to a structural defect, such as a deviated nasal septum or a narrow throat, or to a dynamic factor like the relaxation of the muscles holding the tongue forward. Such habits as sleeping on the back or drinking alcoholic beverages before bedtime can exacerbate structural or dynamic factors. When a significant weight gain combines with a structural or a dynamic defect, a full-blown sleep disorder may emerge. First, the snoring escalates in loudness, and then it is followed by episodes of complete obstruction when no breathing takes place for 10 seconds or more despite vigorous efforts of the chest. These pauses are called apneas, and the condition is known as sleep apnea syndrome. For this subgroup of chronic snorers, the condition poses a significant health risk.

The diagnosis of sleep apnea syndrome must be made with the help of sleep-laboratory recordings showing episodes of respiratory pausing that occur at a rate of more than five per hour of sleep. In some patients this rate can be as high as 100 per hour. When the condition is severe, not only is there a nighttime problem because the affected person must wake up to break out of the obstructed episode many times but there is also a daytime problem—difficulty remaining awake during the following day. Sleep apnea patients often fall asleep while driving, at work, while watching television, or during any other sedentary time. These symptoms come on so gradually that they may not be recognized as anything more than fatigue. Usually the connection between the nocturnal snoring and the daytime sleepiness is not apparent to the affected individual or to others.

Snorers and their spouses need to be treated as a couple. A patient who has sleep apnea at night will often have little energy to engage in family life. The wife needs to be counseled to help her understand the problem and to get her to participate in the treatment plan. This is particularly true if the snorer is obese and needs to change his diet and be encouraged and supported in an exercise program.

An estimated 4 million to 10 million Americans (1–4% of the population) are thought to be affected by sleep apnea. Snoring is considerably more prevalent—as many as 45% of people snore at some time, and as many as 25% are chronic snorers. Because snoring is a prelude to apnea, it should not be ignored; it may be an important warning sign.

Treatments for both conditions range from surgery that removes obstructions or excess tissue in the nose or throat to exercises that improve the tone of the tongue and throat muscles to weight-loss programs. There are also many devices that have been developed to help overcome the noisy breathing. Some of these are dental appliances worn during sleep. One device holds the tongue taut in a forward position to keep it from falling backward and thus obstructing the airway when the patient relaxes into sleep. Another holds the jaw forward to increase the room at the back of the

A man who suffers from sleep apnea syndrome wears a nasal continuous positive airway pressure device that administers pressurized air through his nose and upper airway while he sleeps. The treatment helps him breathe normally and reduces snoring.

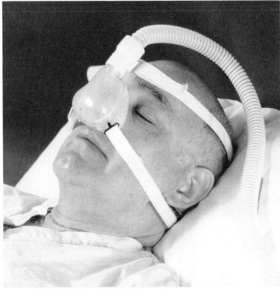

Mayo Clinic Health Letter, Rochester, Minnesota

airway. There is also a palate lifter that holds the soft palate firmly to keep it from vibrating. Other devices train patients to avoid sleeping on their backs. One is a beeper that is worn on the torso and sounds to warn the patient to turn over onto his or her side. Many sleep apneic patients and snorers are entirely relieved of their problems by sleeping in the lateral position (on either side). Another, more inventive, device that accomplishes the same thing is a nightshirt with a vertical pocket on the back that holds four tennis balls. This, too, trains the patient to sleep only in the lateral position.

All of the above devices are helpful for some patients. However, when snoring and apnea are severe, the treatment that has become standard is nasal continuous positive airway pressure, or CPAP. This therapy utilizes equipment consisting of a mask that is worn over the nose and has a hose connected to a compressor; the latter pumps room air under variable levels of pressure, which is inhaled by the sleeper to keep the throat muscles from collapsing. This treatment is highly successful and is often used as an interim treatment while the patient is losing weight, exercising to increase muscle tone, or learning a new sleep position.

Insomnia: psychological and physical causes

Snoring is probably the most common of the problems seen at the specialized sleep centers but not the most frequently heard complaint that patients take to their physician. Insomnia, without doubt, holds that position, with an estimated 15 to 30% of the adult population affected at some time in their lives. Commonly those suffering from inadequate amounts of or poor-quality sleep medicate themselves with herbal teas, over-the-counter preparations, or alcohol. Those who complain to their physician may be given a short-acting benzodiazepine such as temazepam (Restoril) or lorazepam (Ativan) or an antidepressant such as amitriptyline (Elavil). Or they may be told to take a vacation. The medications usually give some temporary relief and are appropriate for only very short-term troubles. Other approaches include muscle-relaxation training to calm the body, visualization techniques to prevent the excessive worry common in insomnia, and psychotherapy to retrain patients in handling their waking tensions more appropriately.

There are many reasons for an inability to fall asleep or stay asleep long enough to wake refreshed. A physical problem that is subtle and can be difficult to diagnose is called periodic movements of sleep, in which there is rhythmic twitching of the feet and legs that prevents sound sleep and may result in multiple arousals. It is sometimes preceded by restless leg or restless limb syndrome. Persons suffering from this disorder are fatigued during the day but are unaware of their sleep problem and thus of the cause of their tiredness. To identify the problem it is usually necessary to monitor their sleep in a sleep laboratory.

One method that has been used as a treatment for leg twitching is the stimulation of the legs *before* sleep by an electric stimulator; this appears to tire the specific muscles of the legs so that they remain calm during sleep. Some patients are treated with the muscle-relaxing drug clonazepam (Klonopin), which does not stop the twitching but tends to enable patients to sleep through the night without being roused by their leg movements.

Sleep–wake cycle disturbances

Another problem that is at the root of poor sleep for some patients is a dysfunction in the basic biological rhythms that underlie the sleep–wake cycle. The most important of these is the body temperature cycle. This rhythm keeps body temperature high during the day, when physical activity is high, and low during the night, when activity is reduced. At night the body's temperature normally drops by one to two degrees Celsius (two to three degrees Fahrenheit). Alertness cycles coincide with body temperature variations. In some people the nighttime drop in temperature is too small at sleep onset, and the temperature remains higher than normal during the whole sleep period. This results in a lighter, more easily disrupted sleep.

An effective treatment for many who have this problem is to take a very hot bath two hours before bedtime. The hot bath drives the body temperature up, which then forces the body's internal regulating mechanism to reduce the temperature to lower than normal levels. Falling asleep while one's temperature is in the process of being adjusted lower will usually result in a deeper and more stable sleep.

There are other sleep–wake cycle disturbances associated with shift work, jet-plane travel across time zones, or times when, for example, students skip nights of sleep and then "sleep in" to recover. Any of these situations can affect the basic body rhythm, with the result that sleep is delayed until very late and waking up at the usual time in the morning becomes very difficult. This condition is known as phase delay. Sleeping medications to hasten sleep onset are not the appropriate solution because they do not correct the underlying problem. Two approaches are generally helpful in these cases.

One is a program called chronotherapy, which progressively delays sleep and wake times by two hours each night. In this way the sleep cycle is adjusted until the desired times are reached. This takes up to 10 days to complete and requires strong motivation on the part of the patient. Chronotherapy has been used with those who work on varying shifts—from days to evenings to all-night shifts.

Another technique for helping those with sleep–wake rhythm problems takes advantage of the fact

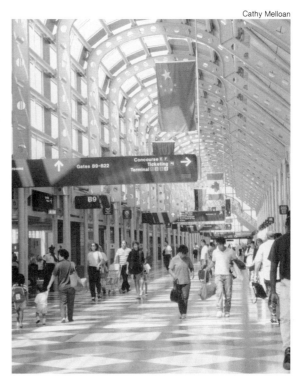

Cathy Melloan

Air travel across time zones upsets the human circadian pacemaker, causing disruption of the sleep–wake cycle. New research is showing that exposure to bright lights can help those who suffer from jet lag by resetting the body's biological clock.

that humans are light sensitive. Sitting near bright lights that mimic the full spectrum of sunlight for an hour in the morning helps set the internal clock back so that earlier timing for sleep is possible. Getting up and taking an early morning walk may do the same thing for those who live in a sunny climate.

The opposite rhythm problem of being phase delayed is to be phase advanced. Phase-advanced patients are too sleepy too early in the evening and wake up too early in the morning. Many elderly patients have this problem. This can be treated by the use of bright lights in the early evening hours and the wearing of eyeshades to block morning light.

The usefulness of bright lights for resetting the human circadian pacemaker (the body clock that primes the human body for restful sleep at night and peak performance during the day) is currently being explored for people who suffer from seasonal affective disorder (SAD). Apparently, these people become depressed in response to the reduction of daylight in the autumn and winter months. The application of this work to helping persons who are suffering from jet lag after international travel or who have difficulty sleeping after changes in work shifts seems very promising. In recently reported experiments, researchers successfully reset the biological clocks in human subjects by exposing them to five hours of bright light; after three cycles of exposure, their circadian pacemakers were reset by up to 12 hours. In essence the brain is "tricked" into believing it is daytime no matter what the actual time is. Intensity of lighting and timing were apparently the keys to the experiment's success.

Depression and dreaming

The most common of the underlying problems that contribute to poor sleep are anxiety and depression. Depression affects waking life as well as sleep and comprises many psychological and physical symptoms. Most patients who suffer from depressive disorders also complain of short and unrefreshing sleep. This sleep disturbance has some unique properties that differ from the characteristics that are typical of other poor sleepers. One feature of depression-related sleep dysfunction is that the time between falling asleep and beginning the first dream period is reduced. The first sleep cycle, therefore, is much shorter than normal—usually by one-third to one-half. Another difference is in the length of this first period of REM sleep, which is often longer than normal and may even be double in length. Even the rapid eye movements are affected; they occur in dense bursts of activity followed by quiet periods. These REM differences have suggested to sleep researchers that there may be some malfunction in the psychology of the dream as well.

Dreaming has remained an area of mystery because of the difficulty most people have in remembering this material. However, in sleep laboratories polygraph recordings can be made of a patient's brain waves, respiration, muscle activity of the chin and legs, and movements of the eyes. Once the REM sleep is over and NREM sleep begins again, the memory of the dream is likely to disappear completely. When people are awakened in the sleep laboratory during their REM sleep, there is very little loss of the memory of the dream. Typically from three to five dreams can be retrieved each night with this technique, and the technique has made it possible to compare the dreams of the depressed with those of persons not suffering from depression.

Recent work has shown that the dreams of depressed persons do have unique properties, which provides sleep researchers with insights into the nighttime psychology of depression and also helps explain why the morning mood of the depressed patient typically is so low upon awakening. Studies of the dreams of those who are going through or recently have been through periods of unusual stress reveal that there is commonly a process of searching through earlier memories that occurs in the minds of these people during sleep. This is seen in people who have experienced natural disasters, in victims of criminal assaults such as rape or kidnapping, in those facing major surgery or going through bereavement, or at any other time of

heightened emotion. The search through earlier memories may produce dream scenarios that are useful in working things through or disastrous in reemphasizing the individual's helplessness. Which of these patterns the dreams follow seems to depend on the individual's personal history of successful coping in the past.

Whether helpful or troubled, dreams provide important information on the structure of the emotional memory system unique to that individual. This can be very useful to the clinician working with the depressed patient. Dreams allow a therapist to work more quickly and with greater assurance in addressing the patient's difficulties in coping with overwhelming stress. Patients can usually understand and accept the dream material as being their own views of their problem better than they can accept a therapist's view of their troubles. Dream therapy, which has been out of fashion for several decades, is beginning to come back into use now that dreams can be retrieved more reliably in the sleep laboratory.

Sleepwalking and acts of violence

Other sleep-related problems presently receiving special attention are somnambulism (sleepwalking) and night terrors—the so-called behavior disorders of sleep. Both are relatively common in young children, although they occur in adults as well.

Recently there have been several reported cases of acts of violence, even murder, taking place during sleepwalking episodes. Although it is hard to be sure after the fact, the persons who have been examined by sleep experts have been found to be profoundly deep sleepers who experience arousals into some kind of confusional state during which they believe they are being attacked and must defend themselves or a loved one. Thus, they lash out without being fully awake. Some of these persons have done severe bodily damage to themselves and to others while in this kind of active dreamlike state—usually without having any memory of these events the following morning. In the cases of murder, the question has been raised: Was the crime an act for which the murderer is "not guilty by reason of insanity"? Or is the individual guilty despite the inability to recall the act or have any motivation for the attack in the waking state?

As better understanding of and better means to diagnose sleep-related problems have accrued, the field of sleep disorders has become faced with new legal and ethical issues. Sleep is a system designed for the mind's and the body's rest and recuperation. It is, however, vulnerable to many kinds of disruption—some transient, some persistent, some benign, and some even lethal. The public should be aware of what these disorders are. For sleep to be restored to its proper state of functioning, the problems need special attention.

—*Rosalind D. Cartwright, Ph.D.*

Four Months in a Cave: Experiment in Chronobiology

by Joseph Degioanni, M.D., Ph.D.

At noon on May 23, 1989, in Carlsbad, N.M., a crowd of reporters and photographers gathered around an opening in the ground, waiting to catch the first glimpse of a woman who had just participated in a most unusual scientific experiment. Some of them may have been surprised by the sight of a slender, unprepossessing young woman, blinking in the bright sunlight as she emerged from the underground habitat in which she had just spent 131 days. The woman, Stefania Follini, was not a veteran scientific investigator but rather an adventurous 27-year-old from Ancona, Italy. Follini, an interior designer by profession and also a brown belt in judo, had volunteered for this mission. The experiment—in which Follini surpassed the previous record for time spent by a woman in "timeless isolation" by 31 days—represented the culmination of many months' work on the part of an international group of scientists.

The timeless isolation project was conceived by an organization called Pioneer Frontier Explorations and Researches, based in Ancona. Its members—psychologists, physicians, geologists, engineers, and other research scientists—share an interest in the burgeoning science of chronobiology, the study of biological rhythms and the mechanisms that govern them. The Pioneer group's main purpose is to investigate the effects on human health and functioning of solitary existence in "clockless" environments. The head of the group, Maurizio Montalbini, a clinical psychologist, holds the world record for timeless isolation; in 1986–87 he remained alone in the Frasassi Cave (near Ancona) for 210 days.

In November 1988 Montalbini and two of the other Pioneer scientists traveled to the U.S. to begin making plans for the project involving Follini. They had gained the attention of this author, who is a medical officer at the Johnson Space Center of the National Aeronautics and Space Administration (NASA) in Houston, Texas, and had been investigating the effects on astronauts of extended-duration space missions. A collaboration ensued in the experiment at Carlsbad, which the Italians dubbed Frontiera Donna ("Pioneer Woman").

A great many other people also lent their support to this unique project. It should be pointed out that the invaluable help provided by individual scientists was not in connection with or financially supported by the institutions with which they are affiliated; their involvement in this experiment was on a strictly personal and voluntary basis.

Studying biological rhythms

Chronobiology as a science truly began in the 20th century, when scientists became generally aware of biological rhythmicity. Since the late 1940s reports on the subject have been produced at an almost exponential rate. Experimental designs have involved all types of species—plant and animal—and have been conducted at all levels—organ, cellular, and biochemical. Chronobiologists have investigated the flowering of the Chinese bamboo (*Phyllostachys bambusoides*), the effect of light on immune function in rats, and the rhythms of the production of the hormone melatonin and its precursors in the pineal gland of humans. Important applications have come out of this research—light treatment for human fatigue and depression, biorhythmically structured schedules for the administration of chemotherapy to cancer patients, and the identification of the phenomenon of morning hypercoagulability (an acceleration in the normal process of blood clotting), which correlates with the peak incidence of strokes and heart attacks in the early morning hours.

Other experiments have been designed to investigate the effects on humans of alterations in the social environment. With the help of volunteer subjects, researchers succeeded in modifying natural biological rhythms such as the sleep-wake cycle and the cycle of melatonin production. Attempts were made to correlate these changes with the subjects' moods and their performance of various tasks. Institutions with an interest in the effects of confinement and isolation on their personnel—among them, the U.S. Navy and NASA—have collaborated in such experiments.

Few experiments, however, have focused on the chronobiological experience of individuals confined for prolonged periods (three months or longer) in a constant environment. Those who have carried out work in this area include Jack Findley, a psychologist at the University of Maryland, who pioneered such an effort in 1963, and two French researchers, Michel Siffre and Jean-Claude Dumas, who have organized a series of underground isolation experiments over the past 25 years.

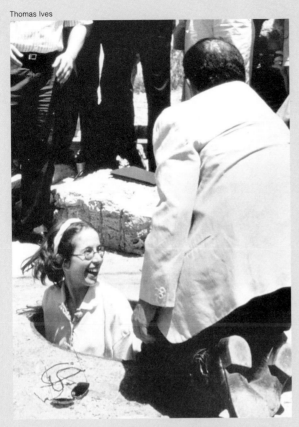

On May 23, 1989, a triumphant Stefania Follini emerges into the brilliant New Mexico sunlight from the underground habitat in which she had spent 131 days participating in a human isolation experiment.

The cave: a "natural" for human isolation

There are many advantages to underground or cave experiments. From a scientific point of view, the cave environment is reliably constant (even the air temperature does not fluctuate perceptibly); total isolation from the surface environment can be promptly achieved; and monitoring of the subjects is relatively easy. From a budgetary point of view, the cave is far less expensive than construction of an artificial environment would be and, furthermore, it has a popular appeal that typically attracts news media interest. In fact, such publicity has, over the years, provided a substantial subsidy to the funding of cave experiments. An important consideration of the Pioneer Woman project was that a long-duration isolation experiment would be more likely to succeed in a natural setting than in an artificial one. The theory behind this approach is simple; it is presumed that human beings feel more at ease in natural surroundings, whereas artificial environments may be psychologically harsh and would not be well tolerated over extended periods of time.

The NASA connection to the cave experiments dates back to a 1972 experiment by Siffre, a speleologist and expert in human chronobiology; Siffre had re-mained in isolation in an underground habitat in Texas for six months. NASA provided Siffre's meals; the agency was interested in developing food that would be palatable to an individual essentially simulating a six-months' space voyage.

Choosing subject and site

Stefania Follini—the "pioneer woman" of the experiment—was primarily interested in surpassing the record for timeless isolation by a woman, which had been established in 1988 by Veronique LeGuen, an underwater speleologist, who had remained for 100 days in a cave in southern France. Volunteers for the experiment had first been recruited by advertisement in Italian newspapers. The field was narrowed to about 12, who were then subjected to a battery of psychological tests, a thorough medical checkup, and a series of interviews. The investigators wanted to make certain they would have a subject who was physically healthy and had no psychiatric problems. In addition, each was taken to the Frasassi Cave in Italy, left alone, and told that someone would return to fetch him or her in a given period of time; it was felt that candidates' responses to this particular stress would be especially revealing. In the end, Follini was chosen over the others primarily because of her extremely high level of motivation—considered by the researchers to be an essential factor. She had read of Montalbini's research and was eager, interested, and determined to succeed.

Lost Cave in New Mexico had been selected by Montalbini during his November 1988 trip with the assistance of Ron Kerbo of the U.S. National Parks Service. Kerbo, a cave expert assigned to the Carlsbad Caverns National Park, was already familiar with Montalbini's work and had participated in Siffre's Texas cave study. A cave in the town of Carlsbad, outside the park itself and away from the tourist traffic, was selected. It satisfied the primary criteria of being totally soundproof and providing a comfortable, "shirt-sleeve" environment (in temperature and humidity). It was also free from bats, and the radon level was acceptably low. The cavern itself is shallow, the floor being about 9 to 12 m (30 to 40 ft) from the surface; it is about 23 m (75 ft) wide and 91 m (300 ft) long.

The Pioneer group brought their own personnel and engineers to build the 9-sq m (100-sq ft) Plexiglas and plywood habitat that Follini would occupy. The habitat was set against the far end wall of the rocky cavern. The city of Carlsbad was immensely supportive of the project and assisted the Italian visitors by supplying the trailers from which they monitored the experiment as well as extra electrical and communication lines. (The city council gave Montalbini a plaque and Follini the city's keys!) The Italian research team worked frantically with a very small budget to put the various components of the investigation into working order.

Monitoring mind and body

Before the experiment began, the aid of Franz Halberg, who is director of the Chronobiology Laboratories at the University of Minnesota, was enlisted to handle the bulk of the chronobiology analyses. Halberg is probably the world's preeminent authority on biological rhythms. In fact, it was he who coined the term *circadian* (meaning "a period of about 24 hours"). The automatic, continuous monitoring of Follini's blood pressure was started about two weeks prior to January 13, the day she entered the cave. This was the first time an experiment had undertaken to measure a free-running blood pressure rhythm. (A rhythm is free running when it drifts independent of the environmental and social cues to which one is constantly subjected in everyday life.)

The equipment and protocol necessary to conduct an ongoing monitoring of Follini's immune system during the isolation was provided by Gerald Sonnenfeld, an immunologist from the University of Louisville, Ky., in collaboration with John Measel of the Arlington (Texas) Cancer Center; Michael Loken of the Becton Dickinson Monoclonal Center, Mountain View, Calif.; and Gerald Taylor of NASA. This protocol required some complicated logistics because blood samples had to be analyzed within 24 hours of drawing. Follini had learned under a physician's guidance how to draw her own blood. A 61-m (200-ft)-long, 15-cm (6-in)-diameter plastic pipeline was set up to deliver samples from the cavern to the surface. A total of 10 blood samples were drawn for this study, including both preisolation and postisolation specimens. These were then shipped for analysis at the three centers—the University of Louisville, the Arlington Cancer Center, and the Becton Dickinson Center.

Electroencephalographic (EEG) equipment, which had been deemed extremely important, was difficult to come by without appropriate funding. Finally, only two weeks prior to the experiment, the research team obtained help from a group of scientists headed by Jon DeFrance, a neurophysiologist at the University of Texas Health Science Center at Houston. DeFrance had been developing a program to correlate behavioral performance with cognitive evoked potentials—that is, electrical activity produced by the brain in the presence of an attention or memory task.

The electrical component that was of most interest to the researchers was the P300 evoked potential, so called because it occurs about 300 milliseconds after the stimulus to the brain and it is a positive (P) electrical signal. The strength and distribution of the P300 evoked potential can be correlated clinically with certain mental dysfunctions, including attention deficit problems (*i.e.*, difficulties in concentrating). Additionally, when administered with a battery of computer tests, the technique can provide an index of the amount of effort expended by the brain in completing these tests.

DeFrance and his associate Chris Hymel transported the computer equipment to New Mexico just two days prior to the start of the isolation. Several dedicated people worked to set up the evoked potential hardware in the cave. Unfortunately, owing to a series of technical problems, an adequate signal was never obtained, and the researchers had to be satisfied with standard EEGs recorded during Follini's sleep. However, they were able to perform the P300 studies shortly after Follini returned to the surface and again six months later when she returned to the U.S. for follow-up tests.

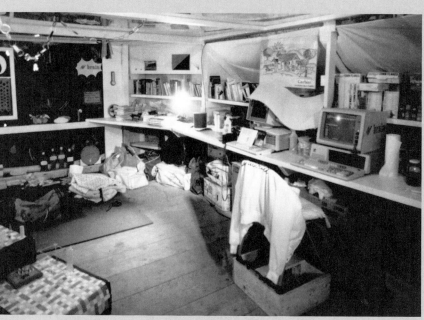

Follini's Plexiglas and plywood habitat was set into a rocky cavern about 10 meters (33 feet) belowground. The computer terminal was her only means of communicating with the outside world. She spent her days reading 200 of the 400 books she had with her, playing her guitar, studying English, and writing in her diary—and, in the process, she lost considerable track of the time; when she emerged late in May, she believed it was about the end of March.

Before, during, and after the experiment, Follini was also required to complete a battery of tests, given by a portable computer called the automated portable test system (APTS), which consists of 21 tasks that address aspects of human performance such as reaction time, memory, and accuracy of response. The APTS has been used in assessing performance decrements in subjects who have taken anti-motion-sickness drugs (used—or for potential use—in spaceflight), in subjects deprived of oxygen in altitude chamber testing, and in other NASA studies. A battery of 11 tests was chosen for the Lost Cave experiment. Each battery took approximately 45 minutes to administer, and Follini did the testing 53 times during the isolation period.

An investigator from the University of Ancona, Andrea Galvagno, was particularly interested in monitoring the depletion rate of the vitamin D stored by Follini's bones. Normally, vitamin D is constantly replenished by diet and manufactured in the skin following exposure to sunlight. In order to accomplish Galvagno's objective, it was necessary that no vitamin D be supplied in Follini's diet or in the spectrum of light to which she was exposed. Both of these requirements were achieved. It was felt that for this and other reasons, the subject's bone mineral density should be measured at least prior to and after the isolation. With the assistance of Victor Schneider, a specialist in bone metabolism and a NASA investigator studying the demineralization of bone in microgravity, the research team obtained measurements of Follini's total bone mineral density before and shortly after the experiment and again six months later.

Passing the time

How does one combat boredom, loneliness, and, ultimately, depression during such confinements? Montalbini's personal approach in the isolation experiments he has completed has been to rely on his own creative potential. For this reason, he chose not to structure Follini's day with any rigid guidelines. She took with her 400 books, a guitar, a tape recorder with English-language tapes, and a diary. She did not have any video or music tapes, which are felt to interfere with personal creativity. Being a vegetarian, she took plenty of cereals, legumes, dried fruits, and seaweed. Her only link to the surface was a table-top computer screen; all communications were transmitted by keyboard. A buzzer sounded in the cave to signal her when people on the surface wished to communicate with her. When not directed to do tests, she studied English from the tapes, made all sorts of drawings, decorated her habitat extensively, and read about 200 of her books.

Two cameras monitored Follini constantly. One was situated about nine meters from the habitat and provided a wide-angle view. Another was inside the habitat and transmitted a close-up picture. Follini could move out of field of the cameras by strolling beyond the wide-angle camera. The toilet facility was private. Waste was treated chemically and stored until removal from the cave at the end of the experiment. She did not have a shower or tub and washed herself with packaged towelettes. She had a small burner and fry pan to cook her own meals. Electric light in the cave was constant, as any alteration could trigger an unwanted biorhythm. She could, however, reduce the intensity of light in the habitat slightly when she went to sleep.

Clockless existence

Follini appeared to have a strong "internal clock" that did not deviate significantly from the normal 24-hour sleep-wake cycle until probably the second half of the isolation period. Later on, however, some of her sleep-wake cycles ranged as much as 40 hours in length. Her average "cave day" was 25 hours long. Thus, in their analysis of her sleep-wake cycle, the researchers recorded 122 cave days for the 131 actual days she spent in the cave. Her own perception of elapsed time was grossly out of line, as she estimated late March or early April to be the date just prior to termination of the isolation on May 23.

In late March Halberg and his colleagues at the University of Minnesota Chronobiology Laboratories reported free-running blood pressure rhythms of about 25 hours' duration from the automatic blood pressure monitoring device Follini wore. They were puzzled by her free-running heart rate, which indicated a circaseptan rhythm (circaseptan meaning "of about seven days"). Follini continued to wear the blood pressure monitor for several months after completion of the isolation. Halberg observed that the circaseptan heart rate persisted until resumption of her menses in mid-September. (Her menstrual periods had stopped about two weeks into the experiment.) After September her body rhythms were reestablished at precisely 24 hours, and Halberg concluded that the longer cycles, or infradians—as exemplified in this instance in particular by the length of time between menstrual cycles—may become dominant in conditions of social isolation and, indeed, may be responsible for lengthening other, shorter cycles (e.g., from 24 to 25 hours).

Physical findings

Follini lost weight during the isolation, from 51 kg (112 lb) on January 13 to a low of 40 kg (88 lb) on May 17. Her appetite decreased, and she began eating less—despite the researchers' admonitions. The APTS tests revealed no decrements in reaction time or accuracy of response. In mid-March DeFrance noticed that REM (rapid eye movement) sleep had begun to occur earlier in her sleep cycle, a symptom sometimes associated with depression. When questioned about her mood, she reported feeling fine and would not hear of early termination of the experiment. Following her exuberant exit from the cave on May 23, however, she became more solemn in mood and withdrawn; a week later De-France obtained an image of the P300 visual evoked topographic map of her brain at the EEG laboratory of Gulf Pines Hospital in Houston. The result was consistent with the presence of an attention disorder. This finding was thought to correlate with the clinical picture of depression evident at that point. Bone-density measurements taken one week postisolation showed a significant calcium loss from the trabecular bone (lumbar spine) of about 8%, compared with the baseline established prior to isolation.

Follini returned to normal life—that is, to her work and her environment in Ancona—after a several-month span of tours, press interviews, and appearances on talk shows in the U.S. and Italy. She regained the lost weight during that time. She returned to Houston from Italy in late November 1989 for one round of follow-up tests. A repeat bone scan showed a persistent 8% loss in bone mineral density. However, since her menses had resumed just two months prior, the researchers felt that additional time should be allowed for possible recovery of bone density, and further bone scans were planned for the future.

The P300 topographic map was recorded again in November, at the six-month interval. It showed a strong, healthy pattern, indicating complete resolution of the isolation-induced deficits. This finding also correlated with Follini's clinical condition; in mood and affect she had returned to her "normal," outgoing self and had without difficulty resumed her social and professional lives. Additionally, she was eager to get back home, as she missed her new boyfriend in Ancona. Analysis of the samples taken by the immunologists is continuing; additional baseline samples were obtained in March 1990. Preliminary results demonstrate that there was a striking increase in the activity of certain cells vital to normal immune function—called natural killer cells—throughout the isolation phase of the experiment.

Conclusions from the Lost Cave experiment

Follini's willingness to collect physiological data allowed the investigators to probe uncharted territory in biological research. Although it is unlikely that an astronaut would ever be sent alone into outer space, Follini's experience has definite and serious implications for the future of efforts in the colonization of space. Perhaps more importantly, it offers a potential new arena of research for investigating human biological makeup and, ultimately, new insights into the various pathological processes that afflict all of humankind.

Because the experiment was poorly designed to evaluate bone mineral loss, it is difficult to draw any firm conclusions from Follini's significant loss of bone density. Probably the loss was a result of one or more factors, including weight loss, nutritive deficit, lack of estrogen due to cessation of menstruation, and physical inactivity. It is possible that a disruption in biorhythms may have so altered the production of hormones by the pituitary gland and ovaries as to lead to the cessation of menstruation. Another possibility is that depression induced an alteration in biorhythms. Whatever the cause, the significant bone-density loss and Follini's ability to reincorporate calcium into her bones over the next few years will have definite implications for the understanding of osteoporosis. It will also have implications for future astronauts on long interplanetary voyages, who will be subjected to microgravity-induced calcium loss during such flights. The massive increase in natural killer cell activity left many of the researchers puzzled but no less firm in their belief that the immune system is extremely sensitive to environmental factors.

Follini's experiment clearly demonstrated free-running rhythms in temperature and, for the first time, blood pressure and pulse. It is becoming apparent that this kind of alteration, or desynchronization, of various cardiovascular and metabolic activities is commonly associated with unusual schedules (as might be imposed by the vagaries of activities in extraterrestrial space). Therefore, it would be interesting to find out to what extent such desynchronization correlates with adverse effects on both health and performance. It might be equally interesting to determine to what degree synchronization by a variety of environmental influences is desirable for optimal performance and maintenance of health.

It would appear that human tolerance to free-running biological rhythms as elicited in isolation experiments is highly individual and variable. Just as some people cope with shift work successfully, others develop insomnia, depression, and alcohol dependence. Some authorities believe that a factor in selection of a crew for a mission to Mars should be tolerance to free-running biological rhythms. Scientists do not yet know what role desynchronization plays in the many physiological changes—musculoskeletal, cardiovascular, neurological—that occur in the microgravity of spaceflight. The Pioneer Woman project certainly demonstrated that desynchronization may play a significant role in the alteration of metabolic, immunologic, and neurological functioning.

This experiment and other single-person isolation studies have yielded "pure" data on biological rhythms; by contrast, group isolation studies add the dimension of intrapersonal dynamics, which have quite different results. At this point very little is known about so-called social chronobiology; its significance, however, is likely to be important in crew selection for and performance potential during long-duration space missions. Clearly there is considerably more to be learned from both single and group social isolation studies in the future.

Surgery

"The higher technology, of which we are so proud, is aimed largely at the salvation of patients who have already traversed a long and downward sloping road." That statement, which was made in 1985 by a surgeon, Edgar Haber, summed up the achievements of the increasingly dynamic specialty of general surgery.

Throughout the late 1980s and entering the decade of the 1990s, the intensity of surgical research has remained at a high level, with continued good results and improved patient care. New horizons have developed, improved technology has emerged, and some of surgery's most cherished concepts have been challenged. The surgical practices of today are dictated by the research of yesterday; so, too, the practices of tomorrow will emerge from present explorations of new surgical possibilities.

A crisis in trauma care

In 1983 the American College of Surgeons designated three levels of trauma care in the U.S. in an attempt to improve the availability of resources and emergency health care for the injured patient. Levels I and II trauma centers have the immediate availability of skilled surgeons, other members of the trauma team, and support services such as computed tomography (CT) scanning, enabling them to provide quality care on the spot for the trauma patient. Level I trauma centers additionally give high priority to training and research. Level III trauma centers do not have all of the necessary resources needed for complete care of the trauma patient, such as thoracic surgeons or neurosurgeons. Ideally, following stabilization at a level III trauma center, a patient would be transferred to a level I or II center, if necessary.

Despite this organization of resources and the initial enthusiasm for the designation of trauma centers, accessibility to health care for the injured patient has declined markedly. Rising costs of health care, coupled with decreased reimbursement for trauma services, have forced many centers to close. Thus, access to trauma care today is less than adequate, as designated centers and their emergency rooms can no longer subsidize care. The depletion of resources will lead to further closure of facilities; already the resources crisis is causing trauma victims to be transported to facilities that are often at great distances from sites where care is most needed and should be available.

Recently a study at the St. Louis (Mo.) University Medical Center, a level I trauma center, highlighted the problem of reimbursement in trauma care. The costs of caring for patients over a 10-month period were evaluated. The total cost for 207 consecutive patients was $4,044,156, or an average of $19,537 per patient. The total reimbursement was only $2,054,090, or 51% of the total cost.

The present situation will ultimately lead to greater health care costs for treating the complications of poor or nonexistent care at the time of injury—the result of a lack of resources. An increase in preventable deaths may be the end result. Clearly, the criteria for reimbursement in trauma care need urgent reevaluation in order to prevent further exacerbation of this emergent crisis.

New approach to breast reconstruction

Women with breast cancer, and their surgeons, face many decisions with regard to the proper treatment of the malignancy. They must consider: (1) what the appropriate type of surgical management is, (2) whether adjuvant treatments such as chemotherapy or radiation therapy will be used, and (3) what the cosmetic appearance of the breast will be following surgery. If the best surgical treatment of a woman's breast cancer is removal of the entire breast (mastectomy), the chest wall can be reconstructed. A "new breast" can be constructed through the use of a variety of prostheses (plastic implants) placed under the skin or by transfer of muscle from the back or abdomen to create a breast mound.

Previously, immediate reconstruction of the breast—*i.e.*, formation of a new breast at the time of mastectomy—particularly when the cancer had spread to the lymph nodes in the axilla (armpit), was discouraged. The conventional teaching was that the breast should not be reconstructed until after a two-year observation period since breast cancer may recur at the site of

Long delays for care in the emergency room at Cook County Hospital in Chicago are typical of the situation that has resulted from the closing of many urban trauma centers across the United States.

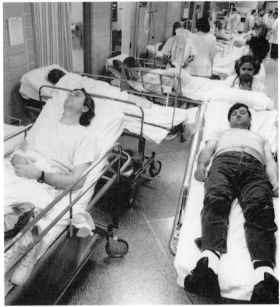

Michael Melford

a mastectomy. It was thought that immediate breast reconstruction could inhibit the detection of a recurrent breast cancer at the mastectomy site by hiding new lumps or concealing small recurrent tumors from detection by mammography (X-rays of the breast).

Recent studies, however, have shown that immediate breast reconstruction does not mask recurrent breast cancers. The freedom from disease and the overall survival of breast cancer patients who have had mastectomy and immediate breast reconstruction have been shown to be similar to those who had mastectomy alone. The investigators in one such study concluded that "in the absence of any apparent negative impact on patient outcome and because of the well documented positive psychosocial benefit of immediate reconstruction, this procedure should be routinely offered to women with operable breast cancer."

Colon cancer: surgery plus chemotherapy

In October 1989 the U.S. National Cancer Institute (NCI) issued an alert to 35,000 oncologists announcing the efficacy of adjuvant therapy using two drugs, levamisole and 5-fluorouracil (5-FU), for patients who have been treated surgically for a particular type of colon cancer. In the United States there will be 150,000 new cases of colon cancer this year. Approximately 21,000 of these patients will have regional lymph node involvement (Dukes' C stage), which carries a relatively poor prognosis, at the time of surgery. Their five-year survival rate is approximately 30–40%, compared with a 60–70% survival rate for those who have a tumor with negative lymph node involvement (Dukes' B).

Positive lymph nodes are a harbinger of widespread microscopic disease. Adjuvant systemic therapy (administered intravenously) attempts to decrease tumor recurrence, thereby prolonging survival and increasing the cure rate. A number of chemotherapy and immunotherapy regimes have been investigated as adjuvant treatment for colon cancer. Until recently, however, most physicians were skeptical about the objective benefits of these therapeutic efforts.

The new, two-drug treatment appears to substantially reduce the risk of dying from recurrent colon cancer. In essence, levamisole plus 5-FU prolongs the time before recurrences appear; in a major clinical study this amounted to 23 months in a treated group, compared with 14 months in a nontreated group. The

Postsurgical chemotherapy for Dukes' C colon cancer				
postsurgical treatment	number of patients	percentage recurring at 5 years	median interval to recurrence	percentage 5-year survival
none	135	55	14 months	37
levamisole and 5-FU	136	41	23 months	49

Source: National Cancer Institute, National Institutes of Health

overall five-year survival rate for Dukes' C cancer was improved from 37% in the nontreated group to 49% in the group treated with 5-FU and levamisole. The investigators and the NCI concluded that postsurgical observation rather than chemotherapy is no longer justifiable. The option of receiving this adjuvant treatment should be discussed with nearly every patient found to have colon cancer with lymph node involvement.

Lung-assist technology: new potential

In recent years surgeons have developed and improved a treatment for neonatal respiratory failure, a common problem that can develop in premature and low-birth-weight babies or can be caused by several conditions affecting newborns. The surgical procedure known as extracorporeal membrane oxygenation (ECMO) entirely bypasses the infant's lungs by connecting one of the carotid arteries in the neck to the heart. ECMO machinery is a modified membrane apparatus that permits the long-term oxygenation of blood with minimal damage to the blood elements, replacing the lungs for a short period of time. The baby's lungs are thus allowed to rest and mature. In one study 50 newborn infants in whom there was a predicted 80% mortality rate were treated through the use of ECMO; the dramatic results showed a survival rate of 90%. This significant technological and palliative advance is now being studied for extension to the supportive care of adult patients. It may be of benefit in treating ventricular heart failure and poor lung function associated with major injuries and as a bridge to lung transplantation.

Shock waves for gallstones

Approximately 500,000 Americans per year undergo cholecystectomy (surgical removal of the gallbladder) as treatment for gallstones. Extensive analysis of patients undergoing this procedure suggests that approximately 95,000 Americans each year are potential candidates for an alternative, noninvasive treatment called extracorporeal shock wave lithotripsy (ESWL), originally developed for treatment of renal, or kidney, stones. ESWL results in the fragmentation of gallstones by ultrasound-guided shock waves.

These procedures are not painless, but the discomfort can be easily controlled by analgesics. Anesthesia is not required, patients return to normal activity within hours, hospitalization is not necessary, and patient acceptance is quite high.

Numerous studies continue to evaluate ESWL with respect to efficacy, safety, recurrence of gallstones, and cost. At least nine manufacturers have produced ESWL instruments; further technical advances will result in improved generations of these devices. Presently, however, the limitations of this technology make ESWL applicable only to a segment of patients with symptoms due to gallstones. Limitations of the procedure are based on the inability of ultrasound to produce images of gallstones in the common bile duct, which drains the gallbladder. Currently, infection of the gallbladder (cholecystitis), obstructions preventing the gallbladder from draining, and multiple stones are contraindications for ESWL.

Although surgical cholecystectomy remains the treatment of choice for gallstone disease, alternate management techniques in addition to ESWL are currently being evaluated. An emerging treatment for gallstones is laparoscopic cholecystectomy, a technique that utilizes the laparoscope (a lighted flexible tube) to enter the abdomen and remove the gallbladder by use of either electrocautery or laser. The potential advantages of this technique are earlier hospital dismissal, fewer complications, shorter postoperative convalescence, and earlier return to normal activity. Long-term results of these newer modalities must await follow-up studies.

Surgery for the youngest and oldest

Age alone is no longer a contraindication to surgical intervention. At the early end of the age spectrum, fetal surgery began to develop in the 1970s with the introduction of fetal ultrasonography, which allowed for accurate visualization of the structure and function of the fetus. The combination of ultrasonography and screening of maternal serum alpha fetal protein (a biological marker) permitted diagnosis of prenatal anomalies. At the other end of the spectrum, surgical procedures in patients 90 years of age and older have become safer and more frequent.

Breakthroughs in fetal surgery. In the 1980s investigators identified several fetal diseases in which a simple anatomic defect that interfered with organ development might be amenable to correction *in utero*. These included hydronephrosis (obstruction of the collecting system of the kidney), hydrocephalus (accumulation of fluid in the head, often due to obstruction of the flow of cerebrospinal fluid), and diaphragmatic hernia. If left uncorrected, each of these anomalies will result in significant damage to the specific organs or possibly death soon after birth.

In the 1980s the International Fetal Medicine and Surgery Society (IFMSS) was formed, and guidelines were issued for fetal intervention. The IFMSS developed a registry to record cases of hydronephrosis and obstructive hydrocephalus in which tubes were inserted into the fetus to relieve the fluid pressure buildup. This procedure is performed by careful insertion of a needle, with the aid of ultrasound, through the mother's abdomen and into the fetus. A tube is then positioned to drain the fluid buildup and is left in place to prevent urine or cerebrospinal fluid from continuing to exert excessive pressure.

More complex operations, such as the repair of diaphragmatic hernias, require an operation on the mother to open the womb and surgically repair the de-

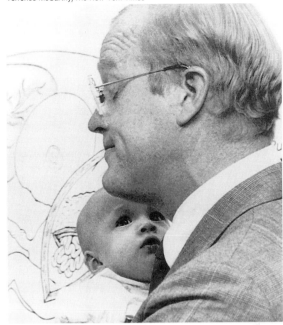

Surgeon Michael R. Harrison holds the baby boy he had operated on as a 24-week-old fetus to repair a diaphragmatic hernia that would likely have been fatal. While such highly experimental procedures involving surgery on the mother through the womb are becoming technically feasible, there remain important ethical questions that must be resolved before the operations are accepted and commonly performed.

velopmental defect. The correction of additional severe fetal abnormalities will require more invasive surgery in both the mother and fetus. These open approaches can be justified only if: (1) the natural history of the human fetal disorder is carefully defined, and it is possible to select only those fetuses with the disorder who are likely to benefit; (2) the pathophysiological structure of the disorder and the safety of intrauterine correction have been previously established in animal models; and (3) the procedure is proved feasible and safe for both mother and fetus in rigorously controlled studies on primate models.

These cases of "open" fetal surgery pose important questions for the surgeon, nevertheless. Often fetal surgery is technically feasible but difficult. Hence, it must be proved safe for the mother and her reproductive potential. The problems of patient selection and diagnostic accuracy will require meticulous surveillance in future years.

Major surgery for the elderly. Demographic data clearly demonstrate a projected increase in surgery for the age group 75 years and older between now and the end of the 20th century. Improvements in anesthetic management and the operative skills of the surgeon have meant that procedures that were previously not even considered for patients advanced in years are now considered feasible—and indeed beneficial.

An extensive study from the Mayo Clinic, Rochester, Minn., compared outcomes for 795 patients 90 years of age and older who underwent major operative procedures with age-, sex-, and calendar-year-matched peers from the general population not undergoing operation. The study revealed that in those having surgery there was a modest decrease in patient survival at one year; this was reversed by two years, with an observed survival at five years being comparable to the survival rate of their non-operated-upon peers.

The surgical procedures included emergency and elective operations on virtually every system of the body. About half required general anesthesia. The data from the Mayo Clinic study suggest that 90-year-old patients are able to tolerate the stresses of surgery well.

"Glue" made from blood

Surgeons are now finding wide use for a product that is made from human blood and applied like epoxy. This substance, known as fibrin glue, is used to stop bleeding and to seal reconnected tissues that have been sutured or is used instead of sutures to close a surgical wound. The glue consists of two components, fibrinogen (the sticky substance) and thrombin (which acts as a hardener). When these blood products are combined, they readily produce a clot. Thrombin is an enzyme that facilitates clotting by catalyzing the conversion of fibrinogen to fibrin. Within seconds the clot adheres to blood vessels, bones, or nerves. Once the bond has served its function, fibrin glue is absorbed into the tissues.

Blood banks in the U.S. produce fibrin glue from the patient's own blood, which prevents the spread of hepatitis, AIDS, and other diseases. Fibrin glue can be produced in a laboratory that has the capacity to remove plasma from the patient's blood and keep it frozen for 12 hours. The plasma is then processed to remove the fibrinogen component and smaller amounts of other proteins. Factor XIII, a blood-clotting protein, strengthens the glue and promotes healing.

In the operating room the fibrinogen is placed into one side of a double-barreled syringe, with the other side containing the thrombin. Both elements are then mixed and used for hemostasis (controlling blood loss). Fibrin glue has been used in ear surgery, reconstructive surgery, and cardiovascular and neurological surgeries and may prove useful in every major type of operative procedure.

Surgeons and HIV infection

Hospital workers have always been exposed to occupational hazards, but in recent years a new risk has arisen in the form of the human immunodeficiency virus (HIV) after accidental exposure to infected blood or blood-containing body fluids. In most studies of HIV infection in hospital health care personnel, data on surgeons have been underreported. One survey, however, at San Francisco General Hospital, found that of more than 200 surgeon exposures, none resulted in infection of the surgeon. Another study involving the risk of HIV infection in surgeons from puncture injuries concluded that if the prevalence of HIV infection in surgical patients is 5%, then the estimated 30-year risk of HIV seroconversion (the presence of antibodies to HIV found in a person's serum, indicating that the virus is or has been in the body) is less than 1% for 50% of the group and greater than 6% for 10% of the surgeons.

Two schools of thought have emerged regarding preoperative screening of surgical patients for HIV infection. Those who favor routine screening conclude that: (1) knowledge of HIV status may allow the surgeon to take precautions to decrease the risk of infection; (2) the patient benefits because HIV infection may alter the risk-benefit ratio of the surgical procedure; and (3) knowledge of the HIV status will not affect how the patient is treated. Those who argue against routine screening contend that: (1) since the risk of the surgeon's acquiring infection during the individual procedure is low, it is unlikely that knowledge of HIV status can reduce the risk; (2) patient care may be negatively affected; (3) screening can produce false-positive results; and (4) screening would violate accepted ethical standards of autonomy, confidentiality, and informed consent.

In a national survey of U.S. hospitals conducted by the University of California at Los Angeles, half of the hospitals did not have a policy for coping with the possibility of AIDS infection in surgeons and other potentially exposed hospital workers, nor was there adequate education of health care staff about risks. The debate over screening of patients is likely to continue, and further study of risk is needed.

Future directions

Ongoing investigations in wound healing, cell and tumor biology, and genetic engineering will increasingly allow the surgeon to extend the limits of surgical care. Technological refinements and advances will allow for more precise operative planning, less invasive surgical intervention, and faster patient recovery. An example of this is the use of endovascular surgical techniques to operate on blood vessels from within their lumen.

Further, understanding of the biochemical and cellular events that lead to recurrent disease will have great importance in determining appropriate surgical treatments, and the advent of biochemical informational systems, which are revolutionizing all of medicine, will have significant impact on surgical care. These are just a few of the roads being explored in surgical research today.

—Claude H. Organ, Jr., M.D.,
and William R. Fry, M.D.

Plastic Surgery: When the Patient Is Dissatisfied

by Robert M. Goldwyn, M.D.

People who elect to undergo cosmetic plastic surgery and then are dissatisfied with their results are fortunately a minority—perhaps about 5%. Nevertheless, the impact on the individual patient is enormous, as indeed it is on the surgeon. No patient would undertake an elective procedure, nor would any surgeon perform it, if either *knew* that the outcome would be unfavorable. Although both may reject the possibility that a mishap will occur, for the patient the fear (perhaps unconscious) of a bad result no doubt lingers.

In general, two types of circumstances resulting in a dissatisfied plastic surgery patient can be distinguished. The first is dissatisfaction with a result that is objectively poor. The second is dissatisfaction with a result that is objectively good, maybe even superior. Dissatisfaction can occur after virtually any type of aesthetic surgery—procedures including rhytidectomy (face-lift), rhinoplasty (nose reshaping), blepharoplasty (eyelid surgery), reduction mammaplasty (breast reduction), augmentation mammaplasty (breast enlargement), mastopexy (breast lift), otoplasty (ear pinning), malar augmentation (cheek augmentation), abdominoplasty ("tummy tuck"), liposuction (removal of fat deposits from the face, thighs, abdomen, or buttocks), collagen injections, and so forth.

Whether dissatisfaction is with an objectively poor result or not, the patient has the right to complain, and the surgeon has the responsibility to listen. If the surgical outcome is realistically below average, the onus is on the surgeon to improve it—if possible. The fact that patients have been informed about possible complications or unfavorable results does not mean that they will accept or should accept an unwanted outcome. An informed patient can still be a dissatisfied one.

In many ways dissatisfaction that is based on reality is less of a problem to manage than when it arises subjectively; *i.e.,* the patient is unhappy with a result that others, who have a more objective view, would rate as good or excellent. That patient unfortunately had expected more than his or her surgeon—or any surgeon—could produce. The time for detecting, and ideally modifying, unrealistic expectations is before, not after, an operation.

Typical unhappy patients

Plastic surgeons have come to recognize—frequently too late—several kinds of patients who may be dis-

satisfied with their operative result even though it would satisfy most others. Some types of patients who should sound an inner alarm for the surgeon and are likely to end up dissatisfied are the following:

The patient who is perfectionistic. The person who is seldom satisfied with anything may not be one who should have aesthetic surgery. The probability is that whatever the surgeon can achieve will still leave that individual unhappy. A problem, however, is that the plastic surgeon, by inclination and training, is usually perfectionistic also. The combination of a perfectionistic surgeon and a perfectionistic patient does not always yield a happy outcome since both have inflated expectations.

The patient with minimal deformity. Patients who have abnormal anxiety about a relatively inconspicuous feature very likely will still be displeased postoperatively with their general appearance and then will focus on another body part.

The patient who overshops. Although every patient has the right to a second or third opinion, there are some who see numerous plastic surgeons not so much to obtain a better doctor or even a better price but to secure a guaranteed result. That patient is liable to settle only for the doctor who promises everything or seems to have promised everything. Occasionally a plastic surgeon is flattered to think that the patient has come to him or her after having seen many other qualified colleagues. In that situation the unwary surgeon may promise more than he or she can deliver.

The patient who seeks an operation to please someone else. Women constitute the greatest proportion of aesthetic surgery patients. Some seek to change an anatomic feature to please a male. Quite often it may be an augmentation mammaplasty—enlarging her breasts—to maintain a male's interest. Interpersonal problems cannot be solved through aesthetic surgery. In this case it may be more appropriate for the plastic surgeon to refer the patient and her spouse or partner for counseling or psychotherapy.

The patient who is a "plastisurgiholic." There are certain patients, usually female and more often than not wealthy, who go from surgeon to surgeon seeking and having various aesthetic operations—on the nose, face, eyelids, breasts (augmentation generally), and buttocks and thighs (liposuction)—and then repeating some or all of these. These perpetual plastic surgery

403

patients undoubtedly have a poor body image and low self-esteem and often are masochistic—submitting willingly and even enthusiastically to surgical procedures that can be painful and risky. Many of these women have poor relationships with peers and crave bonding to a paternal or maternal figure—namely, the surgeon. Because these patients have the time and can afford to pay for repeated cosmetic procedures, they will persist until they find a surgeon willing to operate (or redo a procedure that has already been done). Repeated operations, of course, increase the risks of complications, infections, permanent damage, and, indeed, dissatisfaction. These patients may need psychotherapy more than plastic surgery.

The patient who is depressed. People who have had a recent loss, such as the death of a loved one, a divorce, or even termination of psychotherapy, may be depressed and believe that changing an external feature will improve their inner life. The opposite, unfortunately, occurs; such patients become more depressed after their operation with the realization that their new look is unaccompanied by a miraculous transformation of their emotions.

The "pushy" patient. Patients who are at the outset overly assertive or rude—often in their dealings with a receptionist or nurse in the plastic surgeon's office, insisting on special consideration—may signal trouble. At the same time, they may behave with overt sweetness toward the surgeon. Such patients are often unpleasant afterward, and they are highly likely to complain about a result that would have pleased most others.

The older male patient seeking a "new" nose. The single male over the age of 30 who suddenly wants to change the shape of his nose to alter his appearance (not to correct a breathing problem or to repair a broken nose after an accident) is likely to be dissatisfied

"Okay, you've got your 'nose job.' Now get out there and meet girls."

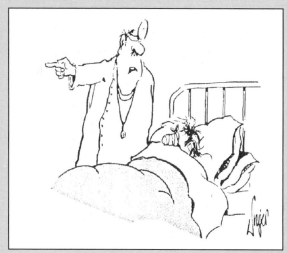

with the result. For unknown reasons these patients are common. Although the phenomenon of men seeking rhinoplasty in middle age has been studied extensively, no clear-cut explanation has emerged; it has been conjectured, however, that may of these patients have long-standing sexual-identity problems and are in conflict about how "masculine" or "feminine" they wish their nose to appear. They frequently complain about the result in a characteristic fashion: "Doctor, you certainly improved my nose, but I really think that you could do just a little bit more." This type of patient may undergo multiple operations but without ultimate satisfaction—perhaps because the identity conflict still lingers.

Happy or unhappy?

Certain operations as well as certain categories of patients are associated with greater patient happiness or unhappiness than others. In contrast to the often unhappy older male rhinoplasty patient, the teenage girl is almost always delighted with her result after nasal surgery. This is often true even if her family, friends, and surgeon thought the surgery was unnecessary or think the "new" nose is not an improvement.

Several recent studies have shown that rhinoplasty produces lasting satisfaction in the vast majority of teenage patients, even when done as young as 13. From a psychological perspective it has been speculated that nasal operations performed on younger (*i.e.,* adolescent) patients may tend to be more successful because they are performed before their self-image, which includes aspects of personal appearance, is fully formed.

On the other hand, most plastic surgeons recognize that in older patients the reactions of intimates can be critical in determining whether they like or dislike the result. A common example is the middle-aged woman who is recovering normally from a recent face-lift but not surprisingly is still black-and-blue and swollen. She may become profoundly depressed and dissatisfied if a friend tells her at this early postoperative stage that she looks "horrible." Immediate reassurance from the surgeon is helpful but not always successful in restoring her emotional equilibrium.

Coping with dissatisfaction

Most plastic surgeons, if willing to follow their observations and intuition, can usually discern the patient who is dissatisfied after an operation. Accordingly, they should let the patient know that they suspect unhappiness. Under these circumstances, most surgeons respond like professionals. Regrettably, however, some surgeons become offended, distant, angry, or unavailable—behavior that destroys rapport and obstructs further treatment if indeed a problem exists objectively. The responsible professional should suggest a plan to correct the problem. In the instance of

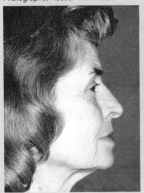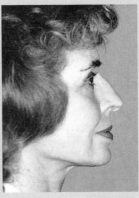

It is important that anyone who undergoes elective cosmetic surgery not have inflated expections. The plastic surgeon must also alert the client to the potential complications that can arise with any surgical procedure. The satisfied patient above is shown before and after undergoing two separate procedures—the first, a chemical peel to remove fine facial wrinkling caused by sun damage, followed two years later by a face-lift to tighten the facial skin.

discrepancy in breast size after a reduction procedure, for example, a further operation, usually under local anesthesia on an outpatient basis, may easily achieve the desired symmetry.

Sometimes, however, the problem is more severe and its solution more difficult. If the surgeon is uncertain about what to do or senses that the patient is uneasy, the surgeon should arrange consultation with a professional colleague for the patient. Although it is better for the doctor to initiate the process, sometimes he or she does not. A patient should then request it. Ideally, the patient would not see another surgeon without telling the first surgeon. Although taking such a step is certainly the patient's right, the second consultation would be more productive for the patient if the surgeon provided the consultant with a detailed summary of the treatment up to that point.

It is common for a patient who has had an aesthetic operation and then has something objective to complain about to experience both guilt and embarrassment. These are sentiments that arise, often prior to the operation, because the contemplated procedure may have been "unnecessary" or seemed "vain" or "frivolous." In fact, no matter how much patients may have wanted or felt the need for the cosmetic procedure, they may have heard from family and friends that embarking on an aesthetic operation was "foolish."

Postoperatively when a complication has occurred, these patients will sense the attitudes of friends who, though they may not say "I told you so" in so many words, will still think it. Not infrequently patients will interpret an unfavorable result as "divine punishment" for changing what God and nature had given them. The surgeon who becomes angry with the dissatisfied patient will increase that person's guilt and misery. The

doctor must appreciate these feelings and should be sympathetic and available for the patient. The focus for both of them should be on remedying the problem and not wallowing in guilt or recrimination.

Realistic expectations

Any surgeon who guarantees a particular result is foolish, and any patient who believes that a surgeon can always produce a specific outcome is naive and uninformed. Factors beyond human control may affect a surgical result—just as they do in every sphere of human activity. In all types of surgery wound healing, for example, is unpredictable. A bad scar is always possible. Although studies are under way on new tests that could predict those who may experience wound-healing problems, at present, there is no way to know in advance which patients are at high risk of developing unsightly scars (*e.g.*, keloids, which are thick masses of tissue that extend beyond the site of incision). Moreover, no operation thus far has evolved that is free of the possibility of infection or excessive bleeding. The occurrence of an infection—for example, after breast augmentation with silicone implants—does not necessarily mean the surgeon or the hospital was at fault.

The patient who has inflated expectations and has not heeded the surgeon's verbal and perhaps even written disclaimers about potential complications is likely to feel betrayed and become angry when something goes wrong. If surgeons have not adequately informed the patient about those possibilities, then they are at fault. Most (but not all) plastic surgeons have the patient sign an "informed consent" form, which carries the statement that the surgeon has told the patient—and the patient has understood—the nature of the contemplated procedure, the type of result that the patient can expect if all goes well, and that no guaranteed result has been given because complications can occur. The informed consent form may specify as possible though unlikely complications death, infection, excessive bleeding, bad scarring, and asymmetry. Frequently, specific complications that are associated with a particular procedure will be mentioned—for example, with correction of baggy lower eyelids the patient could develop an abnormal turning out or "pulldown" of the lids (ectropion), noticeable scars, and even blindness (a rare but not impossible outcome).

Professional responsibility

In most instances the patient and the surgeon should be able to talk about the complication and resolve the problem together. It is extremely important that the surgeon outline a plan of corrective treatment and not leave the patient hanging in ambiguity.

The patient should also understand that good plastic surgeons want the very best for their patients and

405

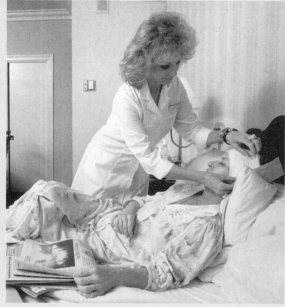

A woman whose cosmetic surgery turned into a 10-year nightmare is comforted by her husband. Her breast reduction, done by a doctor who had no formal training in plastic surgery, resulted in serious infection, loss of a breast, and the need for six more operations.

that, on becoming involved in the operation, they take the outcome personally. Ideally, however, professional training has prepared the surgeon to respond both appropriately and objectively, though also with empathy.

The factor of training is a particularly consequential one. It should be noted that throughout the United States operations considered plastic surgery are frequently done by doctors who are inadequately trained. Dermatologists, otolaryngologists, gynecologists, and internists, for example, may perform some plastic surgery procedures. This does not necessarily imply that only board-certified plastic surgeons (the certifying board in the United States is the American Board of Plastic Surgery, based in Philadelphia) should do plastic surgery, but it does mean that other physicians who undertake a cosmetic surgery procedure should be sufficiently skilled in its execution and in handling complications and unfavorable results should they arise. (The American Society of Plastic and Reconstructive Surgeons, Inc. [ASPRS], the world's largest association of certified plastic surgeons, has a toll-free hot line [1-800-635-0635]; it provides reliable referrals for specific procedures in local areas throughout the U.S.)

The patient should also understand that most surgeons fear that a dissatisfied patient will become a plaintiff in court. While that attitude is unfortunate, such is the ambience of medicine today, particularly in the United States. Sometimes the surgeon reacts too defensively to a patient who is unhappy with the result when, in fact, the surgeon should behave in just the opposite fashion. Patients and surgeons alike may not control their emotions appropriately, although the patient has a right to expect the surgeon to regulate responses to conform to the standards of high professionalism.

Media-promoted miracles

In magazine articles and in advertisements on radio and television, the message conveyed to a gullible public too often is of the "miracles" of plastic surgery. Almost all attention is paid to the faultless transformation of a displeasing or unwanted body feature. Advertisements give disproportionately little emphasis on what can go wrong.

Aggravating this problem of skewed public information, which unrealistically raises the expectations of prospective patients, is the appearance of many plastic surgeons in ads whose message to the audience is, "Look at what a wonderful surgeon I am." Although it is legally permissible for plastic surgeons or other physicians who perform aesthetic surgery to advertise their capabilities, by so doing the effect is to convert a medical procedure (albeit for cosmetic purposes) into a consumer product, available to anyone who can pay. The human transaction between patient and surgeon is thus demeaned. Promoting surgery as if it were a product can backfire, however, because the implication is that if the product (the surgical result) is defective, it can be easily repaired, returned, or replaced. Unfortunately, sometimes it is impossible

Some patients are extremely sensitive to the comments of others who see them just after aesthetic surgery when they are still black-and-blue and swollen. This hotel in Beverly Hills, California, enables those who have had plastic surgery to convalesce in dignity while the bruises heal.

to restore to preoperative status a nose, breast, or face that has been the site of a complication following plastic surgery (either an unavoidable one or one that occurs because of poor execution).

Medically necessary plastic surgery

Thus far, the focus has been on patients who may be dissatisfied following aesthetic surgery. Patients can also be unhappy after reconstructive surgery, where the emphasis is primarily on function and only secondarily on appearance. It has been observed that the more patients consider their operation to be of a "reconstructive" nature, the happier they will be with the outcome. For example, a patient who has had a reduction mammaplasty and viewed her formerly enormous breasts as a deformity or health problem (causing poor posture and neck, back, and shoulder pain) will probably be happier with the result than another patient with a similar problem who seeks surgery purely for appearance's sake (e.g., because she wants to wear fashionable clothes).

The reverse situation has also been noted—the more emphasis that patients who have truly reconstructive surgery give to the "cosmetic" outcome of their operation, the less happy they are likely to be with the result. The patient who has had to have his lower jaw removed because of cancer and then has had it reconstructed (using a graft from a rib) will consider the operation a success if his primary concern had been one of function; now not only has his malignant disease been eradicated but he will be able to swallow and eat better. If, however, he expects that the reconstruction will restore totally his preoperative appearance, then he is likely to be dissatisfied.

The obvious difference between patients who are dissatisfied after reconstructive surgery and those who are unhappy after aesthetic surgery is that for the latter the procedure was elective, sought by the patient and not dictated by unfortunate circumstances, such as trauma or cancer. Few patients following a failed outcome in reconstructive surgery experience guilt or embarrassment. Furthermore, society supports them because their procedure was "medically necessary." They receive additional solace in terms of finances since reconstructive surgery and treatment of complications if they occur are almost always covered by insurance policies, whereas aesthetic surgery is generally not covered. Unfortunately, women who have breast reconstruction after a mastectomy do not always have such support—emotional or financial—the rationale being that the operation is done for aesthetic (and perhaps psychological) reasons rather than for functional ones.

Costs of correcting the problem

From a practical point of view, one of the most onerous of the problems that result when patients are dissatisfied with the outcome of their plastic surgery centers on money: who pays for the correction of the problem? As mentioned, after reconstructive surgery insurance policies are generally liberal in this regard. However, when something goes wrong after an aesthetic operation, it is the patient who usually has to pay the hospital costs, and it is the surgeon who must decide whether he or she will charge the patient for the additional services. These matters should be discussed prior to the operation.

It is much easier for surgeons who have their own operating facilities to correct a problem without the patient paying the costs associated with a hospital operation (whether as an inpatient or outpatient). These surgeons can more easily omit or reduce costs. This is obviously not true for those who operate at a hospital, which determines its own costs.

If the patient chooses another surgeon to remedy the unwanted result, the matter of finances must be decided by the patient and the second surgeon. Most often the patient will have to pay. Some patients, out of frustration, may at that point seek legal recourse because they resent the additional financial burden. Nevertheless, patients who decide to leave the original surgeon, who may have been willing to correct the problem, possibly without charging, will likely end up paying more.

A final word

Finally, some caveats already set forth bear repeating. Plastic surgeons should never guarantee a result, nor should patients expect a guaranteed result. Every operation carries the risk of complication—some serious and some less so—but no undesirable outcome is ever pleasant for the patient to experience, nor is it pleasant for the surgeon to accept and to manage. Surgeons have the responsibility to honor their patients' expectations that they will help to correct the unfavorable result to the best of their ability. Patients have a right to seek additional opinions and consultations, but preferably they should discuss the matter with the original surgeon first and not make these arrangements secretly. Surgeons should understand the patient's emotional distress, and they should make themselves available to the patient who has a postoperative problem; patients should also understand that their complication places an emotional strain on the surgeon. In short, each should recognize the other's vulnerability.

Ultimately, it is to be hoped that the patient and the surgeon, as reasonable and reasoning human beings, will be able to work together. Sometimes when patients have had a complication and their surgeon has stood by them, remaining supportive and understanding and doing everything possible to correct the problem, those patients then have become the surgeon's most staunch supporters.

Transplantation

In dramatic operations that attracted wide public attention, University of Chicago surgeons removed part of a mother's liver and transplanted it to her infant daughter, who was ill with an inevitably fatal liver disease. This double operation in 1989 was followed by others in which parents donated a portion of their own liver as "a gift of life" to a sick child. While the University of Chicago team was the first to perform this surgical feat in the United States, others in Brazil, Japan, and Australia had performed similar transplants. The success of this procedure and other notable achievements—in the transplantation of multiple organs, in donor organ preservation, and in the prevention of rejection of donor organs—are indicative of lifesaving advances that are taking place in the exciting field of surgical transplantation today.

New hope for children needing livers

The live-donor segmental transplant procedure in Chicago followed earlier success, dating from 1984, with segmental transplantation from cadavers. Surgeon Christoph Broelsch pioneered in segmental cadaveric transplants in his native Hanover, West Germany, demonstrating that one lobe—about a third—of an adult liver can be transplanted successfully into the abdomen of a small child. In fact, one liver can be divided between two children or between a child and an adult. A unique feature of the liver is that, unlike other organs, it regenerates and thus will grow with the child or to fit the space left by a resected diseased liver in an adult. Similarly, the portion of the liver resected from a live donor regenerates.

It was Broelsch, now professor of surgery and chief of the liver transplantation service at the University of Chicago, who led the team that removed part of the liver of Teresa Smith, a 29-year-old elementary school teacher from Schertz, Texas, and implanted it in her 21-month-old daughter, Alyssa. Alyssa suffered from the liver disease biliary atresia and was destined to die within a year. The procedure involved the intricate attachment of the child's blood vessels to the new liver and the creation of a new bile duct from part of the small intestine.

About 700 American children a year need liver transplants, primarily because of biliary atresia, a rare congenital, usually fatal condition in which the bile ducts are blocked and bile backs up into the bloodstream and the liver instead of flowing to the small intestine to perform essential digestive work. The condition causes changes in the liver that result in cirrhosis (scarring and degeneration) and loss of liver function. Other conditions affecting children that may put them in need of liver transplants include the so-called inborn errors of metabolism, such as an enzyme deficiency that also results in extreme cirrhosis, and another rare, often familial, disorder, Wilson's disease, which causes excessive copper to accumulate in the liver and other tissues, leading to excessive liver damage.

At the University of Chicago Medical Center, Alyssa Smith, 21 months old, is prepared for the operation in which she received a portion of her mother's liver—the country's first live-donor segmental liver transplant. A week later, recovering, Alyssa is comforted by her parents. Six weeks after the surgery, she was well enough to go home.

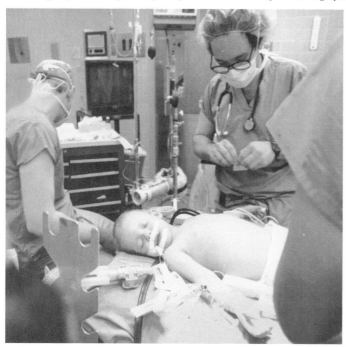
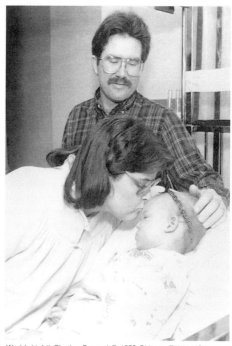

(Left) AP/Wide World; (right) Charles Osgood © 1989 Chicago Tribune Company

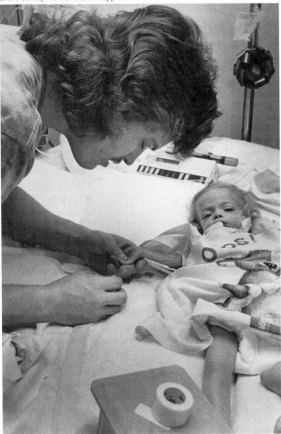

Father and daughter wait to be called to Chicago, where, less than two weeks after Alyssa Smith's transplant, the same surgical team transplanted a portion of Robert Jones's liver into ailing 16-month-old Sarina.

The live-donor operation that appears to have saved Alyssa Smith's life has opened up new possibilities for children who need new livers. Organs to be transplanted had previously come from the bodies of people who had died in accidents, usually from head injuries that did not affect visceral organs. Only a small number of children die under such circumstances, so the shortage of infant-size cadaver organs is acute, and 25 to 50% of children with fatal liver disease die before a suitable organ is available.

Not only does this procedure promise to alleviate the shortage of donor organs but it will improve the chances of the child's surviving the transplant—first, because of better compatibility of tissues resulting from the genetic relationship of blood relatives; second, because the child will be healthier at the time of the operation, since the waiting time for a satisfactory donor is reduced. There is a further advantage in that a liver graft must be implanted within hours of removal from the donor and must be preserved during transfer, which, if the cadaver donor is distant, may result in some damage to the delicate organ.

About 80% of children who receive cadaver liver transplants survive. It is expected that the survival rate will be equally good or better in those select medical centers staffed by highly skilled transplant specialists capable of performing the extremely complex live-donor segmental procedure.

In addition to the complexity of the surgery, another barrier to immediate widespread utilization is cost. At present, the average cost of a liver transplant is $150,000; however, it is expected that this may drop because the recipient will have a shorter presurgical and postsurgical hospital stay in the future. Even so, some ethicists question whether organ transplants are the best use of scarce medical resources and argue that the money could be used to provide care for many more people. The question of rationing also arises, since not all patients who might benefit have these high-technology procedures available to them.

Although critics also argue that taking an organ from a living donor is never completely safe, thousands of living related donors have survived since the first such procedure—a kidney transplant from one identical twin to his brother—was performed in Boston in 1953. The difference in this case is that humans have two kidneys and can function with only one after donating the second. Another, more comparable live-donor procedure involves removing segments of the pancreas to treat a related adult's diabetes. Bone marrow transplants are even more common and have not proved life-threatening to the donor.

A further issue raised by ethicists is whether parents or other close relatives might not feel under pressure to sacrifice part of their liver to save a child. Thus, in addition to the demonstration that live-donor segmental transplants are indeed successful over a long term, many other concerns need to be addressed before the bold new operation is widely performed.

"Cluster" transplants

Within a few days of the first live-donor transplant in the United States, another landmark operation occurred at the University of Pittsburgh, Pa., where Thomas Starzl headed a team of surgeons that performed the first transplant of a heart, liver, and kidney into the same patient. Cluster transplants, as they are called, date from 1966, but this was the first involving these three organs. Cindy Martin, age 26, of Archbald, Pa., received the multiple organs from an Atlanta woman in her twenties who had died in an automobile accident. Martin earlier had received a heart transplant but had developed hepatitis and kidney dysfunction, side effects of the antirejection drug cyclosporine.

Starzl's group also has pioneered in abdominal organ cluster transplantation for the treatment of cancers in the upper abdomen, those affecting the pancreas and duodenum, that have spread to the liver. These patients have had multiple organs of the gastrointestinal

University of Pittsburgh Health Sciences News Bureau

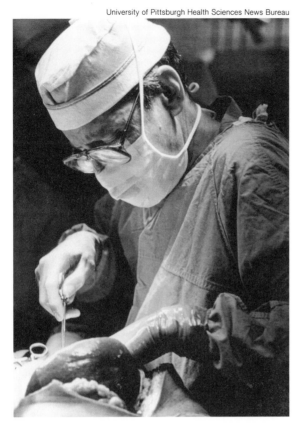

Thomas Starzl has been a pioneer of cluster transplants. Late in 1989 he transplanted a heart, liver, and kidney from a cadaver into a patient who had developed liver and kidney disease after a previous heart transplant.

system removed, including the liver, pancreas, most of the stomach, spleen, duodenum, proximal jejunum, distal ileum, and part of the colon, then replaced by a liver, pancreas, duodenum and, in some cases, the proximal small bowel from a donor.

About 2,000 double or triple organ transplants have been performed over the past decade, primarily for severe diabetes. Recently a few patients have received either four or five organs in a single transplant. If the long-term results of cluster transplantation confirm the initial promise, this procedure too promises new life for many who might otherwise die of diseased organs.

At present, while about 250 transplant teams in the United States are involved in performing about 13,000 transplant operations a year, only a tiny fraction are qualified to perform cluster transplantations. Again, some ethicists question whether a single individual should be allowed to receive multiple organs while at least 17,000 Americans face death while awaiting a single organ.

Single-lung transplants

Another recent transplantation advance has come from Mount Sinai Hospital, Toronto. A surgical team led by

Ronald Grossman has reported promising results in single-lung transplants for patients with bilateral pulmonary fibrosis, a condition marked by scarring of both lungs that is caused by inflammation, pneumonia, or tuberculosis. Between 1983 and 1989, 20 patients with end-stage pulmonary fibrosis underwent single-lung transplants, and nine survived beyond one year. One year after surgery, the surviving patients showed marked improvement in their ability to breathe. In these patients it was found that much of the work of the lung moves from the native diseased lung, which remains in place, to the transplanted lung because the native lung has lost much of its elasticity as a result of scarring, whereas the transplanted lung has normal flexibility.

Transplant specialists say they get excellent results in transplanting just one lung rather than both in selected cases. Some patients do not need replacement of both lungs, and with the shortage of organs available for transplantation, this means that yet another person can benefit. The remaining lung, even though diseased, also serves as a backup in case the transplanted lung is rejected. The native diseased lung serves as well to help diagnose rejection because physicians know that increased blood flow in that lung means the transplanted lung is not doing its work.

Organs from older donors

In order to extend the supply of transplantable organs, another Canadian group, doctors at the University of Western Ontario, are transplanting organs from older cadavers previously thought unacceptable because of the ravages of age on the organs. Until now, the average age considered acceptable has been about 60 for kidneys, 55 for livers, 45 for hearts from women, and 40 for hearts from men. Headed by Calvin Stiller, the university's transplant surgeons have demonstrated that a 75-year-old person can be biologically younger than someone else who is 55. They have performed a number of heart transplants with organs from individuals aged 46 to 58 and transplanted a liver from a 70-year-old man into a 10-year-old boy. The team is also testing the use of human hearts from older donors to keep patients alive while they wait for a younger, better matched organ; thus far, in at least two cases the "temporary" organ functioned so well it was allowed to become the permanent transplant.

New antirejection drug

In 1989 researchers reported that a new drug derived from a fungus found in Japanese soil is markedly better than cyclosporine in preventing rejection of transplanted organs. Cyclosporine itself, which comes from soils in Norway and Wisconsin, revolutionized organ transplantation a decade ago by significantly reducing the high dosages of steroids and other antirejection drugs that transplant recipients were required to take.

Cyclosporine is not entirely benign, however; among other side effects, it can cause kidney damage and elevated blood pressure. In addition, about 20% of liver recipients require a second transplant, and sometimes a third, because cyclosporine does not prevent the failure of the first liver graft. Moreover, with each successive transplant in the same patient, the likelihood of survival decreases because the patients are desperately ill.

The new drug, called FK-506, is said to be 50 times more powerful than cyclosporine and has been found to reverse rejection of livers in some patients. Thus, by reducing the necessity for retransplants, FK-506 has the potential to increase the number of livers available for transplant to those awaiting them.

The drug was developed by Starzl and his team at the University of Pittsburgh after its discovery by the Fujisawa Pharmaceutical Co. Ltd. of Osaka, Japan. It has been used in patients receiving liver, kidney, heart, and pancreas transplants. Apparently, it works by inhibiting production of lymphocytes in the immune system, which, in an attempt to protect the body, seek out and destroy "invading" organisms, thereby causing rejection of "foreign" tissues. FK-506, which Starzl had deemed "a miraculous drug—a wonder drug—one of those drugs that comes along once in a lifetime," was tested on more than 100 organ recipients at Pittsburgh with what has been called stunning success.

Before it can receive approval by the U.S. Food and Drug Administration, and thus become generally available, the drug is being tested further at about 12 medical centers in the U.S. as well as at centers in Europe. The drug is also thought to have potential beyond its use in transplantation—*e.g.,* in the treatment of disorders that affect the immune system, skin, eyes, bowel, kidneys, and brain. Possibilities for such uses are being explored.

Organ preservation

If donor organs could be preserved for a longer period after their removal, a further increase in the supply would result. Until now, the conventional fluid preservation solution in which newly removed organs are kept has been able to preserve a liver for a maximum of 10 hours, requiring the organ transplantation team to obtain the organ from the same geographic region and then rush it back to the hospital and transplant it under emergency conditions. Progress has now been reported with the use of a new solution developed in 1987 by James H. Southard, a biochemist, and surgeon Folkert O. Belzer at the University of Wisconsin Medical Center. Made of starch and lactobionic acid—a milk sugar with an acid attached—the so-called University of Wisconsin solution is designed to prevent the swelling of cold organs in water, a process that kills normal tissue. Prevention is achieved through osmosis, which draws water out of the cells.

The gain from using the preserving fluid is measured only in hours, but this can make a crucial difference because of the time required for matching donor organs and shipping them long distances. About 100 hospitals are using the University of Wisconsin solution; in one case a hospital in Canada was able to ship a preserved liver to France. It also makes possible more complex transplantations that previously had been too time consuming for safe preservation of the organs. In one case a young boy underwent surgery lasting 16 hours and received five organs. The developers report that livers have been successfully transplanted after being preserved in the solution for 33 hours, more than three times as long as was previously possible, and kidneys have been preserved for 60 hours, about twice as long as before. Research is under way to adapt the solution so that it might be used to prolong the viability of donor hearts and lungs as well.

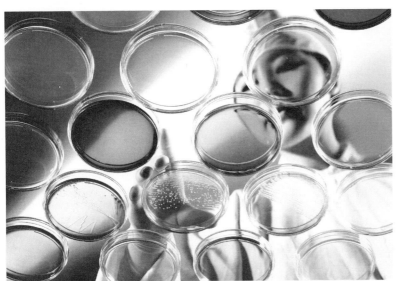

A fungus, derived from soil, ferments in a laboratory at the Fujisawa Pharmaceutical Co. in Japan, an early step in the preparation of a new drug for preventing the rejection of transplanted organs. The drug, known as FK-506, appears to inhibit the white blood cells in the immune system that would ordinarily attack and destroy foreign tissues in the body. In early trials FK-506 has proved to be considerably more effective than cyclosporine and other agents that have been the mainstays of antirejection therapy following surgical transplantation.

Fujisawa Pharmaceutical Co., Ltd.; photograph, Isao Itani

Urgent need for donors

The United Network for Organ Sharing, which comprises hospitals and medical schools where transplants are performed, reported in 1990 that 19,549 Americans were on the waiting list for an organ transplant. This included 16,536 waiting for a kidney, 1,459 for a heart, 885 for a liver, 318 for a pancreas, 245 for heart and lung, and 112 for lung. In addition, the Eye Bank Association estimates that 5,000 patients are on the waiting list for a cornea transplant. One donor, if healthy at the time of death, can provide organs and tissues for as many as 200 people. Skin, heart valves, and bone, in addition to eyes and organs, can be transplanted. However, in 1982, the latest year for which figures were recorded, out of an estimated 20,-000 neurologically dead patients who might have been donors, only 2,500 donations were made.

—*Charles-Gene McDaniel, M.S.J.*

Urology

The last decade has seen major advances in many fields of medicine, and the subspecialty of urology is no exception. There have been exciting developments in the recognition, diagnosis, and treatment of many urologic disorders. Genitourinary cancers, disorders of sexual function, and voiding dysfunction are representative of the broad spectrum of problems encompassed by urology; focusing on the pathology of specific diseases and disorders within each of these categories will provide examples of some of the important diagnostic and treatment modalities that are coming into broad usage for both male and female patients.

Carcinoma of the prostate

The prostate is an acorn-sized male sex accessory gland that adds secretions to the sperm. It surrounds the urethra at the point where it emerges from the bladder. In the United States carcinoma of the prostate gland is the second most common cause of cancer-related deaths in men, exceeded only by lung cancer. In 1990 approximately 100,000 new cases will have been diagnosed.

There has been considerable progress in the management of cancers of the prostate gland. Advances include improved methods of diagnosis, more exact ways to determine the extent of disease (clinical staging), improvements in surgical techniques for potentially curable cancers, and hormonal treatment for tumors no longer curable.

Prostate cancer is conceptually a very complex disease for physicians and patients alike because of the striking variance between the number of patients who clinically develop symptoms of cancer and the number of people with evidence of microscopic cancer in the gland itself. Autopsy studies have shown that 30% of men over age 50 display evidence of prostate cancer,

but fewer than 2% of deaths are due to the cancer. It has been calculated that only one of 380 men older than 50 years with microscopic evidence of prostate cancer will die from the disease each year. Once a prostate cancer has grown large enough to be recognized during life—brought to the individual patient's attention either through routine physical examination or because he experiences secondary symptoms of the disease—it requires treatment to prevent or postpone complications of the cancer and death. But how aggressive the diagnostic modalities used should be is not certain since, as noted, microscopic evidence of prostate cancer seems to be so common in the aging male yet so unlikely to cause disability or death.

Improved techniques for diagnosis and staging. Until recently the mainstays of diagnosis have been the physician's digital rectal examination, biopsy of suspicious (firm or nodular) areas of the prostate (a procedure that uses a thin needle to remove a sample of tissue), and the quantification of acid phosphatase and prostate-specific antigen (substances often elevated in the blood of patients with prostate cancer). Newer modalities have evolved, however. For example, transrectal ultrasound, an essentially painless examination done by placing an instrument slightly larger than the examining finger in the rectum, has recently been introduced into clinical practice. The transducer sends out sound waves and almost instantaneously detects their echoes, which form a picture of the prostate on a television monitor. Areas with a lack of echoes (hypoechoic) are considered suspicious for tumor. Presently, it is generally agreed that transrectal ultrasound aids the urologist in accurately sampling an area that feels abnormal on digital examination. It can also be helpful in determining the local extent of a known cancer and may be useful in making a decision as to whether a curative operation is feasible.

The usefulness of transrectal ultrasound has also raised an important issue: whether it has potential efficacy as a tool for screening large populations for cancers that are not palpable on routine physical examination. The proportion of nonpalpable ultrasound abnormalities that have proved to be cancerous is as low as 10%, and up to 25% of cancers detectable by rectal examination are not visible by ultrasound. Only well-controlled, large-scale, prospective studies conducted over many years will determine whether ultrasound screening for prostate cancer has the necessary accuracy to be of value.

Magnetic resonance imaging (MRI), a non-radiation-based, noninvasive diagnostic study that relies on the magnetic properties of nuclei with protons and neutrons to construct accurate images of organs of the body, will increasingly play a role in the staging of prostate cancer. Further, recent experience with a surface coil, placed like an examining finger in the rectum, has resulted in staging accuracy exceeding 90%.

Because curative treatment is unlikely to be successful if the tumor extends outside the prostatic capsule, this technique may be able to prevent many operations that ultimately would prove to be unsuccessful in terms of cure.

Better treatments, reduced complications. Prostate cancer is potentially curable if it is confined to the gland itself. Aggressive treatment is generally reserved for patients with at least a 5- to 10-year life expectancy, as it takes at least that long to see a difference in survival rates between patients treated for cure and those treated only when symptoms develop. The two most common curative treatments have been radiation therapy and radical surgical removal of the prostate and surrounding tissue. While results with surgery and radiation have been comparable, until recently many physicians and their patients relied mainly on radiation therapy because of potential surgical complications that were not uncommon. These included major blood loss, a 5–10% risk of urinary incontinence (constant leakage of urine), and a 99% risk of impotence. While radiation has other potential complications, the risk of impotence with radiation is about 50%, and blood loss and incontinence are not problems. Fortunately, new surgical techniques have reduced the incidence of all three of these major complications, thus making surgery a more reasonable alternative for cure.

Since the 1940s, disseminated prostate cancer (cancer that has spread to other organs) has been treated with hormonal therapy. While this is not curative, hormonal therapy markedly improves the quality of life of patients suffering from the effects of prostate cancer. Normal prostate cells are dependent on male hormones (androgens) to carry out their metabolic processes. Testosterone is the major circulating androgen, 90% of which is produced by the testes. If androgen is removed, prostate cells atrophy. Almost all prostate cancers have some cells that are androgen dependent and that respond to treatments that result in diminished androgen levels in the body. Unfortunately, eventually the non-androgen-dependent cells proliferate, and tumor growth is uncontrolled.

Until recently the only alternatives to hormonal therapy were surgical removal of the testicles (orchiectomy) and the oral administration of estrogens, female hormones that block testosterone production. Although orchiectomy is safe and effective and has no life-threatening side effects, many men are unable to tolerate the psychological effects. Oral estrogens can result in water retention and painful breast enlargement, and in some cases potential cardiovascular complications can develop that result in death. Moreover, all hormonal treatment results in impotence. Now, however, new forms of endocrine manipulation have been developed that reduce complications. Substances (luteinizing hormone-releasing hormone [LHRH] agonists) that upset the normal pituitary-testicular thermostat and result in the virtual absence of testosterone secretion are now available in preparations that can be injected monthly in a physician's office. This procedure avoids the adverse emotional impact of orchiectomy and the thromboembolic and feminizing side effects of estrogens.

Another new hormonal agent, flutamide, has been found to prolong the survival of patients with fatal prostate cancer. Flutamide is an antiandrogen and acts by inhibiting the cell binding of the active form of testosterone. Thus, it prevents the 10% of androgens produced in the adrenal gland from binding to prostate cells and, when used with other, conventional hormonal modalities, results in a virtually complete androgen blockade, which may help to prolong life. When flutamide therapy is begun in conjunction with but prior to the initiation of the injectable LHRH agonists, it confers the additional benefit of preventing problems from the initial increase in serum testosterone that, while transitory, can result in an increase in symptoms of metastatic prostate cancer in patients who receive LHRH therapy alone.

Male sexual dysfunction

Impotence, the term commonly used to denote a failure of the penile erectile mechanism, affects up to 10 million American men. It is an age-dependent disorder with an incidence of 1.9% at 40 years of age and 25% at 65. The incidence in the male population with the common endocrinologic disorder diabetes approaches 50%. While in the recent past impotence was believed to be largely a psychological disorder, it is now under-

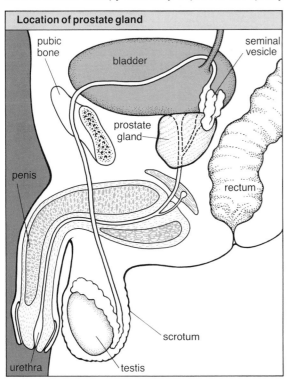

Location of prostate gland

pubic bone

bladder

seminal vesicle

prostate gland

rectum

penis

scrotum

urethra

testis

stood that more than half of erectile dysfunction is at least in part the result of pathological alterations in the normal physiological mechanisms that are responsible for erection. There is now as well an improved understanding of the processes involved in normal sexual function, and new diagnostic tests make possible the recognition of the specific causes of erectile failure in the majority of patients. Treatment options, as a result, have been increased, and almost all patients can be helped to regain the capability for sexual intercourse.

The process of erection. Penile erections are dependent upon a normal nerve supply to the penis. Certain pathways allow for reflex erection upon manual stimulation of the penis; other pathways allow for psychogenic erections from stimulation by a variety of senses (touch, taste, vision, and imagination). Both pathways work together, and the nerves secrete chemical transmitters that cause relaxation of the smooth muscle of the penis and the arteries that carry blood into the two erectile bodies that constitute much of its substance. Dilatation of the arteries and relaxation of the smooth muscle results in a major increase in blood flow to the organ. As the penis fills with blood, it becomes erect. The veins that normally drain the blood are squeezed shut against the firm wall of the erectile bodies, thus preventing a leakage of blood and loss of erection. The process of climax—expulsion of semen (ejaculation) and orgasm—is associated with an outpouring of sympathetic nervous system stimulation; these special nerves send out chemical messengers that constrict the arteries and increase the smooth muscle tone of the penis, resulting in loss of erection. Normal sexual functioning in the male is dependent on the presence of testosterone; while testosterone is definitely involved in stimulating the desire for sex (libido), its effects on erection are less certain.

Impotence evaluation. The evaluation of impotence has many parts. It begins with a history and physical exam. Blood is then drawn for studies to evaluate hormonal status and look for the presence of other diseases that may affect sexual function. Problems such as hypertension, diabetes, heart disease, kidney disease, and vascular disorders can all affect sexual function; many medications can also adversely affect erectile function. At the present time, there is no universally agreed-upon diagnostic approach; many of the available studies are new, and their reliability has not been fully determined.

Nocturnal penile tumescence (NPT) testing is used to document the quality of the normal sleep-related erections that occur three to five times per night and last 25–30 minutes in men from adolescence to old age. The assumption is made that if these erections are normal, then the "equipment works," and the problem is psychological in origin. Sleep testing is commonly done in a sleep laboratory, where the quality of sleep can be monitored; new research suggests that some sleep disorders may directly impair sexual function in the waking state. In addition, poor sleep quality may give unreliable NPT results. A variety of devices to monitor NPT at home are available, but they lack the advantages of evaluation in a sleep laboratory.

Neurological testing can sometimes aid in the diagnosis of primary neurogenic impotence (impotence that originates in the nervous system). However, in practice it is uncommon to subject a patient to a battery of neurological tests unless he has symptoms of nervous system disease (*e.g.,* multiple sclerosis or spinal cord injury).

Of all the tests used in evaluating male impotence, vascular testing has progressed the farthest in the last few years. Given that vascular disease may be the most common contributing factor to erectile problems, studies looking for poor arterial inflow or failure of the veins to trap the blood in the penis are essential in all patients for whom definitive therapy is being considered. The most dramatic development has been the ability to safely and directly inject tiny amounts of drug (papaverine or prostaglandin E_1) into the penis to relax the smooth muscle, dilate the penile blood vessels, and activate the venous blood-trapping mechanism—thereby inducing an almost physiological erection. Tests based on this principle not only can pinpoint the cause of the dysfunction but also allow the physician and patient to determine if a "self-injection" program, wherein the patient is taught to inject his penis with these vasoactive medications, might be an appropriate form of long-term treatment.

In conjunction with penile injection testing, new ultrasound equipment can actually visualize the penile arteries and veins, determine blood flow, evaluate the outer layer and inner substance of the erectile tissue, and predict which patients might benefit from other forms of treatment. X-ray studies can also be done to look for venous leaks and evaluate the adequacy of blood supply to the penis.

Treatment options. Standard treatment for *psychological* impotence is some form of sex therapy. For essentially *physiological* impotence there are now many treatment possibilities. Testosterone can be administered, usually by injection, in patients with low levels of this hormone. Oral medication is sometimes used to treat sexual dysfunction but often is not helpful. The most commonly used drug is yohimbine, an old agent that some studies indicate may improve sexual function, although the mechanism is unknown.

Many patients can resume normal sexual activity by learning to inject their penis with the same medications used in the diagnostic studies described above. This is done about 15 minutes before having sex. While not a cure, this new form of treatment allows for satisfactory intercourse without the need for a surgical procedure. There are uncommon but potentially serious side effects of such injection treatment, however, making it essential that the physician prescribe the therapy only for appropriate patients, who are then carefully instructed and followed up.

Where diagnostic studies show that a patient has a primary abnormality of the veins draining the penis (venous leak), new surgical procedures that seek to tie off the leaking sites can be employed. Young patients who have suffered traumatic injuries to a penile artery are candidates for new surgical procedures that attempt to revascularize the penis, much as coronary bypass operations revascularize the heart. Unfortunately, revascularization has not been as successful in penile arterial disease unrelated to isolated trauma.

Finally, virtually all patients with organic impotence can be helped by a surgical procedure in which a penile implant made of silicone or similar material is placed in the penis to make it rigid. Newer forms of implants allow for manual inflation and deflation of the penis with a very low risk of mechanical malfunction.

Interstitial cystitis: a malady long misunderstood

There are patients who experience symptoms that are often very disabling but for which urologists, until recently, have had no explanation or rational treatment. The majority are women with complaints of urinary frequency, burning on urination, pelvic pain, and pain on intercourse. Only 10% of patients are men. The symptoms, when evaluation failed to reveal an underlying infection of the urinary tract as a cause, had been attributed to psychological problems, neurosis, or a "waste-basket diagnosis" of so-called urethral syndrome. Over the last decade a major advance has been the realization that these unfortunate patients have a real disease that is known as interstitial cystitis (IC).

In large part because of the work of patient advocacy groups, the recognition of this chronic disorder by physicians has increased dramatically, and its seriousness has come to be appreciated. A recent epidemiological study suggests that symptoms of IC may occur in up to 450,000 people in the United States alone. IC can devastate the daily life of those affected. Patients may need to urinate as often as every 15 minutes, day and night, and they are often in pain constantly.

IC is primarily a diagnosis arrived at by exclusion. Patients are evaluated through studies including examination of the bladder through a telescope placed in the urethra (cystoscopy), performed under anesthesia, in order to rule out cancer and infection as well as other less common disorders. A common finding for IC is tiny bleeding points on the bladder wall after it has been distended with fluid; when the distending fluid is allowed to drain from the bladder, it appears tinged with blood.

Patients generally experience an onset over a period of a few weeks, with urinary frequency, pain in the area of the pelvis and bladder, and sometimes pain on intercourse. The symptoms generally manifest themselves like an infection. Despite negative cultures for bacteria, patients are often treated with a variety of antibiotics, but to no avail.

While the cause remains unknown, recent research suggests that the lining of the bladder wall in patients with IC may have subtle abnormalities that either result in the symptoms or leave the bladder vulnerable to some constituent in the urine perhaps unique to IC patients. A major research effort to establish its etiology is presently under way in centers in the United States and Europe.

On the positive side, interstitial cystitis does not lead to cancer and is not a life-threatening disease. Further, many treatments are available to manage the symptoms. These include oral medications such as amitriptyline, an antidepressant, and medications that are directly administered by catheter into the bladder, such as dimethyl sulfoxide (DMSO), which may relieve symptoms by anti-inflammatory or direct analgesic actions. Some patients respond to distension of the bladder under anesthesia. Many patients find relief by avoiding certain foods or beverages that experience has taught them aggravate their symptoms. Another method uses transcutaneous electrical nerve stimulators (TENS)—electrodes that are placed on the back of the leg (over the posterior tibial nerve) or directly over the bladder. The patient wears a compact, battery-powered device (a stimulator) on a belt at the waist. The stimulator is hooked up to the electrodes by wires and is operated by the patient to deliver a mild electrical current to the pain site. It is recommended that patients self-administer TENS for 8–10 hours a day; beneficial results may occur over a two-to-four-month period.

Fully 50% of patients will experience spontaneous remission of their symptoms for varying periods of time with no treatment at all. Ultimately only about 10% of patients will require a major surgical procedure. A procedure known as an ileal conduit urinary diversion attaches the ureters to a piece of bowel that diverts urine from the bladder to the skin; to collect urine, the patient wears a bag on the outside of the body that is periodically emptied. Alternatively, the bladder can be removed entirely and a new bladder constructed from bowel tissue, which does not require wearing a collection device for urine.

Efforts are also under way to discover treatments that not only manage the symptoms of the disease but attack the primary problem causing it. A medication that has been given experimentally, sodium pentosanpolysulfate (Elmiron), may act to replenish the bladder lining. Other medications that stabilize mast cells—*i.e.,* cells that act as chemical factories in the bladder and other tissues and may excrete potentially toxic substances—are being tested in clinical trials.

—Philip M. Hanno, M.D.

HEALTH
INFORMATION
UPDATE

Instructive and practical
articles about common
and not-so-common
health concerns

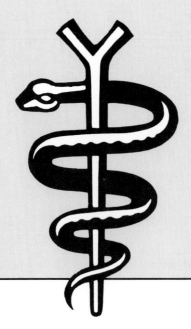

Flu

by Nancy H. Arden, M.N.

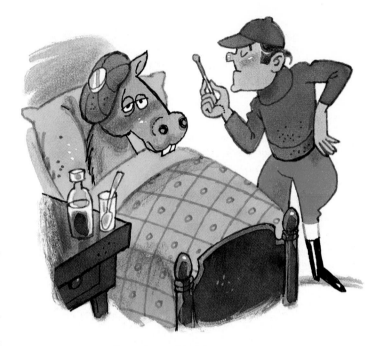

Influenza, commonly called the flu, is caused by viruses that primarily infect the respiratory tract. While many viruses cause respiratory infections, flu viruses are unique in several respects. They often produce a more severe illness than other respiratory viruses and are more likely to result in potentially life-threatening complications. Influenza viruses also have a unique seasonal pattern, causing epidemics that begin and end abruptly and affecting a substantial proportion of the population in a short period of time.

Symptoms, duration, spread

The illness caused by influenza viruses is usually characterized by respiratory symptoms such as cough, sore throat, and nasal congestion, accompanied by fever, headache, muscle aches, and often extreme fatigue. Although gastrointestinal symptoms such as nausea, vomiting, and diarrhea sometimes accompany influenza, especially in children, these symptoms are rarely prominent. "Stomach flu" is a misnomer for gastrointestinal illnesses caused by other viruses or bacteria.

Most people who catch the flu are acutely ill for only two to four days and recover within one to two weeks. Some, however, develop serious complications such as pneumonia. These complications can be deadly, as evidenced by the fact that in the U.S. alone, influenza is associated with an average of about 20,000 deaths each year. There are no exact statistics on the number of people who get the flu each year. One reason for the absence of data is that many people who have influenza do not seek medical care. Epidemiologists estimate that, on average, between 10 and 20% of the U.S. population are affected per year.

Influenza is highly contagious and spreads by transfer of the virus from an infected person to one who is susceptible. The virus is usually transferred by tiny aerosolized droplets expelled by coughing, sneezing, or even just talking. Influenza can spread quickly in closed environments such as classrooms, offices, stores, theaters, and buses. Symptoms usually begin one to three days after infection, but infected persons can transmit the virus before they develop symptoms. Those with some degree of prior immunity can also shed viruses, thus transmitting infection, without having an apparent illness themselves.

Seasonal pattern and circulation

Influenza has a distinctive seasonal pattern. It occurs during the winter in temperate and colder climates, causing epidemics that can affect 10 to 40% of the population in a period of about 6 to 12 weeks. Influenza occurs virtually every winter in these regions, and epidemics occur in about two of every three winters. It is this pattern of activity that gave the virus its name. During the 14th century, because of its sudden and regular appearances, the disease was attributed to the "influence" (from the Latin *influentia*) of certain constellations that were present during epidemics of cough and fever and, later, to the *influenza di freddo* (Italian for "influence of the cold"). In the Northern Hemisphere, influenza usually occurs from about December through April, with peak activity during January, February, and early March. An exception to this pattern has been seen during pandemics (worldwide epidemics), when influenza activity has been detected from early autumn until well into the following spring. Influenza can occur in the tropics at any time of year and most often occurs in the Southern Hemisphere from about April through September.

No regular pattern of worldwide spread of influenza—or of flu viruses—has been observed. In fact, new strains of flu virus are often detected in many parts of the world within a matter of months. Although new influenza strains frequently have been first identified in the Orient, the reasons for this are not clear. The origins of the 1957 and 1968 pandemics were traced to China, and the so-called Russian flu of 1977, which was first detected in the Soviet Union, is also thought to have originated in China. One theory about the origin of flu viruses is that pandemic strains may arise when a human and an animal strain infect a common host (see *Influenza in animals*, below); such an event may be more likely to occur in a country such as China, where in rural areas many

Flu

people live in close proximity to domesticated animals that are known to be susceptible to influenza infection (pigs, ducks, horses), thus increasing the chances for coinfection and genetic reassortment ("reshuffling") between two distinct influenza viruses.

The influenza virus

The influenza virus has a fatty envelope that is studded with two types of protein molecules, called hemagglutinin and neuraminidase. The hemagglutinin molecules attach the virus to its target cell, while the function of the neuraminidase molecules is to free the virus when it has attached itself to a cell or other substance that it cannot infect. Once attached to a susceptible cell, the virus then takes advantage of the cell's normal defense mechanisms to gain entry; as it does when confronted by other small foreign particles, the cell engulfs the virus into a small sac and then attempts to destroy it with enzymes. Instead of destroying the virus, however, the action of these enzymes allows the contents of the virus to pour into the cell. The viral material subverts the cell's normal reproductive mechanisms and uses cellular genetic material to make copies of itself. Progeny viruses bud from the cell and go on to infect others.

The cells that the influenza virus most often infects are the cells of the epithelium (membranous surface tissue) of the nose and throat. These cells have tiny hairlike structures, called cilia, that help keep the respiratory tract clean and protect it from invasion by foreign substances, including bacteria. As a result of the damage caused by influenza infection, these ciliated epithelial cells die and slough off. Depletion of ciliated cells contributes to the development of complications such as bronchitis and pneumonia by allowing infectious agents—usually bacteria—to gain access to the respiratory tract and to proliferate within it.

When people are infected with influenza, they produce antibodies that protect them against future infection by the same flu virus. Thus, influenza occurs less frequently in adults than in children. (Adults are much more likely to get frequent "colds" than flu because there are several hundred viruses than can cause common cold symptoms, while at any given time there are only a few different human influenza viruses in circulation.) Nonetheless, people do continue to fall victim to flu throughout their lives. The reason for the continuing susceptibility to flu is that influenza viruses continually change. Mutations, or in some cases complete changes in the character of the viral genes, result in sufficient alterations in the structure of the hemagglutinin and neuraminidase that the antibodies produced against the "old" proteins no longer recognize the newly "disguised" virus and are, therefore, unable to prevent another flu infection from occurring. However, existing antibodies often help to reduce the severity of the infection.

Emergence of "new" viruses and pandemics

There are three types of influenza virus, designated A, B, and C. Type C influenza has a somewhat different composition than types A and B; it does not cause epidemics and rarely causes severe illness. Influenza A and B cause illnesses that are clinically indistinguishable, and both undergo change while circulating. Influenza A is responsible for epidemics more often than B and, in addition to mutating gradually over time (a phenomenon known as antigenic drift), it can also change abruptly (antigenic shift), which does not occur with type B viruses. Influenza A viruses that undergo antigenic shift emerge with a completely new hemagglutinin, neuraminidase, or both. When shifts occur, large numbers of people—sometimes the entire human population—have no antibody protection. Pandemics are a result of these antigenic shifts.

Three of the most recent antigenic shifts occurred in 1918, 1957, and 1968; each time, the old type A influenza virus disappeared when the new, antigenically shifted virus emerged. However, for reasons that are not completely understood, the impact of each of these newly emerged viruses differed. The 1918–19 pandemic known as Spanish flu was by far the most severe, causing many more deaths than any other influenza pandemic on record; in fact, it ranks second only to the Black Death (the plague) of the 14th century in terms of mortality. In the United States alone, about 500,000 people died from the Spanish flu; more than 20 million deaths occurred worldwide.

The first influenza virus was not isolated until the early 1930s. Thus, there are no samples of the 1918–19 virus for scientists to study. However, information about flu viruses that circulated before the 1930s has been obtained through study of antibodies in the blood of people who were living during that time, a technique known as seroarchaeology. Using a combination of seroarchaeology and analysis of viruses, scientists have determined that viruses similar to the one that caused the 1918–19 pandemic continued to circulate, mutate, and cause smaller epidemics until 1957. For reasons that still are not understood, the viruses that circulated after 1919 were not associated with the extremely high death rates seen during 1918–19.

In 1957 another antigenic shift occurred in the influenza A virus, resulting in the pandemic of so-called Asian flu that was associated with approximately 70,000 deaths in the United States during the 1957–58 flu season. Although high rates of illness occurred among all age groups, serious complications and death were more common among the elderly and people with chronic illnesses—groups that consistently show a greater risk of serious flu-related problems.

Influenza A virus again underwent an antigenic shift in 1968, resulting in the 1968–69 pandemic that became known as Hong Kong flu. About 34,000 deaths in the United States were attributed to this pandemic.

One possible reason for the lower death rate compared with other pandemics is that only the hemagglutinin component of the virus changed; the neuraminidase remained similar to that of the "Asian" strain. Furthermore, seroarchaeological evidence suggested that a virus with a similar hemagglutinin circulated from 1899 to 1917. Thus, older people still alive in the late 1960s may have been protected by antibody acquired earlier. Since 75 to 90% of influenza-related deaths usually occur among people 65 or older, protection of this group should substantially decrease death rates. However, the cumulative mortality due to influenza during epidemics between antigenic shifts is usually higher than that that occurs during pandemics. In the years since the emergence of the Hong Kong strain in 1968, approximately 300,000 U.S. deaths have been attributed to viruses that evolved from this strain. Of the three flu virus strains currently in circulation, this type A strain, designated type A(H3N2)—the H3 and N2 indicating the particular hemagglutinin and neuraminidase—is associated with the highest mortality.

In 1977 an event occurred that took many influenza researchers by surprise and upset some of the theories previously held by epidemiologists; a virus that was virtually identical to one that circulated in the early 1950s reappeared. Adding to this surprise was the fact that the type A virus that had emerged in 1968 continued to circulate rather than disappearing, as previous type A viruses had done following an antigenic shift. Both of these type A viruses have continued to circulate up to the present.

Influenza in animals

Influenza A viruses infect animals other than humans—most often swine, horses, seals, whales, and birds.

Fourteen distinct hemagglutinins and nine neuraminidases have been distinguished among these animal flu viruses, though only three of these hemagglutinins and two neuraminidases have been found in human viruses. Animal viruses are believed to play an important role in the development of human pandemic strains. Antigenic shift may be caused by a "reshuffling," or exchange, of genes between human and animal strains infecting the same cell of a human or animal "host." Animal strains might also undergo changes making them capable of infecting humans.

The impact of influenza in animals varies. The virus can cause respiratory illness in mammals, but mortality is usually low. Influenza infection in ducks is often asymptomatic, but the virus can cause devastating epidemics among other economically important fowl. Influenza is also a threat to the Thoroughbred horse industry.

Some animal influenza viruses can cause illness in humans, and human influenza viruses can also infect animals. While in most cases animal influenza viruses do not appear to cause severe illness in humans, they do have this potential. Seroarchaeological evidence strongly suggests that the 1918–19 pandemic was caused by a virus similar to influenza viruses that have continued to cause flu in swine.

Surveillance and identification of viruses

International surveillance of influenza viruses has been conducted by the World Health Organization (WHO) since 1947. The number of participating laboratories has increased over the years—by 1990 there were more than 200 national influenza centers worldwide, representing every continent and virtually every major geographic area in the world. The main purposes

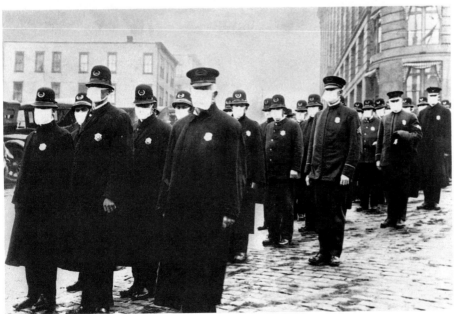

The devastating influenza pandemic of 1918–19 known as the Spanish flu was the most severe in history, causing as many as 20 million deaths worldwide. In the U.S. alone, about 500,000 people died as a result of the disease. Vaccines against the flu virus had yet to be developed; gauze surgical masks like the ones worn by these Chicago policemen were the only available protective measure.

Culver Pictures

of this surveillance program are to determine which virus strains are circulating and to monitor their impact and any antigenic changes that occur. The findings of this surveillance system are used to determine which strains should be included in the current influenza vaccine, which must be updated annually to accommodate the antigenic changes.

Several hundred laboratories throughout the world send virus samples to one of two WHO reference centers located in London and Atlanta, Ga. There the viruses are tested, and each is given a unique name. Viruses are identified according to the virus type, place of isolation (usually a country or a city), and number of isolates of that type of virus from that place and year. If the virus is type A, it is also identified according to subtype. For example, the 10th type A virus of the H3N2 subtype to be isolated in Singapore in 1988 was designated A/Singapore/10/88 (H3N2). It is because of this system that certain virus strains come to be known popularly by such names as Russian flu and Hong Kong flu.

Influenza viruses are isolated by being cultured in the laboratory from specimens obtained from people who have acquired the infection naturally. Specimens are usually taken by a swab from the back of the patient's throat or the inside of the nose. Influenza-infected cells from the surface epithelia are easily obtained. Specimens are then transferred onto a type of culture media where influenza viruses are likely to grow. The types of media used are either thin sheets of living cells (grown from a continuous cell line originally derived from animals) or hen's eggs. (Most influenza viruses grow particularly well in eggs—the viruses used in the commercial influenza vaccine are grown in hen's eggs.)

Of the viruses that are sent to one of the two WHO centers, those that represent different variations of circulating strains are stored in ultralow-temperature freezers (−70° C [−94° F] or below) or in liquid nitrogen. They are stored indefinitely and may be retrieved for a variety of purposes. For example, as more advanced laboratory techniques are developed, studies of viruses that circulated in the past could lead to a better understanding of the evolution and molecular epidemiology of influenza.

Diagnosis and treatment

Although the respiratory symptoms of influenza and the common cold can be similar, flu is generally accompanied by other, severe systemic symptoms, including fever, headache, muscle aches, and extreme fatigue. Flu symptoms develop quite suddenly and usually appear one to three days after exposure to influenza virus. Although flu symptoms are usually more debilitating than cold symptoms, in both cases the duration of symptoms can vary from a few days to two weeks or more. The acute symptoms of influenza usually subside in three to five days, but other manifestations—hacking cough, fatigue—often persist for another week or longer. Secondary bacterial infections are more likely to occur after influenza infection than after a cold.

While it is possible to diagnose influenza in the laboratory, it usually requires several days to a week to obtain results; furthermore, the test is relatively expensive and is not performed in most clinical laboratories. A new test is currently being developed that may allow physicians to diagnose influenza in their offices quickly and inexpensively. However, at the present time physicians usually make a clinical diagnosis of flu

Flu viruses similar to those that infect humans also infect domesticated animals, including pigs, ducks, and horses. According to one theory of the origin of flu viruses, pandemic strains arise when a human and an animal strain infect a common host. Such an occurrence might be likely in rural areas of a country such as China, where people live in close proximity to animals that are susceptible to flu.

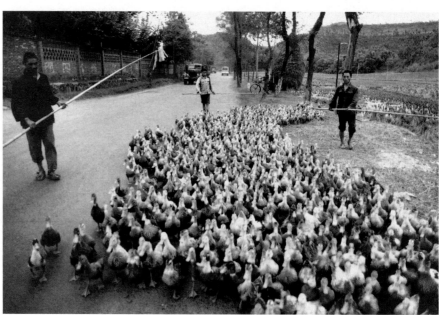

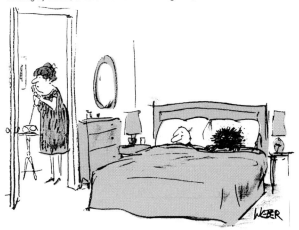

"He won't be in today. He's in bed with a bug."

based on the patient's symptoms combined with the knowledge that influenza tends to occur in epidemics in the coldest months. Thus, during the winter, when they begin to see a sharp increase in the number of patients with acute respiratory illness associated with fever and accompanied by characteristic flu symptoms, doctors are usually correct in suspecting that most of these illnesses are caused by influenza viruses. By keeping informed of the results of state and national influenza surveillance, physicians also know which influenza virus type or strain is likely to be responsible, since one particular strain often predominates in a given flu season.

If the predominant influenza strain is a type A virus, the doctor may prescribe the antiviral drug amantadine (Symmetrel) for patients with influenza symptoms. Its mechanism of action is not completely understood, but the drug appears to inhibit replication of influenza A viruses; it is not effective against influenza B. If taken within the first day or two after symptoms begin, amantadine can reduce the severity of flu symptoms and may also reduce the duration of the illness. Although the drug is usually safe when taken as prescribed, adjustments in dosage are needed for children and older adults, as well as for people with kidney disease and seizure disorders such as epilepsy. Patients should ask their physician about potential side effects and know which symptoms may represent side effects that warrant discontinuing the drug.

People who require regular medical supervision for a chronic disease (*e.g.,* heart and respiratory conditions, kidney disorders) should consult their physician when they develop a flulike illness. However, many otherwise healthy people may not need to see a doctor when they get the flu. Uncomplicated influenza can be treated by bed rest, fluids (hot or cold), and simple home remedies or over-the-counter medications. Gargling with warm salt water can help soothe a sore throat, and sipping fluids can reduce the frequency

and severity of a cough. When a dry, hacking cough is persistent or interferes with sleep, a cough suppressant may be helpful. Decongestants can relieve pressure and congestion in the nasal passages, sinuses, or ears, and antihistamines can help relieve a runny nose or watery eyes. When considering multisymptom preparations, it is important to understand the purpose of each ingredient and to consider whether all are needed. It may be better to treat the most troublesome symptoms with one or two single-ingredient medications.

The choice of medication for treatment of fever, headache, and muscle aches is especially important for children and teenagers with influenza. While most adults can safely take either aspirin or an aspirin substitute such as acetaminophen, children and teenagers (6 months old up to 18 years of age) should never be given aspirin when influenza is suspected. It has been found that children and teenagers who take aspirin during and after influenza infection are at greater risk of developing the rare but very serious illness Reye's syndrome.

While most people recover from influenza with aftereffects no more serious than a tendency to tire easily for a week or two, some develop more serious complications. The most common are bacterial infections. These include ear infections, which occur more frequently in children than in adults; sinusitis; bronchitis; and pneumonia. The severity of these conditions can vary greatly, and while antibiotics have no effect on the influenza virus, they are effective against secondary bacterial infections. People with acute respiratory infections who continue to have troublesome symptoms or significant fever for more than three or four days should see their doctor.

Prevention

For some people, preventing influenza infection is especially important. Annual influenza vaccination is specifically recommended for people who, because of their age or certain chronic health conditions, are at increased risk of serious flu-related complications. These high-risk groups include the following people: (1) adults and children with chronic diseases of the heart or lungs, including asthma; (2) residents of nursing homes and other chronic care facilities; (3) anyone 65 years of age or older; (4) adults and children who have diabetes, kidney disease, severe forms of anemia, or immunosuppression (including those with symptomatic human immunodeficiency virus infection—*i.e.,* AIDS or AIDS-related complex); (5) children and teenagers who are receiving long-term aspirin therapy (for juvenile rheumatoid arthritis, for example) and may, therefore, be at greater risk of developing Reye's syndrome after an influenza infection.

Except during the pandemics of 1918–19 and 1957–58, pregnancy has not been shown to increase the risk of influenza-related complications. However, pregnant women who have any of the chronic medical conditions listed above should be vaccinated since it has been determined that influenza vaccination is safe during pregnancy. Flu vaccine is also recommended for those who are in frequent contact with people at high risk, such as health care providers and family members of those at high risk.

In the United States influenza vaccine is usually given a short time before the influenza season—from about September until December—because the level of antibody is highest about a month after vaccination and can begin to decline several months thereafter. However, people in the high-risk groups should consider receiving influenza vaccine at any time if they plan to travel to the tropics or to the Southern Hemisphere between April and September, when influenza may be circulating.

Influenza vaccine is made from flu viruses that have been killed, or inactivated. The fear that being vaccinated may actually cause a person to get the flu is unfounded; the fact that the vaccine contains only killed viruses makes infections impossible. In the past, however, flu vaccines were not as highly purified as they are now, and reactions to the vaccine, in the form of symptoms such as fever, muscle aches, or headache, were more common. Most people who receive current influenza vaccines have no such side effects; however, because the viruses for influenza vaccine are grown in eggs, people with severe egg allergies can have an allergic reaction to the vaccine and should therefore not take it.

Another reason some people do not get flu shots is that they believe the vaccine is not always effective. In fact, effectiveness can vary from one season to another. Because the virus strains that are used in making the vaccine must be chosen months in advance of the flu season, sometimes one or more of the circulating viruses change between the choosing of the vaccine strains and the actual flu season. However, even when the vaccine does not completely prevent influenza infection, it often decreases the severity of illness and the likelihood of developing complications. For elderly people and those with immune deficiencies, flu vaccine has been found to be more effective in preventing complications and death than in preventing flu itself.

Although amantadine can also be used to prevent influenza A infection—it is 70–90% effective—it is not generally recommended as a substitute for flu vaccine (except in some immunocompromised individuals), as it does not protect against type B influenza, and it must be taken every day over the entire period of potential exposure to influenza. However, it can be a very useful adjunct to vaccine in certain situations.

Another antiviral drug, rimantadine (Flumadine), is also being studied for prevention and treatment of influenza. Rimantadine is chemically similar to amantadine but appears to cause fewer side effects. Like amantadine, it is also ineffective against type B influenza. Another possible limitation of these antiviral agents is the potential for the emergence of drug-resistant viruses. Influenza A viruses resistant to amantadine and rimantadine have been found in some patients treated with these drugs; however, the potential for spread of resistant viruses is not yet known. The vast majority of circulating influenza A viruses that have been tested up to the present time have not been drug resistant.

Ongoing research

Other approaches to preventing influenza are being explored. Researchers have been studying a live influenza vaccine that is administered in the form of nose drops or spray. The vaccine is made from attenuated influenza viruses (*i.e.*, reduced in disease-causing potential) that cannot replicate in the lower respiratory tract and that produce a very mild, often subclinical, infection. These viruses are combined with naturally occurring influenza viruses to create viruses that have the hemagglutinin and neuraminidase of circulating influenza strains but other proteins of the attenuated strain. This process produces a virus that can induce immunity to circulating viruses but causes only a very mild, or subclinical, infection. Among the potential advantages of live influenza vaccines are that they may induce immunity against a broader range of influenza virus variants than vaccines made from killed virus and that they may also induce longer-lasting immunity.

Finally, scientists are continuing to study the virus itself in the hope that a better understanding of its biological properties may lead to the development of even more effective control measures. As the tools of molecular biology become more sophisticated and more widely applied, the structure of influenza virus proteins and the genetic code of the viral genes are being studied in greater detail. For example, researchers not only have identified the gene responsible for amantadine and rimantadine resistance but also have elucidated portions of the gene and the changes in the nucleotide sequences encoding the proteins of this portion. This finding has allowed researchers to characterize resistant viruses, and it may eventually lead to a better understanding of the mechanisms of influenza virus replication; this may in turn contribute to the development of better ways to inhibit replication. Molecular techniques are also being applied to studies of the immune response and show great promise for the development of more effective vaccines.

Gestational Diabetes
by Donna L. Jornsay, R.N.

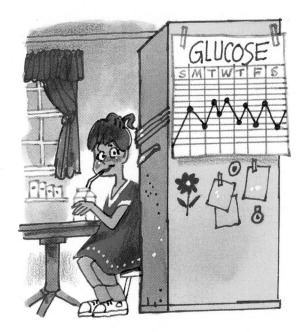

Gestational diabetes is a form of diabetes that develops during pregnancy (gestation) and usually disappears when the baby is born. It affects about 3% of all pregnant women but is much more common in certain ethnic groups, including Hispanics, blacks, Native Americans, and Asian Indians. It is one of the most common complications of pregnancy.

The exact cause of gestational diabetes is unknown. During pregnancy the placenta (the organ nourishing the baby) produces hormones that help the fetus grow but also block insulin's action in the mother's body. This is known as insulin resistance. Insulin is the hormone produced by the pancreas that helps the body's cells use or store glucose for energy. Glucose is the body's simplest form of sugar obtained from digested food.

During pregnancy, all women experience changes in the amount of insulin their bodies produce. This extra insulin is needed to meet the energy needs of both the mother and baby. When there is not enough insulin produced by the pancreas or the insulin is not used effectively, as is the case with insulin resistance, glucose cannot be used for energy and builds up in the bloodstream. These high blood glucose levels during pregnancy constitute gestational diabetes. High blood glucose levels (hyperglycemia) are unhealthy for both mother and baby.

Gestational diabetes usually appears around the 24th week of pregnancy, when the placenta begins producing large amounts of the hormones causing insulin resistance. Women with a family history of diabetes or who are overweight have a greater chance of developing gestational diabetes, although it may occur in any woman. Also, as women age, their chances of acquiring gestational diabetes increase, so even a woman who did not develop gestational diabetes during her first pregnancy may develop it during later pregnancies. Although it cannot generally be prevented, in 98% of the women affected, gestational diabetes goes away after pregnancy. However, statistics show it is likely to recur with subsequent pregnancies.

Screening tests

There are usually no signs or symptoms of gestational diabetes. For this reason, health care professionals recommend that *all* women be screened for gestational diabetes between the 24th and 28th week of pregnancy. Women who have had gestational diabetes in a previous pregnancy or have other risk factors may be screened earlier than the 24th week.

The screening test requires that the woman drink a glucose solution. One hour later, a blood glucose level is measured. If the result is abnormal, a glucose tolerance test is performed. The night before, she consumes nothing after midnight; in the morning a blood sample is taken. She then drinks a larger amount of glucose solution than for the screening test. Blood samples are taken hourly for three hours. If two or more of the four blood test results are higher than established values, she has gestational diabetes. It is not uncommon for women to have abnormal screening tests but normal glucose tolerance tests; these women do not have gestational diabetes.

How the baby is affected

In women with gestational diabetes who maintain normal glucose levels (60 to 140 milligrams per deciliter [mg/dl]), babies are at only slightly higher risk for complications than babies of healthy women who do not have diabetes. Babies of women with gestational diabetes are not born with diabetes regardless of what the mother's blood glucose levels were during pregnancy. If gestational diabetes has been poorly controlled, the following problems can affect infants:

Macrosomia (big body). The term *macrosomia* is used to describe a baby who is abnormally large for his or her developmental age. When a woman has increased blood glucose levels, this "highly sugared" blood crosses the placenta to the baby. The baby is "overfed" by this extra glucose and gets fat. Delivery of a large baby can be difficult for both the mother and the baby. The baby may be too large to be delivered vaginally; a cesarean delivery may therefore be

423

necessary. Large babies who are delivered vaginally have an increased chance of injury to their arms or shoulders during delivery.

Hypoglycemia (low blood sugar). Hypoglycemia is another problem for babies of mothers who have high blood glucose levels in the last few days of pregnancy or during labor. High blood glucose levels cause the baby to produce extra insulin. After delivery, this extra insulin can cause the infant's normal blood glucose to fall to lower than normal levels. Thus, these infants have their blood glucose levels checked frequently in the first few hours after birth.

Jaundice (hyperbilirubinemia). Jaundice (yellowing of the skin) may occur more often in babies born to women with gestational diabetes. In the days following their birth, they may need to be exposed to special lights in the hospital nursery to help break down the extra bilirubin (yellowish pigment) that has built up in their systems as the result of the normal transition from fetus to infant. In most, this treatment is very successful and lasts only a few days.

Other problems. Respiratory distress syndrome is a condition in which the infants' lungs are not mature enough for them to breathe on their own. It occurs most commonly in babies who are born prematurely, and women with poorly controlled gestational diabetes are at greater risk for preterm births.

It is important to stress that gestational diabetes does *not* cause birth defects, as it does not develop until later in pregnancy. The baby's organs are formed before blood glucose levels rise. Birth defects are more common in infants of women with diabetes prior to pregnancy. Only if the mother's "gestational diabetes" is actually previously undiagnosed diabetes and her blood glucose levels are high early in pregnancy will her baby be at increased risk for birth defects.

The mother's health

Women with gestational diabetes and large babies may have prolonged labors. The baby's head can have trouble fitting through the mother's pelvis (cephalopelvic disproportion). There may therefore be a need for a cesarean delivery, which carries an increased chance for maternal complications.

Women with gestational diabetes may have a greater chance of developing infections, especially vaginal, bladder, and kidney infections. These women should have frequent urine cultures to detect the presence of any urinary tract infection that would require treatment with antibiotics.

Toxemia (preeclampsia or pregnancy-induced hypertension) is a potentially serious complication of pregnancy that is more common in women with gestational diabetes. It causes high blood pressure, urine protein spillage, and swelling (edema), especially of the legs and feet. High blood pressures are not healthy for the mother or the baby and can be life-threatening if

untreated. Treatment can vary—from bed rest to hospitalization. Toxemia usually resolves after delivery.

The persistence of diabetes after delivery is the most serious problem for women with gestational diabetes. As indicated previously, this occurs in approximately 2% of women with gestational diabetes. Up to 60% of women who have had gestational diabetes, however, will develop non-insulin-dependent diabetes later in life. Obese women have the greatest risk for the development of lifelong diabetes.

Management of gestational diabetes

The goal of gestational diabetes management is normalization of blood glucose levels. The "tools" that enable women with gestational diabetes to achieve normal blood glucose levels and will help them to achieve the goal of having a healthy baby include:

The health care team. Prior to the diagnosis of gestational diabetes, most pregnant women receive prenatal care only from their obstetrician. Women with gestational diabetes need care from a specialized team that may include an endocrinologist, a dietician, and a nurse educator.

Blood glucose monitoring. In order to monitor how well the treatments are controlling the diabetes, women are frequently asked to test their blood each day. The results of these tests (in addition to the monitoring of urine) provide the woman and her health care team with the information necessary for making adjustments for keeping both mother and baby healthy.

Blood glucose values fluctuate throughout the day; they are lowest before meals and highest one to two hours after meals. Desirable blood glucose ranges for pregnancy are premeal glucose values of 60–90 mg/dl and postmeal values of less than 140 mg/dl. Testing schedules vary, but most health care professionals recommend testing in the morning before eating and one to two hours after each meal. Blood glucose testing may be required more frequently for women taking insulin.

Blood glucose testing can easily be done by the woman herself. It requires only a pinprick to the side of the fingertip to obtain one small drop of blood. There are automatic devices available that do the "sticking" and make the process simple, quick, and painless.

There are several different methods for measuring the amount of glucose in the blood. All methods require a small drop of blood to be placed on the pad of a chemically treated test strip or membrane. One method uses a meter, which gives an automatic and exact readout of blood glucose. Another method uses test strips only (without a meter). Neither method is difficult to perform, but all require the woman to be carefully trained in their use.

Urine ketone monitoring. Ketones are waste products that develop when the mother's body breaks down fat because there is no other energy source available. This happens during pregnancy if there has been a long interval between meals or if the mother is not eating enough for both herself and her baby. Ketones are monitored because they cross the placenta and large amounts may be dangerous to the baby. The mother may be asked to check her urine for ketones every morning before eating. To prevent ketones it is important that she not skip or delay meals and follow the prescribed meal plan.

Healthy eating for two. A healthy meal plan is the key to success with gestational diabetes. Foods the mother eats are broken down into glucose and raise blood glucose levels in varying amounts. Of the three main food types—carbohydrates, proteins, and fats—carbohydrates (starches) have the greatest effect on blood glucose. Most carbohydrates are turned into sugar within one to two hours. Simple sugars such as concentrated sweets and desserts are absorbed even more quickly. Proteins and fats are digested more slowly and have only a small effect on blood glucose.

A well-balanced meal plan includes adequate amounts of all these basic nutrients, including sufficient quantities of carbohydrates to promote the baby's growth. Many women when diagnosed with gestational diabetes try to control blood glucose levels by eliminating starches from their diet. This can be harmful to the developing fetus, who needs these foods to grow. Also, sufficient starches are needed to control glucose levels adequately.

A dietician will design a meal plan that includes all the necessary nutrients for pregnancy and balances meals throughout the day. This alone may be enough to keep blood glucose levels normal. Blood glucose monitoring tells the mother and her health care team how well the treatment is working.

The goals of the diet are: (1) blood glucose values of less than 140 mg/dl one hour after meals; (2) a pregnancy weight gain of 48–59 kg (22–27 lb; obese women may need to gain only 33–44 kg [15–20 lb]); and (3) absence of ketones in maternal urine.

The moderate use of aspartame (*e.g.,* one diet soda or one serving of aspartame-sweetened dessert per day) is considered safe during pregnancy. The artificial sweetener saccharin, however, crosses the placenta and should be avoided during pregnancy. Caffeine, alcohol, and concentrated sweets should also be avoided.

Exercise. Physical exercise lowers blood glucose by making body cells more sensitive to insulin. For this reason, exercise can be very helpful in the management of gestational diabetes. A woman with gestational diabetes may be advised to go for a brisk 20–30 minute walk every day after breakfast, or even after every meal, to control the blood glucose response to that meal.

In general, exercise during pregnancy should be done at a moderate level so that the mother's pulse does not exceed 140 beats per minute, and the exercise should be performed in 20-minute sessions so that the pulse does not stay elevated. Acceptable

2,220-calorie sample meal plan					
	exchanges*	food (amount)		exchanges*	food (amount)
breakfast:	0 fruit	fruit (none)	PM snack:	1 meat	cheese (1 oz)
	1 meat	egg (1) or slice cheese (1)		½ milk	plain low-fat yogurt
	2 starch	whole-grain bread			(½ cup) or skim
		(2 slices) or dry			milk (½ cup)
		cereal (¾ cup)		1 starch	crackers (4) or
	2 fat	margarine (2 tsp)			breadsticks (3)
		or polyunsaturated			
		oil (2 tsp)	dinner:	4 meat	broiled lean fish, chicken,
	½ milk	skim milk (½ cup)			or meat (4 oz)
				1 vegetable	cooked vegetables (1 cup)
AM snack:	½ milk	skim milk (½ cup)		2 starch	rice (1 cup) or pasta
	1 starch	crackers (4)			(1½ cups)
				2 fat	margarine or oil (2 tsp)
lunch:	3 meat	lean fish, chicken,		1 milk	skim milk (1 cup)
		or cheese (3 oz or 3 slices)		1 fruit	fresh fruit (one
	1 vegetable	cooked or raw			small piece)
		vegetables (1 cup)			
	2 starch	bread (2 slices)	bedtime snack:	½ milk	skim milk (½ cup)
	1 fat	margarine, mayonnaise,		1 starch	bread (1 slice)
		or oil (1 tsp)		1 meat	cheese (1 slice) or
	1 milk	skim milk (1 cup)			peanut butter (2 tsp)
	1 fruit	fresh fruit (small piece)			
		or banana (½)			

*based on American Diabetes Association diabetic exchange lists, which divide foods into six groups (meat, starch, vegetable, fruit, fat, and milk)

Source: Pat Anastasio, Diabetes Care and Information Center of New York

forms of exercise include brisk walking, swimming, and prenatal stretching exercises. Activities that may be too strenuous for the pregnant woman include jogging, tennis, racquetball, volleyball, basketball, snow skiing, and waterskiing. These and other forms of exercise should first be discussed by the woman with her health care team.

Insulin treatment. If a meal plan and exercise do not keep blood glucose levels in the desired range, treatment with insulin may be needed. This occurs in approximately 15% of women who develop gestational diabetes. Insulin must be injected; it cannot be taken in pill form because it is broken down during digestion. Oral diabetes medications cannot be used during pregnancy.

A nurse educator teaches women how to give themselves insulin. With the very fine needles available today—and with the proper technique—injections are virtually painless. Women who need insulin will also be instructed in the different types of insulin, how they work, and how to balance the insulin they take with the meals they eat in order to avoid low blood sugar levels. A woman's need for insulin usually increases as her pregnancy progresses. This is *not* a sign that the diabetes is worsening.

Frequently, pregnant women worry that taking insulin may hurt the baby. Insulin does *not* cross the placenta; blood glucose does, however, and high levels are dangerous for the baby. It is therefore essential that blood glucose levels be normalized.

Keeping a log. It is important for the mother to keep some sort of log in which she records blood glucose and urine ketone values, times of the tests, and any changes in diet, exercise, or insulin. These results will need to be reviewed regularly with the health care team so that any necessary adjustments in the treatment plan can be made.

Obstetrical follow-up

Between the 30th and 40th week of pregnancy and until the time of delivery, the obstetrician may recommend some special tests for women with gestational diabetes. These tests measure the growth and evaluate the condition of the baby. Some of the more common tests that may be prescribed are:

Ultrasound. An ultrasound examination is a safe and painless exam of the baby that uses sound waves to produce a picture (sonogram) of the developing baby. Ultrasound is often performed at various times throughout the pregnancy to evaluate the baby's growth. Many obstetricians order an ultrasound to estimate the baby's size when choosing the safest method of delivery.

Kick counts (fetal movement tests). The kicks or movements the mother feels from the baby are good indicators of the baby's health. The mother may be asked to count the number of movements within spe-

cific time periods each day. The doctor or nurse will explain this test, and the mother should notify the doctor if there is any decrease in the number of movements or change in the pattern of movements.

The nonstress test (NST). The nonstress test is an appraisal of the baby's well-being based on changes that occur in the fetal heart rate with the baby's movement. It is a painless test that uses an external monitor attached to the mother's abdomen—without stimuli (stress) to the baby—to record the fetal heart rate, which should accelerate when the baby becomes active. It is usually done for a period of 20–30 minutes in the doctor's office or hospital clinic.

Delivery and postpartum

Most women with gestational diabetes have successful pregnancies and deliver healthy babies. If the gestational diabetes is well controlled and the baby is of a normal size, most women with gestational diabetes can deliver their babies vaginally, and their babies will be perfectly healthy. It bears repeating that babies of women who have had gestational diabetes will *not* have diabetes. Many hospitals still care for these infants in the special-care nursery, however, so they can receive special attention if needed.

Like all women, those who have had gestational diabetes are encouraged to breast-feed their infants. Breast milk is an excellent source of infant nutrition, and it contains antibodies to help fight infections. Breast-feeding can also help mothers in their efforts to lose weight after pregnancy.

Ninety-eight percent of women with gestational diabetes will not have diabetes after delivery. The maternal risks of undiagnosed diabetes make it important that women who have had gestational diabetes have a two-hour glucose tolerance test 6 to 12 weeks after delivery to ensure that their diabetes has resolved. The 2% of women who still have diabetes will need good medical care; prompt diagnosis is essential.

In 60–90% of women who have had gestational diabetes, the condition will recur with subsequent pregnancies. As already indicated, a diabetes screening test is important early in subsequent pregnancies.

Of the women who have had gestational diabetes, 60% will develop non-insulin-dependent diabetes later in life; most will be obese. Of those women who return to ideal body weight after their pregnancy, only 25% will develop diabetes. The healthy eating habits developed during pregnancy should be maintained postpartum, but caloric intake will need to be reduced in order to promote weight loss. Specific caloric needs will depend on the individual woman's height and body size and her activity level. Women who have had gestational diabetes should have an annual fasting blood glucose test to make certain that non-insulin-dependent diabetes has not developed.

Kidney Stones

by Fredric L. Coe, M.D., and Joan H. Parks, M.B.A.

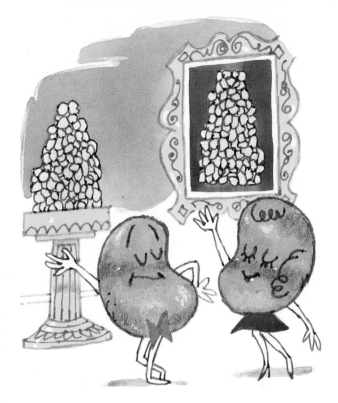

In March 1988 the U.S. National Institutes of Health convened a consensus conference at which experts from the United States and Europe deliberated and came to conclusions about the best and most up-to-date methods of treating and preventing kidney stones. The conference was held partly because new treatments have become available and partly because kidney (or renal) stone disease (nephrolithiasis) is so common; some 328,000 people in the U.S. alone are affected annually, and kidney stones are thought to occur in 1% of adult men in the industrialized countries of the world.

The kidneys and the stones they form

The kidneys are bean-shaped organs that act as chemical filters of the blood. From the food and drink people consume, the kidneys separate chemicals; chemicals the body does not need are drained as urine that flows down through long, narrow tubes—the ureters—into the bladder, which acts as a temporary reservoir until the time of urination. The bladder in its turn drains into the urethra, and the urine is passed out of the body.

Human kidneys have evolved to conserve water so people can live on dry land; they can eliminate essentially all their waste products in as little as 350 ml (10.5 fl oz) of urine a day. This water conservation, with concentration of salts in the urine, a benefit during evolution, has a distinct drawback: it raises the risk of forming stones.

All kidney stones are made of crystals held together by common urine proteins. Most—80%—are made of calcium crystals, most commonly calcium oxalate. These kidney stones form because humans produce urine that contains more calcium and oxalate than can be held in solution. Kidneys normally add more calcium and oxalate to the urine than it can hold, so crystals always can be found in urine; stone-forming people simply exaggerate this tendency and make more crystals than is normal. Their urinary crystals bunch together into stones, which obstruct urine flow and can cause pain and bleeding.

Of the other types of stones, about 5% are made of crystals of uric acid. Rarely, stones are made of cystine, an amino acid normally found in blood, which spills into the urine in certain people who have an inherited kidney abnormality. About 15% of stones are formed in the kidneys by the actions of bacteria that infect the urinary system; some bacteria possess an enzyme that converts urea, a normal urine constituent, into ammonia, which initiates a chain of reactions leading to crystals of magnesium ammonium phosphate, called "struvite" after Heinrich Struve, the mineralogist who first discovered similarly composed crystals in caves. Kidney stones can be a combination of different crystals. The size of stones can range from flecks that can barely be seen on an X-ray to a "staghorn," which can fill up an entire kidney. Stones can be smooth and round or can have sharp, jagged edges.

Factors that increase the risk of stones

A number of factors can contribute to a tendency to develop kidney stones. These include:

Sex and age. Stones most often start in young adulthood, the peak ages being between 20 and 30; rarely, they begin during childhood or in later adult life, after age 50 or 60. Stones are overwhelmingly (80%) a disease of men, though women who form stones tend to experience more trouble from them; *e.g.,* urinary infection and the need for surgery.

High urine calcium losses (hypercalciuria). Over half of the men and three-fourths of the women who have stones have hypercalciuria. Hypercalciuric people are able to absorb more calcium from their diet than most people, and they excrete the excess calcium in their urine. About 10% of the general population are hypercalciuric. This trait, which could have survival advantages in a calcium-poor environment, is inherited in an autosomal dominant manner, like brown eyes; this means hypercalciuria occurs in successive generations of families that carry the trait, and equally in both sexes.

High urine uric acid levels (hyperuricosuria). The diet of some stone-forming people, mostly men, consists largely of meat, fish, and poultry. These protein-rich foods also are high in purines, of which the metabolic by-product is uric acid. Their diets overload their urine with uric acid, which is poorly soluble and forms crystals. Uric acid crystals can grow into a stone or act as seed crystals that promote the crystallization of calcium oxalate. Sometimes the two crystals grow into each other. A minority of patients overproduce uric acid because of hereditary predisposition; they are also prone to mixed stones even though their diets may not contain a preponderance of meats or other high-purine foods.

Low urine citrate levels (hypocitraturia). Citrate is a chemical found in urine that binds with calcium to form a soluble salt, thereby depriving oxalate or phosphate of the calcium it needs for making crystals or stones. The greater the amount of calcium compared with the amount of citrate in an individual's urine, the more likely that person is to form stones. Women who have never formed stones tend to have the highest ratio of citrate to calcium in the urine, about twice that of women who have had stones; men who have not had stones have citrate-to-calcium ratios equivalent to those of stone-forming women; men with stones have the lowest ratio of citrate to calcium of all.

Dehydration. Despite the fact that civilization has provided people in most parts of the Western world with clean water in essentially unlimited amounts, some people decline to drink it, or they work or play in a manner that causes dehydration. People who do not consume enough water produce too little urine to dissolve even normal amounts of materials that form stones.

Symptoms and diagnosis

Kidney stones (or even one stone) usually announce themselves by causing pain, bleeding, or urinary infection. While they are growing, attached to the outer surfaces of the kidneys, just at the openings of the tubules that produce the urine, stones are silent, although there may be occasional bleeding from the damaged kidney surfaces. Such bleeding may escape detection or be so fleeting that it is noticed only at a routine physical examination when a urinalysis is performed.

Some stones pass. When they break loose from the kidney, and then are able to roll about freely in the drainage system of the urinary tract, stones can plug up some portion of the tract, block off the flow of urine, and cause the drainage system upstream of the blockage to dilate and balloon out from the accumulation of urine; this causes the special pain of stone passage called renal colic. Renal colic comes on sud-

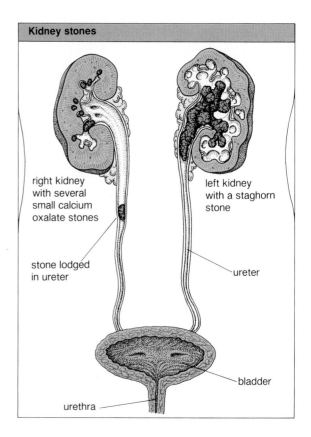

Kidney stones

right kidney with several small calcium oxalate stones

stone lodged in ureter

left kidney with a staghorn stone

ureter

bladder

urethra

denly and increases to maximum severity over about 30 minutes. The pain may begin in the flank, just at the angle formed by the lower ribs and the spine, or lower down in the back. It may gradually shift to the abdomen, and later to the groin, as the stone makes its way down the ureter. Renal colic may be accompanied by blood in the urine; frequent, urgent, or burning urination; and secondary symptoms such as nausea, vomiting, or diarrhea. When the stone passes, the pain stops as suddenly as it started. In some cases stone passage can be confused with gallbladder pain, appendicitis, viral infections, urinary infection, or other abdominal pain.

Not all stones pass, and those that do not require treatment. Various tests can be done to determine if a stone is present. A so-called KUB (kidney, ureter, bladder) X-ray provides a picture of the entire abdominal area and can reveal the general location of a renal stone. An intravenous pyelogram (IVP) is an X-ray in which dye is injected so the drainage of the kidney and its associated structures can be seen. Three-dimensional ultrasound pictures of the kidneys are also useful for determining if the kidney is obstructed by a stone. Urinalysis will often show blood, sometimes in small amounts that cannot be seen by the unassisted eye, and sometimes white cells, which can indicate infection. Urine cultures will generally show if the urinary tract is infected and with what organism.

Today's treatment: innovations replace surgery

Hospitalization (inpatient or outpatient) is needed for about 50% of those who experience kidney-stone attacks, usually because of the severe pain, which is unaffected by position, movement, or anything else the person can do. Some people attempt to drink water to help move the stone, but some are too nauseated to do so. All stone patients should strain their urine when in the midst of an attack (a coffee filter makes a good strainer) so that any crystals that pass can be analyzed.

Open surgery, which until recently was the only treatment for problematic stones, now is needed only when the anatomy of the kidney is abnormal or the stones are very large—i.e., large enough to fill the entire draining system of the kidney. This surgery requires an incision in the side, opening of the kidney or ureter to remove the stone, then suturing the wound closed and placing a temporary drain near the incision to carry urine away from the wound. Usually a patient is hospitalized for 4 to 10 days.

Instead of open surgery, stones can now be fragmented by extracorporeal shock-wave lithotripsy (ESWL), which was introduced into U.S. practice in 1984 and is now recommended for the majority of stones—i.e., those smaller than 2 cm (0.8 in)—that are not in the lower portion of a kidney. ESWL machines generate high-intensity sound waves that pass through the soft tissues of the body and produce violent vibrations that cause the stones to break up. The fragmented sandlike particles then pass through the urinary tract within days or at most a few weeks. ESWL is not indicated for very large stones because

the number of shocks needed to pulverize them would be excessive and the bulk of the resulting fragments would be difficult to pass.

Lithotripsy is a remarkably effective innovation, preferable to open surgery, which results in scars, convalescence, and loss of work time. ESWL is best done in a medical center that has expertise and the latest equipment in place.

Although unusual, the short-term effects of ESWL can be pain or bleeding. In some cases another procedure requiring hospitalization may need to be done if ESWL does not succeed in fully eliminating stones. Elevation of blood pressure may follow ESWL in some patients. The long-term effects on the kidney and the adjacent tissues are unknown. Thus, prudence in using the lowest intensity shocks is recommended. The use of ESWL in children should be carefully evaluated before it is recommended and then should be done with extreme caution.

About 15–20% of stone attacks require cystoscopies—inserting an instrument into the bladder through which thin tubes may be threaded up the ureters to the kidneys—to extract the stone. Stones larger than two centimeters usually require percutaneous nephrolithotomy (creating a surgical opening through the patient's back to reach into the kidney), which is followed by ESWL. Another approach is to create an opening in the patient's lower back about as thick as a pencil, through which an instrument can be passed into the kidney and the stones extracted; or the stones can be fragmented by thin sound-wave generators or lasers at the end of very narrow tubes inserted through the instrument into the kidney.

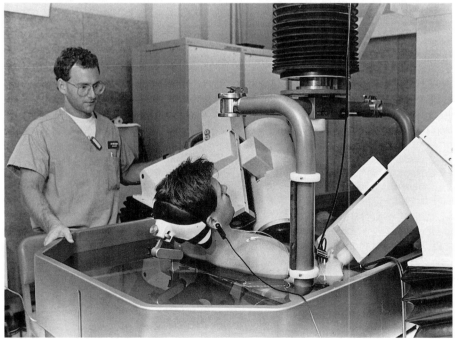

Most kidney stones can be treated by extracorporeal shock-wave lithotripsy, which spares the hospitalization, convalescence, scars, and risks associated with open surgery. This patient undergoing the procedure is immersed in a water bath after having received a local anesthetic; the lithotripter then delivers shock waves to the site of his stones to shatter them. In most cases the treatment is quick, effective, and without complications.

Emory University Hospital; photograph, Nancy Scherm

Preventing new stones

A person who has formed one stone is very likely to form another. Typically, 50% of people who have had one stone produce at least one more by 5 years, and 90% seek care for further stones by 15 years. Anyone who has formed even one stone should be evaluated metabolically (with blood and urine chemistries) to determine the likely causes of the stones so that new stones can be prevented. And all people who have formed stones should drink more water—at least 2 liters (4.2 pt) daily. Water is the fluid of choice because many flavored beverages have substances in them that may actually contribute to stones.

In a minority of people, calcium stones are caused by a systemic disease. Among calcium stone formers about 6% will have primary hyperparathyroidism, which is manifested by high levels of calcium in the blood and urine and low blood phosphorus levels; it can be cured by surgical removal of the abnormal parathyroid gland or glands. Some patients will form stones as a result of intestinal diseases such as ulcerative colitis or regional enteritis; the diarrhea associated with these diseases depletes the body of fluids and also of alkaline salts, causing the urine to be scanty and acidic. Uric acid in particular crystallizes in such urine and can make pure uric acid stones, or stones of both calcium oxalate and uric acid can form. If the small intestine is badly damaged or partially removed so that semi-digested fats from the diet are not absorbed and reach the colon, the lining of the colon can be injured and become porous to oxalate in the diet. The oxalate enters the blood and is filtered through the kidneys into the urine, where it forms calcium oxalate stones. In rare cases a hereditary condition causes people to excrete excess oxalate; this condition can lead to such extreme crystallization that the kidneys are damaged, and kidney failure can occur.

Most calcium stone formers, however, have no systemic disease. They have, instead, increased urine calcium, oxalate, or uric acid; decreased citrate excretion; or low urinary pH, due to a combination of diet and heredity. People with hereditary hypercalciuria are cautioned against consuming more than one gram of calcium per day (a cup of milk or yogurt or 1.5 oz of cheese contain about 300 mg calcium) and against a high salt intake, which increases urine calcium excretion. Thiazide diuretics lower urine calcium excretion by direct action on the kidney; in double-blind randomized studies—the gold standard of clinical studies—the new stone formation rate has been as much as 10-fold lower in people taking thiazide than in those taking a placebo. Other medications that may be helpful, by reducing intestinal absorption of calcium, are cellulose phosphate and inorganic phosphate supplements.

People with high urine uric acid levels due to high purine content in the diet can decrease them by eating less meat (especially organ meats), poultry, and certain varieties of fish (anchovies, herring, sardines, scallops, and mackerel are especially high in purine); for those who cannot manage to change their food habits, the drug allopurinol, which reduces uric acid excretion, is usually prescribed. When hypocitraturia, or low urine citrate, is a cause of calcium stones, oral alkali in the form of citrate or bicarbonate can raise the urine citrate levels.

Diet can raise urine oxalate enough to increase the risk of stones in some people. Most calcium stone formers are cautioned against heavy loads of oxalate in their diet (such foods as colas, chocolate, and peanuts are high in oxalate) as well as against the excessive use of vitamin C.

Infection stones are treated initially by the complete removal of all stone material and by antimicrobial medications. These two forms of therapy are also the best method of preventing regrowth, for if any infected stone fragments are left in the urinary tract, they can regrow rapidly, especially in the presence of an unsuppressed infection. If the patient is not a good surgical candidate, antimicrobial therapy as well as use of the drug acetohydroxamic acid, a urease inhibitor, is recommended.

When cystine stones are present, in order to prevent them from growing or multiplying, the patient must consume enough water to dissolve the cystine, usually three to four liters (six to eight pints) per day. Water must be consumed regularly throughout the day and night for the rest of the person's life so that cystine is always being dissolved. Raising the pH of the urine is of slight help. If necessary, medications such as d-penicillamine or other sulfhydryl agents that make cystine more soluble are used, but they can cause allergic reactions in up to 50% of the people who take them.

A final word

Nature did not intend that people form stones and has defended human kidneys and urinary tracts against rampant crystallization. There remain quite a few unanswered questions about kidney stones and their formation, which are being pursued in basic and clinical research. Two particular urine proteins (nephrocalcin and Tamm-Horsfall protein) are currently being investigated; the former prevents the growth of crystals, and the latter prevents clumping together of crystals. Because both of these have been shown to be abnormal in some stone formers, there is active research to understand their exact roles. Further work is needed to determine why they are abnormal in some people and whether these are genetic abnormalities.

For now, the best general advice to those who may be at risk for stones is to practice moderation in food intake, avoid dehydration, and, most important of all, learn to love water as a beverage.

Skin and Hair Problems of Black People

by Deborah Ann Scott, M.D., and Michael Bigby, M.D.

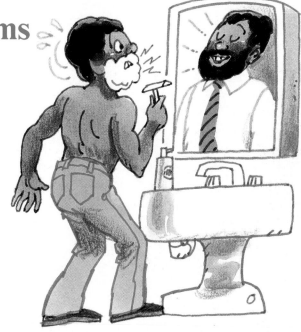

The races have been classified primarily on the basis of skin color and differences in scalp hair. The black race is identified by the presence of brown skin and curly hair, both of which are determined genetically. For an understanding of the differences in skin color and hair types among the races and of skin disorders that occur most commonly in blacks, a basic review of the skin's structure and function is helpful.

Structure and function of the skin

The skin is the largest organ in the body. It weighs 3–4 kg (6.6–8.8 lb), constitutes 6% of body weight, and covers about 2 sq m (about 20 sq ft) of the average adult. It consists of three principal layers: the epidermis, the dermis, and the subcutaneous tissue.

The epidermis is the most superficial layer. It is stratified into four visually distinct layers when viewed in cross section with a microscope. The outermost compartment of the epidermis, the stratum corneum, or horny layer, is very thin but supple and resilient. The stratum corneum acts as the principal barrier for retaining water and interfering with the entrance of microorganisms and toxic substances. Below the horny layer are the granular layer, the spinous layer, and the basal layer. The basal layer contains actively dividing cells that are responsible for constantly generating new cells that migrate upward to replace cells lost from the horny layer. As cells migrate from the basal layer toward the surface, they become flattened and die but remain firmly attached to their neighbors. The basal layer also contains melanocytes (pigment-producing cells) that synthesize the pigment melanin, which protects against ultraviolet (UV) radiation and gives the skin its color.

The dermis consists primarily of connective tissues that protect against trauma and envelop the body in a strong and flexible wrap. Also within the dermis are blood vessels, lymphatics, nerves, and the epidermal appendages: eccrine and apocrine sweat glands, sebaceous glands, and hair follicles. The third layer is the thick, fatty subcutaneous tissue that helps conserve body heat and serves as an additional shock-absorbing buffer.

Origins of skin color

Skin color is determined by the amount of melanin present in the skin and the way in which it is distributed.

The concentration of melanocytes per unit surface area varies significantly in different areas of the body. There are, however, no significant differences among the races in the number or distribution of melanocytes in the skin. The skin of black people is darker than that of the other races because their skin is more efficient at producing, distributing, and retaining melanin. The pigment melanin is produced in pigment granules known as melanosomes. Melanosomes are synthesized in melanocytes but are passed to epidermal cells in the lower layers of the epidermis. Melanosomes in blacks are large, dense, and numerous and are distributed singly to epidermal cells. In Caucasians and Asians melanosomes are small, less dense, and few in number and are distributed in clusters enclosed in a surrounding membrane. Enzymes that degrade the melanosomes are also present within this membrane. Melanosomes in Caucasians are therefore degraded before the skin cells are able to migrate to upper layers of the epidermis. In blacks melanosomes are retained during the cells' migration to the surface. Melanin production increases in response to UV exposure and results in tanning. The ability to increase melanin production in response to UV is genetically determined and is greatest for blacks and for Asians and Caucasians of Mediterranean descent.

Dark skin absorbs and disperses ultraviolet radiation more effectively and thereby prevents much of the damage done by such exposure. Black skin has a natural "sun protection factor" (SPF) of approximately 5. The SPF was devised to measure the relative effectiveness of sunscreens (protective lotions) in blocking the effects of UV irradiation on the skin. The SPF is defined as the amount of time required for producing a mild sunburn in a person wearing a sunscreen divided

431

Cross section of dark skin

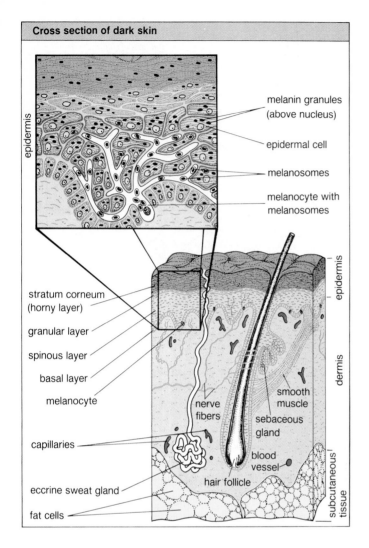

melanin granules (above nucleus)

epidermal cell

melanosomes

melanocyte with melanosomes

epidermis

stratum corneum (horny layer)

granular layer

spinous layer

basal layer

melanocyte

nerve fibers

smooth muscle

sebaceous gland

epidermis

dermis

capillaries

blood vessel

subcutaneous tissue

eccrine sweat gland

hair follicle

fat cells

by the amount of time required for the same person to get a sunburn without sunscreen. For example, a Caucasian who normally would sunburn in 10 minutes would need 150 minutes of exposure to UV light to get an equivalent sunburn when using a sunscreen with an SPF of 15. A person with dark brown skin requires approximately five times as much exposure for sunburning as the "average" Caucasian.

Since erythema (redness) associated with sunburn is often not visible in people with dark skin, there is a mistaken belief that blacks do not sunburn. Sunburn in blacks occurs, however, and is frequently manifested by skin tenderness within 24 hours of exposure and desquamation (peeling) of the skin three to four days after exposure to UV radiation.

Differences in hair types

The phenotypic (visibly characteristic) variations in hair forms among the races are most likely due to differences in the three-dimensional shape of the hair

follicle, through which the hair grows to reach the surface. Four broad hair types have been defined: straight, wavy, helical, and spiral. Black hair is commonly helical (forming coils of constant diameter) or spiral (forming coils that diminish in diameter outward). Black hair has the flattest or most elliptically shaped fibers and is produced by curved hair follicles. The hair follicle in blacks is curved with the concavity toward the epidermis. Asian hair is generally straight, has a circular structure, and arises from a straight hair follicle. Caucasian hair is the most variable; it ranges from straight to wavy or helical and has a round or oval shape and a thin cross-sectional area. Pubic, beard, and eyelash hairs tend to be elliptical in all races.

No biochemical differences have been detected among the various forms of human hair. The physical properties of hair are derived from the central portion, or cortex, which makes up 90% of the hair's shaft. The shape and strength of the cortex are derived primarily from bonds between the amino acids (protein-building blocks) that make up the hair. Disruption and reformation of these bonds by physical, mechanical, or chemical methods cause straightening of the hair shaft. The changes produced by manual stretching and heat are reversible after wetting. Chemical straighteners cause the hair to be permanently restructured. Water weakens some bonds, allowing transient restructuring, which is the basis of "wet setting."

Avoiding arbitrary classifications

The division of people into races is sometimes arbitrary and misleading. Some people classified as Caucasians have darker skin than others classified as black. Many Asians have dark skin but have hair that is very straight. To what race does a person belong whose parents or grandparents are black and Caucasian, Caucasian and Asian, or black and Asian? In trying to understand skin diseases, it is more useful to think of dark skin that is effective in producing pigment in response to UV exposure than to think of racial divisions of people. Dark-skinned Caucasians, Asians, and blacks have most if not all of the problems associated with dark skin that are discussed below. Similarly, problems described that are attributed to tightly curled or spiral hair or to the grooming techniques required for managing the hair will occur in all races of people with curled hair or who use the same grooming techniques. The majority of skin diseases occur with equal frequency among the races. Perceived or real differences in the prevalence of many diseases may be due to socioeconomic or environmental factors.

Normal variations in black skin

Blacks frequently have hyperpigmented (dark) macules (flat spots distinguished from normal skin *only* by being a different color). Such macules are considered normal. Blue-black macules on the gums are com-

432

mon; brown macules are frequently seen on the sclera (whites of the eye) and on the palms of the hands and the soles of the feet in adult blacks. Brown streaks along the long axis of the nails are also common and increase with age. Several normal pigmentary demarcation lines occur. The two most common occur on the upper outer arm (Futcher's line) and on the inner side of the thigh. Dermal melanocytosis (bluish black macules present at or soon after birth) occurs in up to 90% of normal black babies. The areas are usually round or oval and generally fade with age.

Disorders associated with curly hair

Several disorders frequently encountered in blacks are due to grooming techniques used to increase the manageability and to lessen the innate curliness of black hair. In recent years straightening the hair with a hot comb or curling iron has become less popular than it once was. The technique usually involves applying a pomade or oil to the hair and then using a very hot comb or curling iron to straighten it. Hot combing may damage the hair shaft and lead to breakage. Also, hot oil may run down the hair shaft and damage the hair follicle at the base of the hair. In the latter case permanent hair loss may result. One can prevent this "hot comb alopecia" (*alopecia* simply means "hair loss") by avoiding extreme heat and by making sure that the head and hair are always held in a direction that will not allow heated oil to run down the hair shaft to the follicle.

Hair straightening, relaxing, and waving are currently most commonly done with chemicals. Properly applied chemical hair relaxers are usually well tolerated and do not have a tendency to produce complications. Inappropriate use of chemical relaxers or application to hair that has been previously straightened, bleached, or damaged, however, will result in significant hair-shaft breakage. Such breakage may occur immediately or as late as six months after the straightening process and may not become apparent until the addition of another insult to the hair. Hair loss secondary to chemical relaxing is usually not permanent since the hair follicle is usually not damaged.

Traumatic hair loss can occur with both straightened and unstraightened hair. Spiral hair flattens at the points where it bends. The stress of extending the hair during combing may cause breakage. This breakage is seen most commonly in those with "natural" hairstyles who groom their hair with metal combs, in which the hair can become ensnared. The result is a characteristic pattern of uneven hair with frayed ends mixed with patches of shorter hair.

"Traction alopecia" is commonly seen among women and children who braid their hair tightly and often. Hair loss occurs both because hairs are pulled out of their follicles and because traction causes inflammation and atrophy of the follicle itself. If the cause of the

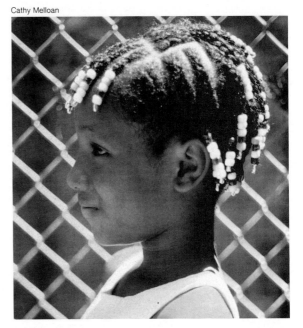

Hairstyles that lessen innate curliness and grooming methods that increase manageability sometimes cause traumatic hair loss—a problem often seen in girls who wear their hair tightly braided. Traction causes hairs to be pulled out of the follicles, and follicles themselves may be damaged.

hair loss is unrecognized and traction continues, traction alopecia may become permanent. The distribution of traction alopecia tends to be quite characteristic; while some of the hair loss varies with the particular hairstyle, there is usually uniform symmetric loss of hair in front of and above the ears.

Pomades are frequently applied to the hair to increase its manageability and to improve its appearance. For reasons that are less clear, pomades are also frequently applied to the scalp. An oil folliculitis of the scalp may result from this practice. Oil folliculitis is manifested by the appearance of clusters of pustules (white bumps filled with inflammatory cells) surrounding the hair follicles. The inflammatory cells accumulate in response to bacteria that are able to proliferate within partially occluded hair follicles. It is important that this infection be recognized and that the causative agent (the pomade) be discontinued. Antibiotics are frequently prescribed by a dermatologist to control the infection.

Application of pomades to the hair and scalp may also result in pomade acne. In this condition pustules, whiteheads, and blackheads form on the temples and forehead. The lesions are indistinguishable from regular acne (acne vulgaris) but generally resolve within four to six months once application of pomades has stopped. Newer liquid "curl activators" that are predominantly composed of water and propylene glycol tend to produce similar effects on the hair but are not associated with acne and folliculitis.

433

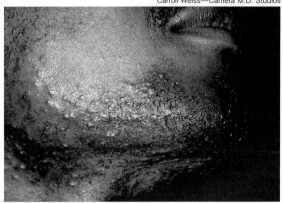

Black men who shave commonly experience some degree of pseudofolliculitis barbae (razor bumps)—small, raised bumps and pustules in the beard area, resulting from curly facial hairs reentering the skin.

Razor bumps

Pseudofolliculitis barbae (commonly referred to as "razor bumps") is a disorder seen to some extent in nearly all black men who shave. Pseudofolliculitis barbae is caused by tightly curled beard hair reentering the skin after it has grown out from the follicle. The reentering hair penetrates the epidermis and enters the dermis, where it causes inflammation. Pseudofolliculitis barbae is characterized by the development of papules (small, raised bumps on the skin) and pustules in the shaved beard area. In severe cases large, red, and tender lesions occur. Ingrown hairs can be identified in most lesions.

Numerous treatments have been recommended for this disorder. The only one that is universally successful is cessation of shaving. Ingrown hairs will spontaneously pull themselves out if the beard hair is allowed to grow. Most lesions will resolve within two months. Therapy for men who must shave or who prefer to is not as successful. Recommendations for men who want to continue shaving include softening the beard with a hot towel prior to shaving, shaving daily but not shaving closely (*i.e.*, leaving hairs approximately one millimeter long), not pulling the skin taut while shaving, shaving with the grain of the hair, using a new razor blade for each shave, and using chemical depilatories. Dermatologists sometimes prescribe topical corticosteroid or tretinoin creams, which have been reported to be helpful. When possible, ingrown hairs should be manually freed from the skin either by a dermatologist or by the affected individual himself, using a clean, tapered-tipped instrument such as a plastic toothpick, a needle, or an instrument specifically designed for freeing ingrown hairs.

Ringworm

For reasons that are unclear, tinea capitis (ringworm of the scalp) has become a disease predominantly of young black and Hispanic children. Tinea capitis is contagious and may become epidemic. It may appear as areas of alopecia associated with scaling of the scalp, as large, tender, pus-filled nodules (kerions), or as areas of alopecia studded with small black dots representing broken hairs. Treatment is with oral griseofulvin for 8–12 weeks.

Most tinea capitis currently encountered in blacks and Hispanics is caused by a soil fungus. In Caucasian children ringworm is usually caused by fungi acquired from household pets. Fifty years ago ringworm occurred with more equal frequency in Caucasians and blacks, and most cases were due to fungi acquired from animals.

Acne keloidalis

A peculiar disorder whose etiology is unknown, affecting the hair follicles in blacks, is acne keloidalis (also called dermatitis papillaris capillitii). Acne keloidalis is characterized by the development of firm papules and pustules on the nape of the neck. In severe cases large lesions can form, and the disease can result in significant scarring and permanent alopecia. No single therapy is effective for all patients. Recommended therapies include corticosteroid injections and topical corticosteroid preparations that may or may not also contain antibiotics. A variety of surgical techniques are also utilized with varying success. These techniques include localized removal of individual papules with scissors, a scalpel, or lasers. In more severe cases the entire affected area is excised, and the wound is closed with sutures.

Seborrheic dermatitis

Seborrheic dermatitis (severe dandruff) is a disorder that occurs with equal frequency in all races. Erythema, scaling, and pruritus occur on the scalp in seborrheic dermatitis. Areas of the face (particularly the eyebrows and skin beside the nose) and the chest may be similarly affected. Seborrheic dermatitis is normally treated by daily hair washing with a shampoo containing tar, selenium sulfide, or zinc pyrithione and by application of a corticosteroid or tar solution, ointment, or gel to the scalp. Many black people, however, are reluctant to wash their hair more than once or twice weekly because tightly curled hair is difficult to manage after washing. (As already mentioned, heat straightening of hair and the effects of "wet setting" are reversed by wetting the hair.) For those patients who wash their hair infrequently and who have difficulty managing their hair after washing, management of seborrheic dermatitis will involve both more frequent washing and management of the hair during more frequent washing. Management of the hair may entail a change in hair style (*e.g.*, a natural hair style or treatment with a chemical relaxer) or the use of a curl-activator containing propylene glycol to make the hair easier to comb.

434

Camera M.D. Studios

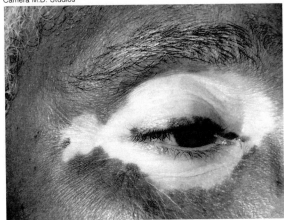

In the disorder vitiligo, stark white areas develop on the skin because melanocytes stop producing pigment and die. All races can be affected, but the hypopigmentation is most visible in those with dark skin.

Disorders of pigment

Alterations in pigmentation occur commonly in blacks. It is estimated that nearly half of all visits of black patients to dermatologists primarily or secondarily involve alterations in pigmentation. This estimate is not surprising since alterations in pigmentation frequently produce dramatic and easily visible contrasts between the appearance of normal and abnormal areas of dark skin.

Hyperpigmentation and hypopigmentation. Dark skin frequently reacts to trauma or inflammation by developing pigmentary changes. When the skin becomes darker than normal, it is known as postinflammatory hyperpigmentation; when the skin becomes lighter than normal, it is known as postinflammatory hypopigmentation. In postinflammatory hyperpigmentation increased amounts of melanin appear in the epidermis or are deposited in the dermis, often in large globules. Hypopigmentation probably occurs because of a temporary defect in the ability of melanocytes to pass melanin to the surrounding epidermal cells. The reasons that some patients respond to inflammation of the skin with hyperpigmentation while others respond with hypopigmentation are unknown.

Postinflammatory hypopigmentation almost always fades with time; although it may take many months, complete resolution usually occurs. Hyperpigmentation, however, is often a much more difficult and persistent problem; dark areas may take years to fade, and in some cases the hyperpigmentation never completely disappears. When postinflammatory hyperpigmentation is due to increased amounts of pigment in the epidermis, bleaching creams can be effective, but when it is due to deposition of pigment in the dermis, bleaching is totally ineffective and may increase the contrast between normal and abnormal areas by lightening the normal skin.

Vitiligo. Vitiligo is a disorder in which melanocytes in certain areas cease making pigment and die. The skin in affected areas becomes increasingly light and eventually completely white. The disease most commonly begins with involvement of the hands, around the mouth, and in the genital region; any area of the body may, however, be involved. The disease affects all races with equal frequency. Because of the sharp contrast produced between normal dark skin and the white, depigmented skin in vitiligo, this disorder tends to be much more distressing for dark-skinned people.

Patients with vitiligo may concurrently have other disorders; the most commonly associated disease involves the thyroid gland, and anemia may also occur. Although the disorder often is a source of significant emotional distress, vitiligo *can* be treated. Repigmentation can be stimulated by exposure of affected areas to long-wave ultraviolet light (UVA) in combination with an oral medication—psoralen—that specifically sensitizes the skin to UVA. This combined therapy, also widely used in the treatment of extensive psoriasis, is known as PUVA.

Melasma. Hyperpigmentation of the cheeks and forehead commonly occurs in blacks and is known as melasma. Melasma occurs in all races, but the degree of pigmentation produced is often greater in dark-skinned individuals, and it is much more common in women than in men. It often appears during pregnancy or while a woman is taking birth control pills. As with postinflammatory hyperpigmentation, excess pigment in melasma may be present in the epidermis,

Earlobes are a common site for keloids, a benign skin disorder. Dark-skinned people may be genetically predisposed to developing these painful, itchy, and often quite enlarged lesions.

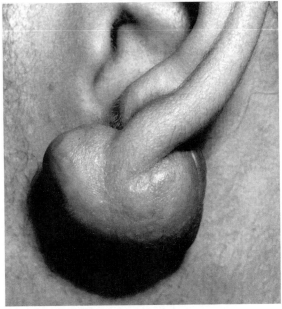

Suzanne Olbricht, Beth Israel Hospital, Boston

in the dermis, or in both areas. Therapy for melasma is directed at bleaching out excess epidermal pigment and in strictly avoiding exposure to the sun.

Ashy skin. Blacks frequently complain of being "ashy." This is not a disease, however. The condition arises because cells in the horny layer of the skin contain less pigment than the cells in lower layers. As horny layer cells normally flake off of the surface of the skin (as they do in all people), their light color contrasts with the darker skin below and gives the skin of dark people an ashy appearance. Wetting or applying oil to the skin obscures the contrast between the horny layer and the skin below. Ash can thus be well camouflaged, or it can be ignored.

Skin cancers

Skin cancer is the most common type of cancer in Caucasians. Malignant tumors of the skin are extremely rare in blacks. As already indicated, the decreased occurrence of skin cancer in blacks is directly attributable to the ability of dark skin to absorb and disperse ultraviolet radiation and thereby prevent the cancer-inducing effects of UV exposure.

Malignant melanoma is the one type of skin cancer that commonly spreads from the skin to internal organs. It is the leading cause of skin cancer-related deaths. Malignant melanomas appear as pigmented areas on the skin that have irregular borders, variegate color (usually some combination of black, blue, red, grey, or dark brown), and an uneven contour (flat and raised areas within the same lesion). The incidence of malignant melanomas is 10 times greater in whites than in blacks. In Caucasians malignant melanomas occur on the face, neck, chest, back, and extremities. Almost all melanomas in blacks occur on the palms of the hands or the soles of the feet.

Early recognition and surgical removal are the mainstays of treatment for malignant melanoma. Patients with melanomas that are detected early and surgically removed when they are still small can be cured by removal of the lesions. Black patients with melanoma generally do poorly; roughly 70% of black melanoma patients will die because of metastasis of the disease within five years.

Keloids

Keloids are a benign condition that appears to be more common in dark-skinned races; it is thought that the propensity to form keloids may have a genetic basis. Keloids result from excessive deposition of connective tissue in the dermis and usually form in response to trauma or in sites of previous acne, but they may occasionally develop spontaneously. Keloids most commonly occur on the central chest, on the back, and on the earlobes at the sites where ears are pierced. Although they generally grow slowly, keloids can achieve enormous dimensions. Pain and itching caused by the lesions are common. Unfortunately, management of keloids is difficult; even with surgical removal they often recur.

Dermatosis papulosa nigra

Dermatosis papulosa nigra is another frequently occurring benign tumor of the skin that affects black people. The face is the most commonly affected area. Lesions consist of warty (rough-surfaced) papules that may be normal skin color but more often are hyperpigmented. Dermatosis papulosa nigra lesions are more common in women than in men, and the number of lesions increases with age. These benign tumors are easily removed by means of a variety of simple techniques, including cryotherapy (freezing), electrodesiccation (treatment with a needle heated by an electric current), surgical removal, and lasers. However, therapy may be complicated by the development of postinflammatory hyperpigmentation or hypopigmentation.

FOR ADDITIONAL INFORMATION:
McDonald, Charles J., and Scott, Deborah A., eds. *Dermatologic Clinics,* vol. 6, no. 3. Philadelphia: W.B. Saunders Co., 1988. This short book was written for dermatologists, but the chapters can be easily understood by nonprofessionals. Nearly every facet of skin diseases in blacks is discussed.
Rosen, Theodore, and Martin, Sandy. *Atlas of Black Dermatology.* Boston: Little, Brown & Co., 1981. This extensively illustrated book is another source of useful information.

Delusions
by Brendan A. Maher, Ph.D.

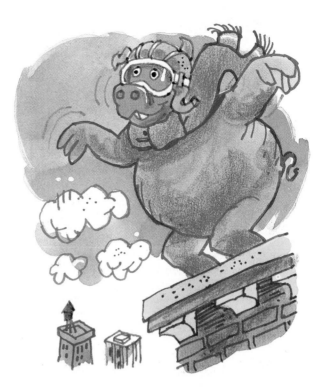

Delusions are found in more than 70 medical disorders. These include not only the well-known psychoses such as schizophrenia, depression, and bipolar affective disorder (commonly known as manic-depressive psychosis) and delusional disorder (formerly known as paranoia) but also with less frequency in a wide range of disorders of the nervous system, of the endocrine system, and arising from substance abuse. Delusions have also been reported in healthy individuals who have been placed in sensory-deprivation chambers or in solitary confinement or who have been exposed to situations or experiences that deviate from the normal, created for the purposes of research.

What is a delusion?

In spite of the fact that delusions are found in so many disorders, the definition of *delusion* is somewhat ambiguous. In the United States the generally accepted formal definition for *delusion* is provided by the *Diagnostic and Statistical Manual of Mental Disorders,* third edition, revised (*DSM-III-R*), published by the American Psychiatric Association in 1987. It reads as follows:

A false personal belief based on incorrect inference about external reality and firmly sustained in spite of what almost everyone else believes and in spite of what constitutes incontrovertible and obvious proof or evidence to the contrary. The belief is not one ordinarily accepted by other members of the person's culture or subculture (*i.e.,* it is not an article of religious faith).

General classification

Delusions are often classified according to the content of the belief involved. Thus, it is customary to refer to delusions under the following headings; the list is not exhaustive but includes the most common types.

Delusions of being controlled. Here the deluded individual experiences his or her own feelings, thoughts, actions, etc., as being controlled by some outside agency. An example is that of a man who believed that his thoughts were not his own but were being placed into his head by somebody using remote radio control. Delusions of control are important in the diagnosis of schizophrenia; in repeated surveys, delusions of being controlled have been found in more than 70% of patients diagnosed as having schizophrenia.

Somatic delusions. A person may believe that some part of his or her body has undergone a significant and sometimes bizarre change. An example: a patient

was convinced that one side of her body had shrunk in size and persisted in this belief even though her reflection in the mirror indicated no abnormality.

Grandiose delusions. Grandiose delusions have content that conveys an exaggerated sense of personal power, wealth, or significance. An example would be a person who believes himself or herself to be the unrecognized heir to a throne or the possessor of hidden millions of dollars. These delusions are found most often in manic episodes of bipolar disorder and in general paresis—a brain disorder arising from prior syphilitic infection. Over the last half century grandiose delusions have been decreasing in frequency in patients with schizophrenia.

Delusions of persecution. Delusions of persecution are those in which the individuals believe that a conspiracy exists to harass, cheat, or otherwise injure them. A woman believed that her fellow workers were conspiring to have her fired by a concealed campaign of complaints of her inefficiency and of general personal harassment. She saw evidence of this in her perception that her coffee tasted unpleasant and had therefore been tampered with and that sometimes the company switchboard delayed putting through her phone calls, among other things. Unfortunately, the behavior of individuals with a delusion of persecution may lead them to behave in a manner that provokes other people to respond in ways that ultimately confirm the originally mistaken belief. The initial delusion thus becomes a valid belief. Delusions of persecution are often found in paranoid schizophrenia.

Delusions of jealousy. The patient is dominated by the belief that a spouse or lover is unfaithful in the absence of concrete evidence that this is so. It is difficult to check the validity of such a delusion, as unfaithful spouses are likely to deny the charge.

Erotomanic delusions. The deluded individual is convinced, without evidence, that some other person is in love with him or her. A young woman approached her male supervisor with a corporate purchase order made out with the wording of a marriage certificate and asked him to sign it. She had previously told her friends that she knew that he was in love with her and that they were going to be married. He had had no personal interactions with her at all before this event. Erotomanic delusions may be accompanied by delusions of jealousy. Clinical conditions in which erotomanic delusions predominate are currently known as de Clérambault's syndrome, named for the French psychiatrist Gaetan de Clérambault, who first described erotomania. The syndrome is defined thus: "characterized by the delusional conviction of being in amorous communication with another person, usually of higher rank."

Delusions of reference. The main theme of delusions of reference is that events, objects, and other people in the environment have an unusual significance, often of a kind that is derogatory to the individual. Thus, a man walking down the street stopped at the corner at 11 AM on November 11, the anniversary of the World War I armistice. He noticed that the street number of the nearest house was 11 and concluded that this signified that he had been responsible for World War I.

Classification ambiguities

The specific content of delusions is generally closely related to the cultural and educational background of the patient. Thus, devoutly religious people are likely to have delusions with religious content; patients with a background in science may have delusions involving the activity of cosmic rays; and so on.

For this and other reasons, definitions based on the specific content of the delusion have proved to be of minimal value. They reveal little about the underlying psychological processes that may be involved in creating delusions and are often ambiguous when one attempts to assign them to actual clinical cases. Other approaches to classification have emphasized the experiential processes that are associated with delusion formation rather than the specific content of the delusion itself.

Kurt Schneider, a leading German psychopathologist, preferred to distinguish two fundamental originating processes in the onset of delusions—*i.e.,* delusional perceptions and delusional intuitions. According to Schneider's classification, patients with delusional perceptions attach unusual significance to a real perception but without any cause that is understandable in rational or emotional terms. The perception itself is accurate, but it is interpreted delusionally. Thus,

the man who concluded that he was responsible for World War I had attached delusional significance to his real perception of the house number, the time, and the date. Delusions with different types of content may all arise on the basis of delusional perceptions. Schneider has described delusional perception as one of the prime symptoms of schizophrenia, the other prime symptoms being certain kinds of auditory hallucinations.

Included in Schneider's category of delusional intuitions are sudden ideas (not arising from delusional perceptions and hence not activated by the process of perception) that one has been summoned by God, is loved by somebody else, has special powers, is being persecuted, and so forth. Clearly, many of the delusions in the previous listing, such as delusions of persecution and erotomanic, grandiose, somatic, and other delusions, can be included in this framework.

Delusions and hallucinations. It is important to distinguish between delusions and hallucinations. Hallucinations are defined as "false sensory perception," such as the experience of people who hear voices speaking to them when there is nobody there. Delusions may arise on the basis of hallucinations, in the form of inferences about the origin and purposes of the voices, their relation to the hallucinating individual, and so on. The transition from hallucination to delusion may be relatively continuous and coherent.

Delusions and true but improbable beliefs. In the course of clinical practice most psychopathologists come across instances where a person firmly expresses a belief that seems to be so improbable as to be obviously false but is later found to be true. Personnel at the United States embassy in Moscow who alleged correctly that they were being subjected to microwave transmissions by Soviet intelligence agencies were expressing a belief that closely parallels in content the kind of complaint made by many psychotic patients. In 1973 Martha Mitchell, estranged wife of former U.S. attorney general John M. Mitchell, made headlines with a bizarre series of late-night phone calls to the press as the Watergate scandal was unfolding and alleged that there were nefarious doings at the Nixon White House. Her charges contributed to the conclusion that she was suffering from a psychiatric disorder, but her allegations turned out to be correct. In 1982 the Miami, Fla., police found a destitute elderly lady wandering on the beach. She stated that she was the sister of a former British ambassador, Sir Neville Meyrick Henderson. Improbable and grandiose though that seemed, her claim turned out to be true. All of these instances are reminders that it is unwise to conclude that a belief is false merely because it seems to be prima facie incredible.

That the seeming falsity of a belief does not qualify it as a delusion is confirmed by many instances in history of individuals who firmly believed something that seemed incredible at the time, that was disbelieved by the majority of their fellow citizens, that seemed to fly in the face of the visible evidence, but that turned out to be quite correct. An obvious example is that the world would appear to be flat when viewed from the perspective most people have from their daily, limited outlook; furthermore, it is easily demonstrated that objects that move over the surface of a sphere fall off. These perceptions, however, proved to be invalid when applied to determining the shape of the Earth. Columbus (and others) who sailed west to reach the East demonstrated that what people see with their eyes is misleading and that the Earth is not flat but round, regardless of the majority opinion of their day.

Popularity of implausible beliefs. Most often the beliefs of the majority are realistic. Many popular beliefs may be true even though the kind of evidence used to justify them may be irrelevant. Nonetheless, a glance at contemporary culture, particularly as reflected in the tabloid publications of the variety displayed at most supermarket checkout counters, indicates that a readiness to believe in improbable notions is not rare. Consider the enthusiastic crazes for believing in the Bermuda Triangle, flying saucers and UFOs, Bigfoot, people returned from the dead, and the survival of a doddering Adolf Hitler in the jungles of South America. Such beliefs seem to be widely held in spite of the lack of adequate evidence to support them, but they are generally regarded not as pathological but as wild, superstitious, or simply mistaken.

The origin of delusions

Psychopathologists have offered several different theories to account for the origin of delusions. These theories can be summarized as follows:

Freud and the Schreber case. Sigmund Freud, the "father of psychoanalysis," offered his most extensive discussion of delusions in his description of a case of severe paranoia in a patient, Daniel Paul Schreber. Freud never met Schreber but based his conclusions on his reading of Schreber's book, *Memoirs of My Nervous Illness.* Freud concluded that Schreber suffered at the same time from both schizophrenia and pure paranoia; it was the mechanism of delusion formation in the paranoid condition that attracted Freud's main interest. Some of Schreber's delusions centered on the belief that he was undergoing a bodily change from male to female. Freud concluded that the fundamental cause of Schreber's delusion was his repression of unacceptable homosexual impulses and their projection onto other people. He asserted that attempts to deny unconscious homosexuality could explain several different kinds of delusion. These included the delusion that one is extremely attractive to the opposite sex, with a resulting hyperactive heterosexuality (erotomania), that one is being pursued by active homosexuals (delusion of persecution), Schreber's own somatic

Cathy Melloan

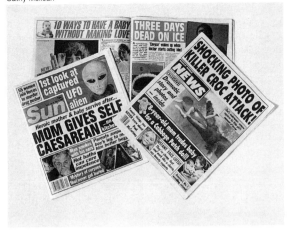

Not all beliefs lacking adequate evidence to support them are delusions. A glance at the headlines of widely circulated tabloids gives a good indication of people's readiness to accept the most implausible kinds of stories.

delusion of bodily change, and so on. Although doubts about bodily structure and personal identity are common in schizophrenia, a substantial body of research has failed to confirm that homosexual impulses have a unique and invariable role in the genesis of psychotic delusions.

Deficient reasoning ability. Because the beliefs expressed by delusional patients seem to be unjustified by the available evidence, many investigators have hypothesized that delusions arise in people who suffer from a fundamental defect in their capacity to reason from evidence. Several studies have compared patients who have delusions with other kinds of patients and with normal persons in tasks involving logical reasoning. No significant differences have yet been found between these groups, and there appears to be no reliable research to support this hypothesis.

Anomalous experience. Delusions are found in such a wide variety of conditions that there are grounds to believe that in many cases (although not all) they may represent a normal human reaction to abnormal experiences or abnormal environments. In such cases the delusional reaction serves the purpose of providing an explanation that reduces the anxiety and perplexity that the anomalous experience creates. Studies of delusional elderly patients, for example, have shown that a significant number of them have undiagnosed hearing loss or undiagnosed visual impairment. As already mentioned, hallucinations can have a role in giving rise to delusions. Many of the neurological disorders in which delusions are sometimes found are disorders in which there are abnormalities of bodily sensation. Otherwise normal individuals who are placed in abnormal environments (*e.g.,* in sensory deprivation chambers) or who endure abnormal experiences (*e.g.,* one who takes a hallucinogenic drug or goes on a hunger strike)

439

sometimes suffer from both hallucinations and delusions. In one study at Stanford University, normal persons were hypnotized and given the suggestion that they suffered from hearing loss. Subsequently these patients showed unusually high scores on the paranoia scale of the Minnesota Multiphasic Personality Inventory—a scale that measures psychopathology. Delusions that arise from these transient conditions generally disappear when the underlying experience is terminated. The gist of this evidence is that anomalies of conscious experience give rise to delusional thinking in a wide range of conditions—strongly suggesting that the presence of delusions in the clinical features exhibited in a patient's condition warrant checking for previous anomalous experiences.

Additionally, there are a significant number of cases of delusions in patients with brain diseases or injuries or where brain malfunction has been induced by repeated abuse of drugs or ingestion of other chemicals. In such cases abnormal experiences may arise directly from the brain pathology.

Transient, crowd-induced "delusions." Historic examples abound of transient false beliefs, or "popular delusions." Because of the frenzied activity that accompanies them, these are sometimes described as "manias." Implausible schemes involving the financial potential of chain letters, investments offering incredible rates of return on small deposits, the fortunes to be made from panning for gold, and so forth appear to influence individuals largely because many other people believe in them. These beliefs, although false, are transient and are abandoned quickly when undeniable evidence of their falsity—often involving substantial financial loss—finally emerges.

Treatment of delusions

In the diagnosis and treatment of delusions, it is first necessary to be sure that the patient's belief meets all of the necessary criteria—*i.e.,* that it is in fact false and is based upon incorrect inference—and that the patient has been presented with incontrovertible evidence of its falsity. While this is generally evident from the content of the belief itself, it is not necessarily so. Careful questioning by the clinician is required at this point. Where the delusion is accompanied by other symptoms of disturbance, such as hallucinations, disorders of motor behavior, and the like, the probability that a stated implausible belief is delusional is high. Where the delusion is not accompanied by clear signs of psychosis, examination of the functioning of the sensory systems is advisable in order to exclude the possibility that sensory impairment is *not* involved.

Clinicians have generally reported that direct attempts to refute delusional beliefs by pointing out the contrary evidence to the patient have little effect. It is not clear, however, that this technique has been tried often or persistently enough to confirm that it is inef-

fective. A few reports have been made claiming that patients who have somatic delusions have abandoned their delusions following pseudosurgery intended to reassure them that the bodily pathology has been cured; this suggests that the provision of counterevidence may be effective in some cases.

Major tranquilizers are widely used in the treatment of schizophrenia and other psychoses; they reliably reduce delusions in a variety of conditions. Medication of this kind is the primary form of treatment. The drugs include the phenothiazines, (chlorpromazine, triflupromazine), the butyrophenones (haloperidol), and the related drug pimozide. Lithium is not generally used with schizophrenic patients but is commonly used with manic patients and reduces the symptoms (including manic delusions) reasonably effectively. However, in the case of major psychoses, the termination of medication is typically followed by a reappearance of the original symptoms of psychosis, including delusions where they were present. Longitudinal studies of delusional psychotic patients indicate that their delusional beliefs remain stable over many years, even though the emotional involvement with the belief may diminish. Where the delusions arise from transient conditions, the termination of the medication does not usually lead to a recurrence of the delusions, provided that the precipitating condition has been eliminated.

Patients whose delusions and other symptoms are controlled by medication can be further helped by being taught to identify the early signs of a recurrence of their delusions. They are then encouraged to seek direct treatment when this happens.

Although interpretive psychotherapy in the form of modified psychoanalytic treatment—group psychodynamic psychotherapy or short-term psychoanalysis—has been tried, no systematic study has reported favorable effects on delusions.

Dealing with another's delusions

Delusions may develop in persons known to abuse drugs, people who report recurring unusual perceptions or other strange conscious experiences, or elderly persons with undiagnosed sensory impairments. The judgment that somebody's stated belief is delusional is complex and should be considered as a possibility only when it is reasonably clear that there is strong evidence against the belief.

Referring delusional persons for professional help may be difficult because they regard their beliefs as true and will be unlikely to see a need for help. The use of deception to induce someone to see a psychotherapist carries with it the risk that this will add elements of persecution to the delusions. In attempting to help someone who appears to be delusional, it is always wise for the concerned layperson to seek consultation with a mental health professional.

Hallucinations
by Manfred Spitzer, M.D., Ph.D.

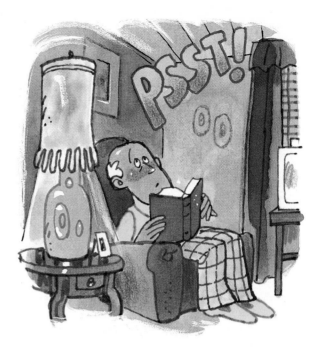

Hallucinations are usually defined as perceptions without object. They are among the most frequent symptoms of mental disorder. Most hallucinations can be classified as visual, "seeing" things ranging from spots and flashes to scenes or other people, or auditory, common in schizophrenia and often consisting of "voices" talking to or about the patient. However, auditory hallucinations may also consist of noises and clicks, and they are not specific to schizophrenia. Less common are hallucinations of smell, taste, or touch.

History

Hallucinations are by no means a modern-day phenomenon; there is ample evidence that people had hallucinations long before they were regarded as a medical problem or termed *hallucinations*. These experiences had great impact on people's lives. Saul, born a Jew around AD 10 in Tarsus, for example, is thought to have suffered from epilepsy. His "visions" on the road to Damascus, resulting in his conversion to Christianity and his becoming the apostle Paul, may actually have been hallucinations during an epileptic seizure. In the 12th century, Hildegard von Bingen (Sibyl of the Rhine) apparently suffered from migraine attacks, accompanied by visions of the Holy Spirit. She was viewed as a visionary mystic and, though never formally canonized, is venerated as a saint. Hallucinations took quite another course throughout Europe from the late Middle Ages to the late 18th century and in colonial America; many schizophrenic women who "heard" or "saw" the devil were burned or hanged as witches rather than treated.

Even without written accounts, it is known that certain native societies of the Western Hemisphere have used plants containing hallucinogenic substances for thousands of years. The Huichol Indians of Mexico use peyote, the cactus that contains mescaline as its active hallucinogenic ingredient and produces visual hallucinations of a distinct kind—certain patterns, textures, and shapes. These patterns have been reproduced in carpets and on pottery made by the Huichol.

The term *hallucination*—whose original meaning was "to wander in mind"—was used as early as 1600. Then in 1838 the French psychiatrist Jean-Étienne-Dominique Esquirol attached a more specific meaning. He defined hallucinations as perceptions without an object, and differentiated them from illusions, the latter being deceptions that occur when some object is really there (*e.g.*, in a dark forest one sees a "ghost," which turns out to be a white tree trunk). Being equipped with an appropriate concept enabled investigators to explore more deeply the phenomena in question.

Theories

Symptoms of mental disorder, and especially hallucinations, have long influenced the theories of philosophers and psychologists. Descartes, for example, asked whether one can really know anything, because it might well be that everything is merely hallucinated.

The two famous psychoanalytic models of the mind—the "structural" model, consisting of the unconscious, preconscious, and conscious, and the "dynamic" model, with the interacting id, ego, and superego—are based on Sigmund Freud's studies of hallucinations. The first model was established to explain why dreams are as alike as they are (Freud equated the visual phenomena that occur in dreams with hallucinations). With the second model Freud tried to account for the voices schizophrenic patients hear.

But theories about the mind have also influenced understanding of hallucinations. Just as there is no single, unifying theory of the mind, there are many competing theories about hallucinations. The most influential model of the mind holds that it consists of "faculties" such as perception, thought, affect, and so forth. Hallucinations are often considered and sometimes loosely called "false perceptions." Hallucinations are not, however, a concrete entity but, like "delusions" and "thought disorders," a concept that is useful for psychiatrists to discriminate aspects of patients' experiences. This is not unlike the concepts of "hue," "saturation," and "brightness," which are useful for artists to communicate about colors.

441

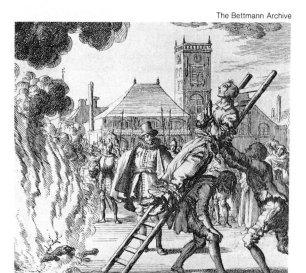

In medieval Europe women who hallucinated were often thought to be possessed by the devil. Probably they suffered from the mental disorder schizophrenia, but they were burned at the stake as witches rather than treated.

Hallucinations in "normal people"

Some researchers have claimed that as many as 70% of a sample of college students who had been asked to fill out a questionnaire reported having had non-drug-induced hallucinations. Other researchers say that, by definition, "normal people" never hallucinate because hallucinations are always a sign of mental or physical disorder. This striking difference in the opinion of experts can be explained by the fact that the investigators had very different phenomena in mind. Some of them were willing to count positive answers to questions like "Have you ever gone to the door because you thought the bell was ringing, but it turned out that nobody was there?" as plain evidence for the presence of hallucinations. Others are more restrictive and call only instances of severely disturbed perceptual experiences hallucinations.

The question whether hallucinations occur under conditions of sensory deprivation also depends on the strictness of the concept applied. For example, those who have spent a couple of hours in the dark, such as during a power outage or in an experimental setting, may report, "I saw some very vivid images." But should such experiences be counted as hallucinations without further questions about what the subjects thought about those images or how they behaved while seeing them? When a strict criterion is applied, hallucinations are not as frequent as has been thought under conditions of sensory deprivation.

There are more myths than facts about hallucinations in children. Freud postulated that children hallucinate the objects of their wishes, thereby getting

easy satisfaction—a claim for which there is no empirical support. Today child psychiatrists are careful to use the term *hallucinations* only in cases of severe disturbance. It is generally agreed that it does not make sense to ascribe hallucinations to children younger than three years of age, who may not be able to distinguish between fantasy and reality. Young children who spend a lot of time alone sometimes have imaginary companions. The child easily distinguishes these imaginary friends from real ones, and most clinicians agree that there is nothing abnormal about such fantasy friends. Hypnagogic and hypnopompic hallucinations (*i.e.,* hallucinations that occur while falling asleep and waking up, respectively—and considered normal) are also common in childhood and have to be distinguished from pathological hallucinations.

Hallucinations in mental disorders

In the realm of mental disorders, there are differences among hallucinations that—taken together with other symptoms—have diagnostic significance. The "voices" that are heard by schizophrenics tend to talk with one another or to make comments about what the patient is doing or thinking. The patients have no control over the voices, and the content is mostly unpleasant. In addition, the content of the "voices" heard by schizophrenics is highly idiosyncratic and varies from person to person as well as with time and culture. A study in Colombia found that modernizations in the early 1960s had a distinct effect on the content of the hallucinations of schizophrenic patients. Cases from 1956–59 were compared with cases from 1964–66. Whereas mainly supernatural elements (spirits, ghosts, etc.) had been the content of hallucinations in the earlier period, elements of "modern reality" (radio waves, X-rays, etc.) replaced them in the later period.

The frequency and type of hallucinations of persons with schizophrenia vary from study to study. Auditory hallucinations have been reported in 50–80%, visual hallucinations in 10–30%, and hallucinations of smell (olfactory hallucinations) and of taste (gustatory hallucinations) each in about 2–15% of patients. Tactile hallucinations and experiences of strange bodily sensations have been reported in 35–70%.

Most clinicians agree that hallucinations may occur in the major affective disorders—particularly depression and bipolar disorder (manic-depressive psychosis)—but only about 10% of patients experience them. These hallucinations tend to reflect the disturbed mood of the patient; they may involve themes of guilt, poverty, and suffering in depressed patients and themes of grandiosity or wealth in manic patients.

In organic mental disorders, two conditions in which hallucinations occur have to be distinguished: delirium and hallucinosis. The delirious patient suffers from clouded consciousness and is unable to distinguish hallucinations from reality. As a result of such "impaired reality testing," a delirious patient may sit on a hallucinated chair (and fall), may talk to hallucinated people, or may stamp on hallucinated bugs.

In contrast, organic hallucinosis is characterized by the presence of hallucinations (as the only or the most prominent symptom) in a state of clear consciousness. The patients may or may not believe in the reality of the hallucinations, which are to some extent determined by the cause of the disorder. In alcoholic hallucinosis, which generally occurs within 48 hours of cessation of alcohol ingestion, the hallucinations—typically auditory—are often threatening and insulting. "Voices" may address the person directly, but usually they discuss him or her in the third person. The condition is dangerous, as the patients may try to defend themselves against intruders or even may want to escape their enemies by killing themselves.

Tactile hallucinations such as bugs crawling on the skin are a characteristic of cocaine-induced hallucinosis. Olfactory hallucinations may occur in temporal lobe epilepsy—a form of epilepsy that is usually considered a psychiatric disorder.

Hallucinogenic drugs

The quality of psychedelic-induced hallucinations is different from that of the hallucinations of patients with schizophrenia; hallucinogenic drugs tend to produce peculiar, colorful patterns and shapes (constant forms) that are further "elaborated" by the mind into all sorts of visual images, from bizarre landscapes to monsters. In small doses these drugs generally cause visual disturbances only of what is really seen (*e.g.,* enhanced and false colors, colored edges, distortions, and movement of objects). With increasing drug doses occur "real" hallucinations; *i.e.,* perceptions of things that are not there. Drug users normally know that they are hallucinating as a result of the drug taken and that the effect will disappear when the drug wears off. Hence they do not experience the kind of anxiety that often accompanies the hallucinations of patients with schizophrenia, especially at the onset of the disorder when they are experiencing the first psychotic episode.

Hallucinations in nonpsychiatric illnesses

Hallucinations are a common feature of migraine; these visual disturbances range from simple blurred vision, which is experienced by almost all patients, to a very characteristic zigzag pattern wandering from the center of the visual field to the periphery over a period of about 20 minutes. This very bright spectacle, experienced by about 40% of all migraine patients during the "aura" that precedes the headache, usually causes a temporary loss of half of the visual field (scotoma).

During recovery from open-heart surgery, patients frequently experience hallucinations as a result of microembolias in the brain. Tiny blood clots that formed during or shortly after the operation, because of alter-

National Migraine Art Competition, British Migraine Association and WB Pharmaceuticals Ltd.

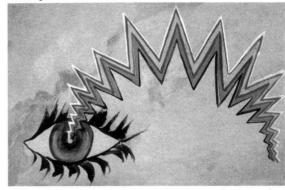

Migraine sufferers commonly experience hallucinations during the aura that precedes their headache. This painting by a migraine patient depicts a typical hallucinated image: bright zigzags of light flashing across half the visual field.

ations of the normally very smooth interior of the heart and blood vessels, are transported with the blood flow into the brain, where they get stuck in small blood vessels (microembolia), causing some neurons to die. While these events may be too small to cause impairment of any major function of the central nervous system, the dying neurons "fire" in unusual patterns, thus giving rise to experiences of hallucinations.

Treatment in an iron lung, which was common with poliomyelitis, sometimes resulted in hallucinations. This may have occurred as a result of sensory deprivation.

Fever, hormonal imbalances, vitamin B_{12} deficiency, loss of hearing or sight, or loss of an arm or leg may also cause hallucinations. Hallucinations have been reported as well with brain tumors, before an epileptic seizure, after a stroke, and shortly before death.

Hallucinations may occur as a side effect of certain drugs taken for therapeutic purposes, such as antiparkinsonian drugs (relatively frequently) and antidepressants (sometimes). Other drugs only rarely cause hallucinations, but this side effect has been reported with quinidine, cimetidine, cyclosporine, digoxin, furosemide, nalorphine, penicillin, pentazocine, primidone, propranolol, and a quite a few other prescribed medications.

The biology of hallucinations

As hallucinations are not a single entity but rather a spectrum of very different phenomena, a single physiological cause can hardly be expected. Indeed, what is known about the biology of hallucinations varies from "literally nothing" to "a great deal," depending on the phenomena in question.

Little, for instance, is known about the origin of the "voices" of schizophrenics. However, the bright zigzag lines and other visual phenomena in migraine and the patterns and shapes seen by psychedelic drug takers are phenomena whose causes are quite well understood; although there is a subjective element in what

Hallucinations

is actually "seen," these two phenomena are due to direct stimulation of certain groups of cells in the visual cortex (the outer layer of a rear part of the brain) that are normally responsible for seeing visual patterns.

The hallucinations of a patient with delirium due to alcohol withdrawal are of a different nature. There is evidence that dream sleep (or REM sleep, as it is called, because of the rapid eye movements that occur) is essential for human beings; the suppression of REM sleep leads to a pressure toward such a brain state. Alcohol has a suppressant effect on REM sleep, and electroencephalogram studies have found that the same brain waves that occur in REM sleep are present in hallucinating alcoholic patients; it is likely that the hallucinations experienced represent some form of dream state while being awake. The hallucinations that occur in narcolepsy—in which there are recurrent brief episodes of daytime REM sleep—can also be explained in terms of REM episodes intruding into waking life.

There is evidence that at least three different neurotransmitters are involved in hallucinations: dopamine, serotonin, and acetylcholine. Dopaminergic substances that are given for the treatment of Parkinson's disease frequently cause hallucinations, and drugs that block dopaminergic pathways also alleviate hallucinations. LSD (d-lysergic acid diethylamide) is structurally related to serotonin and blocks central receptors for that transmitter, as anticholinergic substances like atropine block cholinergic transmissions. At present, however, the exact role of neurotransmitters is far from well understood.

Other biological explanations for hallucinations— e.g., the theory of hallucinations as "output without adequate input" and the theory that hallucinations are a disturbance in the balance of the two hemispheres of the brain—are far too general to lead to testable, empirical hypotheses. This is also true of the "perceptual release" theory, which proposes that the normal waking brain is under constant bombardment by information from the outside world as well as from within the body, but if this input is significantly inhibited (such as in sensory deprivation or as a result of damage to a sense organ), perceptual memories are activated or "released." These released memories are said to take the form of hallucinations.

Individual reactions and coping strategies

To a great extent the circumstances in which one hallucinates determine the reaction to the experience. LSD-abusing persons at least know that they took the drug, while schizophrenics are terrified by experiences they may never have had before. If a person is given a hallucinogenic drug without knowing it, the effect of hallucinations can be so unsettling as to be disastrous.

The reaction of the person who experiences hallucinations can also depend on cultural background.

This can be shown, for instance, by giving subjects the same dose of a hallucinogenic drug (assuming that this will lead to somewhat similar biological changes) and observing the differences in behavior. Members of cultures where it is natural to believe in "spirits" may react calmly; to most people in contemporary Western civilization, however, uncontrolled perceptual experiences are likely to produce anxiety and emotional instability—reactions that exacerbate the experience.

Some people react to hallucinations by wanting to be in a dark or quiet environment; others are most comfortable in a crowded marketplace; some talk back to their voices; others seek conversation with another person. Usually the most a therapist can do is encourage patients to "experiment" to find out what works best to quell their hallucinations.

Treatment

There is no specific antipsychotic drug that has proved to be particularly helpful in the treatment of the hallucinations of schizophrenic patients. It is known, however, that these drugs (called neuroleptics) work better in cases of acute onset of hallucinations, compared with cases where hallucinations have lasted for months or years. In fact, some chronic patients prefer to cope with the voices rather than take the drugs, which can have significant side effects. An appropriate solution must be worked out in close supervision with a skilled psychiatrist.

In patients with organic brain disorders, the actual cause of hallucinations can vary from a worsening of the condition (e.g., the growth of a brain tumor) to an improvement (e.g., in some cases after a stroke, some parts of the damaged tissue in the visual cortex recover, temporarily inducing hallucinations). Treatment, therefore, varies considerably—from surgery to steroids (to relieve effects of a tumor pressing on surrounding tissue) to antipsychotic drugs or mere reassurance of the patient.

In many elderly patients who have to take a number of drugs for several ailments, hallucinations are caused as a side effect of one drug or interacting medications. Depending on the circumstances, the drug or drugs in question should be discontinued or replaced by another drug or the dosage lowered. If none of these options is possible, there are still things that can be done. Hallucinations tend to occur during the nighttime in these cases, and a mild sleeping pill might keep the patient asleep and prevent hallucinations.

The person who has taken LSD or another psychedelic drug and goes to a hospital emergency room for medical help may just need reassurance that hallucinations will abate and will usually not last for more than one or two days. Minor tranquilizers may help, and sometimes neuroleptics are given, especially if the patient is extremely agitated or in a panic.

Eating for Two
by Myron Winick, M.D.

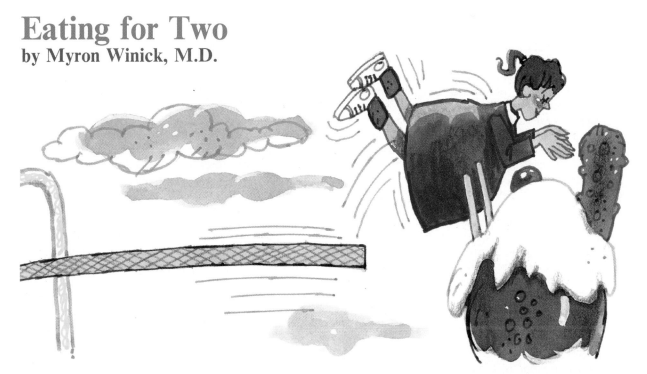

Pregnancy is a natural process that is perhaps the most important biological event in the entire mammalian kingdom. It is certainly the most significant biological event in the lives of those women who experience it. Good nutrition plays an important role both before and during pregnancy, preparing and sustaining a smooth course and ensuring the best chance of a successful outcome for mother and baby. While many of the guidelines followed today seem to be natural, commonsense practices, ideas about diet and pregnancy have evolved considerably over the past 100 years, and the thinking about nutrition during—and before—pregnancy has changed radically.

Historical background

At the end of the 19th century, obstetrics was just emerging as a separate medical specialty. The incidence of maternal death during childbirth was high, and the prime responsibility of the physician was to safeguard the mother's life. One important factor in determining whether the mother would survive labor and delivery was the size of the infant; the bigger the baby, the greater the maternal risk. Although no comprehensive studies were undertaken to test the validity of this observation, physicians began to notice that by restricting the amount of weight a woman gained during pregnancy, they could reduce the average size of the babies they were delivering. Thus, standard obstetrical practice for the first 30 or 40 years of the 20th century was to limit weight gain to 4.5–7 kg (1 kg = 2.2 lb) per pregnancy by placing the prospective mother on a strict calorie-restricted diet.

During the first third of the century, medicine in general and obstetrics in particular underwent dramatic changes. The rate of death in childbirth dropped to very low levels, and maternal mortality was no longer a major danger to the woman receiving good obstetrical care. And yet the practice of restricting weight gain during pregnancy persisted. The rationale often put forth was that limiting weight gain would lower the incidence of toxemia, a serious complication marked by high blood pressure, fluid retention, and sometimes convulsions. It was also believed that women who gained less weight during pregnancy would be less likely to be obese afterward. There are no scientific data to support either of these assumptions.

A wartime lesson: peril of low birth weight

In the 1940s physicians shifted their attention from the health and safety of the mother to the size and survival of the fetus. Data from around the world were demonstrating that if birth weight fell below 2,500 g (5½ lb), infant mortality increased. The time had come to examine in more detail the relation of maternal diet to birth weight. In the winter of 1945 a tragic historical event made such a study possible. The Dutch, expecting an imminent Allied invasion, called a transportation strike. The invasion, however, did not come for nine months, and the Germans retaliated by placing an embargo on all trains to the western part of The Netherlands. In cities such as Rotterdam, caloric intake dropped to 800–1,000 cal per day or less. The Dutch kept meticulous hospital records, and it was later possible to examine the effects of the famine

445

on birth weight and placental weight. Average birth weight dropped about 300 g (¾ of a pound). Subsequent studies confirmed these findings and further demonstrated that in undernourished populations food supplementation will increase birth weight.

The data from the Dutch experience revealed an even more startling fact. While the average mother lost about 2% of her weight during the famine, the fetus lost about 10% of its weight. Thus, the mother seemed to be actively protecting herself at the expense of fetal growth. Although on the surface this observation may seem to contradict basic principles of evolution, it really does not. Pregnancy is a time when the mother's body is not only nurturing the fetus but also preparing for lactation. Part of the body's preparation for lactation involves depositing fat in order to build an energy reserve for the production and delivery of milk. When food is scarce during pregnancy, it is also likely to be scarce during lactation. And it is during lactation that the mother's fat reserve is crucial to the infant's survival. Thus, a woman's body will continue to deposit fat during pregnancy for use during lactation even at the expense of fetal growth.

Recent studies have defined the mechanism by which maternal food restriction reduces fetal growth. Normally, during pregnancy a woman's circulatory system adapts to be able to increase the blood supply to the uterus and the placenta. The volume of blood circulating through her system increases by about 40%, and the blood flow to the uterus and placenta increases even more. If food is scarce, this adaptation is not complete, and the amount of blood perfusing the placenta is reduced. This reduction in placental circulation affects both the growth of the placenta and the quantity of nutrients being passed to the fetus. The result is slower fetal growth and, ultimately, a reduction in birth weight.

Weight gain: how much?

How much weight should the average woman gain during pregnancy to maximize her chance of delivering a normal-sized infant? When allowed to eat as much as they wish, most women will gain between 11 and 13.5 kg during pregnancy. The weight of the fetus, placenta, and amniotic fluid, plus the weight of the increased maternal tissues (uterus, breasts) and expanded maternal blood volume, is calculated to be between eight and nine kilograms. In addition, 2 to 4.5 kg are deposited as fat for use during lactation. In studies that examine the weight gain of a large number of women and correlate this weight gain with birth weight, it has been found that between 11 and 13.5 kilograms is the minimum necessary to deliver an optimal-sized infant. Below this weight gain, infants are smaller, whereas above it, infants do not become larger. On the basis of these data, about 15 years ago the American College of Obstetrics and Gynecology

recommended that the average woman gain 11–13.5 kg during pregnancy.

This recommendation has been refined in recent years to take into account individual differences, including differences in nutritional status before pregnancy. Presently, most physicians believe that women who are either of normal weight or underweight prior to pregnancy should reach 120% of their ideal prepregnancy weight at term. Thus, a woman who should weigh 45 kg and who does weigh 45 kg prior to pregnancy, needs to gain only 9 kg during the pregnancy. By the same reasoning, a normal-weight woman of 68 kg needs to gain 3.5 kg during pregnancy. However, if a woman's ideal prepregnancy weight is 68 kg, but she weighs only 63.5 kg, she needs to gain 18 kg during pregnancy to have the best chance of delivering an optimal-sized infant. Thus, any deficit in weight prior to pregnancy must be made up *during* pregnancy. Obese women, on the other hand, cannot lose weight during pregnancy without compromising fetal growth. The best available data suggest that even women who are 10% or more above their ideal weight should gain seven kilograms during pregnancy. Thus, if possible, it is desirable for underweight women to gain some weight and for overweight women to lose some weight *before* becoming pregnant.

Caloric needs

What modifications must a pregnant woman make in her diet in order to achieve the weight gain necessary to ensure adequate growth of the fetus? How many extra calories must she consume each day to reach the desired weight? The total number of extra calories necessary to account for the weight of the fetus and placenta, the increased size of the uterus and breasts, and the amount of fat that will accumulate, as well as the extra work involved in carrying a pregnancy to term, equals about 80,000 extra calories during the course of pregnancy; this works out to 250–300 extra calories per day. Studies show that when pregnant women are allowed to follow the dictates of their appetites, they consume about 250–300 extra calories daily. Apparently, nature provides for the caloric needs of pregnancy by increasing the woman's appetite just enough to fill those needs. Moreover, the extra caloric intake need not be consumed on a daily or even weekly basis. Typically, if fewer extra calories are consumed early in pregnancy, more will be consumed later to compensate. If extra calories are consumed early, usually fewer will be consumed later.

In other words, the body seems to be able to regulate its caloric intake over the entire course of pregnancy. Thus, women who suffer from so-called morning, or pregnancy, sickness (nausea and vomiting) early in pregnancy will compensate for their low caloric intake later on. Only very severe nausea and vomiting, which is a rare occurrence, need specific medical intervention. The expectant mother should be reassured by the knowledge that if too few calories are consumed at this early stage, the body will compensate later, and the health of the baby will not suffer.

Nutrient needs

The pregnant woman's modest increase in caloric requirement is accompanied by an increased need for most nutrients. In most cases the size of this increase is proportional to the rise in caloric requirement. In the case of certain nutrients, however, the requirement increases far more than the 10–15% increase in caloric intake. For these nutrients to be adequate, special attention must be paid to the quality of the diet, and in some cases routine supplementation may be desirable. The four most important nutrients in this regard are iron, zinc, calcium, and folic acid.

Iron. During pregnancy a woman's iron requirement more than triples. The reason is that the prospective mother's blood volume expands, and more iron-containing red blood cells must be made to occupy this expanded blood volume. In addition, the growing fetus is making an entirely new blood supply of its own, and the iron necessary for this process comes from the mother. Iron deficiency is the most common nutrient deficiency among U.S. women who are not pregnant, and many women, therefore, begin pregnancy with their iron stores already depleted. Because of this widespread deficiency, doctors routinely advise all pregnant women to supplement their diets with 30–60 mg per day of iron. However, even though a woman is taking a supplement, it is prudent for her to consume a diet that is as rich in iron as possible.

Foods rich in iron include lean red meats, dark meat of fowl, liver and other organ meats, leafy green vegetables, iron-fortified cereals, dried beans, and dried fruits such as prunes, raisins, and apricots.

Zinc. Zinc is a mineral that is required for any cell within the body to divide. During pregnancy the rate of cell division increases in certain maternal tissues and in all fetal tissues. Therefore, a woman's normal zinc requirement increases by about 35%, from 15 to 20 mg. In animals severe zinc deficiency during pregnancy results in congenital malformations in the offspring. Zinc deficiency has also been associated with birth defects in humans. Adequate amounts of zinc are usually obtainable through the diet.

Foods rich in zinc include red meats, dark meat of fowl, liver, shellfish, cheese, whole-grain cereals, leafy green vegetables, dried beans, cocoa, and nuts.

Calcium. Calcium is a very important nutrient during pregnancy. The fetus should deposit about 30 g of calcium into its developing skeletal system. In order for this to occur without draining calcium from the mother's bones, she must consume adequate amounts of calcium. At present the Food and Nutrition Board of the U.S. National Academy of Sciences recommends a dietary intake of 1,200 mg or more per day during pregnancy. This is a 400-mg, or 50%, increase over the 800 mg required by nonpregnant women. Many health professionals feel that 1,500 mg per day should be recommended during pregnancy. In order to ensure that adequate amounts of this crucial nutrient are available to meet fetal demands, nature has provided a mechanism whereby the pregnant woman can absorb more calcium than the nonpregnant woman. Therefore, most pregnant women should be able to get the 1,200–1,500 mg of calcium they need from their daily food supply. However, since most of the calcium in the U.S. diet comes from dairy foods, pregnant women must concentrate on getting enough milk (low fat) and cheese or products made with these foods. Women who have an intolerance to lactose (milk sugar) can often substitute low-lactose milk products and yogurt. If this strategy does not work, then a calcium-supplemented food or calcium tablets may be advised.

Foods rich in calcium include milk, yogurt, hard cheese, cottage cheese, sardines (with bones), oysters, salmon (canned, with bones), kale, spinach, greens (mustard, turnip, collard), and tofu.

Folic acid. Folic acid, a B-complex vitamin, seems to be particularly important during pregnancy. The requirement for this vitamin doubles during pregnancy, from 400 to 800 micrograms per day. The increase is necessary because folic acid, like zinc, is essential for cell division. In animals folic acid deficiency produces congenital malformations in the offspring. Recent studies in human populations suggest that folic acid deficiency may be related to a specific group of malformations—the neural tube defects (NTDs). In one study, providing a folic acid supplement to women with a history of giving birth to a child with an NTD completely prevented any recurrence; there were recurrences in about 5% of women not taking such a supplement. The supplement was given for one month *before* conception and throughout the entire pregnancy. Taking a multivitamin containing folic acid both before and during pregnancy has also been shown to prevent recurrence of NTDs. Thus, today any woman who has given birth to a child with a neural tube defect should seek medical advice before trying to become pregnant again. The health professional will advise her to begin taking a multivitamin containing folic acid at least one month before trying to conceive. (Most NTDs probably occur very early in embryonic development, often before a woman knows she is pregnant.)

Foods rich in folic acid include liver, spinach and other dark-green leafy vegetables, broccoli, asparagus, peanuts, and wheat germ.

Preparing for pregnancy: crucial considerations

While it is mandatory that all women who have had complications in a previous pregnancy seek medical advice before becoming pregnant again, it is probably prudent for all women to do so, in order that proper preparation for pregnancy can be instituted for those who need it. Such preparation would include an evaluation of the woman's nutritional status and dietary practices, the development of a plan for losing or gaining weight if she is significantly over- or underweight prior to pregnancy, and the addition to her diet of a multivitamin-iron supplement, again started *before* pregnancy.

No matter how ideal or carefully calculated her diet, a woman cannot ensure delivery of a healthy baby if she does not concern herself with other than strictly dietary habits. The use of substances such as alcohol, tobacco, and drugs should also be discontinued *before* pregnancy begins. Alcohol ingestion has been linked to specific birth defects known as the fetal alcohol syndrome. Although most common among heavy alcohol users, it has been reported in moderate drinkers and even among women who drink only occasionally. Because even small amounts of alcohol can apparently be harmful, complete abstinence is best, ideally even *before* a woman tries to become pregnant.

Cigarette smoking impedes fetal growth and, therefore, results in a lowering of birth weight. Smoking causes repeated constriction of maternal blood vessels, thereby limiting the amount of maternal blood reaching the placenta. These interruptions in the maternal blood supply reduce nutrient availability to the fetus, which in turn results in retarded fetal growth. Further, the effects of smoking are additive. The more cigarettes a woman smokes, the greater the effect on the fetus. The longer she smokes during pregnancy (*i.e.,* for one or two months or for nine), the greater the effect. Thus, cutting down on the number of cigarettes and the duration of smoking both reduce the degree of fetal growth retardation. Of course, complete cessation of smoking even *before* pregnancy begins is best.

Illicit drugs as well as certain prescribed and over-the-counter drugs are harmful to the fetus. All of these should be discontinued *before* pregnancy. If a drug is necessary for the mother's health, it should be used only under strict medical supervision. In addition, some substances that are often ingested with food may not be healthy when consumed in large amounts during pregnancy. Caffeine probably falls into this category. Animal studies have shown that large amounts of coffee or caffeine can retard fetal growth and alter the behavior of the young after birth. Presently, the recommendation is that a pregnant woman drink no more than two to three cups of coffee per day and only an occasional caffeinated soft drink.

Special diets and megadose vitamins

One question that has been arising with increasing frequency as people become more and more nutrition conscious is whether any particular diet (*i.e.,* low fat, low salt, high fiber, vegetarian) is desirable during pregnancy. The answer varies, of course, with the diet in question. The recommended low-fat, low-cholesterol diet, as outlined by the 1988 Surgeon General's Report, the National Academy of Sciences' Committee on Diet and Health, and the American Heart Association, is really not low in either of these substances—it is simply comparatively low in relation to the amounts usually consumed by most people in the U.S. Thus, limiting the amount of calories derived from fat to 30% of total calories and limiting cholesterol to 300 mg per day is not only safe but desirable for pregnant women. Increasing fiber intake to between 20 and 30 g per day is also desirable, particularly during later pregnancy, when constipation can be a problem. A vegetarian diet, even if completely devoid of all animal-derived foods, is acceptable but should be supervised by a nutritionist. Such diets can be low in protein, iron, zinc, vitamin B_{12}, and calcium if the proper foods are not chosen. More restrictive regimens like Zen macrobiotic diets or liquid protein diets should not be followed during pregnancy. Finally, sodium-restricted diets are all right if too much sodium is being consumed—that is, if salt is being added to foods in cooking and at the table. However, overzealous sodium restriction (less than 500 mg per day) during pregnancy is not desirable. Thus, the best advice on sodium is moderation.

An unfortunate recent nutritional trend is the use of certain nutrients in very high doses (megadoses). While there is no evidence of any health benefit for anyone taking megadoses of vitamins or minerals, there is strong evidence that some of these nutrients, when consumed in very high doses, are toxic. Both vitamins A and D, when taken in large doses (3 to 10 times the recommended dietary allowance, or RDA), have been shown to be associated with severe congenital malformations. Any woman who is taking megadoses of vitamin A or D for treatment of a medical problem should consult her physician and tell the physician of her desire to become pregnant so that a plan for discontinuing these large doses can be established *before* conception. There is also some evidence that a pregnant woman's consuming large doses of vitamin C may induce a dependence on larger than normal doses of vitamin C in her offspring, which can persist into infancy. Thus, any woman regularly taking megadoses of vitamin C (500 mg per day or more) should gradually reduce her intake (over several weeks) *before* becoming pregnant. If she does become pregnant while taking large doses of vitamin C, it is not a cause for alarm, however, but both her obstetrician and pediatrician should be informed.

The simple nutritional guidelines outlined above are easy to follow and could prevent problems later on. For the prospective mother, good nutrition should start as soon as she decides to have a baby; for the infant, at the moment of conception.

Heart Murmurs
by Marc K. Effron, M.D.

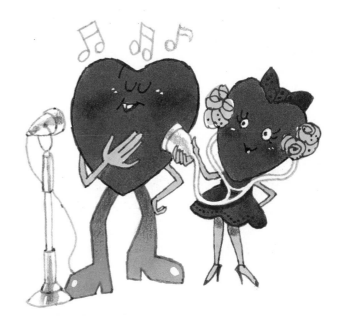

A heart murmur is an abnormal sound beyond the heart's normal "lub-dub." It is usually a prolonged sound produced by turbulent blood flow. As blood in the heart is forced through a narrowed orifice or leaks back across a malfunctioning valve, a sustained murmur is created. A murmur may have a blowing, vibratory course or a musical quality, depending upon the velocity and direction of flow inside the heart.

The physician detects a heart murmur by listening to the heart (auscultation) with a stethoscope, either as part of a screening or routine physical examination or in evaluation of a symptom suggesting heart disease, such as shortness of breath, chest pain, or fainting spells. A murmur is a physical finding that may lead to a diagnosis of heart disease. It is not a symptom; an individual with a heart murmur does not feel the abnormal flow through the heart.

Murmurs are frequently detected in children and in pregnant women. Most of these murmurs represent healthy blood flow and become less audible as a child reaches adolescence or when a pregnancy is completed. Murmurs become somewhat more common in the elderly as well. Calcium deposits on worn cardiac valves after the age of 70 produce turbulent flow and a corresponding murmur, which is usually not serious.

Pathological murmurs, reflecting serious conditions requiring treatment or close follow-up, can occur in all age groups. Congenital defects, inflammatory distortion of the heart valves, bacterial infection of the heart, and advanced degeneration (wear and tear) of the valves may all cause such murmurs.

In 1816 the French physician Réné Laënnec devised the first stethoscope in order to listen to heart sounds without having to apply his ear directly to the patient's chest. He used a sheaf of papers rolled into a tight cylinder; by placing one end on the patient's chest and his ear to the other end, he was able to hear the sounds clearly. Subsequently he devised a 30.5-cm (one-foot)-long durable tube to transmit heart sounds. Cardiac auscultation blossomed in the decades that followed as Joseph Skoda, a Viennese physician, and others correlated the sounds and murmurs of the heart with anatomic findings. Cardiac auscultation remains a focal point of cardiology practice today. Appropriate interpretation of a heart murmur enables the physician to either reassure a healthy patient or choose the most expeditious, noninvasive test to provide a prognosis and guide treatment.

Identifying murmurs

Heart murmurs are characterized by their location on the chest wall (see Figure), intensity, timing in the cycle of the heartbeat, and quality of sound. The range of murmurs includes those originating from the aortic valve, best heard at the upper right border of the sternum; murmurs involving the pulmonary valve, heard at the upper left sternal border; tricuspid valve murmurs heard at the lower left sternal border; and mitral valve murmurs heard at the lower pointed end of the heart on the left side (cardiac apex).

Murmur intensity is determined by the velocity of blood flow, the distance from the stethoscope, and the type of tissue between the site of origin and the surface of the chest. Murmurs can be louder in children and adults with thin chest walls. Murmurs are muffled by the presence of fluid around the heart (pericardial effusion) or in the chest cavity (pleural effusion), produced by inflammation or malignancy. Obesity and overinflation of the lungs in patients with emphysema also dampen murmurs. Murmurs are commonly graded on a scale of I to VI, grade I denoting a barely detectable murmur and grade VI denoting an extremely loud murmur that is audible even without a stethoscope.

The timing of a heart murmur in the cycle of the heartbeat is a major identifying feature. The cardiac cycle is the rhythmic sequence of the heart's chambers contracting and filling, heart valves opening and closing. The first and second heart sounds are brief and distinct sounds that outline the systolic (contracting) and diastolic (filling) phases of the cycle. The first heart sound correlates with the closure of the mitral and tricuspid valves; the aortic and pulmonary valves

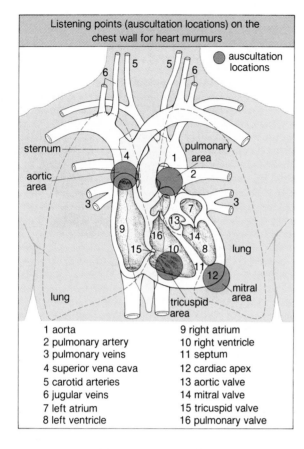

Listening points (auscultation locations) on the chest wall for heart murmurs

● auscultation locations

sternum

aortic area

pulmonary area

lung

tricuspid area

mitral area

lung

1 aorta	9 right atrium
2 pulmonary artery	10 right ventricle
3 pulmonary veins	11 septum
4 superior vena cava	12 cardiac apex
5 carotid arteries	13 aortic valve
6 jugular veins	14 mitral valve
7 left atrium	15 tricuspid valve
8 left ventricle	16 pulmonary valve

then open, and blood is ejected from the ventricles into the aorta and pulmonary artery during systole. The second heart sound correlates with closure of the aortic and pulmonary valves at the end of systole. The mitral and tricuspid valves then open and, during diastole, blood from the atria fills the ventricles. Diastole ends with the next first heart sound.

Murmurs are usually either systolic or diastolic. Some patients have separate murmurs in both systole and diastole. In rare cases a murmur is continuous, spanning both the systolic and diastolic phases of the cardiac cycle.

Auscultation of a pathological murmur may be only a first step in the cardiac evaluation. An electrocardiogram and chest X-ray may be performed. The echocardiogram uses ultrasound waves that bounce off structures in the heart's interior in definable patterns to create an image of the chambers and valves of the heart. The more sensitive Doppler echocardiography records the turbulent and high-velocity flow across obstructed valves; it also maps in color the back-and-forth flow of blood from valves that fail to close properly. These noninvasive techniques may be used serially, along with auscultation, to follow the course of a valvular heart problem. Cardiac catheterization and angiography, invasive methods that accurately assess heart anatomy and function, are usually reserved for

evaluation before surgery. The nature and extent of the special tests performed are ultimately determined by the physician's interpretation of the heart murmur.

Systolic ejection murmurs

Systolic ejection murmurs are generated by forward blood flow in systole at or adjacent to the aortic and pulmonary valves. This kind of heart murmur starts with the first heart sound and ends clearly before the second heart sound. Their intensity increases and decreases in a crescendo-decrescendo pattern during each systole.

Fortunately, in a majority of cases, individuals with a systolic ejection murmur have no structural abnormalities of the heart, and their murmur must be considered a variant of normal. These benign murmurs, most often detected in children and young women, are called *innocent* (or *functional*) *murmurs.* Such murmurs are typically heard best at the mid- and lower left sternal border, and they have a mixed frequency or vibratory quality. They may appear or become louder during pregnancy, upon exercising, with a fever, or if the individual is anemic. An innocent murmur detected by the pediatrician in a young girl during a routine checkup may disappear by adolescence but then be observed later by an obstetrician at the time of a prenatal exam. Innocent murmurs probably are generated from blood flow out of the right ventricle and into the pulmonary artery. Familiarity with the characteristics of these murmurs enables the examining physician to identify a benign physical finding and to avoid inappropriate diagnosis of valvular heart disease.

As individuals surpass age 50, there is an increasing incidence of systolic ejection murmurs arising from the aortic valve. These murmurs are most often attributable to *aortic sclerosis,* scarring of the three cusps (flaps) of the valve. Degenerative scarring and deposits of calcium cause a turbulent blood flow without significant valvular narrowing. Such murmurs are usually only grade I or II in intensity and are heard at the upper right sternal border.

Louder systolic ejection murmurs from the aortic valve may represent true *aortic stenosis* (narrowing). The murmur is usually louder in intensity and harsher in quality, and the peak intensity is later in systole than with simple aortic sclerosis. The murmur radiates to the carotid arteries at the sides of the neck— the two main arteries that supply blood to the head. Aortic stenosis may result from congenital deformity of the valve, from gradual scarring and the presence of calcium deposits on a valve with a mild deformity existing since birth, from rheumatic fever, or from various degenerative changes that occur with aging. Classic symptoms of chest pain, breathlessness, and sudden loss of consciousness usually appear with very advanced stenosis. Severe aortic stenosis can lead to sudden death. The murmur is important because it is a signal that can be detected early in the disease process, permitting close clinical observation.

Treatment of severe aortic stenosis is generally accomplished by surgical repair or by replacement of the valve. In congenital cases the valve tissue may remain pliable and can be salvaged by surgical repair early in life known as valvuloplasty. In cases in which there is advanced scarring and calcification, the valve can be surgically replaced with either a mechanical prosthesis, a specially treated pig valve mounted on supports, or a cryopreserved (frozen) human valve.

Pulmonary stenosis, involving the valve that allows blood flow to the lungs, is a congenital disorder. The systolic ejection murmur of pulmonary stenosis is loudest at the upper left sternal border and, like most murmurs originating from the right side of the heart, becomes more intense with inspiration. As with the murmur of aortic stenosis, the intensity peaks later in systole if the stenosis is more severe. Pulmonary stenosis is usually detected in childhood. Mild pulmonary stenosis is well tolerated and does not require surgical intervention. More severe pulmonary stenosis is treated by surgical enlargement of the valve or by balloon valvuloplasty, a technique in which the valve is permanently enlarged with an inflated balloon.

Hypertrophic obstructive cardiomyopathy, also known as *idiopathic hypertrophic subaortic stenosis* (*IHHS*), is a genetically determined disorder of heart muscle characterized by an increased bulk that can cause severe obstruction of the outflow of blood from the left ventricle as well as abnormal filling of the ventricular chamber. IHHS can cause chest pains, congestive heart failure, and serious ventricular arrhythmias, including ventricular fibrillation with sudden death. The murmur associated with this condition typically has a harsh systolic ejection quality at the lower left sternal border and cardiac apex. A maneuver that causes a decrease of blood in the chamber of the left ventricle (*e.g.,* standing up) results in the murmur's becoming louder, while a maneuver that increases the volume of blood in the left ventricle (*e.g.,* squatting or clenching the fists) will reduce the murmur's intensity. In diagnostic evaluation of IHSS such maneuvers are performed by the patient during auscultation. This is called dynamic auscultation and aids the examiner in distinguishing between various types of heart murmurs. Certain drugs used in the treatment of hypertrophic obstructive cardiomyopathy (beta blockers and calcium antagonists) reduce the forcefulness of ventricular contraction, thereby reducing both the muscular obstruction that inhibits blood flow and the intensity of the murmur. In cases that do not respond to drug therapy and in which the obstruction of blood flow is severe, a segment of muscle from the septum (the dividing wall between the heart's ventricles) can be surgically excised (a procedure known as septal myectomy) to alleviate the inhibited flow of blood.

Systolic regurgitant murmurs

Mitral regurgitation describes a leakage of blood from the mitral valve during systole. Because the valve fails to close correctly, blood flows back and forth between the left ventricle and the left atrium. The murmur is typically "holosystolic"; *i.e.,* it begins with the first heart sound and continues to or beyond the second sound. The intensity may be uniform for the duration of the murmur, known as a "plateau" pattern. The murmur of mitral regurgitation is best heard at the cardiac apex and often has a blowing quality. A maneuver that impedes blood flow out of the heart and through the arteries (*e.g.,* fist clenching) augments the amount of regurgitant blood, intensifying the murmur.

Causes of mitral regurgitation include rheumatic fever, scarring caused by calcium deposits, rupture of the tough, strand-like chords that support the flaps of the valve, dysfunction of the muscle attached to the chords (papillary muscle), and perforation of a valve caused by a bacterial infection. Mild to moderate degrees of mitral regurgitation are well tolerated and do not usually cause symptoms. Severe mitral regurgitation can lead to enlargement of the heart and progressive cardiac failure.

Mitral valve prolapse describes a syndrome of bowing back of the mitral leaflets into the left atrium as they close together during systole. This prolapse movement often generates a brief and crisp systolic sound—a click. If the prolapse also causes the mitral valve to leak, there may be a late systolic murmur. Patients may have no abnormal sounds, an isolated click or group of clicks, a click followed by a murmur, or a late systolic murmur without a click. These sounds are best heard at the cardiac apex with the patient upright. The abnormal finding may come and go.

Although initially defined by auscultation, the syndrome of mitral valve prolapse has been clarified by the use of echocardiography. Mitral valve prolapse is found in all age groups but most often in young women (up to 10%, according to some surveys). A lower rate of occurrence in older age groups emphasizes the somewhat reversible nature of this valvular dysfunction and its generally favorable prognosis. Mitral valve prolapse is not associated with any cardiac symptoms in the vast majority of cases. One study compared the occurrence of breathlessness, chest pains, and palpitations between individuals with mitral valve prolapse and their relatives without it. No differences were observed.

Most cases of mitral valve prolapse have a favorable prognosis and require only simple observation over time. Patients with systolic regurgitant murmurs should receive antibiotics at the time of dental work or when having invasive gastrointestinal, genitourinary, and upper respiratory tract procedures. As with other valvular heart disease patients, they may be at increased risk for infective endocarditis, a serious bacterial infection of the valve. For those without any abnormal physical findings or with only a systolic click, prophylactic antibiotics are generally not needed.

In rare cases, mitral valve prolapse leads to serious heart problems. Life-threatening arrhythmias, infective endocarditis, progressive mitral regurgitation, and abrupt regurgitation from rupture of the mitral chords are infrequent complications of the condition. The clinician's challenge at the time of initial diagnosis of mitral valve prolapse includes distinguishing between the benign variant of normal and cases of more distinct valvular dysfunction that require close follow-up.

Other systolic regurgitant murmurs are less commonly found. *Tricuspid regurgitation* describes a leak of the tricuspid valve. This holosystolic murmur is best heard at the lower left sternal border and increases with inspiration. Severe tricuspid regurgitation causes prominent pulsations of the jugular veins at the sides of the neck. A *ventricular septal defect,* or hole through the dividing wall between the ventricles, causes a holosystolic murmur at the lower left sternal border that can be harsh in quality. Blood flows directly from the left ventricle into the right ventricle. A ventricular septal defect is usually diagnosed in childhood and, unless the defect is quite small, requires surgical closure. Ventricular septal defects can occur in adults as a complication of a heart attack. Damaged ventricular muscle gives way under the force of ventricular contraction, and a hole develops across the intraventricular septum. When these murmurs are detected, surgery is often performed to repair the defect, resulting in improvement of cardiac function.

Diastolic murmurs

The murmur of *mitral stenosis* is a very low-pitched diastolic murmur (often called a mitral rumble) heard over the cardiac apex. This low-frequency sound is best detected with the bell of the stethoscope rather than with the flat diaphragm. With the exception of rare congenital or degenerative cases, mitral stenosis is a consequence of rheumatic fever. An episode of acute rheumatic fever can include a rash, arthritis, cardiac inflammation, and occasionally a neurological disorder of movement known as chorea. Progressive mitral valve deformation caused by inflammation and scarring may continue for years, leading to valvular narrowing. Diastolic blood flow from the left atrium to the left ventricle becomes restricted and leads to elevated pressures in the left atrium and pulmonary veins. In such cases congestive heart failure often develops insidiously, and tolerance for exercise is limited.

Mitral stenosis is more common in women than in men. Symptoms usually appear in early adulthood. Some patients with the condition display a distinct opening snap in early diastole, heard best at the lower left sternal border. The opening snap correlates with the abrupt halt in the opening of the mitral leaflets

due to the restrictive scarring. The two leaflets of the valve open quickly and then suddenly stop. An opening snap is sometimes present without a diastolic murmur. When both are present, the opening snap precedes the mitral rumble.

Aortic regurgitation produces a high-pitched blowing diastolic murmur, often quite faint, at the upper right or left sternal border. Blood leaks back from the aorta into the left ventricle. The "diastolic blow" is most easily detected when the patient leans forward, holding the breath in expiration. A leak of the aortic valve may result from a congenital deformity, excessive calcium deposits, rheumatic fever, bacterial infection, or distortion of the aorta by either an aneurysm or a tear of the aortic wall. Mild aortic regurgitation causes no symptoms but must be followed over time. If aortic regurgitation gradually progresses from moderate to severe, the heart enlarges and congestive heart failure gradually intervenes. Acute, severe aortic regurgitation is not tolerated nearly as well as the chronic condition; acute congestive heart failure and circulatory collapse can require emergency valve replacement.

Pulmonary regurgitation (a leaky pulmonary valve) also produces a high-pitched blowing diastolic murmur, most often at the upper left sternal border. This murmur increases in intensity during inspiration. Pulmonary regurgitation is usually well tolerated. The importance of the murmur is as a diagnostic clue as to the presence of pulmonary vascular disease. Pulmonary hypertension, or high blood pressure in the circulation to the lungs, can develop without identifiable cause. Primary pulmonary hypertension typically affects young to middle-aged women and, if severe, can lead to heart failure and sudden death. Secondary pulmonary hypertension results from chronic lung disease such as emphysema or pulmonary fibrosis. A pulmonary regurgitation murmur may not appear until late in the course of these conditions.

Continuous murmurs

Continuous murmurs (spanning both systole and diastole) are not often observed. A *cervical venous hum* is the most common continuous murmur and does not actually arise from the heart. Such a hum may be heard at the base of the neck just above the collarbone, a site that overlies the jugular vein. A particularly loud hum may also be heard at the upper chest on either side of the sternum. Cervical venous hums are loudest when the patient is upright and may disappear when the patient is supine. This quite benign continuous murmur is most commonly present in children or during pregnancy when the cardiac output is accentuated. The specific features of a cervical venous hum must be recognized by the examiner so that an incorrect diagnosis or unnecessary diagnostic tests can be avoided.

Special Camps for Special Kids
by Ruth Andrea Seeler, M.D.

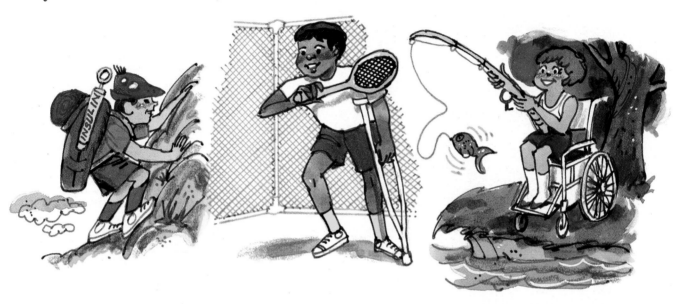

Summer camps are places where youngsters go to make new friends, share experiences, grow, and gain independence under careful guidance. Most important, perhaps, children also go to camp just to have fun. Like all youngsters, those with chronic medical disorders or physical handicaps can derive many benefits from attending residential (overnight) camps.

The American Academy of Pediatrics encourages appropriate camping experiences for children with chronic disorders. There is, however, no one "right" model of residential camping for all children who have chronic diseases or even for those who have the same disease. It is essential that parents do a bit of research to determine what is best for their child. However, parents of children with chronic diseases—and, indeed, the children themselves—may have qualms about the camping experience. Parents need to investigate the options available and, once having chosen a camp, satisfy themselves that the medical and support staffs are well trained. They also need to be reassured that having a chronic disease need not preclude a child's being safe or having a good time.

A growing time for families

Growing up is a two-way affair. It involves the increasing separation of children from their parents, and it requires parents to gradually "let go" of their children. Whereas this separation may be a natural process for children, parents often find it very difficult. At first the separation is for short periods of time, as when parents go out to dinner and leave the child with a babysitter. Then follow bigger separations—children go to school,

get involved in outside activities, meet friends on their own, and so forth. As a child grows up, parents must begin to show increasing trust in their child's judgment and use of independence. For parents of a child with a chronic disease or disability, it is frequently harder to stand back and take an honest look at the child's need for growth and autonomy. Sending the child to camp can be a crucial step in the process of accepting the youngster's need for independence.

Not uncommonly, when parents send their child with a medical problem to camp, they find that during the first summer they stay close to the telephone, certain it is going to ring—a medical emergency. The next year they begin to look forward to their son or daughter going to camp; by the third or fourth year the parents begin to view the child's time at camp as a special time for themselves, to do things such as take a long-deferred vacation. It is only in retrospect that the parents recognize how overprotective they were at first. As this typical scenario suggests, often the camping experience represents a turning point for families in learning to live with a child's disease or disability.

Sponsors, setting, and staff

Out of fear that the medical problem will make the experience too risky, many camps do not permit children with chronic illness to attend. Therefore, special camps have been established for youngsters with specific medical problems, often coinciding with the development of effective medical therapy for the disorders. There are now camps for children with hemophilia, asthma, diabetes, cancer and leukemia, AIDS, cere-

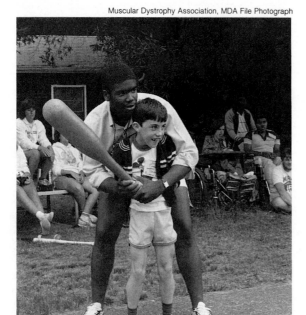

A youngster with muscular dystrophy gets ready to take a swing—with a little help from a friend. Participating in sports and other regular camp activities fosters a "can do" attitude among children with disabilities.

bral palsy, cystic fibrosis, sickle-cell disease, epilepsy, muscular dystrophy, orthopedic handicaps, deafness, emotional handicaps, and mental retardation. Sometimes a special camp may be a stepping-stone to a regular camp that youngsters can attend when they reach adolescence, have mastered their disease, and are ready for the next phase of earned independence.

Camps for youngsters with medical problems are sponsored by a variety of organizations, ranging from local treatment centers and support groups to national foundations such as the Easter Seal Society, which may also foster public education about therapy and raise funds for treatment and research. In most cases the sponsoring group rents space from an existing children's camp. A variety of crippled children's camps are set up for children with disorders of physical mobility, such as cerebral palsy, muscular dystrophy, and various orthopedic handicaps—each of the individual groups of youngsters attending specific one- or two-week sessions. The duration of the camping season—usually one to two weeks—may vary according to who owns or sponsors the camp and how many different groups of youngsters are served.

During the time that a camp is attended by children with a specific condition, also in residence are physicians, nurses, social workers, and, when appro-

priate, physical therapists. Thus, a particular camp facility might serve youngsters with hemophilia one week, children with cancer the next week, followed by campers who have epilepsy, asthma, or sickle-cell disease—each rotation of campers having its own appropriate medical and support staff.

In yet other situations children with special needs attend camp with "normal" children at the same time; the regular staff is supplemented by counselors who themselves have the disease in question and thus serve as role models for the campers. This fosters a "can do" attitude rather than one that says, "I can't because I have x-y-z disease."

Campers' camaraderie

Some critics of the special-camp concept hold that such camps are artificial in that they are unlike the "real" world, where most people do not have disabilities or chronic illnesses. Still, it is better for a child to be able to go to a special camp than to miss out on the experience altogether. Moreover, attending a special camp provides many rewards that are virtually the same as those derived by children who go to regular camps. For example, when the children return to school in the fall, they can wear their camp T-shirts and talk about their camp experiences just as children who attend normal camps do. They too can join in the conversation about the housing, food, new friends, their favorite counselors, their personal feats as well as amusing mishaps, and special events such as a skit night or a scavenger hunt. And, of course, songs sung around the campfire are universal.

Decreased self-pity is a quintessential benefit for children who attend a specialized camp. At camp the children complain to each other about their troubles at home and are reassured to discover that others have a brother or sister who is a "pain in the neck." They learn that everybody has chores at home as part of the family unit. They realize that other children have similar limitations placed on what they can and cannot do. Living and playing with other children who have the same problem proves that they are not "the only one." Nowhere is this more true than in the camps that have been established for children with AIDS and their parents and siblings. Freed for one or two weeks from the web of secrecy, suspicion, and prejudice that surrounds the disease, they can form friendships with other families who share their problems. There is no need to explain; all understand and find mutual support and understanding. As has been observed at other disease-specific camps, the participants increase their factual knowledge of their disorder—and how to cope with it—in a friendly, supportive atmosphere.

Frequently at special camps there develops lasting camaraderie among campers; in this case it is the disease—rather than ethnic background or religious affiliation—that is the common denominator. The ca-

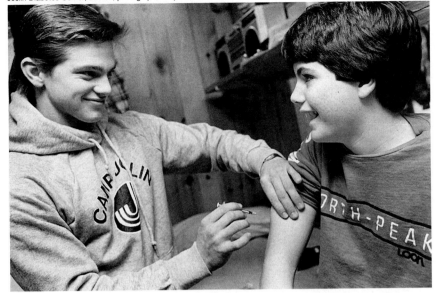

A counselor at the Elliott P. Joslin Camp for Boys with diabetes, in Charlton, Massachusetts, helps one of his young charges with an insulin injection. Camps for children with chronic diseases typically have educational programs that teach the youngsters about their disease and encourage them to take responsibility for self-care.

maraderie starts almost at once. As at all camps, long-lasting friendships form among children who otherwise quite probably would not have met. Campers may become long-distance pen pals during the year, then bunkmates the next summer at camp; they may even double-date as teenagers or become roommates when they go off to college.

During a break in the day's activities, a camper takes her asthma medicine via an aerosol inhaler. One lesson children with asthma learn at camp is the importance of taking their medication regularly—even when they are feeling fine.

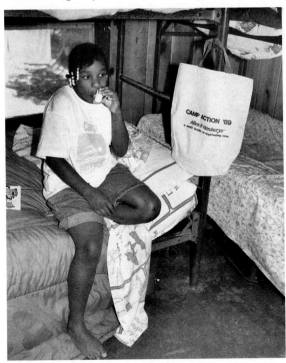

Diabetes camps

Many camps have a specific educational agenda that focuses on learning about the medical condition in question and accepting responsibility for self-care. Children with insulin-dependent (juvenile) diabetes are thus taught about regular self-testing of their blood sugar level, nutrition and good dietary habits, and the self-administration of insulin. There is emphasis on the fact that they will have diabetes all their lives and the sooner they adjust and, above all, learn not to feel sorry for themselves, the happier and healthier they will be.

A registered dietitian is a must at camps for children with diabetes. It is important that the amount of sugar in the children's meals be kept in proper balance while they are at camp. If a camp for children with diabetes uses a regular camp's facilities, most authorities would agree that the canteen should be open—at camp, just as in the outside world, these children need to learn to resist "pigging out" on candy bars and other "forbidden" indulgences.

In 1989 the American Diabetes Association listed 51 camps specifically set up for children with diabetes in 37 states in the U.S. as well as residential camping programs overseas. (In addition to summer camps for children with diabetes, there are also camps for adults with this very common affliction, providing appropriate camplike activities such as weekend retreats.)

Asthma camps

Children with severe and sometimes life-threatening asthma go to special camps where one of the many things they learn is the importance of taking their medicine on schedule (even when they feel well). The regular self-monitoring of pulmonary function with readily available, easy-to-use peak flow meters proves

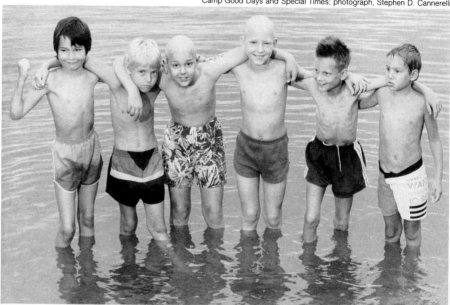

Having cancer has not kept these boys from any of the pleasures of going to camp. Those who have temporarily lost their hair as a side effect of treatment feel no need to hide their heads; living and playing with others who have the same disease reassures each that he is not "the only one."

to the children the differences that taking their medication can make. Typically, nurses, a pharmacist, a respiratory therapist, and an allergist are on the asthma camp's staff.

Epilepsy camps

Children with epilepsy who have infrequent seizures and are not mentally retarded can usually be accommodated by regular camps that have a nurse in residence. However, for children who do have frequent seizures, there are special epilepsy camps; some of these youngsters may be able to go to camps that accept children with multiple handicaps.

Swimming is one camp activity that may pose a potential problem for these children. Seizures may be precipitated by the so-called flicker phenomenon—a fluttering visual sensation—which frequently occurs when sunlight reflects off water. Also, swimming can cause hyperventilation, which in turn may precipitate seizures. This may occur in children who are not strong swimmers or in those who overexert themselves. Whenever children with epilepsy are swimming, there must be additional water safety personnel present who are trained not only in lifesaving but also in handling sudden seizures in a young person with epilepsy. If the children are swimming in open water, such as a lake, or taking part in other water activities, such as fishing, sailing, rowing, or canoeing, there are additional precautions that must be taken. It is imperative in all water activities that children with epilepsy wear life jackets (a special type that is designed to flip a person who becomes unconscious face up).

Camps for children with epilepsy generally have a pediatric neurologist, social workers, psychologists, pharmacists, and nurses in residence.

Cancer and leukemia camps

Camps for children with leukemia and other types of cancer have provisions that allow a youngster to attend camp while undergoing chemotherapy. In many ways the campers with cancer are among the easiest to accommodate at a "regular" camp. For those whose disease is not in remission, often the only special provision necessary is that the kitchen staff prepare foods low in salt for those taking the drug prednisone. The children enjoy all of the usual camping activities, restricted only by their endurance.

Several years ago the Children's Oncology Camps of America, Inc., was established. It lists camps, raises funds to send children with cancer to camp, and helps new groups start special camping programs. Cancer camps have pediatric hematologists and specially trained nurses, as well as medical technologists, on-site so that blood counts can be readily obtained. Many cancer camps have as counselors teenagers who have survived childhood cancer. This is greatly inspiring to those undergoing the rigors of treatment because they have visible proof that the acute discomforts of therapy are worthwhile. The cure rates for childhood cancers today are among the highest of those for all cancers.

The effects of chemotherapy can be difficult for any cancer patient, regardless of age, to endure. The problem of hair loss is common to almost all; at camp the children do not need to feel embarrassed and can enjoy their days without hiding their heads under a cap. They swap stories about chemotherapy and how they have handled a variety of problems imposed by it; they are frequently amazed to find out how many other youngsters have cancer and have been through treatment.

Hemophilia Foundation of Illinois

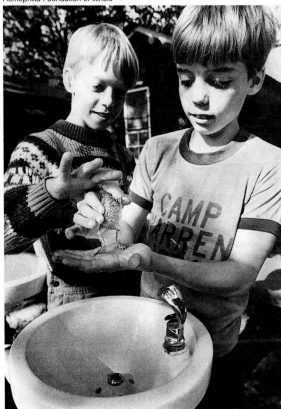

Momentarily fascinated by a frog, these boys with hemophilia seem just like any other campers. Limitations on the campers are few, and should a child experience a bleed, counselors and doctors are there at all times to handle it.

Adaptive rules are quickly developed for those with special problems. For example, in a baseball game a boy who has lost a leg to cancer will take his turn at bat, but someone else will run for him. (When it comes to sweeping the cabin floor, however, everyone takes his or her own turn.)

Hemophilia camps

At hemophilia camp the importance of treatment at the first indication of a bleeding episode is the paramount lesson. Even a relatively minor trauma can cause extensive tissue damage and, if not properly managed, can result in crippling musculoskeletal deformities. Therefore, learning to administer their own coagulant medications is for these youngsters a rite of passage. At a hemophilia camp swimming and water games are especially important activities. For boys with hemophilia water sports provide both recreation and active, hard physical therapy. Running in water strengthens the leg muscles and increases the range of motion of the joints.

Nevertheless, these youngsters can also enjoy most of the regular activities offered by camps. Especially important are team sports, captained by older chil-

dren with hemophilia. There are some adaptive rules needed because of the wide age range of those who usually attend hemophilia camps. For example, in chase games such as "capture the flag," the rule is that a boy can be tagged out only by someone his own size or smaller. Therefore, the team that has the smallest children has an advantage, which requires careful strategic planning on the part of the bigger, older boys. In games and other group activities, boys who have temporary but severe restrictions in physical mobility because of a recent bleeding episode can act as umpires or referees until they are well enough to take a more active part.

Temporary problems in mobility caused by sore or swollen joints are a fact of life for those with hemophilia, which is taken into consideration when campsites are selected. Most of these camps can accommodate children who need to be on crutches or in wheelchairs. The National Hemophilia Foundation publishes a list of more than 20 accredited camps in the United States.

Camps for the physically handicapped

Perhaps the greatest challenge for professional camp directors is the development of programs for children who are wheelchair-bound—*e.g.,* those with cerebral palsy, spina bifida, muscular dystrophy, or traumatic paraplegia. Nevertheless, there are many special camps for these children.

Two young cancer patients say a tearful farewell at the end of camp. One of the best things about special camps is that the friendships that develop often continue long after the camp session is over.

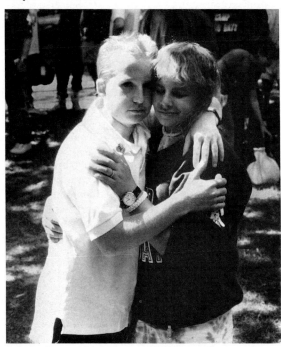

Camp Good Days and Special Times; photograph, Neal Haddad

Special camps for special kids

A camp's natural terrain and rustic facilities need not impede the handicapped camper's full participation in most activities. As in the case of camps for children with hemophilia, the physical setting of these camps is chosen with the youngsters' special needs in mind—thus permitting access for those campers who are in wheelchairs, on crutches, or using walkers. The grounds are usually fairly compact, with manageable distances between the dining room, dormitories, bathrooms, recreation halls, swimming facilities, playing fields, and so forth.

Camps for youngsters with physical disabilities tend to have a larger-than-average number of staff members and supplement the staff with facilitators—personal aides, assigned on a one-to-one basis to provide disabled individuals with any necessary physical help. The staff is typically composed of occupational therapists, physical therapists, and those specializing in physical education of the handicapped (often teachers in training). Facilitators are generally teenagers or young adults who want to help youngsters with disabilities. Occasionally an individual with a chronic disease may become a facilitator—one young hemophiliac, for example, worked for many summers as a facilitator at a muscular dystrophy camp.

Are there risks?

Many people assume that the residential camping experience will pose undue risks for children with medical disabilities. On the contrary, because of the intense educational programs directed at teaching the campers to be responsible for their own health care, the children are not apt to have an exacerbation of their medical problem at camp. Furthermore, because of the presence of the expert medical staff, any problems or emergencies that do arise are handled promptly and on-site by experts. After all, when else in their lives do these children have access 24 hours a day to doctors and nurses who are specialists in treating their illness and are but minutes away? Most camps also have emergency arrangements with nearby hospitals during summer camping sessions.

In short, camping is a celebration of accomplishments that brings out the "champion" in every child. Special camps are places where everyone is equal and the prevailing mood is one of joy. Indeed, the thrill of the summer camping experience is as open to most children with medical disabilities today as to other children, and they, too, can have fond camp memories that endure for a lifetime.

FOR FURTHER INFORMATION:
Many special camps are sponsored by lay support groups or national foundations; local chapters can usually can provide information about specific camps. Social workers at local treatment centers may also provide help in locating camps.

Foundations and support groups for the more common chronic diseases and disorders are generally listed in the telephone book. The following is a guide for finding such organizations in the local phone directory.

asthma:
    Lung Association
    Asthma and Allergy Foundation

cancer and leukemia:
    local pediatric cancer treatment center
    American Cancer Society

cerebral palsy:
    United Cerebral Palsy

cystic fibrosis:
    Lung Association
    Cystic Fibrosis Foundation

diabetes:
    American Diabetes Association

epilepsy:
    Epilepsy Foundation

hemophilia:
    Hemophilia Foundation

muscular dystrophy:
    Muscular Dystrophy Association

orthopedic handicaps:
    medical center specializing in rehabilitation

retardation:
    Association for Retarded Citizens

sickle cell anemia:
    Sickle Cell Anemia Association

spina bifida:
    Spina Bifida Association

Sjögren's Syndrome: The Dryness Disorder

by Steven E. Carsons, M.D.

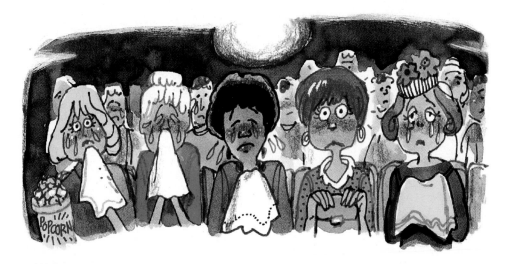

Consider the experience of walking in the desert during a dust storm. The wind blows hot sand against one's face. One's mouth is parched, one's throat is dry, and one's eyes burn and sting. Unfortunately, the person with Sjögren's syndrome (pronounced shō'-grenz) experiences these unpleasant sensations daily. Initially described by Henrik Sjögren, a Swedish ophthalmologist, in 1933, this disorder is characterized by chronic, progressive dysfunction of the glands that produce tears and saliva. Known as the lacrimal and salivary glands, respectively, these and other moisture-secreting glands become the target of an attack by the body's own immune system. Thus, Sjögren's syndrome is considered an autoimmune disorder.

The true incidence of Sjögren's syndrome is unknown, owing at least in part to underrecognition of its symptoms by patients and physicians alike. Estimates suggest that 1% of the U.S. adult population may be affected to some degree. The disorder has been reported in all parts of the world. Sjögren's is predominantly a disease of women rather than men: more than 90% of patients are female. Symptoms usually begin between the ages of 20 and 60, with an average age of onset of 45–50 years.

Types and features

There are two types of Sjögren's syndrome, primary and secondary. Approximately 50% of patients have primary Sjögren's syndrome, with clinical manifestations generally limited to dryness of the eyes and mouth. The remainder (with secondary Sjögren's) are additionally affected by an autoimmune connective-tissue disorder, most commonly, rheumatoid arthritis.

Less often the coexisting disorder is systemic lupus erythematosus or scleroderma.

Typically, the person with Sjögren's syndrome experiences symptoms of dryness involving the eyes, nasal passages, mouth, and throat. This constellation of symptoms is sometimes referred to as the sicca complex (from the Latin *siccus,* meaning "dry").

Dry eye. The discomfort felt by the patient with dry eyes is not always immediately recognized as being caused by dryness. The problem is commonly perceived by the patient as a feeling of constant irritation, as if there were some foreign body in the eye. The eyes may also burn and be unduly sensitive to light. Some patients awaken feeling as if their eyelids have been glued shut, a consequence of reduced tear formation. Although dryness is disturbing in itself, the chronic absence of tears can result in the much more serious condition of inflammation of the cornea. If inflammation is present for extended periods of time, the cornea may become scarred. When corneal inflammation complicates the problem of dry eye, the condition is known as keratoconjunctivitis sicca (KCS). Evaluation of KCS by an ophthalmologist is essential, as advanced scarring, and the increased risk of bacterial infection that accompanies it, may threaten vision.

Dry mouth and related discomfort. Although people with Sjögren's syndrome may be aware of the unpleasant sensation of their mouths being dry and parched, severe dryness may first be clinically recognized with the onset of rampant tooth decay. The tongue may be chronically sore and painful, and cracking at the corners of the mouth—a condition known as cheliosis—may occur. Along with dry mouth, patients may also

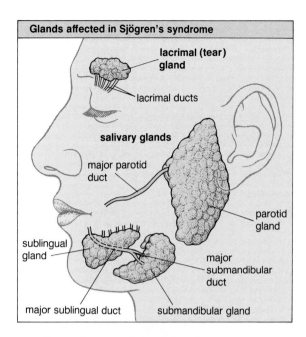

Glands affected in Sjögren's syndrome

lacrimal (tear) gland

lacrimal ducts

salivary glands

major parotid duct

parotid gland

sublingual gland

major submandibular duct

major sublingual duct

submandibular gland

experience dryness of the throat, larynx (voice box), ears, and nasal passages. The inside of the nose may become scabby and crusted. Some patients suffer from a diminished sense of taste. The oral symptoms of Sjögren's syndrome may contribute to difficulty in chewing and swallowing.

Oral symptoms are usually accompanied by mump-like swelling of the parotid glands, located in front of the ears, and the submandibular glands, located under the jaw. The swelling can occur on one or both sides of the face, may be associated with facial discomfort, and may fluctuate over time.

Manifestations in other parts of the body. Sjögren's patients frequently have dry skin, resulting in cracking, peeling, and itching, especially in cold, dry weather. Women frequently experience vaginal dryness, making intercourse painful. Dryness in the bronchial tubes, due to abnormal function of mucus-secreting bronchial glands, may lead to a dry cough. Inflammation of the lungs may be associated with coughing, shortness of breath, and structural abnormalities visible on a chest X-ray. Kidney inflammation secondary to Sjögren's syndrome may result in frequent urination and abnormalities in the acidity or alkalinity (pH) of the blood. However, frequent urination in Sjögren's patients may simply be due to their drinking more fluids in order to soothe a dry mouth.

Occasionally, the syndrome is complicated by another autoimmune disorder called vasculitis (inflammation of the blood vessels), which is caused by deposition of antibody-protein complexes in the capillary walls. Vasculitis can result in the appearance of raised red spots on the legs or feet. Because autoimmune disorders affect the body as a whole, generalized symptoms, such as fatigue, are common.

Less common manifestations. In 1935 Sjögren himself described neurological complications of the syndrome. Recently, an expanded spectrum of neurological features has been identified in a small number of patients. The most common type of neurological involvement is peripheral neuropathy—a dysfunction of nerves supplying the arms and legs. Symptoms include the tingling "pins-and-needles" sensation, burning, pain, numbness, and sometimes weakness of the involved extremity. Painful neuralgia of the face caused by neuropathy of the trigeminal nerve is another of the more frequent types of nerve involvement.

A rare complication of Sjögren's syndrome is lymphoma, a malignancy of the lymphatic system, which may develop in patients whose glands have been massively enlarged for long periods of time. It is characterized by swollen lymph glands in multiple areas, weight loss, night sweats, and pulmonary symptoms.

Medical evaluation

Because Sjögren's syndrome is not the only cause of dryness, diagnosis may be problematic. For one thing, tear and salivary gland function tends to decline with age. Additionally, dry mouth and dry eye are very commonly caused by prescription and nonprescription medications. Diuretics (used to treat high blood pressure and heart disease), antihistamines, and antidepressant medications are among the most common offenders. Climate is another factor that may affect moisture levels of the mucous membranes of the eyes and mouth. For women, hormonal status may affect the tissues lining the vagina—the increasing absence of estrogen causing progressive dryness. Other medical conditions, including viral infections, may cause swelling of the salivary glands.

Depending on the most prominent symptoms or complaint, the patient with Sjögren's syndrome may be initially seen by any one of several medical specialists. Patients with primary eye, dental, or oral problems are likely to first consult an ophthalmologist, a dentist, or an otolaryngologist (ear, nose, and throat specialist). If Sjögren's syndrome is suspected, the patient should be referred to a specialist for a thorough evaluation. The specialists with the most experience in this area are rheumatologists and clinical immunologists.

The physician evaluating a patient with suspected Sjögren's syndrome has four aims: to assess the general health status of the patient; to determine whether the person has an associated connective-tissue (rheumatic) disorder; to search for signs of other autoimmune disorders that may also be associated with Sjögren's, such as thyroid problems; and to ascertain the patient's baseline immunologic status.

Complete patient history. The evaluation begins with the compilation of the patient's complete medical history, in which the patient recounts all of the symptoms and signs leading up to the visit. The physician may

460

inquire about such symptoms as joint aches, skin rashes, numbness of an extremity, unusual bruising or bleeding, and so forth. Because autoimmune and connective-tissue disorders may be influenced by genetic factors, the physician will want to know if others in the patient's family have been diagnosed with any such disorders. The patient will also be asked about smoking, drinking, and use of both prescription and nonprescription medications.

Physical exam. The physician will then perform a general physical exam, including careful inspection of the patient's eyes and mouth and of the glands of the face and neck. The skin, joints, and scalp will be examined, as well as the heart, lungs, abdomen, and extremities. A chest X-ray is performed to check the lungs for subtle signs of inflammation.

Laboratory tests. The physician will also order routine blood tests to obtain counts of white and red blood cells, measures of liver and kidney function, glucose level, and other potentially important indicators. Because some patients with Sjögren's may have inflammation of the kidney, it is important that a urinalysis be done.

Over the past several years, the finding of certain unique antibodies (substances normally produced in response to infection) in the blood of Sjögren's patients has been diagnostically helpful. The physician will usually order a number of tests for such substances as a part of the initial evaluation, including tests for antinuclear antibody and rheumatoid factor. None of these is diagnostic in and of itself, but in conjunction with the clinical exam they are helpful to the physician.

Recently a specific group of antibodies has been found to occur with a relatively high frequency in patients with Sjögren's syndrome. These are most often referred to as Sjögren's antibodies A and B or SS (for Sjögren's syndrome)-A and B. SS-A antibodies occur in 60–70% of Sjögren's patients but can also be seen in people with other rheumatic or connective-tissue disorders. SS-B antibodies are seen in approximately 40% of patients with Sjögren's syndrome, more commonly in those with the primary form.

In order to make a definitive diagnosis, the physician may recommend one last test—a small biopsy of the inner portion of the lower lip. This can usually be performed on an outpatient basis, often in the dentist's office. The lip tissue contains minor salivary glands. If these are found to be infiltrated by lymphocytes (white blood cells active in defending the body against infection), the diagnosis of Sjögren's syndrome is generally confirmed. Because lymphocytic infiltration in a salivary gland biopsy is not unique to Sjögren's syndrome but may appear in other autoimmune diseases, making the final diagnosis ultimately depends on the physician's careful evaluation of all of the signs, symptoms, and test results.

Treatment

While Sjögren's syndrome is rarely fatal or completely disabling, there are periods when patients experience extreme discomfort, which can be incapacitating to various degrees. Although there is no cure for the disorder, the physician with interest and experience can often counsel patients on measures that can help them feel more comfortable.

The mainstay of treatment is moisture replacement. To relieve dry eyes, artificial tears—liquid tear substitutes applied in the form of eye drops—should be used as often as necessary. Tear preparations containing no preservatives are now available for patients who may be especially sensitive to these substances. Lubricating ointments are used at night for longer-acting tear replacement. Eye drops containing natural substances such as gum cellulose, hyaluronic acid, and a protein known as fibronectin are being developed in an attempt to more closely simulate real tears. Dryness of the vagina can be treated by local application of water-soluble lubricating creams or jellies.

For relief of dry mouth, there are several types of artificial salivas that can be sprayed or squeezed into the mouth. Most are water based and contain many of the constituents of natural saliva, but they are short acting and must be reapplied frequently. Some patients prefer to carry a squeeze bottle filled with plain water. Nasal dryness can be relieved with a variety of nonprescription saline-based sprays. Emollients such as petroleum jelly, vitamin E oil, or other suitable oils can be applied to the lips and, with a cotton swab, to the inside of the nose.

Another treatment approach is stimulation of secretions from glands that contain some residual fluid. Chewing gum and sucking hard candy help to stimulate secretion of saliva; because these products have a heightened potential for tooth decay, however, patients should use only sugarless items. (One artificial sweetener, Xylitol, used in some gums and candies, may actually act as a stimulant of saliva.) The drug pilocarpine (Almocarpine) used as drops or in pill form stimulates saliva, but it may have adverse side effects so should be used only if prescribed by a physician. A drug used in Europe, bromhexine, has been found in some studies to stimulate tears and saliva, but its efficacy has not yet been proved, and it is not available in the U.S. An electronic device that stimulates the flow of saliva may be useful in certain cases. Patients who have no residual salivary function do not benefit from any of these forms of salivary stimulation, however.

Simple manipulation of the patient's environment may afford significant relief. Dryness is greatly exacerbated by evaporation caused by central-heating systems. Gas forced-air systems are probably the most drying. Increasing humidity by means of an ultrasonic cool mist humidifier or simply by placing pans of water in the bedroom and other often-used rooms can be very helpful. In the summertime air-conditioning removes moisture from the air; this effect can be reversed by a humidifier. (If a humidifier is used, it should be cleaned regularly to prevent the growth of bacteria, fungi, and other infectious agents, which may cause disease or aggravate allergies.) Wind causes surface evaporation, which results in accelerated drying; protection of exposed surfaces, especially the skin, mouth, and eyes, is important in the wintertime or in windy weather. Plastic moisture-chamber eyeglasses or sunglasses can be helpful in retarding evaporation of moisture from the surface of the eye. These glasses, which can be specially made by optometrists, have clear plastic side pieces that fit snugly against the face, thus sealing out wind.

Aches and pains in salivary glands and joints may respond to aspirin or the newer nonsteroidal anti-inflammatory drugs such as ibuprofen. The antimalarial drug hydroxychloroquine (Plaquenil) may be useful for these symptoms but has not been as yet systematically studied. Corticosteroids (steroid agents) should be reserved for patients with more severe disease in which internal organs such as the lungs and kidneys are involved. Conditions such as vasculitis and lymphoma may require the use of immunosuppressants or drugs used in cancer chemotherapy.

Search for a cause

The precise cause of Sjögren's syndrome is unknown. Research, however, has demonstrated that abnormalities in the immune system play an important role. In autoimmune processes, antibodies that normally serve to protect the body from infection are directed instead against its own tissues—hence the term *autoantibody*. The result is inflammation and tissue damage. Lymphocytes, which are a component of normal immune function, also participate in the autoimmune process. As noted earlier, the blood of Sjögren's patients reveals the presence of multiple types of autoantibodies, including those known as SS-A and SS-B, which are fairly specific for Sjögren's. Autoantibodies that specifically bind to salivary gland tissue, known as antisalivary duct antibodies, are also found in the blood of Sjögren's patients. In the salivary gland biopsy, in which the lip tissue is examined under the microscope, normal glandular tissue is seen to have been invaded by large numbers of lymphocytes. A large proportion of these lymphocytes belong to a category known as "helper" T cells. These helper cells induce and promote immunologic reactions, and they are responsible for sustaining the autoimmune process in the glands. One mechanism by which helper cells promote autoimmunity is by stimulating another group of lymphocytes, known as B cells, to produce autoantibodies.

While no one is sure what actually triggers autoimmunity, many researchers suspect that viruses may play a role. The viral hypothesis is especially attractive in Sjögren's syndrome for several reasons. One is that the salivary glands are natural reservoirs for many viral infections, including the mumps virus and the virus that causes infectious mononucleosis, which is known as the Epstein-Barr virus (EBV). Furthermore, Sjögren's syndrome has been known to develop after mononucleosis, and EBV is capable of activating B cells to produce some of the autoantibodies typically seen in Sjögren's syndrome.

EBV is a very widespread virus, however, so it seems logical to ask why only certain individuals develop Sjögren's syndrome. One possibility is that genetic predisposition plays a part. Although Sjögren's syndrome is not a trait that is passed on directly from parent to child, it appears that certain segments of the population do have an increased risk of acquiring this illness.

Clearly, there is still much to be learned about Sjögren's syndrome. Scientists are currently attempting to trace the complex process by which abnormalities of immune regulation in Sjögren's syndrome lead to the production of the characteristic autoantibodies. Other researchers are seeking ways to identify the genetic factors that may predispose an individual to developing the syndrome. Still others are trying to identify the immediate cause of the illness. If a virus is found, the development of a vaccine might be feasible. In the meantime, a high priority is to find better treatments for patients, including drugs to suppress glandular inflammation and stimulate secretion of existing tears and saliva.

Sources of help

People with a chronic disease often benefit from the support of both health professionals and other patients who are similarly affected. Such emotional support helps patients cope with the burden of living with chronic discomfort that is not medically curable. This is especially true in the case of Sjögren's syndrome— patients often experience long periods of uncertainty as they wait for the diagnosis to be established and, once diagnosed, they may get little practical information from traditional medical sources. Self-help groups provide a forum for patients to share experiences, practical information, and tips for making life more comfortable. These groups often invite specialists as speakers who can keep patients advised of developments in treatment and research.

The Sjögren's Syndrome Foundation, founded in 1983 by a patient, Elaine K. Harris, sponsors meetings and publishes *The Moisture Seekers,* a monthly newsletter. Further information may be obtained from the Sjögren's Syndrome Foundation, Inc., 382 Main Street, Port Washington, NY 11050, and from the Arthritis Foundation, 1314 Spring Street, N.W., Atlanta, GA 30309.

The Pap Smear
by Leopold G. Koss, M.D.

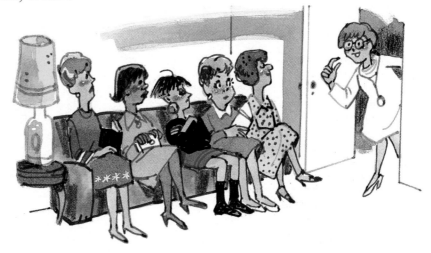

The Papanicolaou, or Pap, smear is an important but not very well understood laboratory procedure widely used for detection and prevention of cancer of the uterine cervix (neck of the womb). The procedure is named after an American researcher of Greek origin, George N. Papanicolaou, who, working at the Cornell Medical School in New York City in the 1930s and 1940s, was instrumental in the development of this test and its subsequent extensive clinical application.

Over the past 40 years in the U.S., the test has resulted in a 70% reduction in the death rate from cancer of the cervix. Prior to mass screening by Pap smears, cervical cancer was the second most common cause of cancer death in U.S. women; today it is not even included among the five leading causes. Nevertheless, although the value of the test has been proved and cervical cancer is now considered preventable, the American Cancer Society anticipated that in 1990 alone 13,000 new cases would be diagnosed in the U.S. and 6,000 women would die of the disease.

Why are American women still dying of an essentially preventable disease? The reasons are complex. Many women who develop cancer of the cervix either have never received a Pap test or have neglected to have the test repeated at regular intervals. Because of errors in the testing process itself or in the interpretation of the results, however, still others will develop the disease in spite of having been tested. It is important, therefore, to examine the rationale behind the Pap test, the achievements of the test, and the reasons for its occasional failures.

How cervical cancer develops

Early in the 20th century, medical scientists studying cervical cancer observed that the disease develops in stages. In the first stage the cancerous change is limited to the cervical epithelium (*i.e.*, surface lining tissue). This stage of the disease was named carcinoma *in situ*. (The term *carcinoma* means a cancer that originates in epithelial tissue.) Carcinoma *in situ* is composed of abnormal cells but is, in itself, harmless. After some years, however, the cells of carcinoma *in situ* become capable of penetrating into the underlying tissue, a process known as invasion. Invasive cancer grows rapidly, spreads to the blood vessels, and becomes capable of sending out cancerous cells to more distant sites, where new colonies of cancer cells are established. This process of spread is known as metastasis. Quite contrary to carcinoma *in situ*, invasive cancer represents a major threat to the woman's life.

It became evident to early researchers in the field that the development of invasive cancer could be prevented if the precursor lesion could be identified and eliminated. Unfortunately, carcinoma *in situ* cannot be identified in the course of a routine gynecological exam because it does not produce any clinical changes visible to the naked eye. In the 1940s Papanicolaou and others investigating the smear technique noted that abnormal cells derived from carcinoma *in situ* could be identified under the microscope in samples of cells obtained from the uterine cervix. Since successful treatment of the precancerous lesions was already available at that time, the Pap test was widely adopted as a tool for the prevention of invasive cervical cancer. Starting in the 1950s, the test began to be used for the mass screening of many millions of women.

Misconceptions about the test

The enthusiasm with which the Pap test was accepted in the 1950s precluded one important step that would be mandatory today, namely a controlled study of its

463

efficacy—*i.e.,* a study in which groups of tested and untested patients are followed and compared. Thus, today there is no objective statistical analysis of how well the Pap test performs.

There are also some widely held misconceptions about the test itself. The primary misconception is the notion that the Pap test is the equivalent of other simple laboratory procedures. This is not the case. The Pap test is a uniquely labor-intensive process, the outcome of which is not machine generated but depends entirely on human observation and judgment. Yet the accuracy of this test, which leaves so much room for error, rarely has been questioned. In 1987 and 1988, however, several articles appeared in the lay press, raising doubts about the usefulness of the test. Out of this grew another misconception; many women concluded that because the Pap test was not 100% accurate, it was not worth doing.

Obtaining the sample

To maximize the chances that precancerous abnormalities will be recognized, an adequate Pap smear must be representative of the epithelium of both the cervix and the endocervical canal, a narrow passage leading from the cervix to the main cavity of the uterus. To ensure that the test is properly performed, the physician first inspects the cervix visually, with the help of a vaginal speculum. To avoid contamination of the cell sample with foreign material, the speculum must be introduced without a lubricant. Once the cervix has been visually examined and found to be free of suspicious abnormalities, a wooden or plastic spatula is applied to the cervix and rotated around its contour with considerable pressure. (This may be uncomfortable for the patient but is rarely truly painful.) An additional cell sample from the endocervical canal is often obtained with a special brushlike instrument. In menopausal and postmenopausal women, a separate smear should also be obtained from the vagina. Cancers of the endometrium (lining of the womb), fallopian tubes, and ovaries are increasingly common in women over age 50, and cancerous cells from these organs may sometimes be present in the vaginal smear.

The sticky material obtained by the spatula is spread onto a glass slide in the form of a smear. To prevent air drying, which might distort the cells, the smear is preserved by a chemical process known as fixation. The laboratory where the slide will be examined must be provided with a summary of essential clinical data, such as the name and age of the patient, her obstetrical and gynecologic history, and a description of the examining physician's clinical findings.

Screening

In the laboratory the smears must be entered into a recording system, given an identifying number, and stained in preparation for the initial microscopic exam-

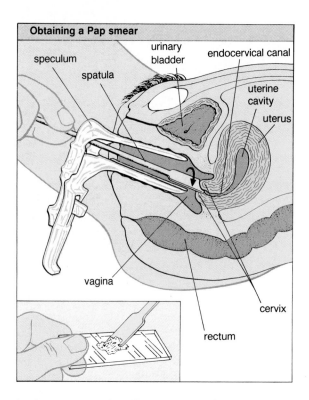

Obtaining a Pap smear

speculum · spatula · urinary bladder · endocervical canal · uterine cavity · uterus · vagina · cervix · rectum

ination, or screening. The purpose of screening Pap smears is to identify among the very large numbers of cells—each smear contains from 50,000 to 300,000 cells—those that may reflect cancerous or precancerous changes. Screening may also disclose other important conditions, such as bacterial or viral infections or parasitical infestations.

The task of screening is delegated to trained technicians called cytotechnologists, most of whom are college graduates who have attended a special school for one or two years and have passed a qualifying examination. Anyone who has not screened a large number of cervicovaginal smears can have only a limited notion of the physical and mental effort required. To do this well, the technician must look at every cell in the smear and record any abnormality. If one considers that each smear contains thousands of cells and that the number of abnormal cells in this material may be only one or two dozen, the quality as well as quantity of observations required is stupendous. The process may be compared to the recognition of a single known face in a crowd of thousands of people. Thus, screening of Pap smears is a difficult, demanding, and time-consuming process. There are obvious limitations in the number of smears that even the most efficient technologist can examine without becoming overly fatigued. The difficulty of the task is such that occasional errors are virtually unavoidable.

These errors are of two types. The first is the error that occurs when evidence of abnormalities is missed, either because the smear contains only scanty evidence that is easily overlooked or because a trivial abnormality goes unrecognized. The result is a so-called false-negative report that may give both the physician and the patient a false sense of security. It is variously estimated that 10 to 30% of abnormal smears are not recognized. The second type of error is based on misinterpretation of benign abnormalities as possible cancerous changes. The result is a false-positive report that may cause the patient unnecessary anguish. The rate of such reports is fortunately small.

In well-run laboratories every effort is made to reduce the number of these errors by a system known as quality control. Rescreening of a certain percentage of smears, close supervision of the cytotechnologists, and creation of the best possible working conditions for the very demanding work of screening are some of the measures implemented in many laboratories.

Interpreting the findings

All Pap smears in which an abnormality is observed are referred to a pathologist, a trained medical specialist who is in charge of the laboratory. It is the pathologist's task to interpret the cytological evidence, to render a final diagnosis, and, if warranted, to alert the referring physician that further examination of the patient should be performed. The interpretation of Pap smears belongs to the most difficult area of microscopic diagnosis. While obvious cases of cancer and precancerous lesions are usually recognized without difficulty by experienced observers, often the evidence of abnormalities is scant and may pose significant difficulties of interpretation.

Furthermore, the smears, even if carefully obtained, do not always reflect the existence of underlying disease. This problem may be particularly troubling in cases of invasive carcinoma, where the surface of the lesion is often covered by cellular debris, and the smear may fail to reveal obvious cancer cells. Another source of error is that precancerous lesions may be represented in a smear by only a few cells with relatively trivial abnormalities.

Since the goal of the Pap smear is to detect precancerous abnormalities and occult (invisible) small carcinomas, the pathologist is obligated to report the presence of any cellular abnormalities, even if they are relatively minor, and refer the woman for the next step in the cancer-detection process; namely, further clinical assessment.

Reporting of test findings

Papanicolaou himself created a system of reporting that was based on numerical assessment of abnormalities, described in a ranked order of classes. In this system a class I smear indicated total absence of abnormalities, and a class V smear denoted unequivocal presence of a cancerous process. A class II smear indicated minor benign abnormalities; classes III

and IV indicated major abnormalities requiring further scrutiny. This manner of reporting is still widely used, but it must be considered obsolete.

With the passage of time and growing experience, pathologists have been able to identify several varieties of precancerous abnormalities. Besides carcinoma in situ, discussed above, other types of precancerous abnormalities, called dysplasias, have been described. Dysplasias have been further subdivided into "mild," "moderate," and "severe." An underlying assumption of this classification was that each of these lesions had a different prognosis and that so-called mild dysplasias were less threatening to the patient than severe dysplasia or carcinoma in situ. While some differences in the behavior of these various lesions have been recorded, the classification is not specific enough to be universally valid. The consensus today is that all of these lesions must be investigated and treated. The term cervical intraepithelial neoplasia, or CIN, has been recommended to describe all of these lesions, which, regardless of name, do not constitute a threat to the woman's life if appropriately treated.

Further investigation and treatment

The Pap smear does not replace a careful clinical examination. Any patient with visible suspicious abnormalities of the uterine cervix should be investigated further, not only by Pap smear but also by a sample of tissue (a biopsy). The biopsy is particularly important if the patient has symptoms, such as vaginal bleeding, that may preclude obtaining a good cell sample. In view of the possible failure of the Pap smear to disclose an abnormality, the biopsy may be essential to the diagnosis of an important lesion.

On the other hand, if an abnormality has been identified in the Pap smear, the recommended investigative procedure is examination by colposcopy. Basically, a colposcope is a magnifying glass mounted on a tripod. The colposcope is used to examine the surface of the cervix under high magnification, after removal of mucus by a mild solution of acetic acid. Colposcopy leads to the clarification of the nature of most cytological abnormalities. If an abnormality is identified on colposcopy, a biopsy is usually obtained to define the lesion better. Still, some lesions located in the endocervical canal are beyond the reach of the colposcope and cannot be seen. In such cases an endocervical tissue sampling (endocervical curettage) or an excision of a small segment of the cervix (conization) must be performed. The purpose of these procedures is to rule out invasive cancer. In the absence of invasive cancer, the treatment consists of local destruction of the lesions by heat (cautery), freezing (cryosurgery), or laser. These procedures usually preserve the woman's reproductive function. In some cases, however, the removal of the entire uterus (hysterectomy) is the treatment of choice.

The Pap smear

In the absence of invasive carcinoma, the treatment of precancerous lesions assures a cure rate of nearly 100%, although in some cases a second treatment may be required. The treated patients must be followed medically for many years, as some may be prone to a relapse of the disorder. If an invasive cancer is identified, other means of treatment, such as more extensive surgical treatment or radiotherapy, ensure the best chance of a cure. The success of the treatment will depend on the degree of spread—or, in technical terms, the stage—of the disease.

Precancerous lesions: unpredictable behavior

Only a relatively small proportion of precancerous lesions, even if untreated, will go on to become invasive cancers. The reasons for the unpredictable behavior of these lesions remain enigmatic. It is clear, therefore, that some women will receive unnecessary treatment. Unfortunately, it is not yet possible to predict with any degree of certainty which lesions will progress to invasive carcinoma and which will not. Thus, as a precautionary measure all lesions must be treated.

Epidemiological studies show that there are certain risk factors associated with precancerous lesions and cervical carcinoma; the most important among them are early onset of sexual activity and multiplicity of sexual partners—although there are clear exceptions to these rules. Cancer of the cervix has often been compared to sexually transmitted diseases, in which disease-causing agents are transmitted to a woman by her male partner. There is now satisfactory evidence that a virus, the human papillomavirus (HPV), may be this agent in the case of cervical cancer. HPV has a clearly documented association with both precancerous states and invasive cancer in the uterine cervix. At least 50 different types of HPV have been identified. Most occur in the skin, where they cause common skin disorders such as warts.

A handful of HPV types have been shown to be associated with lesions of the female genital tract, some of which are benign (*e.g.,* vulvar warts, or condylomas) and some of which are precursor lesions of cervical or vulvar cancer. Most often associated with invasive cancer are types 16, 18, 31, and 33, which are considered high-risk types. The identification of these high-risk types initially raised the hope that the behavior of specific virus types might explain the apparent unpredictability of precancerous lesions. However, this hypothesis has not been proved. Further, within the normal, healthy, sexually active population there is a very large group of individuals, perhaps 30% or more, who have been infected with HPV. About half of this group are carriers of the high-risk types of virus. Thus, HPV infection must be considered to be virtually universal in sexually active women, and the presence of the virus per se is not likely to be the cause of either precancerous lesions or invasive cancer.

There is, nevertheless, a group of susceptible individuals who are more likely than others to develop cancer of the cervix. The search for additional risk factors has not been successful as yet. Cigarette smoking and lowered resistance to infections probably play a role in some, but not all, cases. Until specific causes are established, the best method of prevention remains early detection by means of the Pap smear.

Guidelines for maximal success

Every sexually active woman, regardless of age, should take advantage of the benefits of the Pap test. The test should be performed yearly for at least three consecutive years to ensure that a single false-negative report will not allow an existing lesion to remain undetected. Fortunately, for the vast majority of women the development of precancerous lesions of the cervix is a very slow process, in many cases stretching over a period of several years. Thus, a single failure in detection may be remedied by subsequent annual examinations. After the third negative smear, the length of time that may elapse between tests should be established on an individual basis by the woman's doctor, who will take into account any risk factors that might affect her vulnerability to the disease.

Because douching may remove important cells, it should be avoided for 24 hours before the smear is obtained. The smear should not be taken during a woman's menstrual period because the presence of blood in the sample renders it useless. The best time to obtain a Pap smear is at the midpoint of the menstrual cycle.

As cancer of the cervix may also occur in women over age 50, postmenopausal women should have Pap tests at reasonable time intervals. Further, women with prior hysterectomy—particularly if the hysterectomy was performed because of existing cervical cancer or a precancerous lesion—should have regular examinations and Pap smears, which could aid in the discovery of lesions of the vagina or other genital organs.

Finally, women themselves should take an interest in the laboratory where the smear will be screened. It is appropriate for a woman to ask her physician the name of the laboratory the smear will be sent to. It is also appropriate for her to check the credentials of the laboratory to determine whether it is supervised by a qualified pathologist and staffed by certified cytotechnologists and whether it has a quality-control program in place. In the U.S. all laboratories that perform medical tests are certified by the appropriate local boards or commissions. However, the requirements for quality control vary considerably from state to state. Recent congressional action to improve the performance of cytology laboratories may ultimately result in national standards of excellence, supervised by the U.S. Centers for Disease Control.

466

Boaters Beware!
Perils of Cold Water
by W. Moulton Avery III

When warmer air arrives in spring, many lightly dressed recreational boaters blithely venture onto cold water. In northern latitudes, where water is cold throughout the year, most people dress for the air temperature and assume that they will not fall in. On ocean liners the odds are in their favor, but the reverse is true for craft like canoes, kayaks, rowboats, and small sailboats.

Especially when the air is warm, it is common for the avid recreationist to underestimate the danger of cold water—a miscalculation that proves fatal for thousands each year. Unlike exposure to 10° C (50° F) air, immersion in 10° C water is quite painful; immersion in 1.6° C (35° F) water is excruciating. Water is effectively colder than air because of its higher capacity to steal body heat. Its thermal conductivity is 25 times greater than that of air, and its liquid nature enables it to penetrate clothing quickly. During the first 20 minutes of immersion, the greatest threat to life is drowning due to shock.

Real-life scenarios
At 4 PM on Wednesday, March 6, 1968, nine U.S. marines were nearing the end of a 3.25 km (2 mi) canoe crossing of the Potomac River 40 km (25 mi) south of Washington, D.C. The air temperature was above 5° C (41° F), and a light breeze created small ripples on the water. All the men were excellent swimmers and trained water-survival instructors. Each man had a seat-cushion-type life preserver.

Shortly after 4:15 PM they capsized about 90 m (100 yd) from shore. Whether they attempted to right the canoe and reenter it will never be known. They did make a valiant attempt to swim to safety; not one of the nine made it. The water temperature was 2.2° C (36° F).

On a March night in 1984, the nets of a 23-m (75-ft) fishing boat with a crew of five got caught on the sea bottom, causing the vessel to capsize in the freezing water of the North Atlantic, about five kilometers (three miles) off Heimaey Island in the Vestmannaeyjar archipelago, a string of volcanic islands just south of Iceland. Two crew members never surfaced. The remaining three, soaking wet, managed to climb onto the hull.

It was a clear night; distant lights could be seen shining in Heimaey Harbor, but the three men had no way to reach the ship's life raft, no life preservers, and no way to signal or call for help. After some discussion, they elected to swim. The truly remarkable thing about

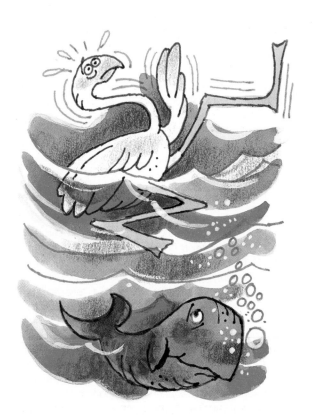

their ensuing struggle is that one of them, Gudlauger Fridthorsson, actually made it to shore and survived.

These two incidents indicate the range of human response to cold-water immersion and underscore the fact that sheer physical prowess is no match for Mother Nature. The vigorously fit marines all failed in their attempt to swim 90 m in 2.2° C water. Fridthorsson was not a particularly good swimmer. Despite this obvious handicap, he successfully swam for about six hours in even colder water than that encountered by the marines. To fully appreciate these examples, it is necessary to understand the effect of cold-water immersion on the human body.

The shock of immersion
The skin is normally quite sensitive to temperature, and immersion in water below 15.5° C (60° F) will immediately trigger a number of cold-shock responses in the average adult (the colder the water, the more intense the response). The most important shock response involves loss of the ability to control breathing, with the dire but likely consequence of drowning. Loss of breathing control begins the moment water makes contact with the skin, triggering a series of huge, involuntary gasps for air, which are followed immediately by uncontrolled hyperventilation. Within 15 seconds, hyperventilation can measurably reduce blood levels of carbon dioxide, causing respiratory alkalosis—a state that can diminish blood flow to the brain, resulting in

467

confusion, dizziness, and possible loss of consciousness. Hyperventilation can also cause tetany, a tingling and numbness beginning in the hands and feet that can progressively develop into severe cramping of the extremeties. Paradoxically, coinciding with hyperventilation is subjective dyspnea, a claustrophobic feeling of not being able to get enough air. This frightening sensation of breathlessness, which continues for up to three minutes before gradually declining, increases the potential for panic and disorganized behavior in the water and makes hyperventilation even more difficult to control.

Typically the cold-water-immersion victim's eyes are about 15–23 cm (6–9 in) above water level, limiting the view of the surrounding water. Many people find this situation disorienting, and it can adversely affect their ability to remain calm and perform even simple tasks. Additionally, within 30 to 60 seconds of immersion, hyperventilation increases the rate of breathing four to five times the normal resting rate. In cold-water-immersion experiments it generally takes up to five minutes for relaxed volunteers to stabilize their breathing to around twice the preimmersion rate. It is probable that victims in real survival situations experience greater difficulty stabilizing breathing since fear and panic resulting from the pain and disorientation of immersion aggravate this shock response.

A further survival threat is the dramatic reduction in the length of time that the breath can be held in cold water. In particular, this phenomenon diminishes the prospect of underwater escape from a capsized vessel. Breath-holding ability falls with water temperature. The ability of an average person to hold breath in water colder than 15.5° C is about one-third of what it is normally in warmer water. Loss of breathing control and reduced breath-holding time make it especially difficult to synchronize breathing while swimming, which can result in water inhalation.

Immersion in cold water also has profound cardiovascular effects. Within several seconds of immersion, heart rate, cardiac output, and blood pressure increase. These changes strain the cardiovascular system and heighten the risk of heart failure and stroke.

The body fat advantage

What saved Fridthorsson? At 1.9 m (6 ft 4 in) and weighing 125 kg (275 lb), Fridthorsson possessed an important asset: he was fat—and that saved his life. Fat is nature's preferred way of insulating warm-blooded animals from the cold—the fatter, the better. Every warm-blooded mammal that thrives in cold water, whether whale, walrus, or seal, has a thick layer of protective fat to insulate the muscles and warm body core.

Fridthorsson's fat did not entirely protect him from the shock of immersion, but its buoyancy helped keep him afloat and over the next six hours provided enough

insulation for him to continue swimming. In fact, by the time he reached the island he was hypothermic. This would not have been the case for a seal under the same conditions.

Being prepared

For the individual who engages in recreational activities on or around cold water, it is important to consider the risks of accidental immersion. Since most victims of immersion succumb to cold shock long before hypothermia can develop, the former presents the premier survival challenge.

Protecting against shock. The best way to minimize the possibility of cold shock, should one become immersed, is to be dressed properly. This means warm clothing covered by a specially designed, waterproof suit for protection in cold water. This combination insulates the body from the cold and prevents water from entering the clothing and making contact with the skin. Insulation of the head and neck are particularly important. In order for manual dexterity to be preserved for self-rescue, it is also necessary for the hands to be insulated because they can rapidly become numb and useless even though the remainder of the body is well protected.

Without the protection of a survival suit, dry suit, or wet suit, a person forced to enter cold water should, if possible, do so gradually to reduce the intensity of the initial immersion shock. The torso is particularly sensitive, so any means for its protection is beneficial.

White-water rafters, like other small-craft boaters, should always consider the risks of accidental immersion. A good life jacket ("personal flotation device") will keep the head above water and help insulate the torso against cold water.

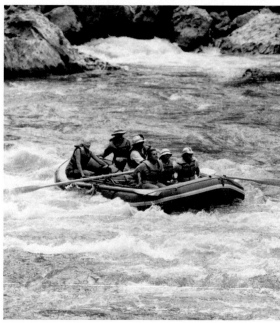

A good life jacket is a definite asset during the early phase of immersion because it helps to keep the head above water. Most jackets, however, will not keep the face out of the water if consciousness is lost because of water inhalation or hyperventilation.

The U.S. Coast Guard uses the term *personal flotation device* (PFD) and classifies six basic types according to various performance characteristics. The type V hybrid will provide enough flotation material to give the adult wearer minimum buoyancy if he or she is suddenly immersed with the PFD uninflated. These devices should be tested in water in an uninflated condition so the user can become familiar with how to inflate them while in the water. Some people find it preferable to wear this kind of PFD partially inflated onboard a boat. Hybrid PFDs are not suitable for children, who may not be able to quickly inflate the devices in an emergency. When worn over clothing, a PFD reduces water circulation next to the skin and provides additional insulation for the torso, which delays the onset of hypothermia. Despite these thermal benefits, it is no substitute for a survival suit, dry suit, or wet suit.

Survival suits afford the greatest thermal protection and are designed to cover the entire body, including the head and neck. Only the face is exposed. They are commonly made of neoprene rubber and are designed to be worn over clothing. Because of their bulk and the fact that they cover the hands, they are cumbersome garments in which to work. Dry suits are coverall-type garments that do not provide insulation for the hands, head, or neck. They are designed to be completely waterproof, and their thermal protection depends on the amount of insulating clothing worn underneath the suit. They are less bulky and easier to work in than survival suits. Wet suits, favored by scuba divers, are generally made of neoprene rubber. They achieve their thermal protection by trapping a thin layer of water next to the skin, where it is warmed by the body, providing a protective "microenvironment." Wet suits need to be snug to work effectively and consequently are more difficult to work in than dry suits. They also do not insulate well when the wearer is out of the water and can actually contribute to heat loss if they are wet and the wind is blowing.

Protecting against hypothermia. A popular but misleading maxim states that if the combined water and air temperature add up to less than 37.8° C (100° F), there is a risk of hypothermia upon immersion. On the basis of this curious formula, a person might conclude that immersion in 4.4°–10° C (40–50° F) water poses no danger if the air temperature is 24° C (75° F), or that immersion in 1.7° C (35° F) water carries little risk if the air temperature is 26.7° C (80° F). In fact, air temperature has no bearing on cold shock or the length of time required for immersion hypothermia to develop. When one is immersed, it is the water tem-

Adapted from
Hypothermia, Frostbite, and Other Cold Injuries by James Wilkerson, Cameron Bangs, and John Hayward; © 1986 The Mountaineers, Seattle

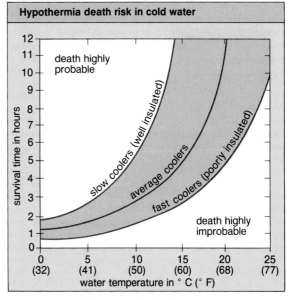

Graphs showing predicted survival times in cold water before hypothermia sets in do not account for cold shock, which can occur during the first minutes of immersion. If not read with proper understanding, they may give the unwary boater a false sense of security. The colored zone in the graph above shows risk of death from hypothermia only for about 95% of lightly clothed, nonexercising teenagers and adults.

perature alone that counts. Regarding hypothermia, the U.S. Coast Guard considers water below 21° C (70° F) to be cold enough to warrant special caution.

For the average person, hypothermia becomes an issue after about 20 minutes in the water. Hypothermia develops gradually. The rate at which body temperature falls is determined by variables such as water temperature, water movement (*e.g.,* currents, waves), physical movement in the water, body type, protective clothing, and length of time in the water.

A number of survival graphs or charts have been developed to show the relationship between water temperature, immersion time, and the probability of surviving hypothermia. These charts are not designed to account for the incapacitating effects of cold shock and the danger of sudden drowning that occur during the first minutes of immersion. Most such charts show an average survival time in excess of one hour for lightly clothed subjects. Without some understanding of the scientific method by which these survival times are calculated, the recreationist can develop a false sense of security. The survival time for "average coolers" on the survival graph shown above is based on a rate of heat loss at which the victim's core body temperature would fall to 30° C (86° F). Any point on the "average" line represents a core temperature of 30° C—a stage at which the heart is vulnerable to fatal arrhythmias (abnormal heart beats), and the person is presumed to be semiconscious and therefore in danger of drowning. It should be readily apparent to the person interpreting a survival graph in this informed context that average victims removed from 0° C (32° F) water at the one-hour mark or 7° C (45° F) water at the two-hour mark are on the brink of death. Without superior medical intervention, they will not survive.

Saving a victim's life

In 1955 Arthur Moffat, a highly experienced canoeist and wilderness explorer, capsized in very cold water on the Dubawnt River in Canada's Northwest Territories. He insisted repeatedly to his concerned companions, "I'm okay, I'm okay." They were not entirely convinced and placed him in a sleeping bag inside a tent, where he died of hypothermia.

Those who participate in recreational water activities should be prepared to help companions if accidental cold-water immersion occurs. There are a number of essential things to know in these life-or-death situations. Among these are that children cool much faster than adults, and thin people cool faster than those with greater body fat. If more than one person is immersed, fast coolers should be removed first, average coolers second, and slow coolers last. In addition to body size and composition, consideration should be given to the insulation provided by clothing.

Following the removal of victims from the water, rescuers need to assess a victim's physical condition on the basis of both environmental circumstances and any obvious symptoms of hypothermia such as shivering, mental confusion, or apathy. It is common for victims to underestimate the seriousness of their own condition and, upon having been removed from the water, to insist, as Moffat did, that they will soon be okay. Rescuers should *always* view such claims with skepticism.

The Moffat tragedy provides a valuable lesson. A person may not technically be hypothermic, with a "deep body," or core, temperature below 35° C (95° F), but the extremities can be severely chilled, with 15.5° C blood in arm and leg muscles and 5° C blood in the skin. In Moffat's case simply providing insulation from the surrounding cold environment was not sufficient to counter this chill. In such cases hypothermia will result unless external heat is added to the system.

Physical movement, particularly walking, can also force the circulation of chilled blood from large muscles to the warmer body core, causing a rapid drop in temperature and possibly sudden heart failure; the heart is weak when the body is cold. It is consequently important to remove people from the water in a manner that involves as little exertion on the victims' part as possible. If brought on board a large vessel, they should be carried below deck even if they are physically able to walk. The same principle applies to people who make it to shore following prolonged immersion in a cold river. It is prudent also to bear in mind that the cold associated with immersion can inhibit the swelling and pain associated with injuries such as an ankle fracture.

The best place for a victim of cold-water immersion to be treated is in a hospital; it is always reasonable to summon professional help even before the person has been removed from the water and his or her condition fully assessed. While waiting for help to arrive, companions should be gentle and avoid unnecessary movement of the victim. Insulation should be devised that will protect the victim from cold surroundings, including wind and cold ground or other surfaces. Particular attention should be paid to insulating the head and neck, which can account for over half of body heat loss. Warming the skin with an electric blanket or placing the victim in a tub of hot water can cause rewarming shock and sudden heart failure; such techniques should not be attempted without professional medical support. Neither should food or fluids be given, as they could cause choking.

If help is completely unavailable or hours or days away, gradual rewarming may be the only option available to the party. The first responsibility of companions is to ensure that the victim does not get any colder. This can best be accomplished by placing the victim in a sleeping bag with an insulating pad under the bag and, if available, hot-water bottles around the chest and neck. Water can be heated on a camp stove and poured into canteens or plastic water bottles, which then should be put into thick wool socks or something similar so that the victim is not burned. If the air temperature is below freezing, care must be taken that the extremities are protected against frostbite. This usually means providing extra clothing and a hot-water container around the victim's feet at the foot of a sleeping bag. Rewarming will probably take many hours. Although the victim will feel better as soon as the skin is warm, the body temperature will still be quite low; rewarming must therefore continue until the entire body has been warmed.

Middle-Age Spread
by William D. McArdle, Ph.D.

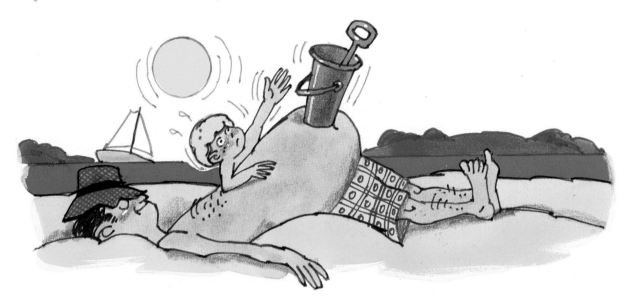

The chances of a person's becoming obese as an adult are three times greater if excessive fat accumulation begins early in childhood—as it often does. There are many people, however, who never experience a weight problem until middle age. For these previously lean men and women, the early to mid-thirties are a time of life associated with the onset of "middle-age spread"—the slow addition of excess weight that tends to accumulate on the hips, buttocks, and abdomen. In the Western world the average 35-year-old gains about 0.45 kg (one pound) of fat each year until the fifth or sixth decade of life; this occurs even with decreased food intake. In one study that followed the progress of 27 men over a 12-year period, from ages 32 to 44, the average weight gain was 6.4 kg; this weight gain represented *accumulated fat*.

Is middle-age spread inevitable? Most researchers note that there are certain age-related physiological and hormonal changes that often predispose people to accumulating some excess fat in middle age, as well as a tendency for this fat to be deposited in specific areas of the body. Moreover, middle-aged men and women invariably weigh more than their college-aged counterparts of the same height. It appears, then, that some change in body shape and composition with age is probably unavoidable. However, the extent to which this "creeping obesity" reflects a normal biological pattern is unknown. More than likely, this trend should *not* be interpreted as being "normal," and adults should *not* necessarily expect their bodies to gradually soften and enlarge, especially if they watch their diets and maintain good exercise habits.

Contributing factors

While the inevitability of middle-age spread may remain in doubt, there is considerable agreement about the factors that contribute to its development. For one thing, in industrialized societies men and women tend to reduce their active pursuits to a significant extent as they grow older. An increasing reliance on other individuals and machines to perform daily tasks such as housework and yard work results in decreased muscular activity and therefore the need for fewer calories. If food intake is not reduced accordingly, a slow and steady increase in body fat occurs. At the same time, underused muscles begin to shrink and lose their tone. Although the exact reasons are not completely clear, for many adults the added corpulence will be concentrated in the hips, thighs, or abdomen. Abdominal muscles that gradually weaken as a consequence of a lack of exercise further contribute to the emergence of that all-too-familiar hallmark of middle-age spread, the potbelly.

The tendency for middle-aged men and women to gain weight may also be due to a progressive change in the metabolic rate during the adult years. For each person a minimum level of energy is required for sustaining the body's vital functions in the waking state. This energy requirement is called the basal metabolic rate (BMR). Studies reveal that the BMR gradually declines about 2% per decade after age 25. Much of this decrease can be attributed to the change in body composition generally associated with growing older; *i.e.*, increased fat and decreased muscle mass (or lean tissue). This change reduces the lean-to-fat ratio,

471

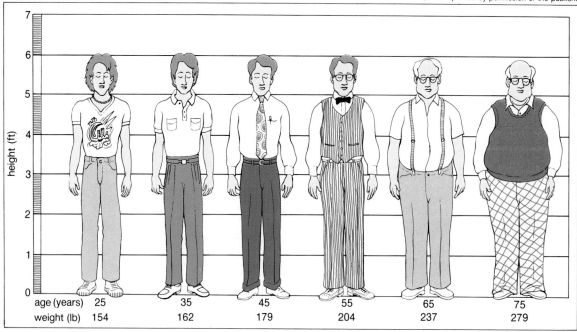

age (years)	25	35	45	55	65	75
weight (lb)	154	162	179	204	237	279

A man who has the same caloric intake and maintains the same level of physical activity at age 75 as he did at his ideal weight at age 25 will steadily gain excess fat, amounting to a weight gain of as much as 57 kg (125 lb). It is possible, however, to prevent this "creeping obesity" by making appropriate adjustments in caloric intake and activity level.

which in turn slows the body's level of metabolism; this occurs because muscle is much more active metabolically than fat and thus requires more energy. The alteration in body composition is further magnified for women after menopause, as hormonal changes and, perhaps, changes in activity patterns accelerate the loss of lean tissue. Such bodily adjustments related to aging reduce the individual's daily caloric needs, making it all too easy for people to put on extra weight if appropriate adjustments are not made in either food intake or energy output—or both.

The good news for those trying to ward off middle-age spread is that the undesired alterations in body composition are probably more a matter of life-style than a true phenomenon of aging. In persons of any age, when muscle is used in physical activity, its components are conserved and even increased; disuse, on the other hand, brings about an actual shrinkage, or atrophy, in muscle tissue. A man or woman who becomes progressively more sedentary loses metabolically active muscle and replaces it with more dormant fat. This form of creeping obesity can occur even without an increase in body weight. One may consider two men of the same height, each of whom weighs about 82 kg. One is a young, athletic individual, who possesses a considerable muscle mass with little fat accumulation. The other is a sedentary older man. In the case of the latter, the chances are that fat makes up a much larger proportion of his total body mass. At rest the energy needs will be lower for the older

individual with the smaller quantity of muscle. Furthermore, because muscle is more dense than fat, it is smaller in volume than a similar quantity of fat. For this reason the younger man has a trim, firm, and fit look, while his older counterpart, although weighing the same, appears larger and somewhat softer.

Research indicates, however, that the age-associated cycle of decline in metabolic rate, loss of muscle, and increase in fat is not universal. In comparisons of young and middle-aged endurance-trained men, for example, there was no difference in lean body mass, and measures of BMR were similar. In other studies elderly people who began exercising regularly actually showed increases in muscle mass when compared with sedentary peers. It is the documented role of exercise in conserving lean tissue, and thus blunting the tendency for metabolism to decrease with age, that explains why maintaining an active life-style makes it easier for people to control their body weight in middle age and after.

Men and women of any age who exercise regularly can alter their body composition in the direction of increased muscle and reduced fat. Even though their body weight is not always reduced, these individuals often report a discernible reduction in body measurements and clothing size.

Energy balance: crucial equation

The energy-balance equation states that body weight remains constant when caloric intake equals caloric

472

expenditure. Any imbalance on the output or input side of the equation causes the body weight to change. The "formula" for the onset of middle-age spread is simple: when the number of calories ingested exceeds the daily energy requirement, the excess calories are stored as fat in cells called adipocytes, largely in the subcutaneous deposits directly beneath the skin. To eliminate unwanted fat, an energy deficit must be created through decrease of energy intake (dieting), increase of energy output (exercising), or both.

Until recently, it was commonly believed that the major cause of progressive weight gain among the middle-aged was overeating. However, if gluttony and overindulgence were the only factors contributing to the development of middle-age spread, the easiest way to combat it would simply be to reduce food intake. Of course, this is not the case. In fact, in terms of caloric balance, since 1900 the number of overweight men and women in the U.S. has nearly doubled, while average caloric intake has dropped by 10%!

In view of all the factors that predispose people to gaining weight, it is truly remarkable that the body weight of most adults in the U.S. fluctuates only slightly during any given year—despite their annual per capita food intake of about 900 kg of food! The relative constancy in body weight then is impressive, considering that only a slight but consistent excess in food intake can cause weight to increase substantially over time if there is no compensatory increase in daily energy expenditure. For example, a person who eats just one extra handful of peanuts (100 cal) each day for a year consumes 36,500 (100 × 365) surplus calories. Because 0.45 kg of body fat equals 3,500 excess calories, this surplus is equivalent to a gain of about 4.5 kg of fat in a single year.

In a 1987 study of middle-aged men and women who exercised regularly, researchers at Tufts University, Boston, found that time spent in physical activity was inversely related to level of body fat—the more activity, the leaner the individual. Surprisingly, no relationship emerged between body fat and food consumption. The researchers concluded that the greater proportion of body fat seen in active middle-aged individuals as compared with their younger, active counterparts was attributable more to a considerably lower activity level than to greater food intake.

Regional fat distribution

The pattern of distribution of body fat in middle age differs between the sexes. In men excess fat usually accumulates in the abdominal region. This form of fat gain, which is often highly resistant to treatment, is referred to as central or android obesity—or more commonly "apple-shaped" obesity or "potbelly." For adult women two patterns of fat distribution emerge. One is the central pattern common in men; the other, more prevalent type is termed peripheral or gynoid fat patterning—or "pear-shaped" obesity. This female fat accumulation is typically distributed in the lower regions of the body, resulting in overample hips, buttocks, and thighs. In both men and women the regulation of local fat accumulation is governed by the regional activity of lipoprotein lipase, or LPL, the enzyme that stimulates fat uptake by cells in specific body regions. The influence of sex hormones—more specifically, of estrogen and progesterone in females—on the local activity of this enzyme probably accounts for the general gender difference in fat storage and distribution.

Role of heredity. Analyses of identical and fraternal twins strongly indicate that genetic factors influence

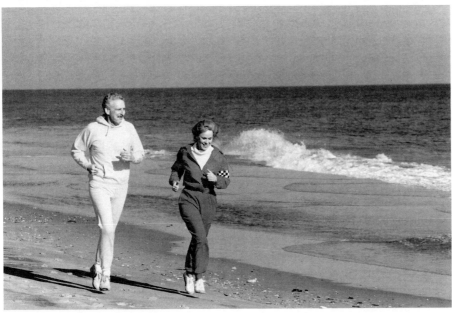

Maintaining an active life-style that includes aerobic exercise is the best way to control body weight during middle age and beyond. Exercise conserves lean tissue and blunts the decrease in basal metabolic rate that inevitably occurs with aging.

Henley and Savage—TSW-Click/Chicago Ltd.

not only total body weight but also the pattern of fat distribution. This suggests that while a reduction in one's total body fat will certainly reduce regional fat, it may not alter a person's basic body shape. Thus, while one is not necessarily predetermined to develop a potbellied physique, if that predisposition exists, the individual may find it virtually impossible to attain a very small waistline or a flat stomach.

Changes during pregnancy. Hormonal changes in pregnancy increase the local activity of LPL, causing the deposition of fat to become more accentuated in the hip region. Presumably this added fat is to be used as a caloric source for milk production during lactation. However, when a woman substitutes formula feeding for breast-feeding, it becomes more difficult for her to lose this excess fat. Thus, fat accumulation in the lower body region is likely to become magnified with repeated pregnancies.

Menopausal changes. In postmenopausal women the specific reproductive functions of fat cells in the hip region are eliminated, local LPL activity is no longer elevated, and these cells are reduced to a size similar to abdominal fat cells. This adaptation in fat cell activity is probably related to the large decrease in estrogen production associated with menstrual cessation. Such observations suggest that after menopause it may be easier for a woman to reduce body fat that has accumulated in the hips, thighs, and buttocks—although this has not been demonstrated scientifically.

Health risks and fat distribution. Although some authorities have maintained that a moderate excess of body fat is not in itself harmful, a 1985 report by a panel of the U.S. National Institutes of Health, entitled "Health Implications of Obesity," concluded that obesity (defined as 20% or more over "ideal" weight) should be viewed as a disease. The report showed that there are numerous health hazards associated with surprisingly low levels of excess fat, even as little as two to five kilograms above ideal body weight.

More recent research has shown that the patterning of regional fat distribution—regardless of the total amount of body fat—significantly alters the health risks associated with obesity. This research has identified centrally located fat—that in the abdomen and midriff—as being a more serious health problem than fat that accumulates below the waist, on the hips and thighs.

Furthermore, the health risks of abdominal fat increase as the ratio of waist circumference to hip circumference increases. A thickening of the torso that causes the waist-to-hip ratio (calculated by dividing waist measurement by hip measurement) to exceed an average of 0.9 is associated with an increased risk of death from heart disease, as well as an increased risk of developing non-insulin-dependent diabetes, elevated blood triglyceride levels, and hypertension (high blood pressure), and a higher overall death rate. Recent data also show that overweight women with the so-called android pattern of obesity are at greater risk of heart disease than those who carry the extra weight on their hips and thighs.

Combating unwanted spread

There are two approaches that may be recommended to counter middle-age spread. The first is to tip the energy-balance equation in a direction that will bring about fat loss. (For the younger adult who does not yet have a weight problem, the tendency for weight gain in later life can be offset simply by maintenance of the proper energy balance.) The second approach is to engage in appropriate exercise to firm, tone, and strengthen muscles for both improved function and overall appearance.

Diet plus exercise: ideal combination. Approaches that combine diet and exercise offer considerably more flexibility for achieving a negative caloric balance and accompanying fat loss than either strategy offers alone. With a weight-loss program that includes

Fat that accumulates in middle age is not evenly distributed on the body but tends instead to be concentrated either centrally, in the abdominal region—the pattern typical in men—or on the hips, thighs, and buttocks— creating the pear-shaped body more common among women. Recent research indicates that the central pattern, in which the waist is larger than the hips, is associated with increased risks of high blood pressure, non-insulin-dependent diabetes, and death due to heart disease. Pear-shaped obesity, with its lower waist-to-hip ratio, carries a lower risk of these conditions.

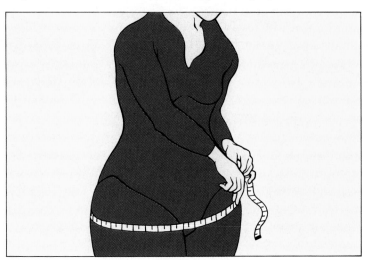

regular exercise, the feelings of intense hunger and other psychological stresses of reduced caloric intake may be minimal, compared with a similar program that relies exclusively on dieting. Exercise also provides protection against the loss of lean tissue that tends to occur throughout middle age and that also occurs when a person attempts to lose weight by dieting alone. This "exercise dividend" occurs because moderate physical activity enhances the breakdown of body fat for energy while at the same time causing muscle to conserve its protein component. The protein-sparing effect of exercise causes a greater portion of the caloric deficit to be made up through the breakdown of body fat. Exercise also combats the body's tendency to slow its metabolism as it attempts to defend against weight loss.

Spot reduction: does it work? The promise of localized fat loss, or spot reduction, with exercise is especially attractive to those whose extra weight is distributed disproportionately in certain body areas. The theory is that exercising a specific body area or muscle group causes fat to be selectively reduced from that area. Thus, to get rid of excess fat in the abdominal region, a person would perform a large number of sit-ups or side bends. Similarly, according to such a theory, bicycling movements and other leg exercises would be the cure for overample thighs.

There is no doubt that localized exercise of, for example, the abdominal area contributes to the firming and strengthening of these important muscles and may even result in an actual reduction in girth. However, there is simply no evidence that fat is released to a greater degree from the fat pads directly over an exercising muscle than from fat deposits in other locations. Scientific understanding of the mechanisms of human energy supply holds that exercise stimulates the mobilization of fat through hormones delivered by the blood to act on the fat deposits throughout the body—not simply in those areas exercised. The areas of greatest fat concentration probably supply the greatest amount of energy.

In one study of this phenomenon, researchers compared the girth and subcutaneous fat stores of the right and left forearms of highly trained tennis players. As expected, the girth of the playing arm was larger than that of the nonplaying arm, owing to the modest exercise-related muscular development of the playing arm. Measurements of fat thickness, however, showed that there was no difference between the arms in the quantity of subcutaneous fat. Other studies have produced similar findings. The conclusion of these studies is that a negative caloric balance created through regular exercise contributes significantly to a reduction in total body fat. Fat, however, is reduced *not* selectively from the exercised areas but rather from total body fat reserves and from the areas of greatest fat concentration.

Exercise guidelines
Regardless of one's present physical condition, there are basic guidelines for embarking on an exercise program. These are especially important for the previously sedentary, middle-aged man or woman who, after a decade or so of the "couch potato" life-style, decides that it is time to shape up, slim down, and regain a youthful appearance. Of course, everyone embarking on a new exercise program should first check with their physician.

Aerobics: essential and effective. Aerobic exercise is the key to combating middle-age spread. Continuous aerobic activities (*e.g.,* running, cycling, swimming) exercise a relatively large muscle mass. These forms of moderate, sustained exercise burn considerable numbers of calories, favorably modify lipid metabolism and blood pressure, and generally promote cardiovascular fitness. No single aerobic exercise is best; each can be equally effective in altering body composition. It is of primary importance, however, that each individual choose an activity that is safe, is pleasurable, and can, if necessary, be adapted to any personal physical limitations. Moreover, very few people will continue to participate in exercise that is so taxing that little or no enjoyment is possible. A good example is running. It is not much fun to run if the end result is shortness of breath, wobbly legs, and a stitch in the side. Even jogging for five minutes at a relatively slow pace is not easy, especially for people who have been sedentary.

A program for increasing one's level of physical activity is most likely to be enjoyable if the probability of success is maximized. What is needed is a planned, systematic approach with long-term rather than short-term goals. Ideally a person should spend 30 minutes exercising aerobically at least two, but preferably three, times a week. More frequent exercise will be even more effective in reshaping the body. As physical conditioning improves, more or longer workout periods can be added. From a calorie-burning standpoint, it is much better to continue an activity for a prolonged period of time at a reasonable pace than to perform the same activity at maximum pace for a short time.

It is important for the beginning exerciser to start slowly and not to overdo. The person who starts out too vigorously is likely to end up with aching muscles and joints, painful cramps, injuries, and, possibly, excessive strain on the cardiovascular system—all powerful deterrents to continued exercise. Instead of starting by walking a couple of kilometers, the beginner might initially walk only a few blocks. The beginning cyclist, instead of trying to go 16 km, might set a goal of 3.

Proper warm-up and cooldown are essential to preventing soreness and injury. The warm-up gets muscles, joints, and the cardiovascular system ready for action. It should include gentle stretching and light calisthenic exercises, such as jogging in place, for the cardiovascular warm-up. The cooldown period allows the body to return gradually to its preexercise state.

An exercise routine is more enjoyable if it includes some variety. Ideally, a person might engage in different aerobic activities on different days of the week—for example, cycling once a week and attending an aerobic dance class on two other days. A person performing calisthenics or jogging can also introduce variety into the activity by interspersing other forms of exercise. For example, instead of jogging continuously around the track, one might jog for 2 minutes, skip for 1 minute, hop on the right foot 20 times and then on the left foot 20 times, jog for 3 minutes, and so forth. The fitness walker might choose a course that includes flat stretches interspersed with steeper ones or find a route that includes some flights of steps between different street levels.

Running, swimming, cycling, aerobic dancing, and other more standard types of "training" are not the only ways to increase daily activity. For most previously sedentary adults, a start-up program need only produce changes in the existing level of physical activity sufficient to burn fat and tone muscle. There are many simple ways to increase energy expenditure while going about one's daily routines. For example:

● When driving to work, park a few blocks away and walk the remaining distance.

● When taking public transportation, get off a few stops early and walk the remaining distance.

● When traveling relatively short distances, allow time to walk instead of driving or taking a bus.

● Replace the cocktail hour with 20 minutes of exercise; replace coffee breaks with exercise breaks.

● Substitute an exercise video for a regularly watched TV program.

● Instead of hiring helpers, expend some energy several days a week in housecleaning, gardening, washing and waxing the car, walking the dog, and the like.

● During television commercials run in place, jump rope, do some sit-ups, jog up and down stairs, or perform calisthenics.

Benefits of resistance exercise. By modifying standard strength-training methods so that muscles are not greatly overloaded, one can develop a form of resistance exercise that increases the caloric cost of exercise while at the same time helping to firm, tone, and strengthen the major muscle groups of the body—a necessary component in a program to combat, or ward off, middle-age spread. As originally conceived, this kind of exercise routine, called circuit training, provides aerobic benefits for people exercising with free weights and weight machines such as are typically found in health clubs. The "circuit" consists of a series of resistance exercises designed to build major muscle groups; by going from one exercise—or exercise machine—to another in quick succession, the exerciser derives aerobic benefits while building muscle.

For those who do not want to join health clubs or invest in costly home exercise machines, it is possible to set up a simple, inexpensive circuit at home. Many household items can be used to provide resistance to muscular contraction. For example, one can make weights by filling buckets or plastic cleanser containers with water or filling socks with sand. A broom or mop handle can serve as a bar to which these heavy objects can be attached (securely, of course). Ski boots, telephone books, bricks wrapped in a towel, or any other objects that can be grasped with the hands and lifted can also serve as "weights." Of course, barbells and dumbbells are the easiest kinds of weights to use—providing that one knows some simple rules for avoiding injury—and they are relatively inexpensive. Chairs, table tops, and other household furnishings can take the place of standard gymnasium equipment. A piece of clothesline can be used as a jump rope. The various items are then arranged around the room, to be used in a certain predetermined order. Making the "circuit" simply consists of performing each action or lifting each weight a given number of times. The goal is to complete all of the exercises in the time available for the workout. As the individual's speed and strength improve, and the target number of repetitions is achieved, more resistance can be added to increase the difficulty of the workout. Another objective might be to perform the required number of repetitions of each exercise in the sequence within a shorter period of time.

Even exercises that require little or no equipment can be modified so that they have a progressive effect on firmness and muscle tone. Increasing the difficulty and thus the strenuousness of the exercise will accomplish this. For example, the conventional push-up can be made more difficult by a change in the body position from horizontal (starting position on the level) to diagonal by placement of the feet on a 30–40-cm (12–16-in)-high bench. One can similarly modify sit-ups by placing the feet and calves on the seat of a chair so that the lower legs are at about a 90° angle to the thighs. This type of "incline" sit-up can be made even more strenuous if a small weight is held across the chest or behind the head.

Pregnancy and the Older Woman

by Bruce D. Shephard, M.D.

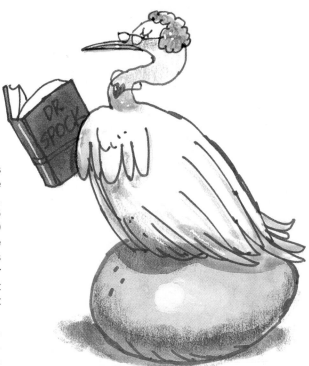

One of the most striking social and demographic trends in the U.S. in recent years has been the increase in the number of babies born to women in their thirties and, in particular, to women 35 and older. Between 1976 and 1987 the birthrate for women 35–39 rose from 19 live births per 1,000 to about 28. In contrast, the rate for women under 30 remained fairly stable during this period. The birthrate among women aged 40 and over has also been nearly constant since 1976—at about 4 live births per 1,000—and is projected to remain at that level through the year 2000.

The proportion of pregnant women in their thirties, especially those in their late thirties, has also increased. The proportion of births to women over the age of 35, which was approximately 5% of total births in 1982, is expected to reach 8.6% by the turn of the century. In 1987 pregnancies among women in the 35–39 age group accounted for 6.5% of all pregnancies. Women over 40 accounted for less than 1% of the total.

The various reasons cited to explain the increasing numbers and proportions of births to women over 35 can be reduced, essentially, to two factors: delayed childbearing and the so-called baby boom that occurred between 1947 and 1965. The baby boom years were marked by the highest numbers of births ever recorded in the U.S. Many women born during this post-World War II era reached their thirties and early forties during the 1980s or will do so in the early '90s. There will, therefore, be a larger population of women in this age group than ever before and a corresponding increase in births.

Accompanying this population shift has been a dramatic trend toward delayed childbearing, indicated not only by higher birthrates among women over 35 but also by higher rates of first births to these women. The rate of first births among women in their thirties more than doubled between 1970 and 1986; the rate of first births to women 40–44 increased by about 50% during this time.

A combination of social and economic factors is responsible for the trend toward delayed childbearing. These include the high costs of childbearing and child rearing and the need for both members of the couple to work before starting a family. Some women delay having children in order to further their educations or their careers. Others marry late or remarry and choose to start a second family in their later reproductive years. Improved contraception—most notably safe and effective oral contraceptives—and the availability of therapeutic abortion have been additional factors contributing to delayed childbearing.

Fertility of older couples

It is a sometimes underappreciated fact that couples over 35 may take longer to conceive than younger couples. Fertility gradually declines with age, so that impaired fecundity (ability to have a live-born child) is three times as likely for prospective parents aged 35 to 39 compared with those aged 20 to 24.

In women this declining fertility results from a decreasing number of available ova and from complex hormonal changes involving the pituitary, hypothalamus, and ovaries. These normal physiological changes during the thirties and early forties lead to a decrease in the regularity of ovulation and menstruation. Approximately one-third to one-half of couples in this age group consult a fertility specialist to determine which of them may have a problem and what the exact nature of the trouble may be. Among the more common findings associated with infertility in women are pelvic inflammatory disease and endometriosis (abnormal growth of the uterine lining). Both conditions may cause infertility (as well as pelvic pain) due to blockage of the fallopian tubes by adhesions. (Tubal adhesions occur when tissues stick together during postsurgical healing or as a result of infection or endometriosis.) In men, decreased sperm counts due to conditions such as varioc0cele (varicose veins of the scrotum) may cause decreased fertility. Overall, however, male factors contribute less than female conditions to infertility in older couples. *Fortunately, most couples with an infertility problem can be helped.* In addition to drugs that stimulate ovulation, there are also promising techniques involving laser surgery and microsurgery to restore tubes that have become blocked.

Age—a risk in itself?

The question of age as an independent risk factor, for either the mother or the fetus, is beset with controversy. Traditionally, age 35 has been considered a "watershed" year, beyond which obstetric complications were believed to increase considerably. This has been the prevailing view since at least 1950, when two U.S. obstetricians, E.G. Waters and H.P. Wager, in an article published in the *American Journal of Obstetrics and Gynecology,* appended the adjective *elderly* to the standard medical term *primigravida* (a woman pregnant for the first time) in referring to pregnant women aged 35 and older. (Today such women are more likely to be characterized as "reproductively mature.")

Waters and Wager were not the first—nor were they the last—to investigate the maternal and fetal risks associated with delayed childbearing. Many of the previously determined risks, however, were called into question in 1986 when Phyllis Kernoff Mansfield, an assistant professor of nursing at Pennsylvania State University, reviewed more than 100 studies on the subject and found inconsistencies and methodological flaws in most studies that linked maternal age to various maternal or fetal risks. Mansfield identified four factors that often had not been considered in evaluating the results of these studies or that had not been controlled for in the studies themselves. These factors were: (1) failure to take into account that earlier investigations often involved disproportionate numbers of older or infertile women, who represented a preselected group somewhat prone to complications; (2) failure to recognize that earlier studies often included relatively more births to women who already had several children, thus overrepresenting pregnancies of poor women with large families and at increased risk for unfavorable outcomes; (3) failure to take into account the fact that the older women in these studies were more likely to have developed a chronic illness such as hypertension; and (4) failure to consider that medical management of older patients is often intensive and usually involves more tests than is the case with younger patients, thus making the finding (and subsequent reporting) of an abnormality more likely. The evaluation of previous research is also complicated by changes in technology and medical management.

Mansfield's view that risks associated with late childbearing were overestimated by earlier research is reflected in other, more recent studies, which have tended to refute the notion that age itself necessarily affects pregnancy adversely. These studies indicate that it is not age but rather the presence of chronic illnesses, which are more common in older women,

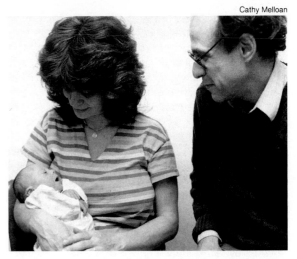

The faces of these proud parents, both in their early forties, leave no doubt that this baby was worth waiting for.

that leads to complications associated with pregnancy after age 35. (These complications, both maternal and fetal, are discussed in more detail below.)

An interesting question concerning the effect of maternal age is whether the risks and complications for older women giving birth for the first time are different from those for women having their second, third, or a subsequent child after the age of 35. No large-scale study has yet resolved this question. *In general, however, whether an older woman has a chronic illness is a far more important determinant of risk than whether she is a first-time mother.*

Potential maternal risks

Perhaps the single greatest maternal risk after the age of 35 is that of hypertension. As the incidence of hypertension naturally increases with age, it is not surprising that hypertensive disorders of pregnancy are more common in older women. Women over age 35 have two to four times the incidence of toxemia of pregnancy than women in their twenties. In earlier studies the term *toxemia* often referred to various pregnancy-related hypertensive disorders, including both preeclampsia, in which there is a sudden development of high blood pressure occurring after the 20th week of pregnancy, and complications due to chronic hypertension predating the pregnancy. Because of inconsistent use of the terms *toxemia* and *preeclampsia* by different investigators, overall frequency of chronic high blood pressure in pregnant women over age 35 is uncertain, but it appears to be at least 10%. Maternal complications of high blood pressure, while less common than fetal problems, can be serious; they include seizures, damage to the kidneys and liver, stroke, and heart attack.

Another medical complication often reported in studies of delayed childbearing is diabetes. The frequency of adult onset, or non-insulin-dependent, diabetes increases directly with age and is found twice as often among pregnant women over the age of 35 as among those in their twenties. Likewise, diabetes that develops during pregnancy, known as gestational diabetes, is twice as common in older patients. Overall, in various studies of pregnant women over the age of 35, the incidence of some form of diabetes ranges from 1 to 6%. For the pregnant woman, the primary risks of preexisting diabetes are high blood pressure and increased difficulty in controlling blood sugar levels. The primary maternal consideration of gestational diabetes is that the woman may later go on to develop insulin-dependent diabetes.

Many other medical complications of pregnancy are age-related, among them connective tissue disorders such as systemic lupus erythematosis, heart disease, neurological conditions, various forms of cancer, and alcoholism. Increased rates for these conditions, as well as for certain obstetrical complications, account for the additional diagnostic tests and more frequent hospital admissions among pregnant women over the age of 35. A number of postpartum complications, including blood clots, heart failure, and complications related to hypertension, are also more frequent among patients in this age group. Other postpartum complications, such as uterine and urinary tract infections, are not increased in older patients.

Bleeding in late pregnancy is usually associated with one of two placental abnormalities, placenta previa (in which some or all of the placenta covers the cervix) or abruptio placenta (in which some part of the placenta separates from the wall of the uterus). Either condition may cause slight, moderate, or severe hemorrhage in the last 12 weeks of pregnancy. The incidence of bleeding has been reported to be two to three times more frequent among women over age 35 than among younger women. Of the two types of abnormalities, abruptio placenta is most clearly associated with maternal age because this condition is closely associated with high blood pressure, particularly chronic hypertension. In one recent case review, the overall incidence of third-trimester bleeding was 1% for women over the age of 35, doubling to 2% after age 40.

Women over 35 are more likely than their younger counterparts to have a cesarean delivery, which, as a major surgical procedure, is in itself a risk to the woman's life. In trying to account for this trend, some researchers cite the relatively higher incidence of fetal distress, preexisting medical conditions, and abnormal labor patterns (especially in first-time mothers) in women over 35. Others believe that the increase in cesarean births among older women reflects a more intense approach to the medical management of labor in the older woman. Generally speaking, however, a woman's chances of having a cesarean delivery are influenced less by age than by birth order—the high-

est rates of cesarean birth in older as well as younger women occur among those giving birth for the first time.

A review of maternal death rates during the 1960s and 1970s showed significantly higher rates of death during pregnancy and childbirth among older women. Between 1968 and 1975, for example, overall maternal mortality was five times higher for women aged 35 to 39, who had a mortality rate of 60 per 100,000 live births, compared with 12 per 100,000 for women in their early twenties. Women aged 40–44 had an even greater risk, with 102 deaths per 100,000 live births. These figures improved between 1974 and 1978, during which time the comparable rates for women aged 35–39 and 40–44 were 51 and 86 per 100,000 live births, respectively. *More recent statistics are encouraging:* maternal deaths for women over age 35 decreased 50% in the mid-1980s compared with the rate during 1974–78. Major causes of maternal death were complications related to high blood pressure, complications related to bleeding, and blood clots. Ectopic pregnancy (*i.e.,* one not implanted within the uterine cavity), the incidence of which also increases with advancing maternal age, is another significant cause of maternal death in the U.S. today.

Fetal risks

Compared with the risks of pregnancy and childbirth faced by older mothers, the risks to the fetus are more numerous and occur more frequently. In the first half of pregnancy, these risks are predominantly higher rates of miscarriage and of developmental defects arising from chromosomal abnormalities. In the second half of pregnancy, most studies indicate an increased risk of birth defects, growth retardation, and preterm delivery, as well as higher rates of fetal distress during labor and a slightly increased incidence of deaths in newborns.

Studies that have examined the relationship of maternal age to the risk of having a miscarriage, or spontaneous abortion, often have been flawed by methodological problems. It is true that numerous studies show a consistent, positive association between age and miscarriage—women in their thirties have a 50% higher rate of miscarriage than women in their twenties; the rate for women over the age of 40 is two- to fourfold higher than that of women in their twenties. However, the relationship of age to miscarriage does not appear to be simply one of cause and effect. For example, some older women who miscarry are women who have a biological predisposition toward miscarriage. It is precisely because of the failures of previous pregnancies that they have continued their attempts to have a child despite their own advancing age. Likewise, some older women conceive late in life because of an ongoing problem of infertility, which itself may have been a contributing cause of miscarriage, quite apart from age. Further, comparisons based on miscarriage rates from earlier studies may be invalid because of changes in medical technology. It is now possible to confirm pregnancy—and miscarriage—much earlier than in previous times. Thus, many early miscarriages that might have gone unnoticed are now known to occur—and are therefore recorded.

The association of advanced maternal age with chromosomal abnormalities is well known and well substantiated. One of the most frequent examples is trisomy, in which one of the 23 sets of paired chromosomes is joined by an additional, third chromosome. Most trisomies involve chromosomes 13, 18, or 21. The most common of these, trisomy 21, is also known as Down syndrome. Down syndrome occurs in only one pregnancy out of 1,000 among 30-year-olds but is found in 11 per 1,000 pregnancies (about 1%) among 40-year-olds. The overall risk of a 35-year-old woman giving birth to a child with some chromosomal abnormality is estimated to be 0.6%, increasing to 1.6% at age 40 and to 5% at age 45. (These rates do not reflect genetically abnormal fetuses that either are lost as miscarriages or are stillborn.) While statistics do show a dramatic increase in abnormalities with age and may be alarming to women contemplating pregnancy after age 35, a more hopeful—and equally realistic—view can be derived by turning the numbers around: *a woman of 40 has a better than 98% chance of having a chromosomally healthy child. Moreover, nonchromosomal birth defects in babies of older women are only slightly increased, if at all.*

There is good evidence that perinatal mortality (the sum of the stillbirth and newborn death rates) is higher for older mothers, predominantly because, compared with overall rates, stillbirths occur twice as often among women aged 35–39 and three to four times as often among women in their forties. Stillbirths occur more often among indigent women and among those receiving no prenatal care, as well as among women with complications of pregnancy such as hypertension and diabetes. High blood pressure—which predisposes to fetal growth problems, preterm labor, and bleeding complications such as abruptio placenta—is perhaps the most important age-associated (*i.e.,* over age 35) factor contributing to perinatal loss.

The incidence of low-birth-weight infants—those weighing less than 2,500 g (5½ lb)—is also increased about twofold among pregnant women over age 35. Low birth weight may result from either preterm labor (*i.e.,* prematurity) or growth retardation or from a combination of the two. Like the stillbirth rate, the incidence of low birth weight is strongly influenced by socioeconomic status and medical factors such as hypertension. The results of a large-scale study published in 1990 looking at the pregnancies of 3,917 women giving birth for the first time showed that of the 799 women who were 35 or older (many of whom were college educated and mostly nonsmokers), there was only a very slightly increased risk of bearing a low-birth-weight infant (1.3 times more likely than women in the study who were in their twenties), and they had no increased risk of preterm delivery. As a result of improved perinatal care in recent years, fetal risks during labor and delivery have been minimized. This study also found that infants born to women aged 35 or older did not have lower Apgar scores than babies born to younger women. (The Apgar score is an index of the health status of the infant at birth.) Despite these recent encouraging reports on fetal outcome, most current research shows that overall these infants have more complications than average during their first year. In 1988 the U.S. government published a report of a study that analyzed data from 1.6 million births that had occurred in 1980. This report showed that compared with death rates for babies born to women under 35, infant mortality was 18% higher among babies born to women in the 35–39 age group and 69% higher for offspring of women over age 40.

Older pregnant women are likely to have more frequent office visits, tests, and hospital admissions than younger ones. This reflects not only the current medical-legal climate but also the belief on the part of physicians—and women themselves—that more intensive health care is beneficial in these pregnancies. One of the most important tests recommended to pregnant women over age 35 is amniocentesis, a procedure usually performed in the second trimester. Newer versions of the technique, which samples fetal cells for chromosomal defects, include early amniocentesis at 13–14 weeks and chorionic villus sampling at 9–11 weeks of pregnancy. Previously, when amniocentesis was the only such procedure available, it was not performed until the 16th week.

In the second half of pregnancy, usually in the 8 to 10 weeks prior to delivery, weekly tests of fetal well-being may include the nonstress test, or NST (a form of fetal monitoring done in the doctor's office), and ultrasound (an imaging technique that uses sound waves rather than X-rays). The basic test, the NST, is usually sufficient. However, if more information is needed, it can be obtained from a test called the biophysical profile, or BPP, which uses ultrasound. The BPP is a more complex test than the NST; it is usually performed by a perinatologist (a specialist in the care of the newborn) or radiologist. Its purpose is evaluation of several aspects of fetal development and activity, including fetal movement and breathing, and of the amount of amniotic fluid. The BPP is quite expensive—costing about $300—but it is particularly helpful in twin pregnancies and in pregnancies that are complicated by growth retardation or placental bleeding problems.

If tests indicate the pregnancy is not perfectly normal, often the woman over 35 must decrease her phys-

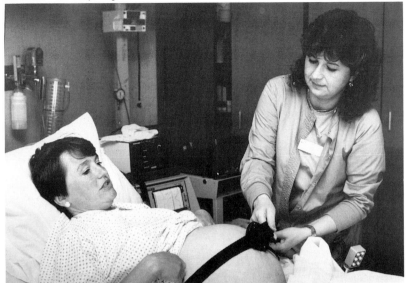

A woman, age 37, in the early stage of labor is prepared for electronic fetal monitoring, which will record both the baby's heartbeats and the strength and frequency of her contractions. Compared with their younger counterparts, older mothers are likely to have more intensive medical management of pregnancy and delivery.

ical activity and modify working conditions to avoid heavy lifting, prolonged standing, or an overheated environment, especially in the last trimester. When birth complications seem probable, or if there are maternal complications such as hypertension, many obstetricians attempt to induce labor before the pregnancy becomes overdue (*i.e.,* more than two weeks past the due date). Labor is started by means of the drug oxytocin, which stimulates contractions; if the attempt to induce labor is unsuccessful (on the basis of the condition of either the mother or the fetus), delivery may be accomplished by cesarean section.

Pregnancy after 40

In the U.S. in the 1990s, about 20,000 women each year are expected to give birth at or after age 40 (some even in their mid- or late forties). Many of the fetal and maternal risks discussed above increase gradually with age, so it is not surprising that compared with those in their thirties, women in their forties have higher rates of high blood pressure, third-trimester bleeding, and cesarean delivery, as well as increased rates of perinatal and maternal mortality. The incidence of birth defects increases significantly in the forties—a 40-year-old woman has 3 times the chance of giving birth to a baby with a chromosomal defect that a 35-year-old has, and a 45-year-old has 10 times this risk. Women 40 and over tend to undergo more intensive medical testing during pregnancy and have higher cesarean birthrates compared with women in the 35–39 age group. Some investigators, Mansfield among them, believe that the higher cesarean rates in women over 40 reflect a self-fulfilling prophecy: obstetricians have come to expect more complications in their older pregnant patients and are therefore more cautious in their medical management of these patients.

Older parents—making the adjustment

Considering the medical risks of older childbearing says nothing about the economic and social adjustments required in child rearing. Older parents may be less flexible emotionally than younger ones and have less physical stamina for dealing with the almost constant demands of a new infant. Such demands may strain the marital relationship, especially if there are other children from an earlier marriage. The requirements of parenting may also conflict with the older mother's career goals, perhaps requiring her to choose part-time employment over a full-time commitment to her work. Other matters that older prospective parents must weigh include financial obligations such as the cost of college. These may come due just when they would be likely to wind down their careers or even retire. Older parents may have to deal with their own elderly parents' health needs at a time when their children are still young and have many needs of their own.

Notwithstanding the above considerations, later life may be the perfect time for some couples to have a child. Having waited longer to become parents, they may be more willing to make the sacrifices—of both time and money—that parenthood often involves. Other advantages favoring older parents-to-be include increased maturity, greater financial security, and high motivation to be parents. Such factors may help older couples to savor the joy of parenthood more than younger couples and to cope more effectively with the problems that parenting almost inevitably entails.

In the final analysis, from a strictly medical point of view, *the great majority of women over 35, and even those over 40, can have a safe and successful pregnancy.* Certainly the odds favor the older patient and her baby, especially if she is in good health.

Contributors to the World of Medicine

Edmund L. Andrews, M.S.J.
Special Report Biomedical Patents: Profits and Pitfalls
Patents columnist, the *New York Times;* free-lance business and technology writer, Washington, D.C.

David Bellinger, Ph.D., M.Sc.
Environmental Health Special Report Children Exposed to Lead—Clear and Present Danger
Assistant Professor of Neurology, Harvard Medical School; Research Associate, Neuroepidemiology Unit, The Children's Hospital, Boston

Diana Brahams, Barrister-at-Law
Special Report Computer Consultants: The Future of Medical Decision Making? (coauthor)
Editor, *Medico-Legal Journal;* Legal Correspondent, *The Lancet,* London

George A. Bray, M.D.
Obesity
Professor and Executive Director, Pennington Biomedical Research Center, Louisiana State University, Baton Rouge

Rosalind D. Cartwright, Ph.D.
Sleep Disorders
Professor and Chairman, Department of Psychology and Social Sciences, and Director, Sleep Disorders Service, Rush-Presbyterian-St. Luke's Medical Center, Chicago

James I. Cleeman, M.D.
Heart and Blood Vessels (coauthor)
Coordinator, National Cholesterol Education Program, National Heart, Lung, and Blood Institute, National Institutes of Health, Bethesda, Md.

Elizabeth B. Connell, M.D.
Obstetrics and Gynecology
Professor, Gynecology and Obstetrics, Emory University School of Medicine, Atlanta, Ga.

Joseph Degioanni, M.D., Ph.D.
Special Report Four Months in a Cave: Experiment in Chronobiology
Medical Officer, Johnson Space Center, National Aeronautics and Space Administration; Adjunct Assistant Professor of Environmental Sciences, University of Texas Health Sciences Center at Houston School of Public Health

Stephen E. Epstein, M.D.
Heart and Blood Vessels (coauthor)
Chief, Cardiology Branch, National Heart, Lung, and Blood Institute, National Institutes of Health, Bethesda, Md.

Kathy A. Fackelmann
AIDS (coauthor)
Life Sciences and Biomedicine Editor, *Science News,* Washington, D.C.

Lameh Fananapazir, M.D.
Heart and Blood Vessels (coauthor)
Senior Investigator and Director, Clinical Electrophysiology Laboratory, National Heart, Lung, and Blood Institute, National Institutes of Health, Bethesda, Md.

George A. Freedman, D.D.S.
Dentistry
Dentist in private practice, Montreal; President-elect, American Academy of Cosmetic Dentistry; Contributing Editor, *Dentistry Today*

William R. Fry, M.D.
Surgery (coauthor)
Assistant Professor of Surgery, University of California at Davis-East Bay School of Medicine

Richard M. Glass, M.D.
Mental Health and Illness
Clinical Associate Professor of Psychiatry, University of Chicago; Deputy Editor, *Journal of the American Medical Association*

Robert M. Goldwyn, M.D.
Special Report Plastic Surgery: When the Patient Is Dissatisfied
Clinical Professor of Surgery, Harvard Medical School; Head, Division of Plastic Surgery, Beth Israel Hospital, Boston; Editor, *Plastic and Reconstructive Surgery*

Philip M. Hanno, M.D.
Urology
Professor and Chairman, Department of Urology, Temple University School of Medicine, Philadelphia

David B. Herzog, M.D.
Eating Disorders (coauthor)
Director, Eating Disorders Unit, Massachusetts General Hospital; Associate Professor of Psychiatry, Harvard Medical School, Boston

Alan M. Hughes, M.A.
Special Report The New Oxford English Dictionary: Keeping Up with Medicine
Senior Editor (Science), *New Oxford English Dictionary;* Associate Editor, *New Shorter Oxford English Dictionary,* Oxford University Press, Oxford, England

Louis A. LaMarca, M.A.
Drugs
Capitol Hill News Editor, *F-D-C Reports: "The Pink Sheet,"* and Senior Editor, *Weekly Pharmacy Reports: "The Green Sheet,"* F-D-C Reports, Inc., Chevy Chase, Md.

John H. Laragh, M.D.
Hypertension
Hilda Altschul Master Professor of Medicine; Chief, Division of Cardiology; and Director, Cardiovascular Center and Hypertension Center, New York Hospital-Cornell Medical Center, New York City

Claude Lenfant, M.D.
Heart and Blood Vessels (coauthor)
Director, National Heart, Lung, and Blood Institute, and Chairman, Coordinating Committee, National Cholesterol Education Program, National Institutes of Health, Bethesda, Md.

Carole Lieberman, M.D., M.P.H.
Mental Health Special Report Shopping Out of Control
Assistant Clinical Professor of Psychiatry, University of California at Los Angeles

Robert L. Lindsay, M.D., Ph.D.
Osteoporosis
Chief of Internal Medicine, Helen Hayes Hospital, West Haverstraw, N.Y.; Professor of Clinical Medicine, Columbia University College of Physicians and Surgeons, New York City

Jean D. Lockhart, M.D.
Pediatrics
Editor-in-Chief, *Current Problems in Pediatrics;* San Rafael, Calif.

William D. McArdle, Ph.D.
Physical Fitness (coauthor)
Professor, Department of Health and Physical Education, Queens College, Flushing, N.Y.

Gail McBride, M.S.
Genetics Special Report Of Mice and Maine
Free-lance medical journalist, Chicago

Charles-Gene McDaniel, M.S.J.
Mental Health Special Report Anniversary Reactions: Not Just Coincidence; Transplantation
Professor and Chairman, Department of Journalism, Roosevelt University, Chicago; Chicago Correspondent, *The Medical Post,* Toronto

Robert Keene McLellan, M.D., M.P.H.
Environmental Health Special Report Drinking Water: What's on Tap?
Director, Center for Environmental Medicine, and Vice-President, Ecotek Corp., Hamden, Conn.; Assistant Clinical Professor of Medicine, Yale University School of Medicine, New Haven, Conn.

Beverly Merz
Genetics
National Editor, Science and Technology, *American Medical News,* American Medical Association, Chicago

Thomas H. Murray, Ph.D.
Genetics Special Report Unraveling DNA: Knotty Issues
Professor and Director, Center for Biomedical Ethics, School of Medicine, Case Western Reserve University, Cleveland, Ohio; member, Working Group on Ethical, Legal, and Social Issues for the Human Genome Institute

Tom D. Naughton
Accidents and Safety
Free-lance health and science writer, Chicago

Michael E. Newman
Environmental Health Special Report Electromagnetic Fields: Tempest in a Charged Teapot?
Free-lance medical and science writer, Gaithersburg, Md.

Claude H. Organ, Jr., M.D.
Surgery (coauthor)
Professor and Chairman, Department of Surgery, University of California at Davis-East Bay School of Medicine

David B. Reuben, M.D.
Aging
Associate Director, Multicampus Division of Geriatric Medicine and Gerontology, and Assistant Professor of Medicine, University of California at Los Angeles School of Medicine

F. Clifford Rose, M.D.
Headache
Director, Academic Unit of Neuroscience, Charing Cross and Westminster Medical School, London

Sami I. Said, M.D.
Asthma
Professor of Medicine and Associate Head for Research, Department of Medicine, University of Illinois at Chicago College of Medicine

Lee M. Sanderson, Ph.D.
Disasters
Chief, Behavioral Surveillance Branch, Center for Chronic Disease Prevention and Health Promotion, Office of Surveillance and Analysis, Centers for Disease Control, Atlanta, Ga.

David S. Stasior, M.D., M.P.P.
Eating Disorders (coauthor)
Researcher in medicine and public policy, John F. Kennedy School of Government, Harvard University, Cambridge, Mass.

Janine K. Stasior, M.S.
Eating Disorders (coauthor)
Projects Coordinator, Eating Disorders Unit, Massachusetts General Hospital; researcher in eating disorders, University of Massachusetts, Boston

Michael M. Toner, Ph.D.
Physical Fitness (coauthor)
Associate Professor, Department of Health and Physical Education, Queens College, Flushing, N.Y.

D.A.J. Tyrrell, M.D., D.Sc.
Common Cold
Director, Medical Research Council Common Cold Unit, Salisbury, England

Elliott P. Vichinsky, M.D.
Sickle-Cell Disease
Associate Director, Department of Hematology-Oncology, and Director, Sickle Cell Program, Children's Hospital, Oakland, Calif.

Rick Weiss
AIDS (coauthor)
Life Sciences and Biomedicine Editor, *Science News,* Washington, D.C.

Jeremy Wyatt, M.A.
Special Report Computer Consultants: The Future of Medical Decision Making? (coauthor)
Lecturer in Medical Informatics, National Heart and Lung Institute, London

Contributors to the Health Information Update

Nancy H. Arden, M.N.
Flu
Senior Research Associate, Department of Epidemiology, University of Michigan School of Public Health, Ann Arbor

W. Moulton Avery III
Boaters Beware! Perils of Cold Water
Executive Director, Center for Environmental Physiology, Washington, D.C.

Michael Bigby, M.D.
Skin and Hair Problems of Black People (coauthor)
Associate Dermatologist, Beth Israel Hospital, Boston

Steven E. Carsons, M.D.
Sjögren's Syndrome: The Dryness Disorder
Chief, Division of Rheumatology, Immunology, and Allergy, Winthrop-University Hospital, Mineola, N.Y.; Assistant Professor of Medicine, State University of New York at Stony Brook School of Medicine

Fredric L. Coe, M.D.
Kidney Stones (coauthor)
Professor, Medicine and Physiology, and Chief, Nephrology Program, University of Chicago Pritzker School of Medicine

Marc K. Effron, M.D.
Heart Murmurs
Cardiologist, Scripps Memorial Hospital; Clinical Instructor, University of California at San Diego School of Medicine, La Jolla

Donna L. Jornsay, R.N.
Gestational Diabetes
Director of Education, Diabetes Control Foundation, Flushing, N.Y.

Leopold G. Koss, M.D.
The Pap Smear
Professor and Chairman, Department of Pathology, Montefiore Medical Center and Albert Einstein College of Medicine of Yeshiva University, Bronx, N.Y.

William D. McArdle, Ph.D.
Middle-Age Spread
Professor, Department of Health and Physical Education, Queens College, Flushing, N.Y.

Brendan A. Maher, Ph.D.
Delusions
Dean, Graduate School of Arts and Sciences, and Edward C. Henderson Professor of the Psychology of Personality, Harvard University, Cambridge, Mass.; Chairman, Panel on Behavioral Sciences, Commission on Human Resources, National Research Council-Institute of Medicine

Joan H. Parks, M.B.A.
Kidney Stones (coauthor)
Research Associate (Assistant Professor) and Administrator, Kidney Stone Program, Section of Nephrology, Department of Medicine, University of Chicago Pritzker School of Medicine

Deborah Ann Scott, M.D.
Skin and Hair Problems of Black People (coauthor)
Clinical Instructor of Dermatology, Boston University School of Medicine; Staff Dermatologist, Massachusetts Institute of Technology, Cambridge, Mass.

Ruth Andrea Seeler, M.D.
Special Camps for Special Kids
Pediatric Hematologist and Director, Pediatric Education, University of Illinois at Chicago College of Medicine

Bruce D. Shephard, M.D.
Pregnancy and the Older Woman
Clinical Associate Professor of Medicine, Department of Obstetrics and Gynecology, University of South Florida College of Medicine, Tampa

Manfred Spitzer, M.D., Ph.D.
Hallucinations
Visiting Associate Professor, Department of Psychology, Harvard University, Cambridge, Mass.

Myron Winick, M.D.
Eating for Two
President, University of Health Sciences/The Chicago Medical School, North Chicago, Ill.

Title cartoons by Phil Kantz

Index

This is a three-year cumulative index. Index entries to World of Medicine articles in this and previous editions of the *Medical and Health Annual* are set in boldface type; *e.g.*, **AIDS**. Entries to other subjects are set in lightface type; *e.g.*, astigmatism. Additional information on any of these subjects is identified with a subheading and indented under the entry heading. The numbers following headings and subheadings indicate the year (boldface) of the edition and the page number (lightface) on which the information appears. The abbreviation *il.* indicates an illustration.

All entry headings are alphabetized word by word. Hyphenated words and words separated by dashes or slashes are treated as two words. When one word differs from another only by the presence of additional characters at the end, the shorter precedes the longer. In inverted names, the words following the comma are considered only after the preceding part of the name has been alphabetized. Examples:

      Lake
      Lake, Simon
      Lake Charles
      Lakeland

Names beginning with "Mc" and "Mac" are alphabetized as "Mac"; "St." is alphabetized as "Saint."

503

N ow there's a way to identify all your fine books with flair and style. As part of our continuing service to you, Britannica Home Library Service, Inc. is proud to be able to offer you the fine quality item shown on the next page.

B ooklovers will love the heavy-duty personalized embosser. Now you can personalize all your fine books with the mark of distinction, just the way all the fine libraries of the world do.

T o order this item, please type or print your name, address and zip code on a plain sheet of paper. (Note special instructions for ordering the embosser). Please send a check or money order only (your money will be refunded in full if you are not delighted) for the full amount of purchase, including postage and handling, to:

Britannica Home Library Service, Inc.
Attn: Yearbook Department
Post Office Box 6137
Chicago, Illinois 60680

(Please make remittance payable to: Britannica Home Library Service, Inc.)

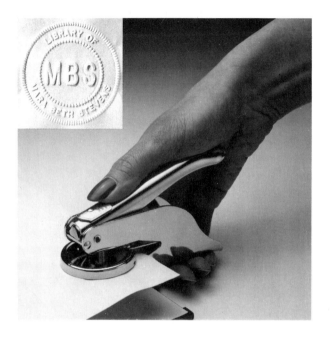